Stereo Operative Atlas of Micro Ear Surgery

Pu Dai • Dong-yi Han • Vincent C Cousins
Yue-shuai Song
Editors

Stereo Operative Atlas of Micro Ear Surgery

Springer

Editors
Pu Dai, MD, PhD
Department of Otolarygngology Head
and Neck Surgery
Chinese PLA General Hospital
Beijing
China

Vincent C Cousins, BMedSci, MBBS, FRACS
Department of Otolarygngology Head
and Neck Surgery
Alfred Hospital
Melbourne
Australia

Dong-yi Han, MD, PhD
Department of Otolarygngology Head
and Neck Surgery
Chinese PLA General Hospital
Beijing
China

Yue-shuai Song, MD
Department of Otolarygngology
Head and Neck Surgery
Beijing Friendship Hospital
Capital Medical University
Beijing
China

ISBN 978-981-10-2088-9 ISBN 978-981-10-2089-6 (eBook)
DOI 10.1007/978-981-10-2089-6

The print edition is not for sale in China Mainland. Customers from China Mainland please order the print book from:
People's Medical Publishing House

Library of Congress Control Number: 2016962211

Printed on acid-free paper
Springer Singapore Heidelberg New York Dordrecht London

This Springer imprint is published by Springer Nature
The registered company is Springer Nature Singapore Pte Ltd.
The registered company address is: 152 Beach Road, #22-06/08 Gateway East, Singapore 189721, Singapore.

Preface

Auditory perception is one of the most important human senses and this is self-evident to all mankind. Structural and functional lesions causing hearing loss are mostly located in the middle and inner ear, which makes them the main targets in microsurgery of the ear and lateral skull base. The temporal bone contains many important structures which are small and delicate and have complex relationships, thus representing one of the most intricate and complicated areas in the human body. Visualization of these structures and their spatial relationships is beyond the ability of the unaided eye, making our understanding of ear anatomy a difficult task. The invention and application of the zoom stereo binocular microscope have opened a new chapter for microsurgery, providing excellent stereo vision and stimulated further development of modern otology.

Microsurgery of the ear is still known as a challenging field due to its delicate nature and its demands of meticulous technical ability. Young trainees starting in the field are faced with significant difficulty in acquiring the surgical knowledge and techniques of the ear and lateral skull base procedures they see demonstrated by their experienced otology and neurotology mentors. This is in part due to the inability of observers to have the same stereo vision as the operating surgeon.

Generally, beginners gain their surgical knowledge of the ear and lateral skull base by studying anatomic drawings, photographs, videos, etc. The learner's personal understanding, spatial imagination, and 3D imaging of the anatomical relationships need to be synthesized in the mind. Inevitably, an incorrect impression may often be generated during this process.

Traditional textbooks cannot provide the 3D features of a surgical field to learners. The trainee has the difficult task of learning and comprehending 3D information based only on 2D images. This has stimulated a drive to develop an innovative method to change this sometimes ineffective learning method.

Twenty years ago, we began to consider reproducing the anatomy and surgical field of ear surgery using computer technology with the aim of providing effective technological support for anatomical research, teaching, and microsurgical training. In the early stages, we achieved computer-aided 3D reconstruction from serial sections of the temporal bone, and this laid the foundation for 3D morphological research of the ear. Based on this technology, we obtained paired stereoscopic images of reconstructed structures with different rotating angles observed with a stereoscope to generate real 3D images. Building on this experience, we collaborated with Dr. You-jun Yu from Foshan Hospital, to publish our first 3D atlas, the *stereoscopic Anatomic Atlas of Temporal Bone* in 2006. That book contains 76 pairs of stereoscopic images and readers can obtain vivid stereovision of anatomic fields with a custom-made stereoscope, which improves the efficiency of learning temporal bone anatomy.

Due to technical limitations, the asynchronous manual exposure technique adopted at that time was unable to address the 3D synchronous photography requirement of the dynamic and ever-changing operative surgical field. For this reason, we invented a stereoscopic photo capture system based on a binocular microscope, which can capture surgical scenes of the right and left light paths without interrupting surgical operations (Chinese Patent number: ZL2008 2 0078610.3). The images taken by this system provide the same authentic 3D surgical scene as observed by the operating surgeon. Based on this breakthrough, we set up a 3D image bank of ear microsurgery, collecting some ten thousand pairs of 3D images from hundreds of ear and lateral skull base surgeries. In this book, we have selected 418 pairs of stereoscopic images from 43 operations, covering a variety of common ear and lateral skull base surgeries. Each set of stereo pictures gives a strong sense of layering and depth, with realistic stereognosis when using an inexpensive folded stereoscope designed for the purpose. Even without the stereoscope, observers can achieve stereo vision by staring at the pairs of 3D images for a period of time. The detailed notes and legends accompanying the stereoscopic images help readers better understand the important surgical procedures, including the spatial relationship of key structures and handling skills required. We believe this technology has great potential to change teaching and training methods of ear and lateral skull base microsurgery, and improve the effectiveness of teaching and academic exchange.

We are keen to share this exciting new technological achievement with colleagues around the world. This is our first publication of a 3D atlas of ear and lateral skull base microsurgery. There will inevitably be some deficiencies and errors in this book and we invite your valuable feedback and advice to help improve the stereo atlas of microsurgery and related technology in the future.

Pu Dai
Dong-yi Han
Vincent C Cousins
Yue-shuai Song

Beijing, China
Melbourne, Australia

Contents

Contributors

Pu Dai, MD Department of Otolarygngology Head and Neck Surgery, Chinese PLA General Hospital, Beijing, China

Dong-yi Han, MD Department of Otolarygngology Head and Neck Surgery, Chinese PLA General Hospital, Beijing, China

Vincent C Cousins, MBBS, FRACS Department of Ear Nose and Throat Surgery, Alfred Hospital, Melbourne, Australia

Yue-shuai Song, MD Department of Otolarygngology Head and Neck Surgery, Beijing Friendship Hospital, Capital Medical University, Beijing, China

Song Gao, MD Department of Otolaryngology, The 175th Hospital of Chinese PLA, Zhangzhou, China

Xue Gao, MD Department of Otolaryngology Head and Neck Surgery, The General Hospital of the Chinese PLA Rocket Force, Beijing, China

Bing Han, MD Department of Otolarygngology Head and Neck Surgery, Chinese PLA General Hospital, Beijing, China

Ming-yu Han, MD Department of Otolarygngology Head and Neck Surgery, Chinese PLA General Hospital, Beijing, China

Wei-ju Han, MD Department of Otolarygngology Head and Neck Surgery, Chinese PLA General Hospital, Beijing, China

Zhao-hui Hou, MD Department of Otolarygngology Head and Neck Surgery, Chinese PLA General Hospital, Beijing, China

Sha-sha Huang, MD Department of Otolarygngology Head and Neck Surgery, Chinese PLA General Hospital, Beijing, China

Yi Jiang, MD Department of Otolaryngology, Fujian Provincial Hospital, Fuzhou, China

Jia-nan Li, MD Department of Otolarygngology Head and Neck Surgery, Chinese PLA General Hospital, Beijing, China

Jian-zhong Li, MD Department of Otolaryngology Head and Neck Surgery, Fuzhou General Hospital of Nanjing Command, Chinese PLA, Fuzhou, China

Jun Liu, MD Department of Otolarygngology Head and Neck Surgery, Chinese PLA General Hospital, Beijing, China

Wei-dong Shen, MD Department of Otolarygngology Head and Neck Surgery, Chinese PLA General Hospital, Beijing, China

Yi Sun, MD Department of Otolaryngology, Chinese PLA Wuhan General Hospital, Wuhan, China

Guo-jian Wang, MD Department of Otolarygngology Head and Neck Surgery, Chinese PLA General Hospital, Beijing, China

Shi-ming Yang, MD Department of Otolarygngology Head and Neck Surgery, Chinese PLA General Hospital, Beijing, China

Fei Yu, MD Department of Otolarygngology Head and Neck Surgery, Chinese PLA General Hospital, Beijing, China

Rui-li Yu, MD Department of Allergy, Beijing Shijitan Hospital, Affiliated to Capital Medical University, Beijing, China

Yong-yi Yuan, MD Department of Otolarygngology Head and Neck Surgery, Chinese PLA General Hospital, Beijing, China

Jian-dong Zhao, MD Department of Otolarygngology Head and Neck Surgery, Chinese PLA General Hospital, Beijing, China

Yu-hua Zhu, MD Department of Otolarygngology Head and Neck Surgery, Chinese PLA General Hospital, Beijing, China

Yi-hui Zou, MD Department of Otolarygngology Head and Neck Surgery, Chinese PLA General Hospital, Beijing, China

Biographical Information

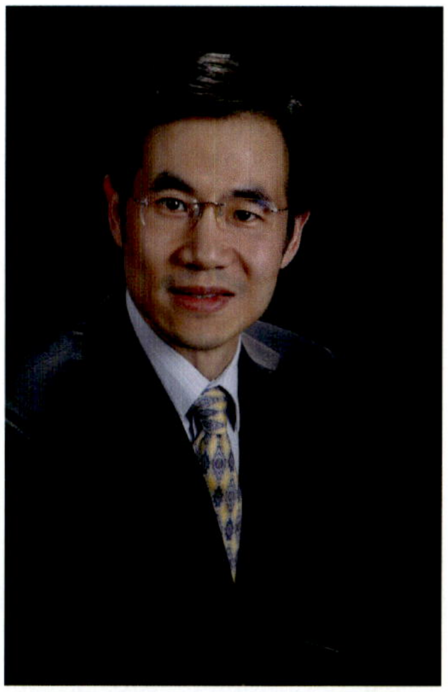

Pu Dai graduated in Medicine from the Second Military Medical University, Shanghai, China, in 1986 and later completed Otolaryngology training, being awarded a Masters and a Doctoral degree from the Chinese People's Liberation Army (PLA) Medical College, Beijing, in 1991 and 1998, respectively. He has practiced as an Ear-Nose-and-Throat doctor in the same hospital since 1991. He undertook a further two-and-a-half years of postdoctoral training at Georgetown University in the United States from January 2000 to August 2012. His current appointments are Associate Chairman and Full Professor in the Department of Otolaryngology Head and Neck Surgery of the Chinese PLA General Hospital. He has a great deal of experience with ear, skull base, and cochlear implantation surgery. His research has focused on minimal access cochlear implantation surgery, hearing preservation, and the genetics of hearing impairment. He has led most of the pioneering three-dimensional (3D) morphological research on the temporal bone in China since 1990 and published the first 3D atlas of micro ear surgery in the world.

Dr. Dai has published more than 40 peer-reviewed journal articles worldwide and 120 journal articles in Chinese. He is the chief editor of four textbooks in the field of Otolaryngology Head and Neck Surgery. Some of his honors include a Second Grade Prize of the National Science and Technology Progress Awards (for controlling birth defects causing severe-to-profound hearing impairment); a Seeking Truth Award; and nomination as a National Distinguished Young and Middle-Aged Specialist. He was the chairman of the Organizing Committee and the conference secretary for the Asia-Pacific Symposium on Cochlear Implantation and Related Science (APSCI) (2015) and became a committee member of APSCI at this meeting.

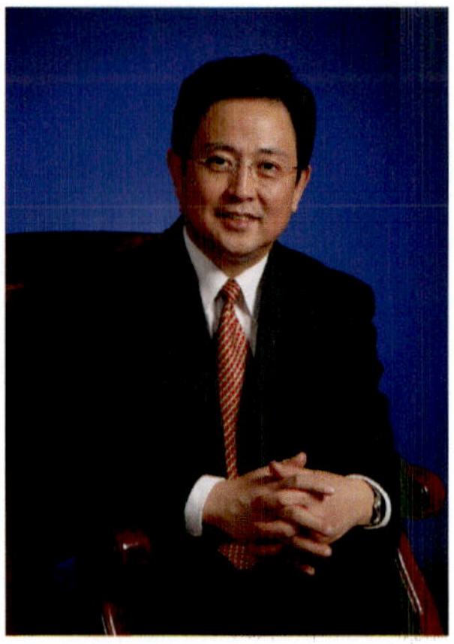

Dong-yi Han, MD, PhD, is a Professor in the Dept. of Otolaryngology Head and Neck Surgery and the Vice Director of the Institute of Otolaryngology at the Chinese PLA General Hospital. He is also the Past President of the Chinese Otolaryngology Head & Neck Surgery Society.

Prof. Dong-yi Han places a great deal of importance on clinical research in ear microsurgery, otoneurosurgery, and skull base surgery. He has made an intensive study of the anatomy of the middle and inner ear, and of the clinical characteristics of cranial nerve lesions, to improve the ability of patients with severe sensorineural deafness to achieve hearing and speech. He introduced the concept of minimally invasive surgery for all types of surgery for diseases of the ear and improved surgical approaches.

Prof. Dong-yi Han has received several key research grants from the National High Technology Research and Development Program of China (863 Program), the National Science Fund for Distinguished Young Scholars, and the National Natural Science Foundation of China. He has been the first or corresponding author of more than 100 papers published in top journals in China and abroad. He has also trained approximately 20 doctoral students and seven postdoctoral fellows. In recognition of his outstanding achievements, he has been awarded the second prize for National Scientific and Technological Progress, the first prize for Military Scientific and Technological Progress, and the second prize for Scientific and Technological Progress from the Chinese Medical Association.

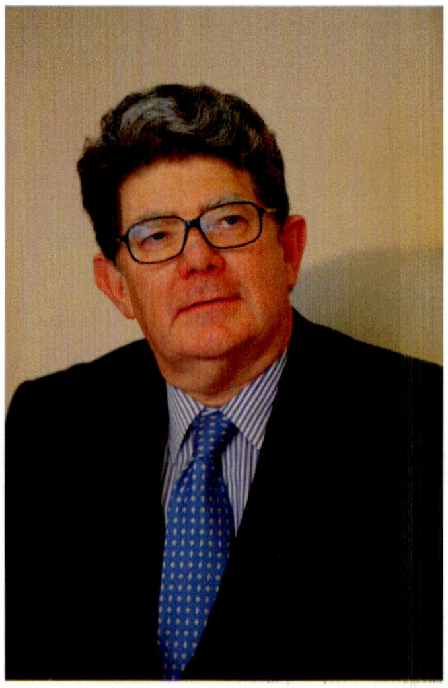

Vincent C Cousins graduated in Medicine from Monash University, Melbourne, Australia, in 1974.

He completed his advanced surgical training in Otolaryngology Head & Neck Surgery in Melbourne (FRACS) in 1984. He then undertook a Head and Neck & Skull Base fellowship with Professor Donald Harrison in London, England, in 1984/1985, and an Otology fellowship with Professor Dietrich Plester in Tuebingen, Germany, in 1986. He has practiced in Melbourne in Otology and Neurotology since then. He is currently Principal Specialist and Head of the ENT-Otoneurology Unit at The Alfred Hospital, Melbourne, and Adjunct Clinical Associate Professor in Surgery at Monash University.

He is Past President of the Australian Society of Otolaryngology Head & Neck Surgery. He has served the Royal Australasian College of Surgeons as Councillor, Chief Examiner (OHNS), and Board Chair of the Academy of Surgical Educators. He has been awarded Distinguished Service Awards from both of these organizations. He is a Life Member of the Neurotology Society of Australia.

He was Visiting Professor in the Dept. of Otolaryngology, Sun Yat Sen University, Guangzhou, China, from 2003 to 2009. He was the Wong Hua Yuen Distinguished Scholar, Hong Kong University in 2004.

He was appointed as the JLO Visiting Professor of the Royal Society of Medicine, London, UK, in 2007. He is a member of the Executive of the International Federation of Otolaryngological Societies.

His research interests include the Management of Acoustic Neuroma, Paragangliomas of the Head and Neck, Facial Paralysis and Temporal Bone Trauma as well as Outcome Measures and Quality of Life in Otology and Lateral Skull Base Surgery. He has published more than 40 peer-reviewed journal articles and book chapters. He is on the review panel for six international journals. He has a particular interest in surgical education and skills training in Otology and Lateral Skull Base Surgery and has directed and instructed on temporal bone dissection and skull base surgery courses in Australia, Africa, and China. He has been part of the Organizing and Scientific Committees and invited faculty member of numerous international Congresses on Otology and Skull Base Surgery.

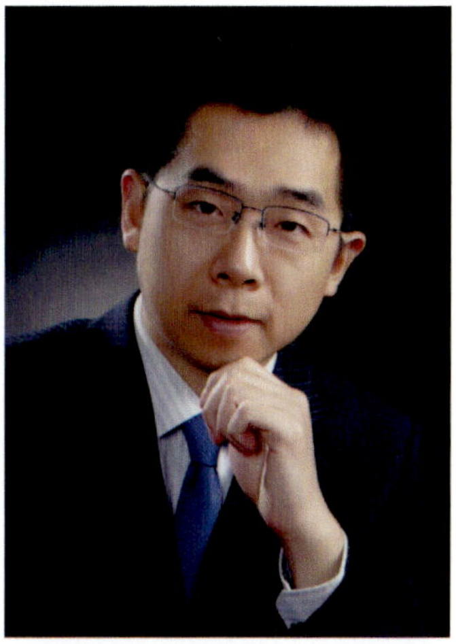

Yue-shuai Song is a junior otolaryngology head-neck surgeon. He graduated from the Nankai University Medical School, in Tianjin, China, in 2009 and later completed his otolaryngology training and was awarded a doctoral degree from the Nankai University Medical School in 2012. He undertook a further 3 years of postdoctoral training at the Chinese PLA General Hospital from 2012 to 2015. He has practiced as an otolaryngology head-neck surgeon in Beijing Friendship Hospital since 2015. He has a great deal of experience with the anatomy of the temporal bone and skull base and has focused his research on cochlear implantation and the three-dimensional (3D) morphology of the temporal bone. He participated in the publication of the first 3D atlas of micro ear surgery and anatomy as vice and chief editor in 2009 and 2016, respectively. Yue-shuai Song has published seven articles in international peer-reviewed journals and seven articles in Chinese journals. He holds six national patents. He is in charge of the anatomy training program in ear surgery at Beijing Friendship Hospital.

1 General Introduction

Yue-shuai Song, Song Gao, and Pu Dai

A Brief History of the Development of Stereoscopy in Ear Micro Surgery

Yue-shuai Song and Pu Dai

Our knowledge of the anatomy of the temporal bone can be dated back to Hippocrates who understood the tympanic membrane to be part of the acoustic apparatus, and Aristotle who recognized the cochlea as part of the hearing organ. Later in 1860 Toynbee studied 2000 temporal bones and published his findings in the classic work Disease of the Ear. So techniques especially modern techniques of dissection have greatly improved our abilities to study the temporal bone, and among them, Computerized Tomography (CT Scanning) has added to this.

The basic threads of three dimensional (3D) spatial shape research of otology came from Newton. In 1879 he suggested reconstructing the temporal bone using contiguous sheets, but this was not available until 1968, when an English engineer Hounsfield invented the first CT machine. With this technique Harada (1988) made some particular observations of the temporal bone, including the external auditory canal, tympanic membrane, carotid artery, vestibule, labyrinth and internal auditory canal. In 1989, Lutz reconstructed the facial nerve and carotid artery and made a 3-D measurement of anatomical structures. He also discussed the anatomical basis of various otologic diseases. In China, the work of Professor Pu Dai (1991) on temporal bone reconstruction based on extensive anatomic data hasn't only expanded the study but also enriched the knowledge of stereo reconstruction in China.

Computer aided temporal bone reconstruction has become a landmark in Medical studies, while it still has some defects, the images which are created by this technique are only an abstraction of the real anatomic structures, far different to real surgical images. Considering this, Professor Dai has further developed a way to capture and save stereo images. He has combined binocular vision theory, the stereoscope and the operating microscope in an ingenious way. This has provided a much more realistic representation of micro ear surgery.

Y.-s. Song, MD (✉)
Department of Otolarygngology Head and Neck Surgery, Beijing Friendship Hospital, Capital Medical University, Beijing 100050, China
e-mail: thinkmed@126.com

S. Gao, MD
Department of Otolaryngology, The 175th Hospital of Chinese PLA, Zhangzhou 363000, China

P. Dai, MD (✉)
Department of Otolarygngology Head and Neck Surgery, Chinese PLA General Hospital, Beijing 100853, China
e-mail: daipu301@vip.sina.com

P. Dai et al. (eds.), *Stereo Operative Atlas of Micro Ear Surgery*, DOI 10.1007/978-981-10-2089-6_1

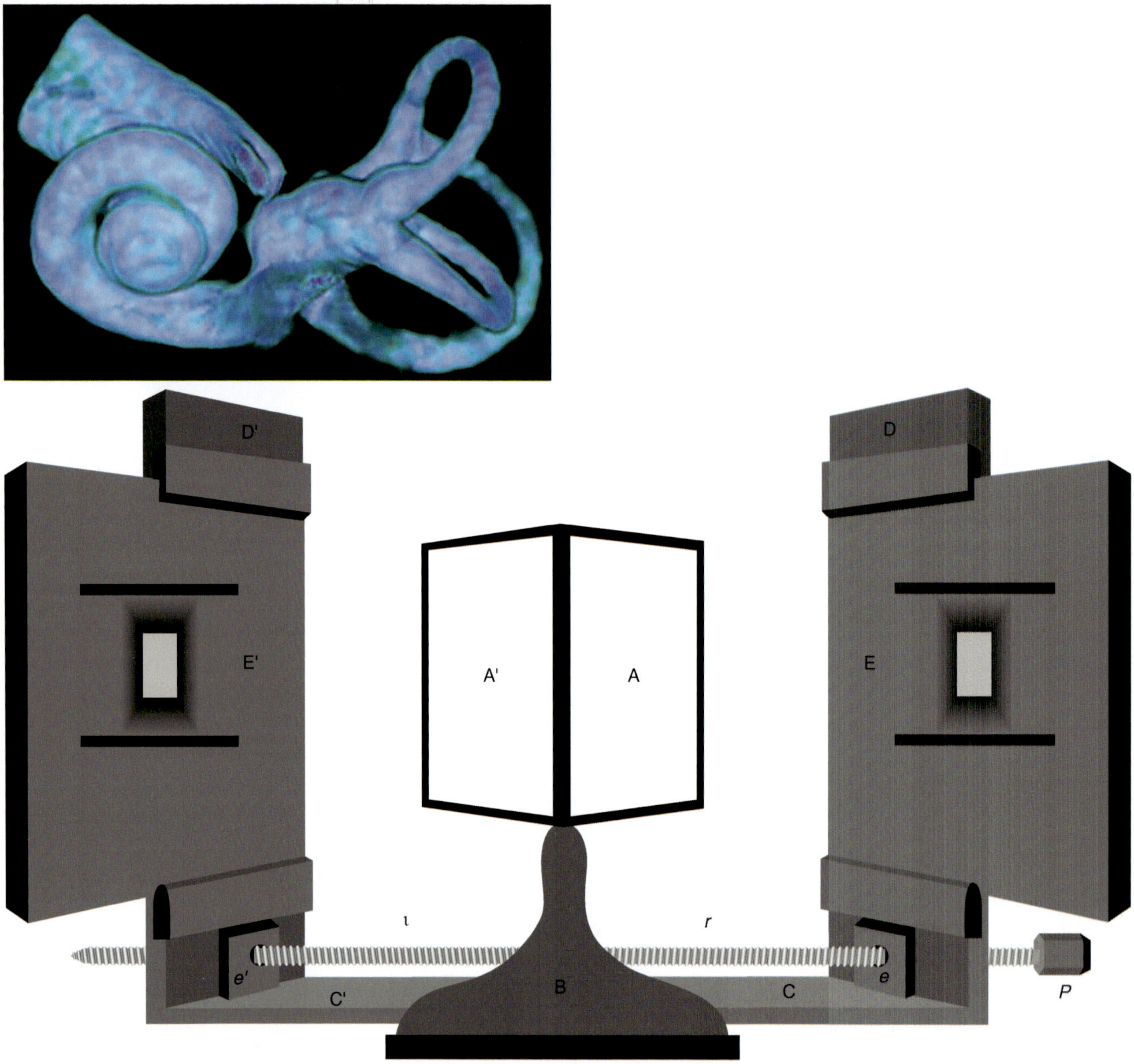

Fig. 1.1 Reconstructed 3D cochlea and reflecting mirror stereoscope
The wheatstone stereoscope (1838): to view images using the stereoscope (Reprint from Volume 68 of the series Intelligent Systems, Control and Automation: Science and Engineering pp 97–130, Springer, 2013)

Stereo Operative Photography of Micro Ear Surgery

Song Gao and Pu Dai

What Is Stereo Images of Micro Ear Surgery and How to Capture Them?

Micro Ear Surgery is routinely performed with the help of the operating microscope which gives true stereo vision through the two eye lens (just like we watch things through our two naked eyes). Traditionally this level of stereo-vision has not been available outside the Operating Room and we have had to bear standard 2D pictures, losing a lot of important spatial information, but now we have used a side-by-side stereoscopic system to address this deficiency. We use two separate Digital Single Lens Reflex (SLR) Cameras attached to an operating microscope to simultaneously capture left and right pictures of the same object as shown in the picture below.

Equipment and Specifications

The following equipment is required to record the ideal paired photographs:

1. Operating microscope with two side ports for attachment of two digital SLR cameras. Each side of the system, including eye-lens and camera, must have the same optical pathway;
2. The two cameras should be controlled by one manual key or pedal so that the left and right photographs are taken simultaneously by two cameras separately;
3. Adequate light: Sufficient light is always very important, especially when you want to capture images of very tiny structures in a very deep situation;
4. Two Hi-Q Digital Single Lens Reflex Cameras, and make sure they share the same settings.

In our department, we use two Canon EOS 5D digital cameras, one Carl Zeiss Pentero microscope with a foot control pedal connecting to it, which is used for image capture. Correct focus is controlled via a video monitor that has the same optical pathway to the right eye-lens.

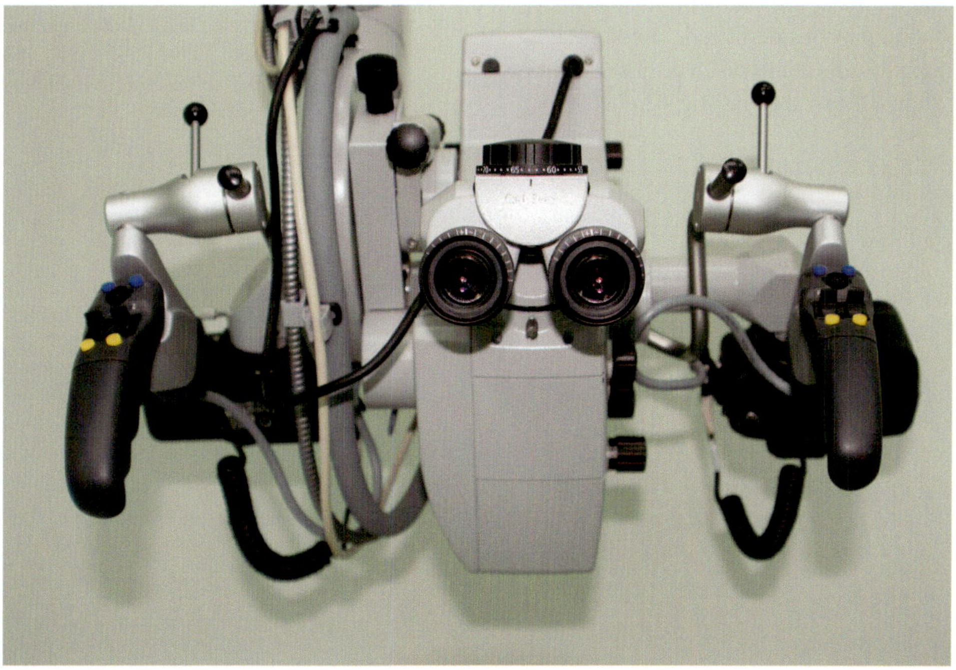

Fig. 1.2 The microscope with stereoscopic photo system

Stereo Image Production

Step 1: Open a pair of photos, captured during surgery in Adobe Photoshop software;
Step 2: Overlap the paired left and right side photos, make sure the structure in the focus of these two pictures can be completely matched.
Step 3: Crop photos to a standard measurement, and keep the observation target in the middle of the field;
Step 4: Position the edited photos side by side in their original side position;
Step 5: Save the side-by-side stereo-images in Hi-Q JPEG format;

The following steps are necessary to ensure effective stereovision:

1. Make sure the structure in the focus of these two pictures can be completely overlapped;
2. Side cannot be exchanged.

How to View the Stereo Images

Step 1: Unfold the stereoscope;
Step 2: Place the two feet of stereoscope in the both lateral margins of side-by-side stereo-image;
Step 3: Adjust lens distance of stereoscope;
Step 4: Enjoy the realistic stereovision!

Suggested Reading

A Brief Development History of Stereoscopic in Micro Ear Surgery

Beckmann EC. CT scanning the early days. Br J Radiol. 2006; 79(937):5–8.

Dai P, Jiang SC, Gu R. Computer assisted three-dimensional (3D) reconstruction and mechanical model establishment of Ossicular chain. Chin J Otorhinolaryngol. 1991;26:272–4.

Dai P, Shi LY, Liu Y. The study and application of the three dimensional anatomical atlas of temporal bone. Med J Chin People's Liberation Army. 2004;29(5):392–5.

Hoffmeister JW, et al. Comput Med Imaging Graph. 1990;14:35–42.

Luo SQ, Zhou GH. Medical images processing and analysis. Beijing: Science Press; 2003. p. 282–7.

Schultheiss D, Denil J. History of the microscope and development of microsurgery: a revolution for reproductive tract surgery. Andrologia. 2002;34(4):234–41.

Wheatstone C. Contributions to the physiology of vision-part the first. on some remarkable, and hitherto unobserved, phenomena of binocular vision. Phil Trans R Soc London. 1838;128:371–94.

Stereo Operative Photography of Micro Ear Surgery

Dai P, JIANG SC, Gu R. Computer assisted three-dimensional (3D) reconstruction and mechanical model establishment of Ossicular chain. Chin J Otorhinolaryngol. 1991;26:272–4.

You-jun Y, Pu D, Zhen L, et al. Application of three dimensional view fixture in temporal bone anatomy. Chin J Otol. 2006; 4(3):231–3.

2 Mastoid and Middle Ear Surgery

Pu Dai, Yue-shuai Song, Rui-li Yu, Yi Sun, Zhao-hui Hou, Fei Yu, Ming-yu Han, and Bing Han

Tympanostomy Tubes

Rui-li Yu and Yue-shuai Song

Indications

1. Refractory secretory otitis media, without improvement after conservative treatments, such as antibiotics, Eustachian tube inflation or previous tympanostomy alone.
2. Glue ear or severe atelectasis.
3. Severe conductive hearing loss due to negative middle ear pressure and having an effect on language development.
4. Recurrent acute otitis media.
5. Abnormal patency of Eustachian tube.
6. Hyperbaric oxygen therapy.

Contraindications

Systemic conditions with patient not suitable for local or general anesthesia.

P. Dai, MD (✉) • Z.-h. Hou, MD • F. Yu, MD • M.-y. Han, MD
B. Han, MD
Department of Otolarygngology Head and Neck Surgery, Chinese PLA General Hospital, Beijing 100853, China
e-mail: daipu301@vip.sina.com

Y.-s. Song, MD (✉)
Department of Otolarygngology Head and Neck Surgery, Beijing Friendship Hospital, Capital Medical University, Beijing 100050, China
e-mail: thinkmed@126.com

R.-l. Yu, MD
Department of Allergy, Beijing Shijitan Hospital, Affiliated to Capital Medical University, Beijing 100038, China

Y. Sun, MD
Department of Otolaryngology, Chinese PLA Wuhan General Hospital, Wuhan 430070, China

Operative Procedures

1. Remove cerumen, then sterilize EAC with 0.1 % thimerosal solution.
2. Tympanic membrane is incised full-thickness under the operating microscope. The length of the incision is about 2–4 mm, and should match the diameter of the inner flange of ventilating tube. Considering manubrium of malleus as vertical axis, umbo of tympanic membrane as horizontal axis, tympanic membrane can be divided into four quadrants, anterior-superior, anterior-inferior, posterior-superior and posterior-inferior. The incision is usually located in the anterior-inferior quadrant of the membrane for better drainage.
3. Drainage of middle ear fluid, and lavage the cavity with the mixed solution of dexamethasone and α chymotrypsin.
4. Tympanostomy tube in position.

Special Comments

1. It is necessary to inspect the tympanic membrane under the microscope preoperatively. A blue or red color of the membrane may indicate a high jugular bulb (more common on right side) or glomus tumor. One should also look for pulsation behind the tympanic membrane.
2. It is better to use a ventilating tube made of Teflon for less infection and less occlusion. Caution: a silicone tube may result in the formation of granulation tissue after prolonged intubation. Shepard and Armstrong Grommets are suitable for most cases, while Goode T Grommet have an increased risk of residual tympanic membrane perforation after long term use ventilation.
3. The incision should avoid the posteriorsuperior quadrant of the drum in order to protect the ossicular chain. In case of long-term intubation, it is better to place the incision in front of the malleus handle.

P. Dai et al. (eds.), *Stereo Operative Atlas of Micro Ear Surgery*, DOI 10.1007/978-981-10-2089-6_2

4. The incision should not be too close to the tympanic annulus or umbo of tympanic membrane for most stable placement.
5. The incision should be made and the drainage tube should be placed in a healthy segment of the tympanic membrane.
6. The EAC should be kept dry. The ear should be reviewed regularly. Avoid any kind of fluid, and apply antibiotic ear drops for infection or apply heparin if the tube is occluded.

Complications

1. Injury of ossicular chain: this is uncommon if the ventilating tube is placed in the antero-inferior quadrant under operating microscope.
2. Otorrhea after tympanostomy tube placement: Avoid infection by sterilizing the operating field carefully and lavaging the external canal with a solution containing antibiotics and glucocorticoid. Otorrhea may occur in some children despite these measures. If otorrhea occurs, apply antibiotic ear drops. Refractory otorrhea requires regular cleaning of the external canal and aspiration of middle ear fluid.
3. A residual perforation following tube removal may take 1 or 2 years to fully heal spontaneously.
4. Tube displaced into the tympanic cavity: this may be caused by an oversized incision or drum atrophy. If this occurs, the tube may be removed via the original or an extended incision.
5. Bleeding from high jugular bulb: A high bulb appears as a dark red structure beneath the tympanic membrane and should be identified before tympanostomy, to avoid injury. If bleeding occurs, stop the operation immediately and pack the canal with gelfoam and antibiotic gauze for hemostasis.

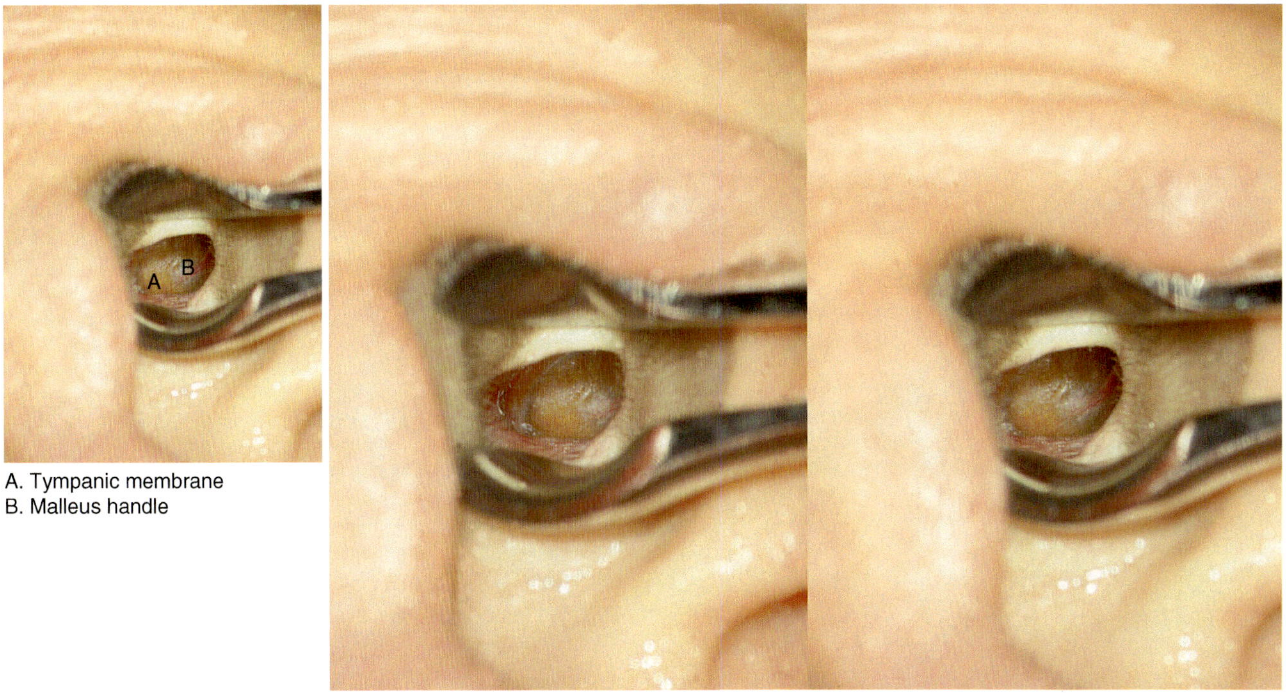

Fig. 2.1 Exposure of tympanic membrane
Remove cerumen from the external canal, sterilize the operation field with 0.1 % thimerosal solution. Expand external canal by otoscope or nasoscope, expose tympanic membrane under operating microscope. The tympanic membrane has lost it's normal gloss and appears yellow. A dilated capillary can be seen on the pars tensa, and the tympanic cavity contains fluid

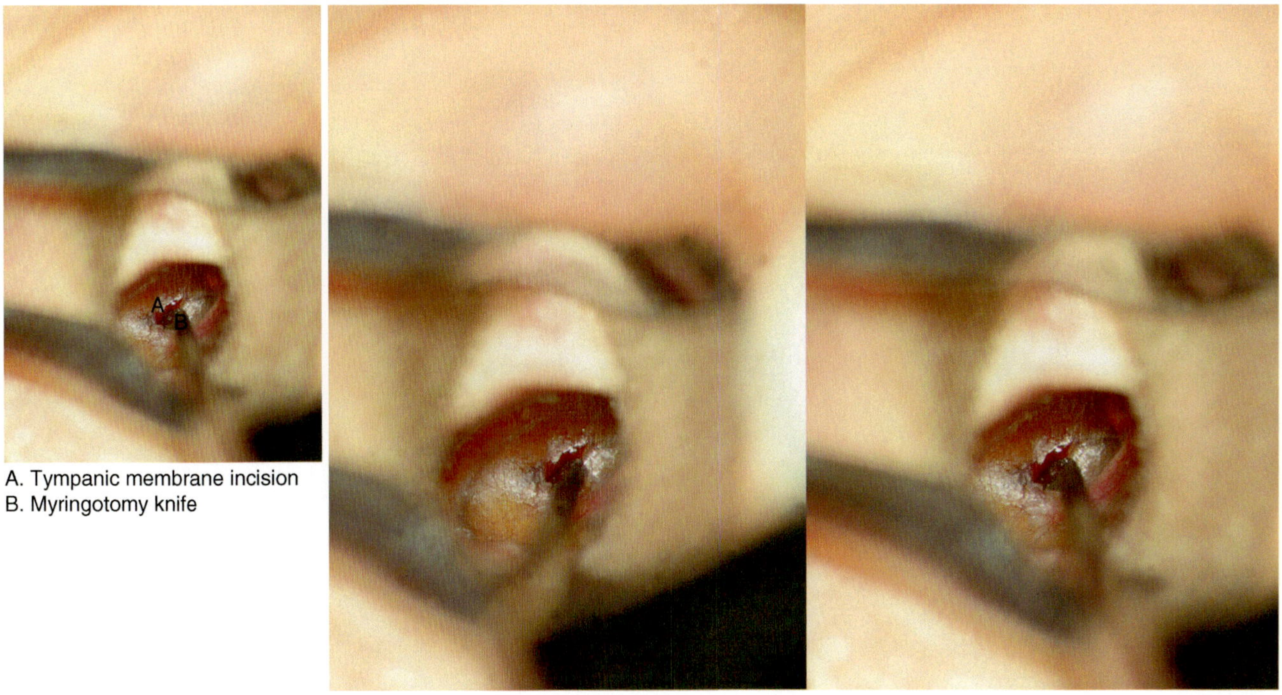

Fig. 2.2 Myringotomy
The myringotomy is carried out with a myringotomy knife in the anteroinferior quadrant of the drum, remaining 3 mm away from the tympanic annulus. The length of the incision should match the diameter of the inner flange of the ventilating tube. In cases of atelectasis, the myringotomy should be made over the deepest possible region of the hypotympanum

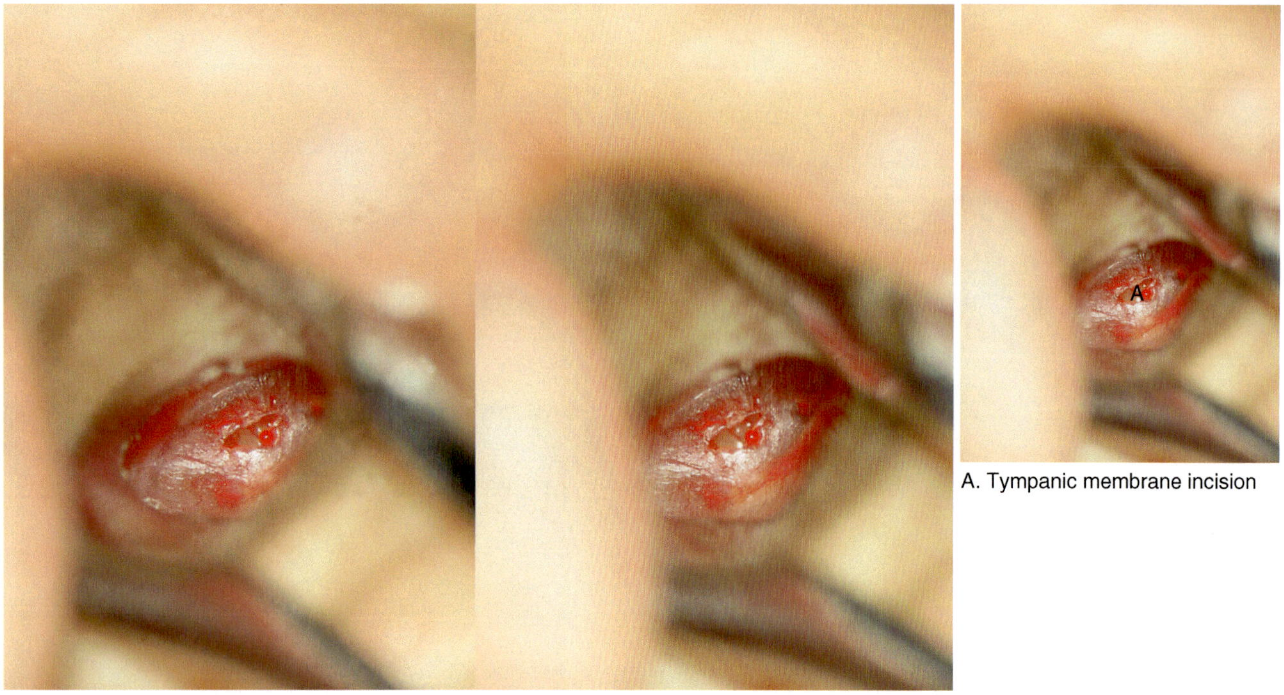

A. Tympanic membrane incision

Fig. 2.3 Drainage of middle ear effusion
After the effusion is aspirated using the smallest possible suction tubes, the inner wall of tympanic cavity is exposed. If the secretion is viscous, an adjuvant incision may be performed at the posteroinferior quadrant to aid aspiration

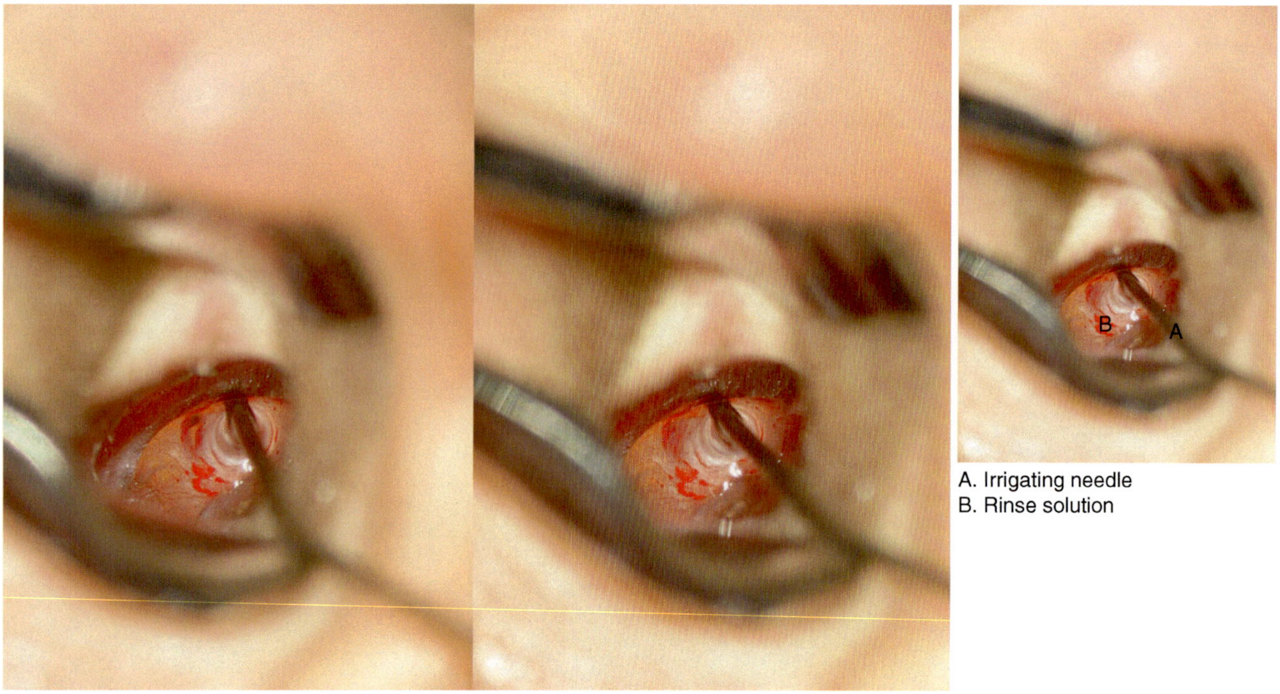

A. Irrigating needle
B. Rinse solution

Fig. 2.4 Tympanic cavity irrigation
Irrigate and aspirate the tympanic cavity with a mixed solution of dexamethasone and α chymotrypsin gently and repeatedly

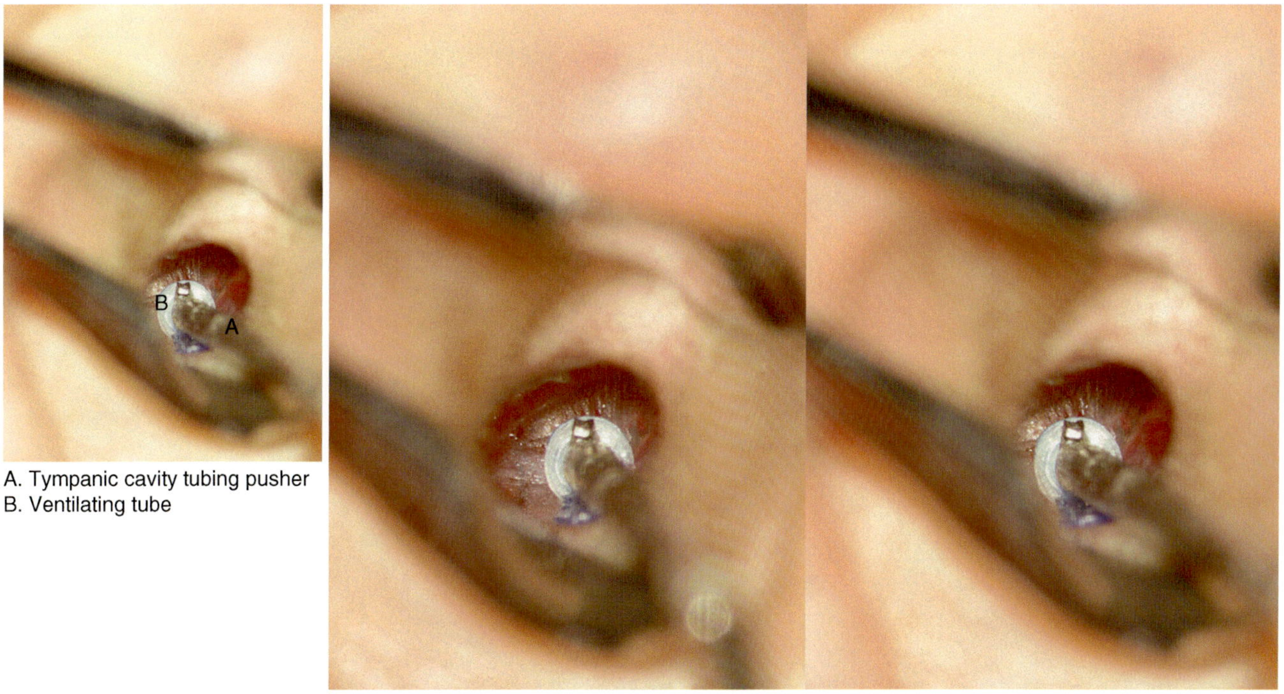

Fig. 2.5 Placement of the ventilating tube
A ventilating tube is introduced into the external auditory canal carefully with a specialized tympanic cavity tubing pusher. One side of the tube is inserted into the incision first, then it is rotated into the tympanic cavity. Finally, adjust the position of the ventilating tube with a 1.5 mm, 45° hook

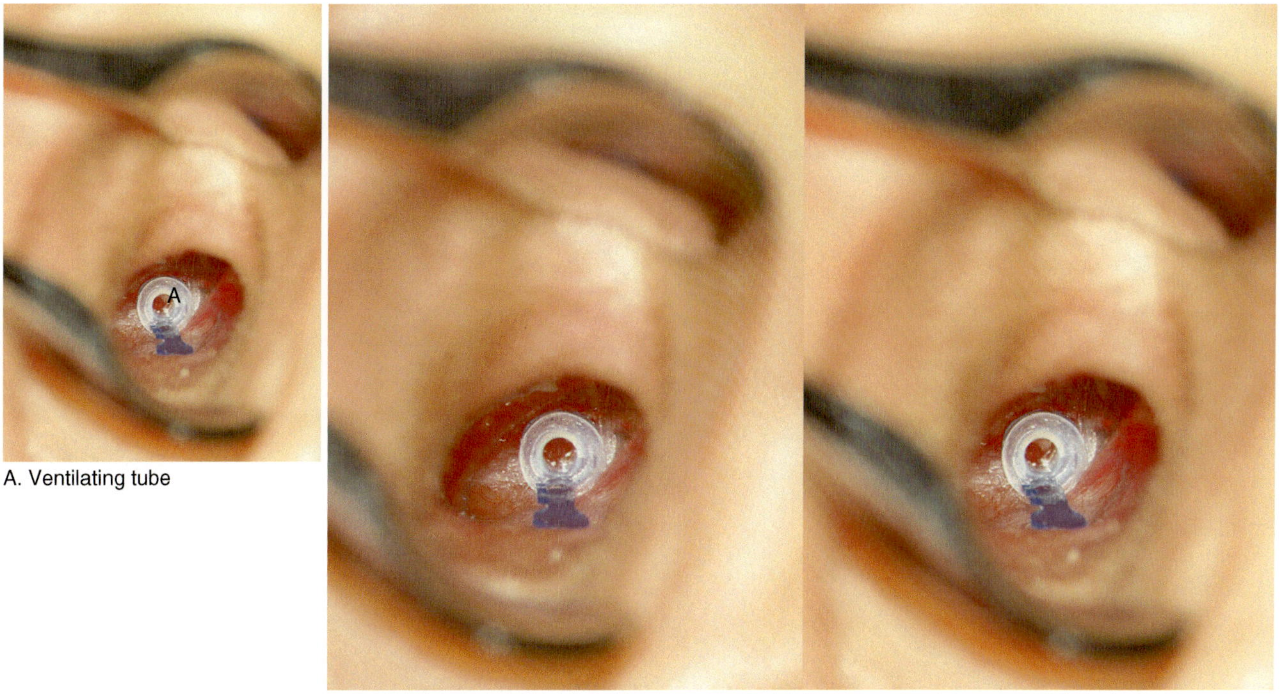

Fig. 2.6 Check the position of the ventilating tube
After the placement of the ventilating tube, its position and stability should be checked. In this case, there is some clear liquid in the tube lumen, the length of the incision is appropriate, and the tube is correctly positioned

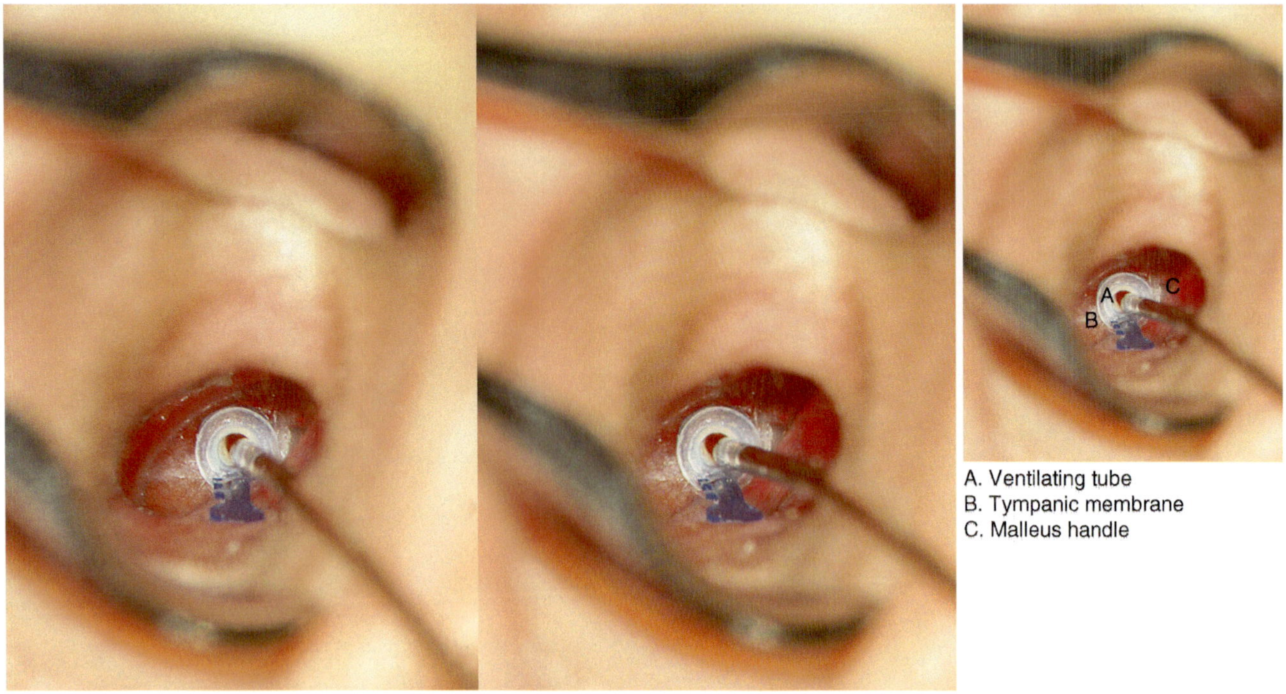

A. Ventilating tube
B. Tympanic membrane
C. Malleus handle

Fig. 2.7 Adjust the position of the ventilating tube
Aspirate blood and liquid from around the ventilating tube, and adjust the position of the tube if necessary. If the tube is displaced into the tympanic cavity, grasp the blue strap on the tube and remove it using a large straight alligator forceps, then reposition the tube correctly

Myringoplasty

Rui-li Yu and Yue-shuai Song

Indications

1. The conducting function of ossicular chain is normal.
2. The size of the perforation is medium or large
3. Small perforation but the residual drum is atrophic
4. The edges of the perforation are infolded.
5. Persisting perforation despite cautery and application of ointment
6. The ossicular chain should be evaluated when a preoperative patch test fails to improve hearing.

Contraindications

1. Middle ear cholesteatoma.
2. Acute suppurative otitis media.
3. Acute infection or active chronic suppurative otitis media.
4. Ear Pseudomonas aeruginosa infection disease in diabetes mellitus patients.
5. Patient unfit for surgery.

Operative Procedures

1. Anesthesia: General or local anesthesia is used in adults, and general anesthesia is used in children. The local anesthesia is injected in four quadrants just lateral to the bone external canal and 2% tetracaine solution is instilled in the tympanic cavity for surface anesthesia during surgery.
2. The preparation of the graft: the temporalis fascia is harvested from the side of the affected ear. A horizontal incision approximately 2.5 cm long is made, 2–3 cm above the auricle. After separating the subcutaneous tissue, the tough white fascia close to the temporal muscle is exposed. The fascia is separated from the underlying muscle. The graft has a diameter of 1.5–2 cm. The graft is spread on a block and any excess fat and muscle are removed. The fascia is placed in the 75% alcohol until it is used.
3. The first skin incision starts from the 12 o'clock position of EAC and carried down to the bone. It is extended laterally between the tragus and the crus of helix for about 1.0 cm.
4. The second incision is semi-circumferential and performed just medial to the bony-cartilaginous junction. It starts from the 6 o'clock position of EAC, and remains 5 mm lateral to the tympanic annulus along the posterior meatal wall in an ascending spiral fashion to meet the first incision. The edges of the perforation are freshened with a straight needle before the tympanomeatal flap is elevated.
5. Elevation of meatal skin flap: An articulated retractor is introduced to expose the operating field. The skin and periosteum of EAC are separated from the underlying bone to the level of the tympanic annulus. The overhanging suprameatal spine is removed using a diamond burr or osteotome.
6. The epithelial layer of the tympanic membrane remnant is separated from the fibrous layer, superiorly, anteriorly and inferiorly in sequence. This prepares the bed for the total overlay grafting technique. However if one edge of the perforation is close to the tympanic annulus, the tympanomeatal flap is raised lifting the annulus to enter tympanic cavity for the combined underlay grafting technique.
7. In the combined underlay grafting procedure, one should inspect the tympanic cavity and ossicular chain after the tympanomeatal flap is elevated when an ossicular problem is suspected. Care should be taken to protect the chorda tympani nerve when separating the fibrous tympanic annulus.
8. The long process of the incus and the incudostapedial joint are exposed with removal of some bone from the postero-superior canal wall.
9. After aspiration of blood, the condition of the tympanic cavity and the mobility of the ossicular chain are examined. Any infected material is removed. Gelfoam pledgets soaked in antibiotic solution are placed in the tympanic cavity.
10. The temporalis fascia is introduced between the epithelial and the fibrous layer of the tympanic membrane remnant (for the total overlay grafting technique); or placed between the tympanomeatal flap and the bony canal wall. If there is little or no anterior tympanic membrane remnant, the graft is inserted against the anterior wall of the tympanic cavity and pledgets of gelfoam are placed in the middle ear to support it. The graft is placed lateral to the malleus handle.
11. Repositioning the meatal skin flap: the meatal skin flap and tympanic membrane remnant are replaced in their original position, covering the fascia. The graft should not extend beyond the external canal incision. The fascia is adjusted to cover the perforation.
12. The external canal is packed with gelfoam and a strip of iodoform gauze.
13. Incision closure.

Special Comments

1. The condition of the middle ear should be explored in cases with a marginal perforation.
2. The epithelial layer of the drum must be preserved during its elevation. If this is not achieved, the combined underlay grafting technique will be used.

3. Removal of epithelial remnants: after the tympanomeatal flap is elevated, care must be taken to remove any residual epithelial remnants on the surface of the fibrous layer of the tympanic membrane to prevent inclusion under the graft.
4. Protection of the chorda tympani nerve: The chorda tympani nerve should be preserved while elevating the posterior tympanomeatal flap and separating the tympanic annulus. The nerve is identified as a cord-like structure along the tympanic sulcus. It should be carefully dissected free from the sulcus and the bone.
5. Care should be taken not to damage the ossicular chain.
6. Ensure that the graft covers the perforation completely. Gentle even pressure should be used when filling the external canal with the gelfoam and gauze.

Complications

1. Incomplete closure of the perforation: this complication may result from the inadequate separation of the epithelial layer from the fibrous layer of the tympanic membrane remnant. The local anesthetic should be injected deep to the epithelial layer to make the separation easier. One must ensure a strict intraoperative aseptic technique. The ear canal packing should be removed within 2 weeks of surgery.
2. Formation of Cholesteatoma deep to the repaired tympanic membrane: this complication occurs when remnants of epidermis have been left on the margin of perforation. The growth of these remnants leads to the formation of the new cholesteatoma lateral to the fibrous layer of the tympanic membrane.
3. Retraction pocket: this complication results from the inadequate Eustachian tube function or tympanic membrane adhering to the medial wall of the middle ear. This complication can be avoided by placing gelfoam pledgets soaked in the antibiotic solution in the tympanic cavity.
4. Thick tympanic membrane: this complication occurs if the graft is too thick. Excess fat and muscle tissue must be removed from the fascia prior to its insertion.
5. Blunting of the anterior tympanomeatal angle: This can occur due to the inadequate fixation of the anteroinferior graft by gelfoam pledgets.

   Incomplete fusion of the drum to the manubrium of malleus: this complication is often seen in the total overlay grafting procedure, and occurs when the graft shrinks and becomes detached from the malleus handle.
6. Stenosis of the external auditory canal: this complication can occur due to extensive injury to the canal skin, postoperative infection and proliferation of granulation tissue.

Surgery 1: Myringoplasty

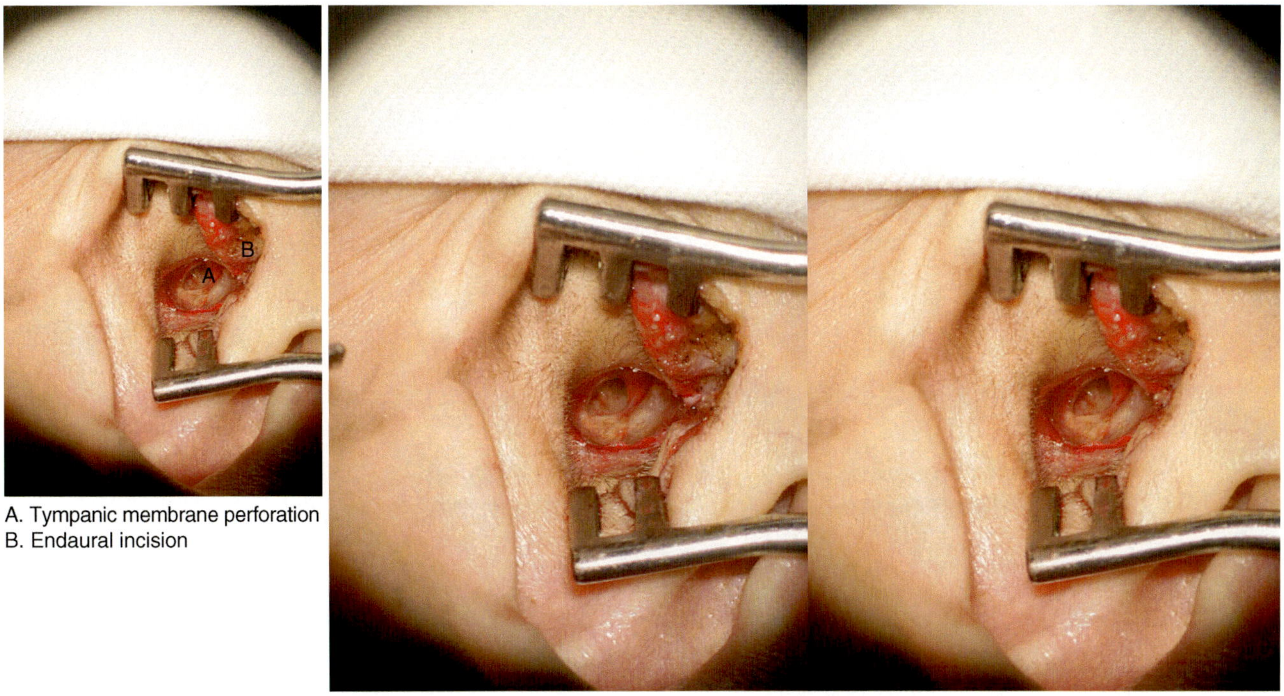

A. Tympanic membrane perforation
B. Endaural incision

Fig. 2.8 Endaural incision
The fascia is harvested from the temporal muscle above the affected ear and dried in 75 % ethanol. The first skin incision is made at the 12 o'clock position of EAC just lateral to the bony-cartilaginous junction and carried down to the bone. An outward prolongation of about 1.0 cm in length is made between the tragus and the crus of helix, and then under the operating microscope the first incision is extended inward to a point about 0.8–1.0 cm lateral to the tympanic annulus. The second incision starts from the 6 o'clock position of EAC, and remains 5 mm lateral to the tympanic annulus along the posterior meatal wall in an ascending spiral (or curved) fashion to meet the first incision. The soft tissue in the junction of these two incisions often needs to be cut with a sharp knife

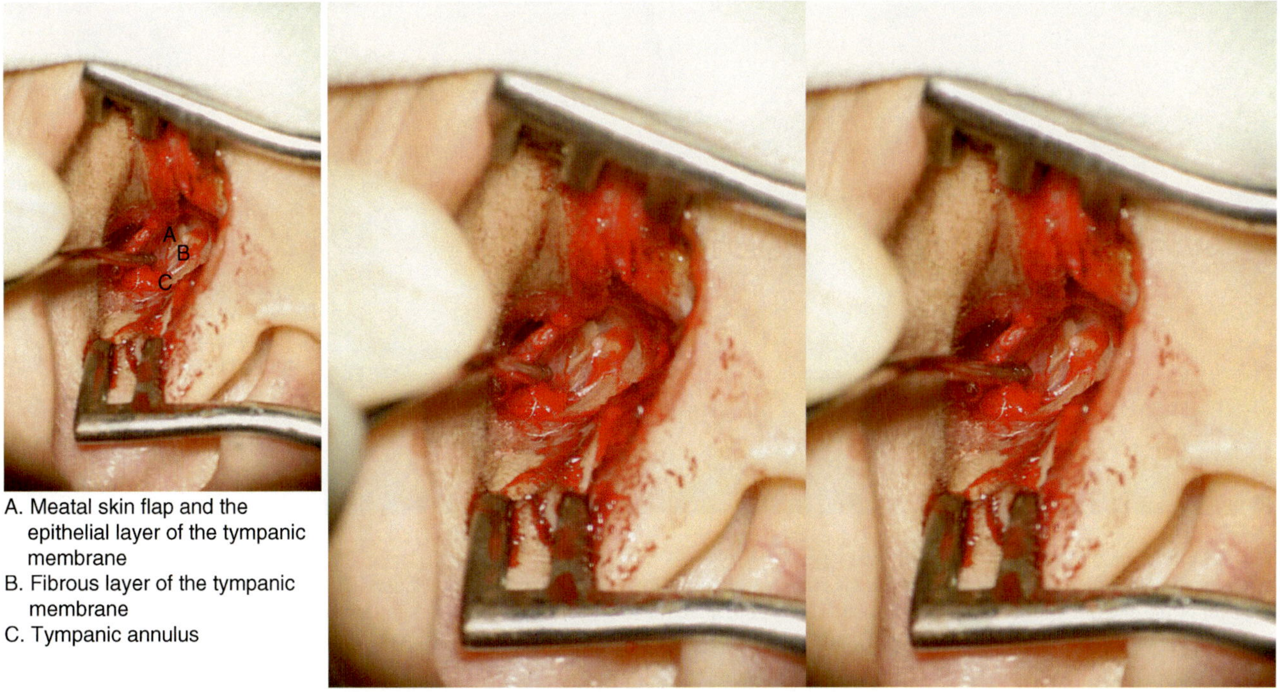

A. Meatal skin flap and the epithelial layer of the tympanic membrane
B. Fibrous layer of the tympanic membrane
C. Tympanic annulus

Fig. 2.9 Elevation of the meatal skin flap and the epithelial layer of the posterior tympanic membrane
Remove the overhanging suprameatal spine using a diamond burr or chisel. Separate the skin of EAC to the level of the tympanic annulus and elevate the epithelial layer of the remnant tympanic membrane across the tympanic sulcus. Expose the lateral process of malleus by separating the epithelial layer from the fibrous layer covering this process

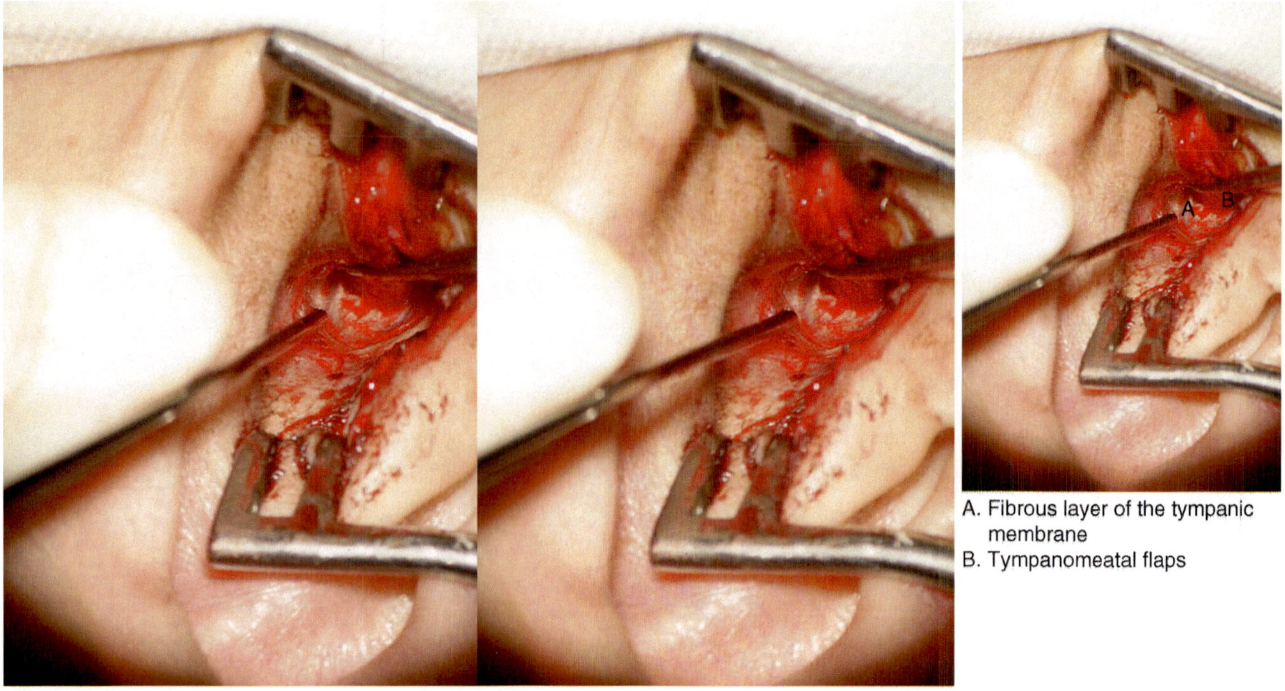

Fig. 2.10 Separate the epithelial layer from the inferior remnant of tympanic membrane
Separate the epithelial layer from the fibrous layer of the tympanic membrane postero-inferiorly, inferiorly and antero-inferiorly, respectively. Then, the epithelial layer is separated from the fibrous layer totally and the tympanomeatal flaps are elevated anteriorly like a swinging door

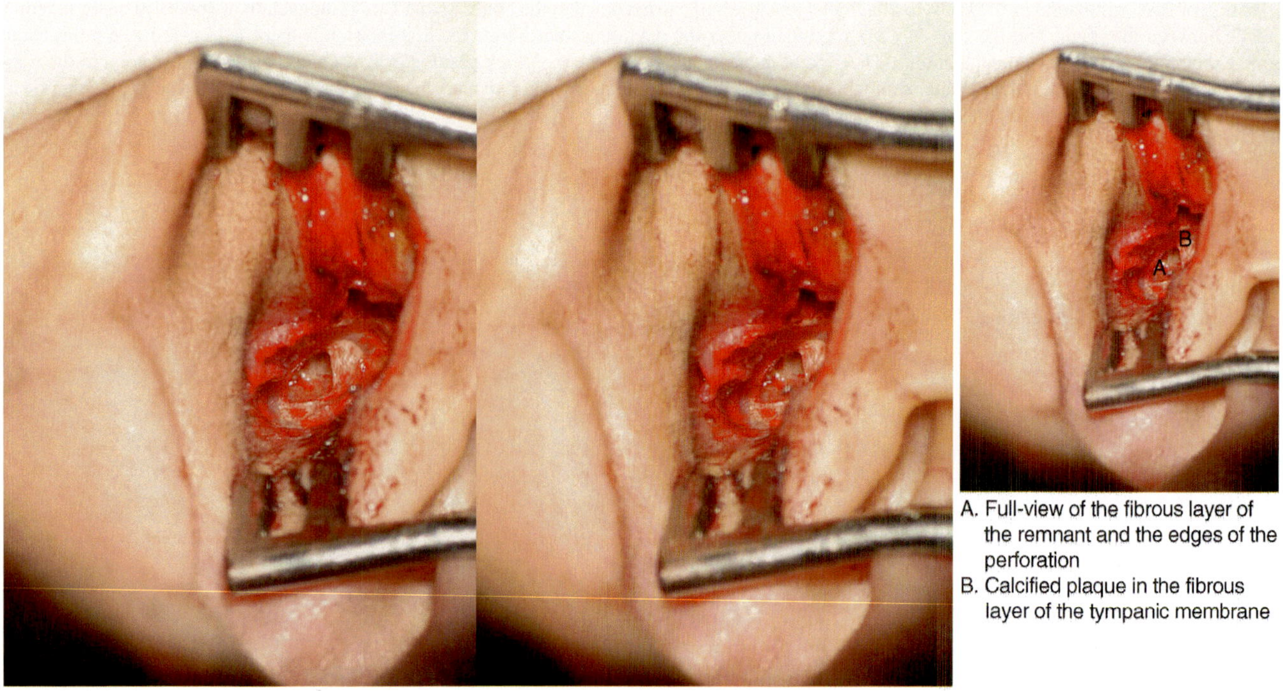

Fig. 2.11 Elevation of the tympanomeatal flaps
After the meatal portion and the tympanic portion of the flap are raised totally, the tympanomeatal flap is completed. Preserve the pedicle including the skin of the anterior wall of the external canal. This will prepare the bed to accept the graft. A posterosuperior tympanomeatal flap is raised, exposing the full-view of the fibrous layer and perforation edges, including the calcified plaque in the fibrous layer of the tympanic membrane in this case

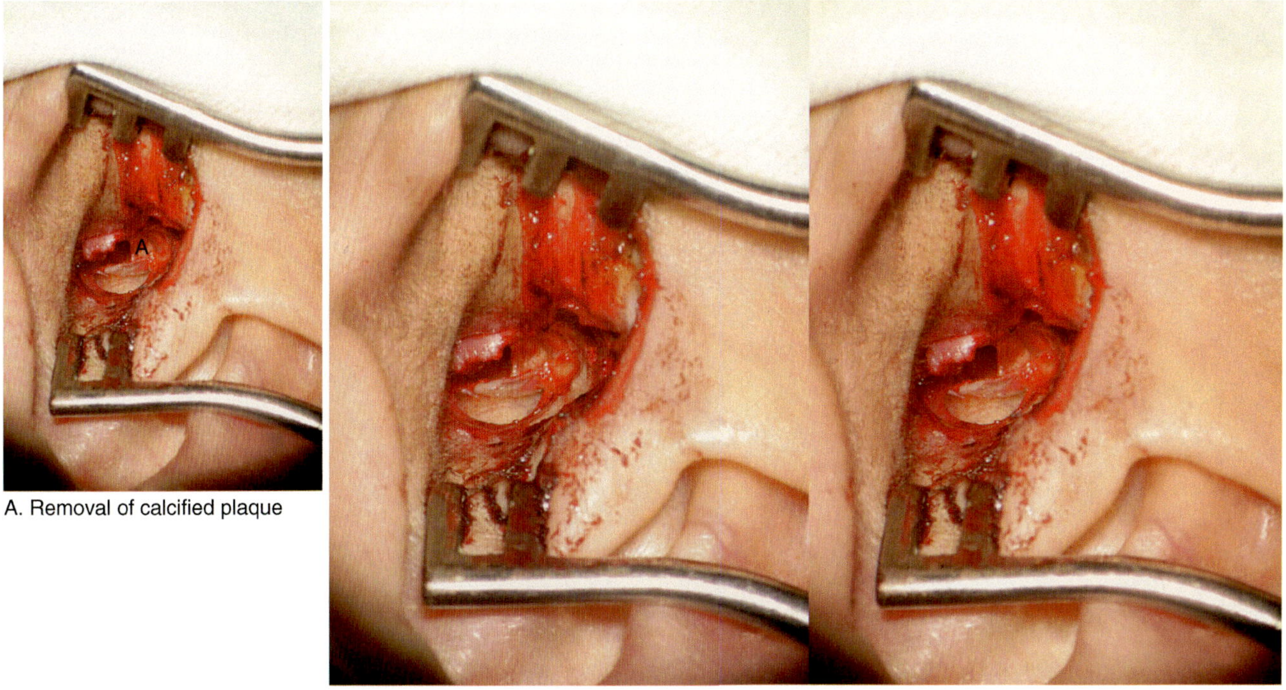

A. Removal of calcified plaque

Fig. 2.12 Removal of calcified plaque in the fibrous layer of the tympanic membrane
Pierce around the margin of the calcified plaque in the tympanic membrane remnant and remove the plaque intact

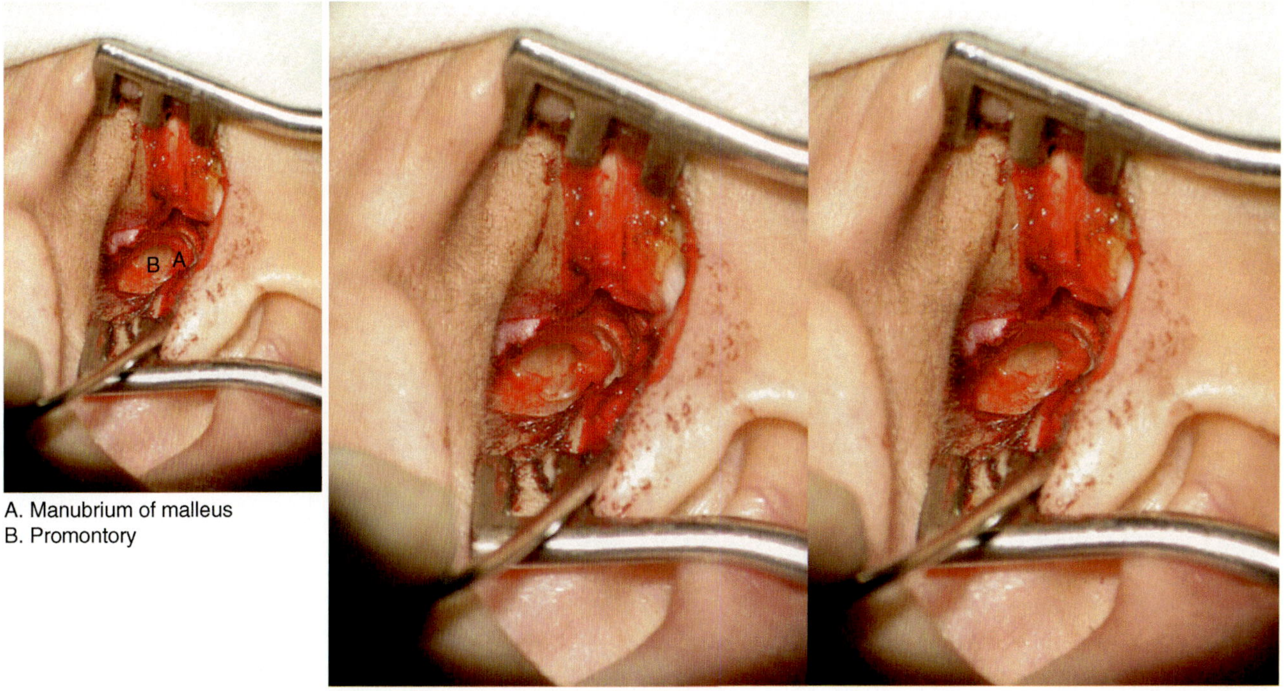

A. Manubrium of malleus
B. Promontory

Fig. 2.13 Expose the manubrium of malleus after removing the calcified plaque
Remove the calcified plaque in front of the manubrium of the malleus to expose it completely. Care should be taken to avoid altering the position of the normal fibrous layer

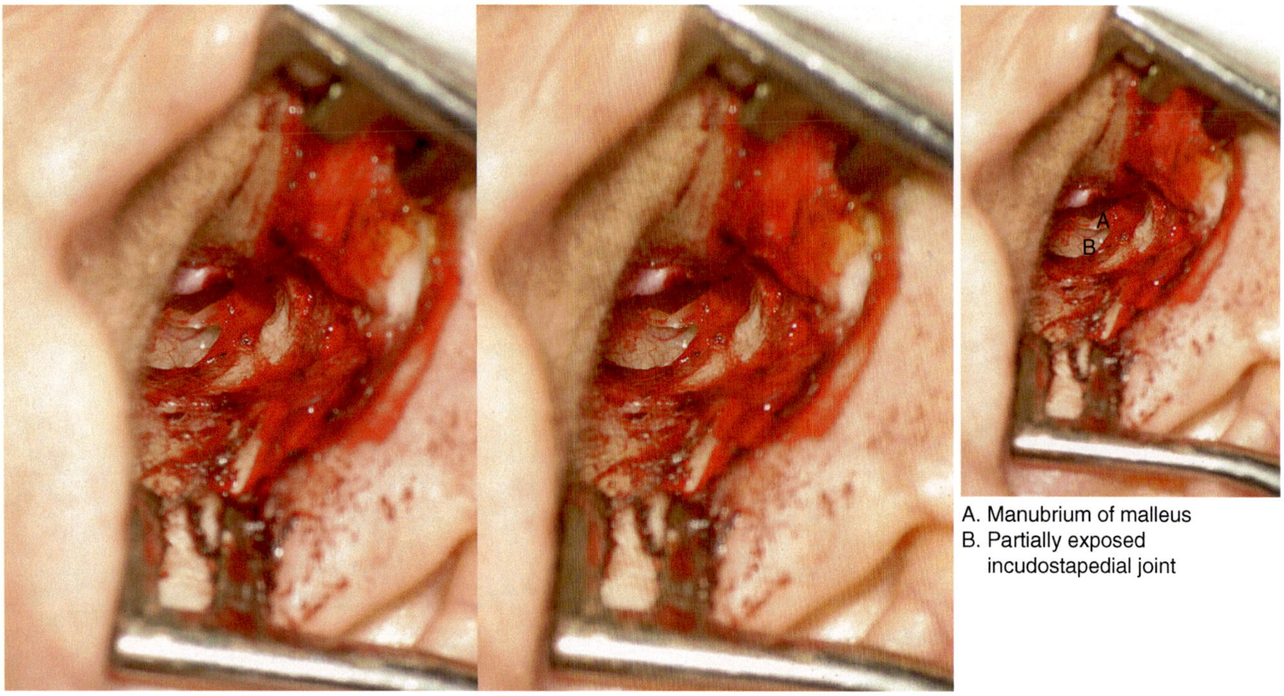

Fig. 2.14 Inspecting the incudostapedial joint
After removing the sclerosis of the fibrous layer, the incudostapedial joint is exposed. The mobility and integrity of the ossicular chain is tested and no abnormality was found in this case

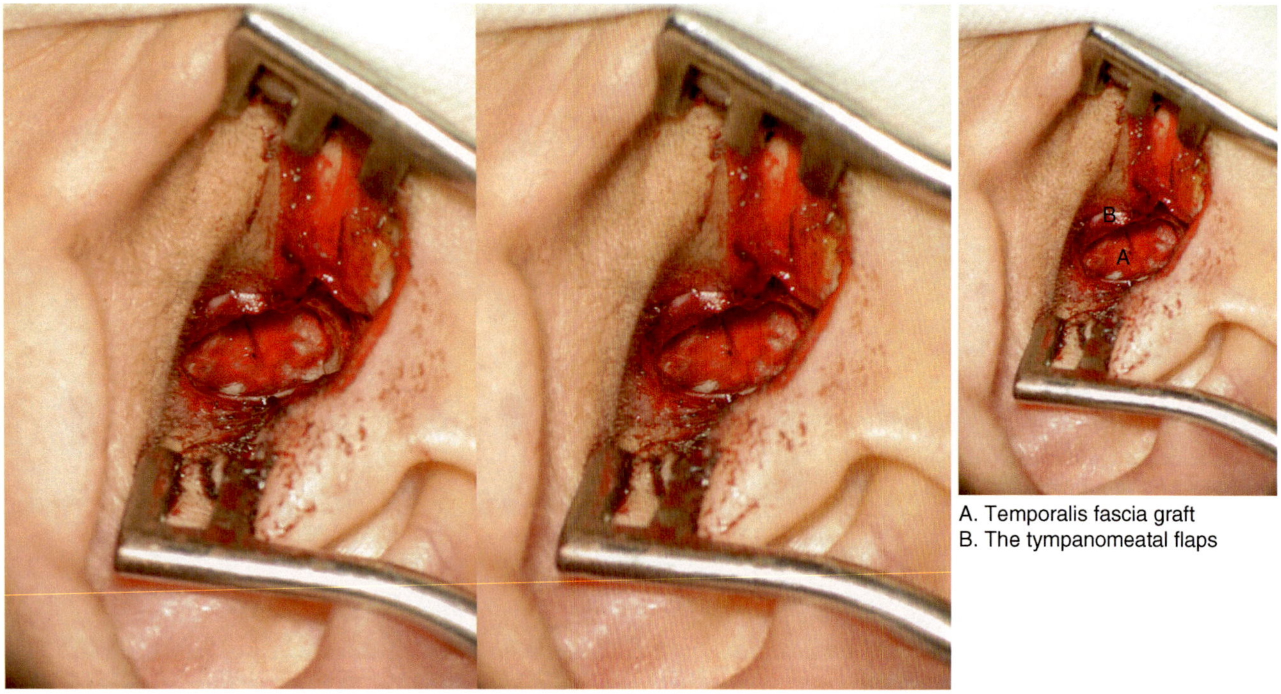

Fig. 2.15 Introduction of the temporal fascia
The graft is cut with scissors to the appropriate size to cover the perforation. The graft is introduced between the tympanomeatal flaps and the fibrous layer of the tympanic membrane. Care should be taken to ensure that the posterior edge of the graft does not protrude posterior to the line of the second incision. The fascia should be placed flat, without folds, bulges or indentations

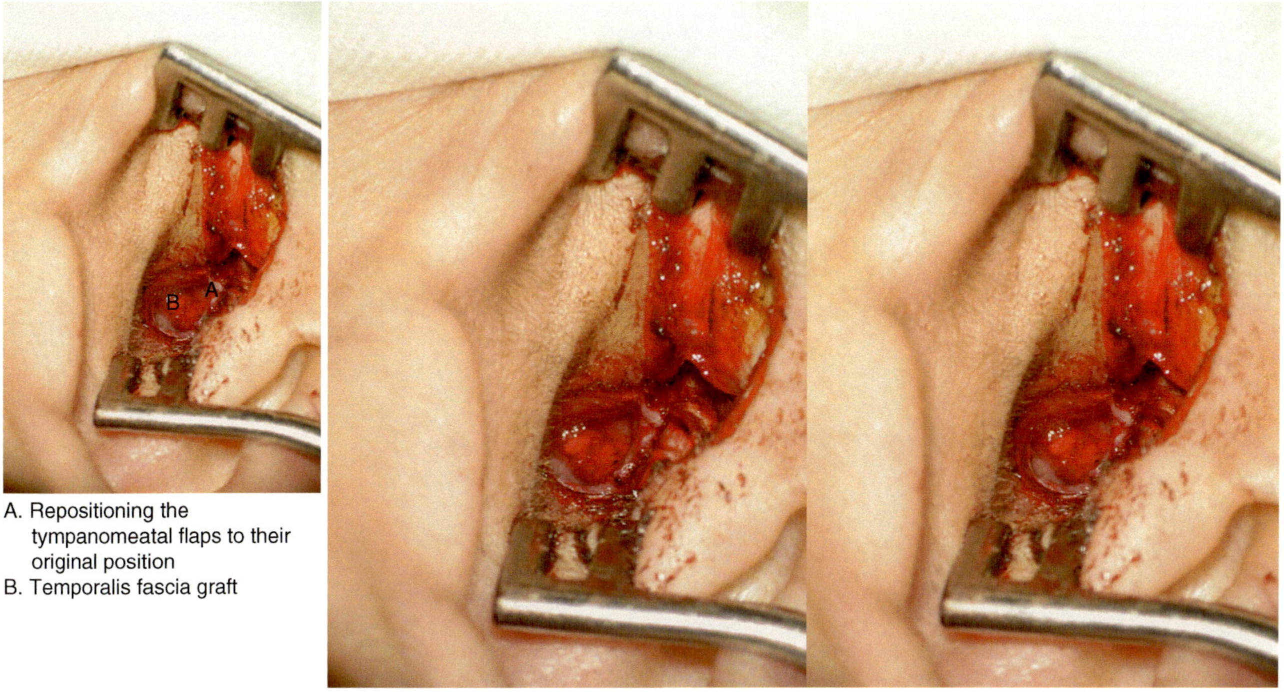

A. Repositioning the tympanomeatal flaps to their original position
B. Temporalis fascia graft

Fig. 2.16 Repositioning the meatal skin flap and the epithelial layer of the drum
The tympanomeatal flaps are repositioned, keeping the fascia in contact with the tympanic annulus and between the epithelial layer and fibrous layer of the drum

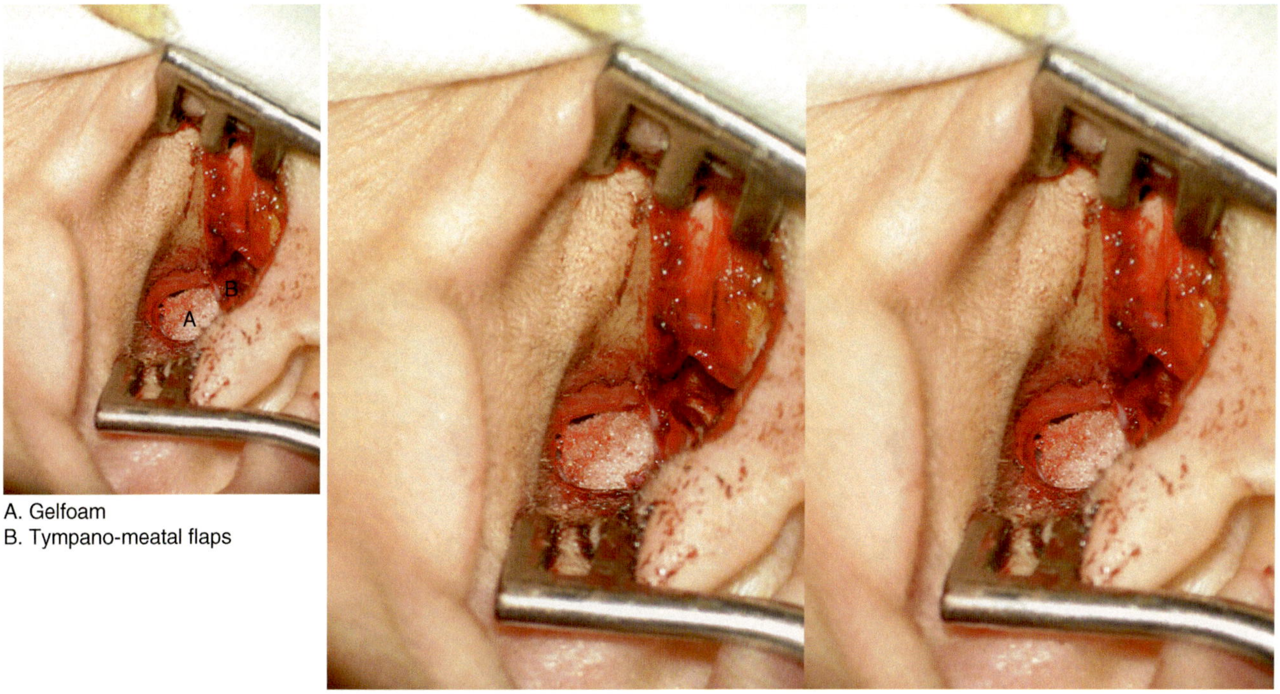

A. Gelfoam
B. Tympano-meatal flaps

Fig. 2.17 Placing the gelfoam on the surface of the drum
Gelfoam pledgets soaked in antibiotic solution are placed in the external acoustic meatus, on the lateral surface of the tympanic membrane and covering the second incision

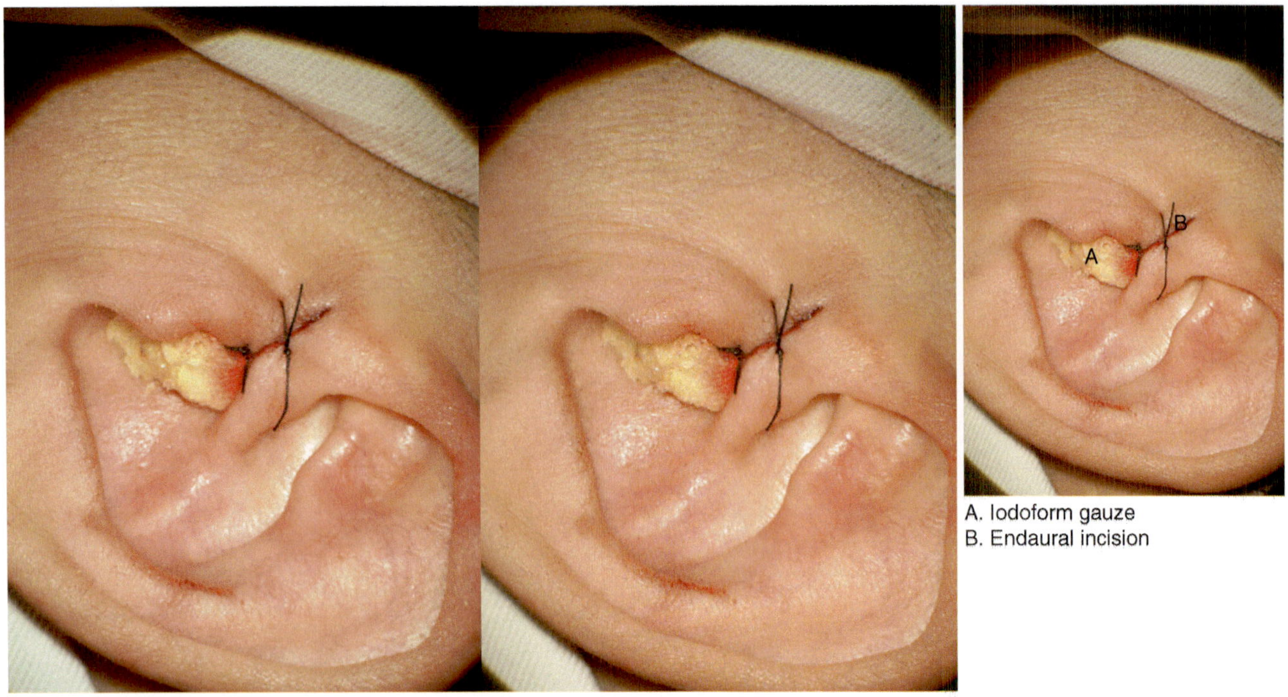

A. Iodoform gauze
B. Endaural incision

Fig. 2.18 Packing the external meatus with a strip of iodoform gauze and closing the wound
The external canal is packed with 0.5–1.0 cm strip of iodoform gauze, and the incision is closed

Surgery 2: Myringoplasty

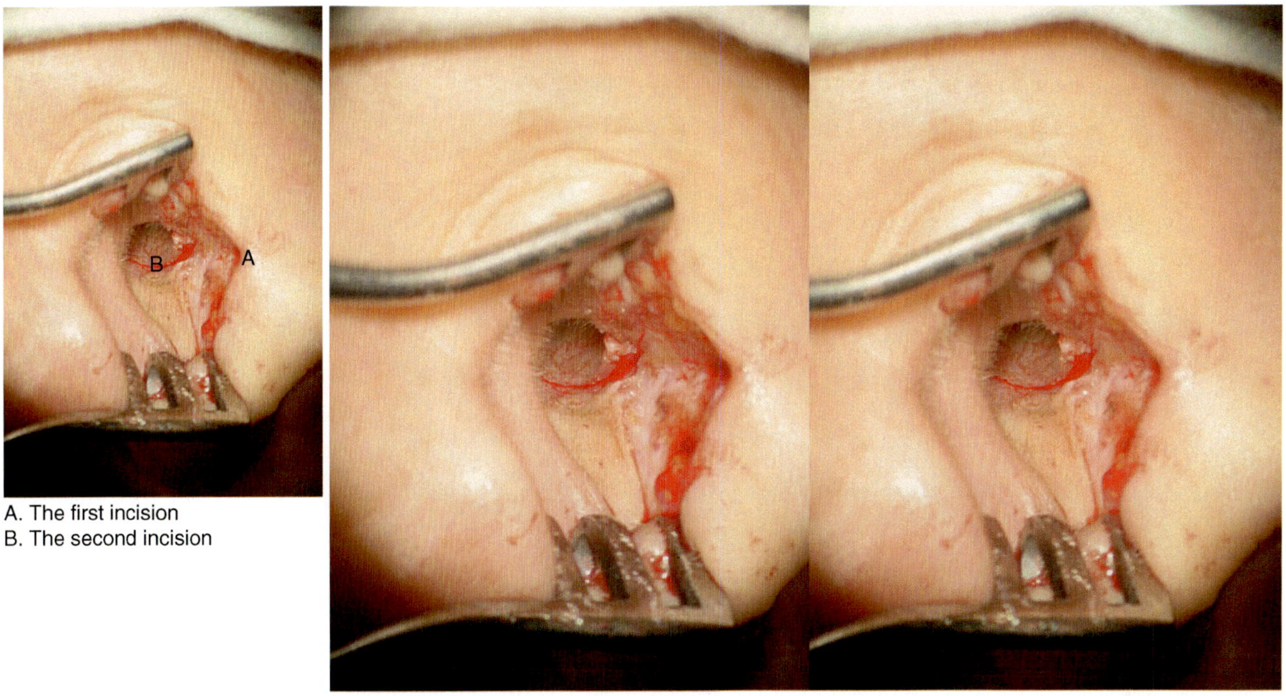

Fig. 2.19 Endaural incision
The fascia is harvested from the temporal muscle above the affected ear and is dried in 75 % ethanol. The skin incision is made between the tragus and the crus of helix and an inward extension is made to a point about 0.8–1.0 cm lateral to the tympanic annulus. The second incision starts from the 6 o'clock position of EAC, and remains 5 mm lateral to the tympanic annulus along the posterior meatal wall in an ascending spiral fashion to meet the inner part of the first incision

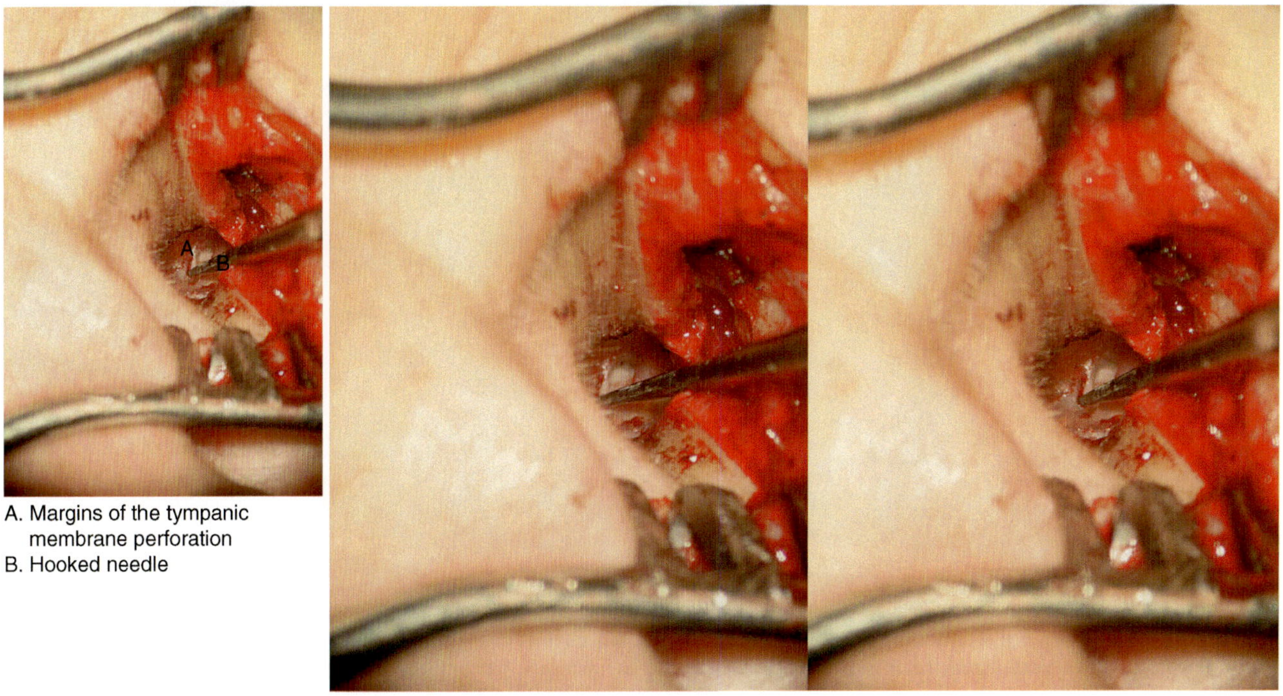

Fig. 2.20 Excising the perforation margins
The edges of the perforation are freshened with a hooked needle 3 mm away from its margin. Care must be taken to remove all epithelial remnants from the rim of the perforation

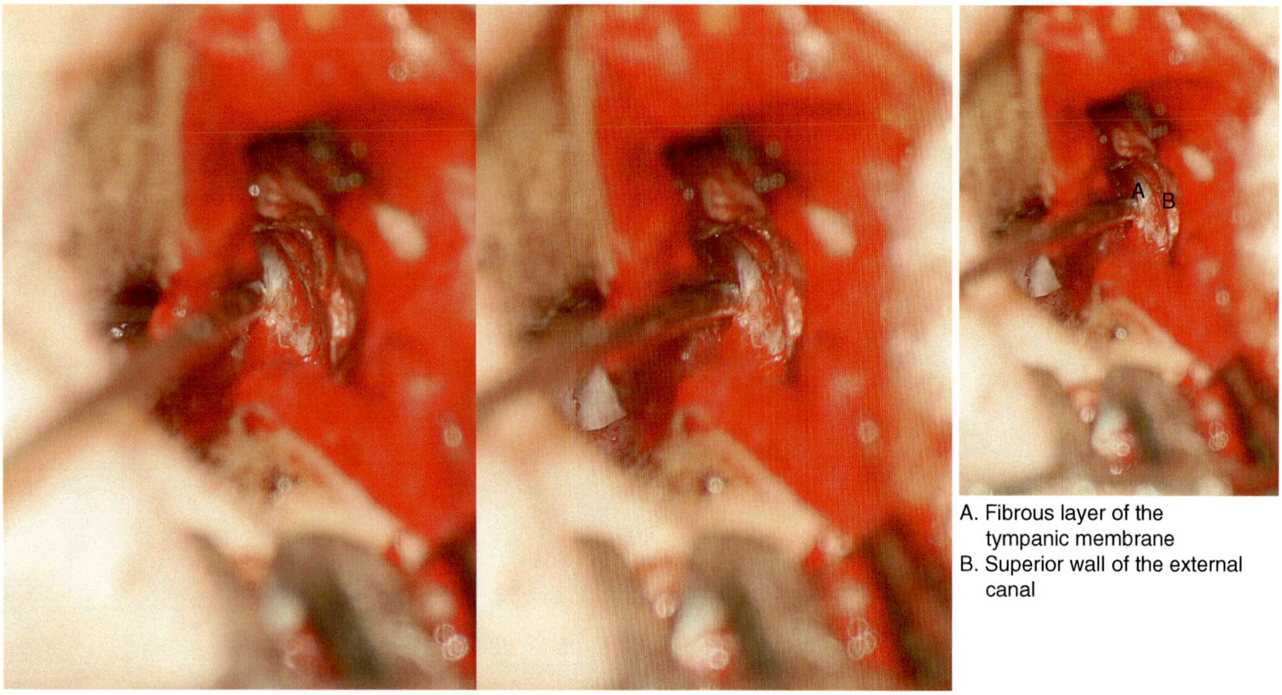

Fig. 2.21 Separate the posterior epithelial layer of the tympanic membrane
Remove the overhanging suprameatal spine using a sharp diamond burr or chisel. Separate the meatal skin flap as far as the tympanic annulus and elevate the epithelial layer from the posterior remnant of the tympanic membrane across the tympanic sulcus. Then separate the epithelial layer from the fibrous layer of the tympanic membrane anteriorly to the manubrium of malleus

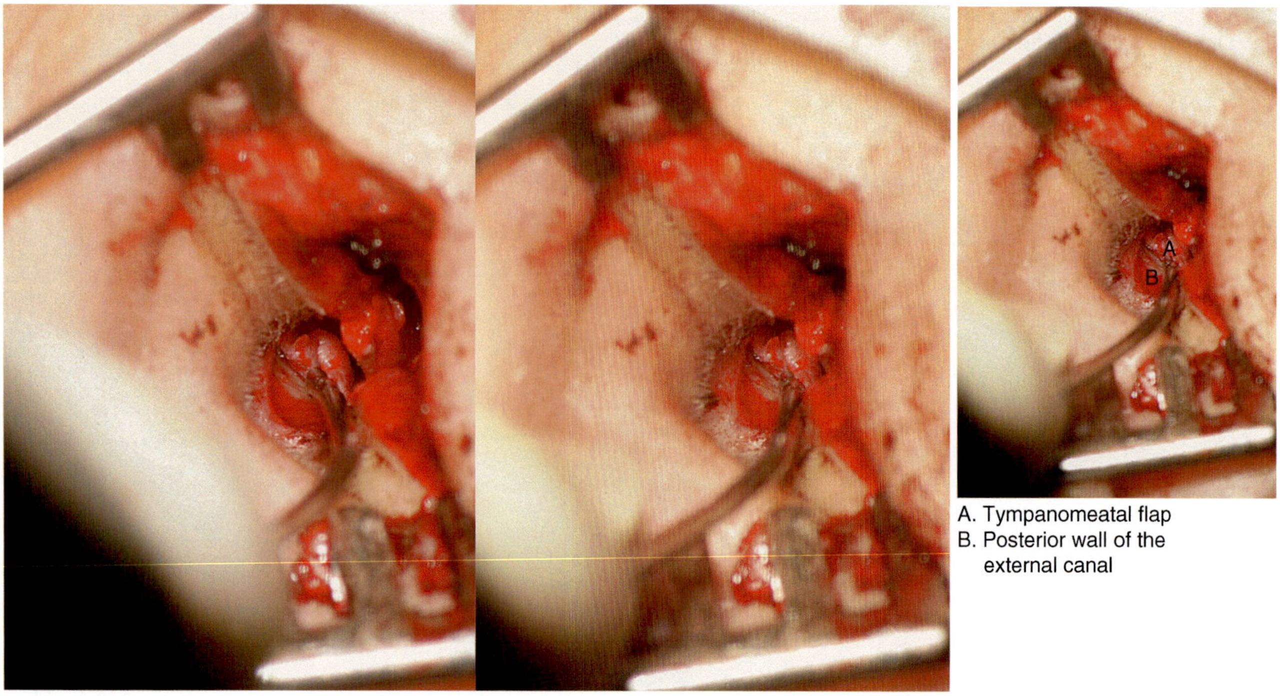

Fig. 2.22 Separate the epithelial layer from the anterior part of tympanic membrane
The epithelial layer is separated from the fibrous layer, then the edges of the tympanic membrane perforation are excised

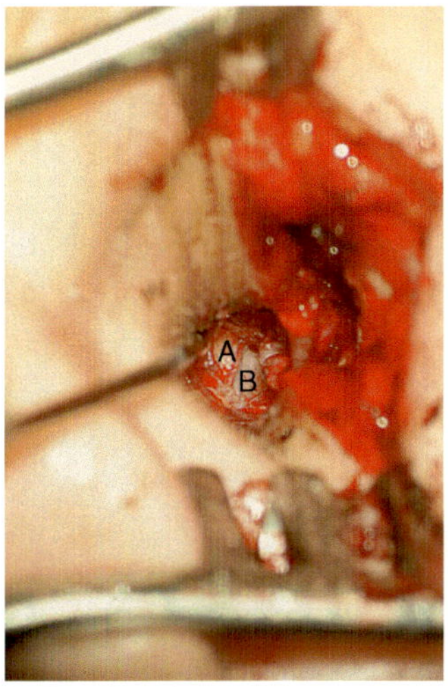

A. Calcified plaque
B. The fibrous layer of the tympanic membrane

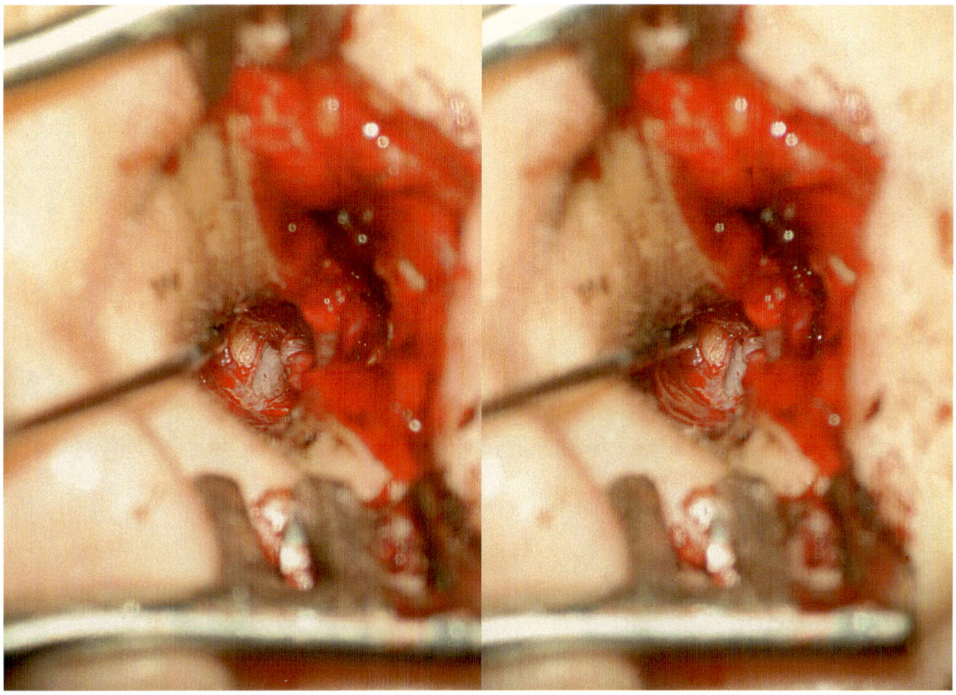

Fig. 2.23 Remove the calcified plaque
Remove a calcified plaque in the fibrous layer posterior to the malleus

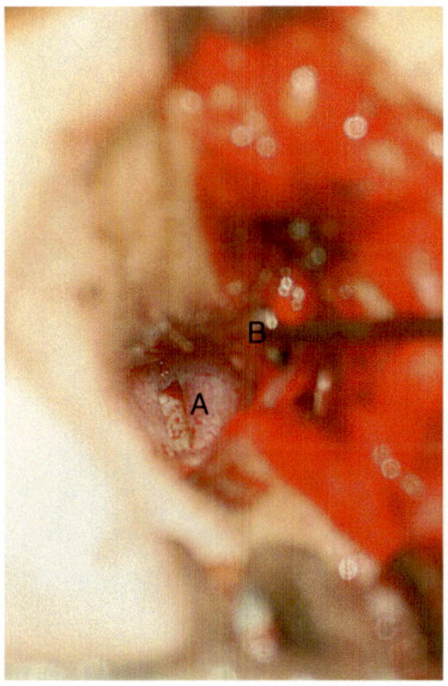

A. The completely separated epithelial layer of the tympanic membrane
B. Meatal skin flap

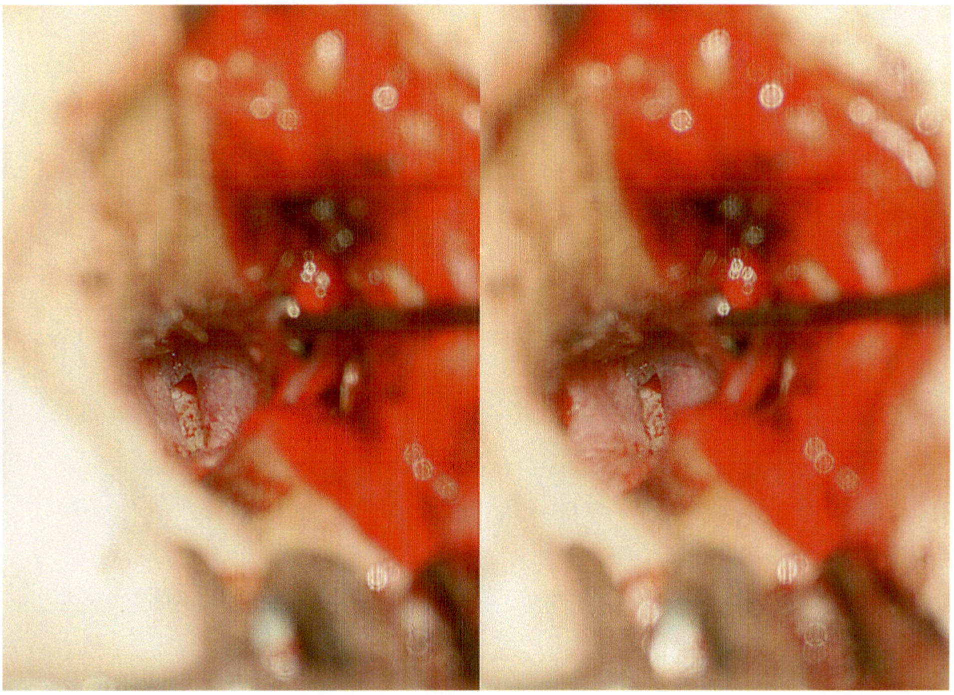

Fig. 2.24 Repositioning the epithelial layer of the tympanic membrane
The transplant bed of tympanic membrane is created, and the epithelial layer of the tympanic membrane is repositioned. Inspect the edges of the perforation again

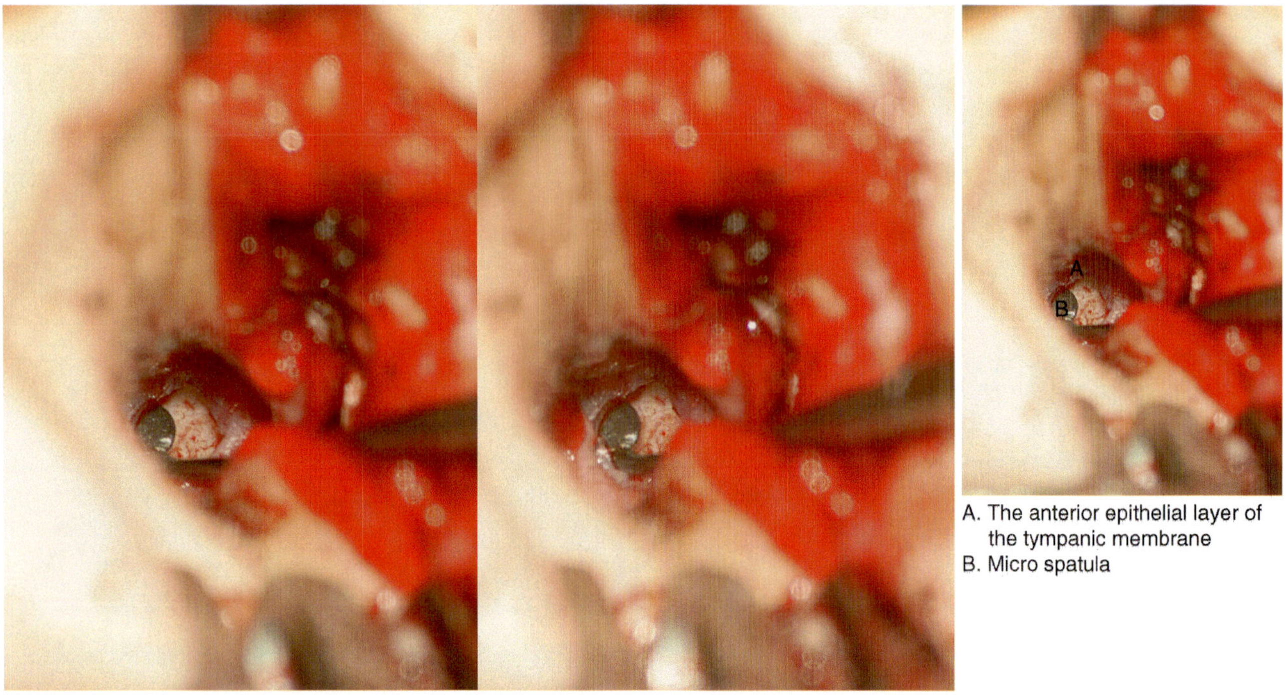

A. The anterior epithelial layer of the tympanic membrane
B. Micro spatula

Fig. 2.25 Check the extent of separation of two layers of the tympanic membrane
Use micro spatula to check separation of the epithelial layer and fibrous layer of the tympanic membrane remnant

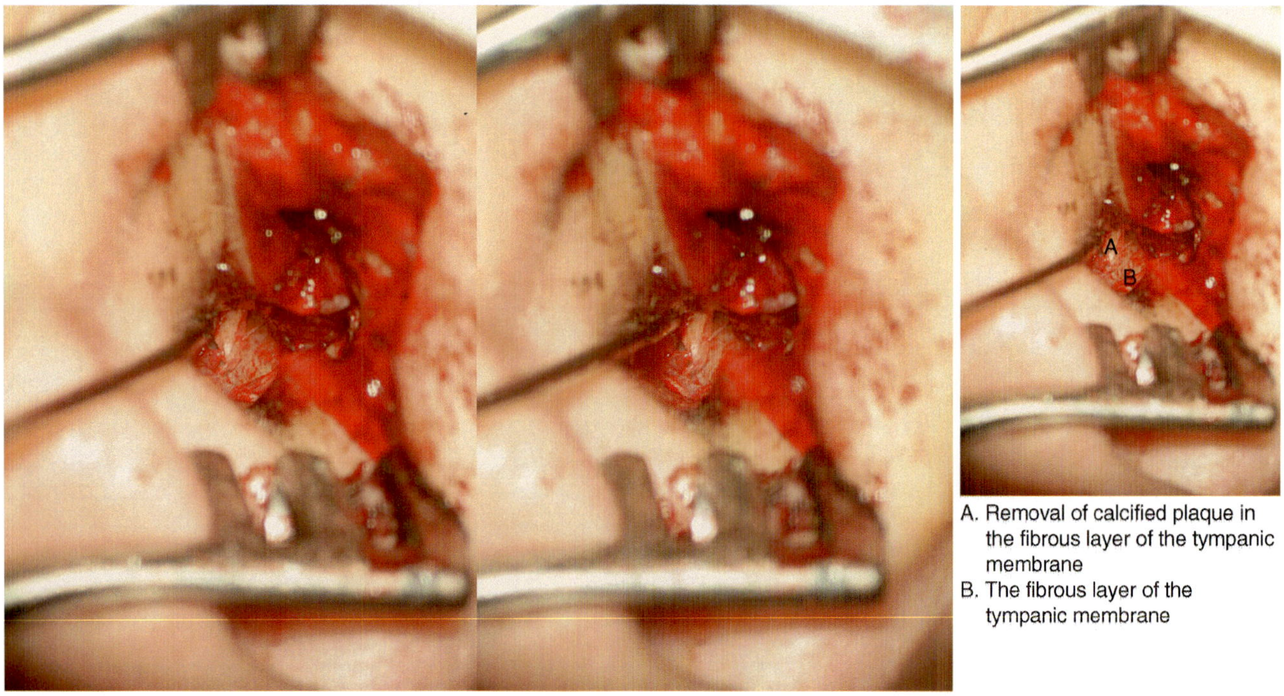

A. Removal of calcified plaque in the fibrous layer of the tympanic membrane
B. The fibrous layer of the tympanic membrane

Fig. 2.26 Inspecting the tympanic cavity
The postero-superior part of fibrous annulus is raised from the tympanic sulcus, and the excess bone of the posterosuperior meatus is removed. The tympanic cavity and part of ossicular chain are visible. Pierce around the edge of the calcified plaque in the tympanic membrane remnant successively and remove the calcified plaque. Take care to preserve the normal fibrous layer as much as possible

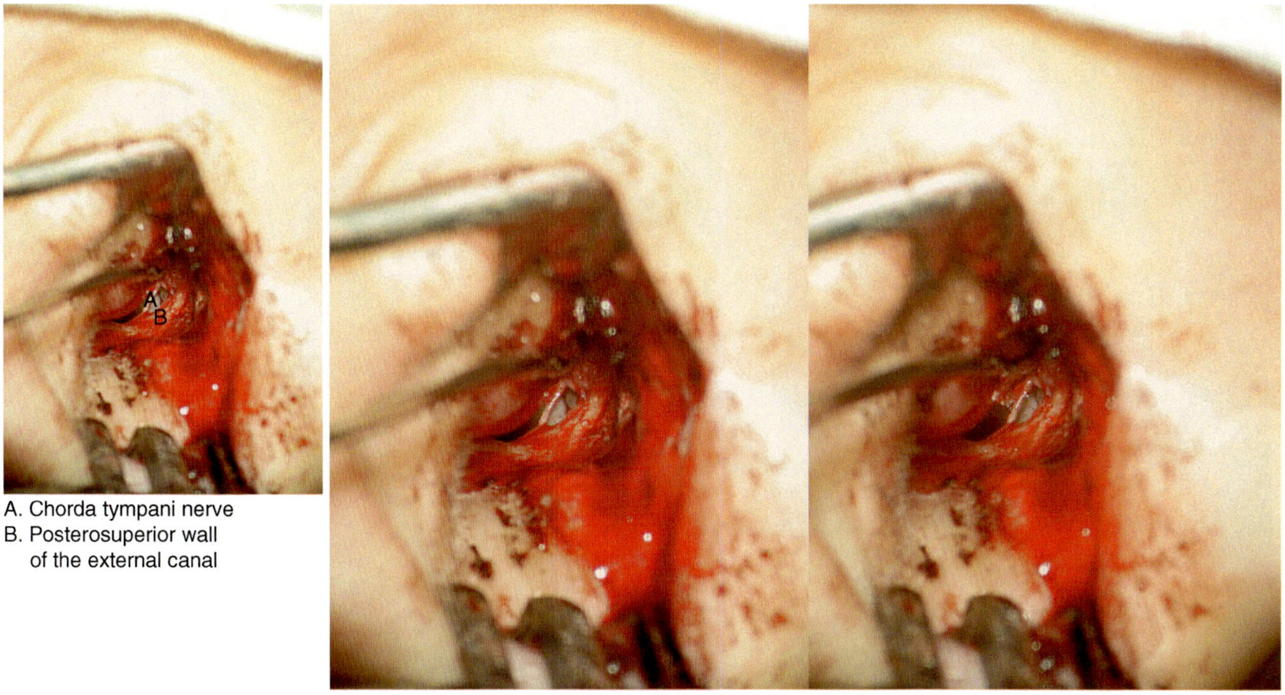

A. Chorda tympani nerve
B. Posterosuperior wall of the external canal

Fig. 2.27 Exposure of the chorda tympani nerve
The chorda tympani nerve is identified between the manubrium of malleus and the long process of the incus, along the line of the tympanic sulcus. Take care to separate the nerve along the tympanic sulcus to protect it from injury

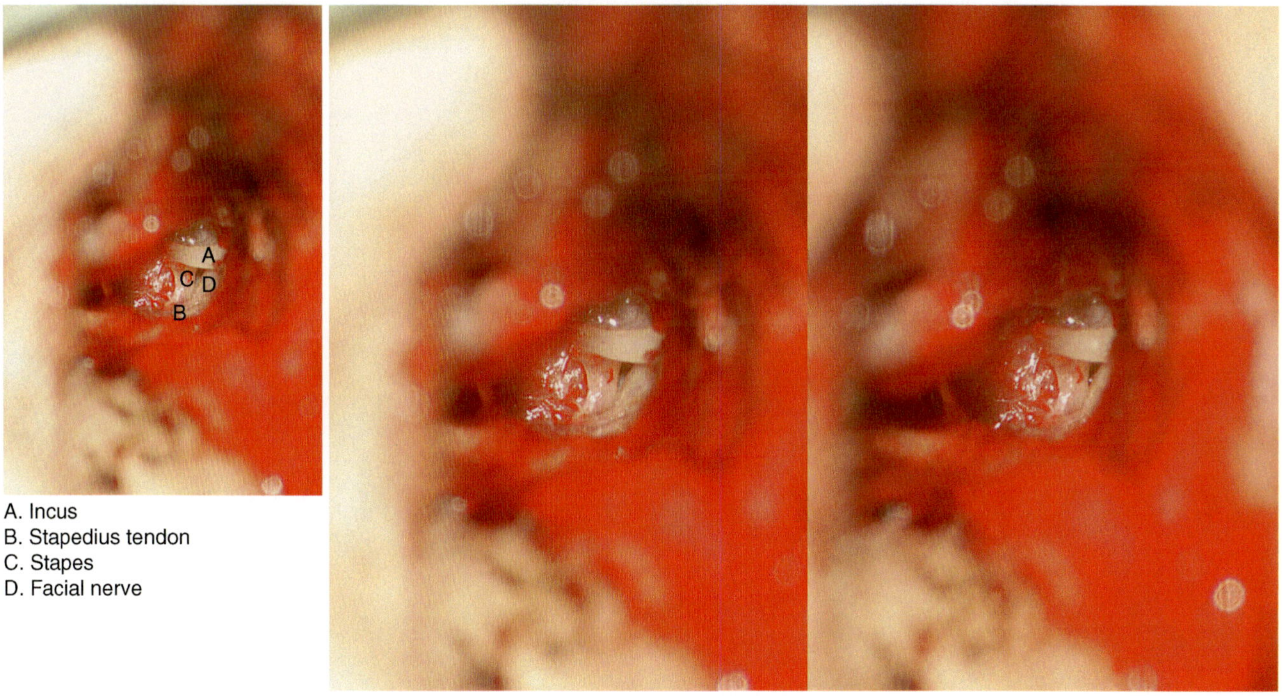

A. Incus
B. Stapedius tendon
C. Stapes
D. Facial nerve

Fig. 2.28 Checking the auditory ossicles
After the excess bony overhang of the posterosuperior meatal wall is removed, the integrity of the incudostapedial joint and the mobility of the ossicular chain are tested (or inspected). They are both normal in this case

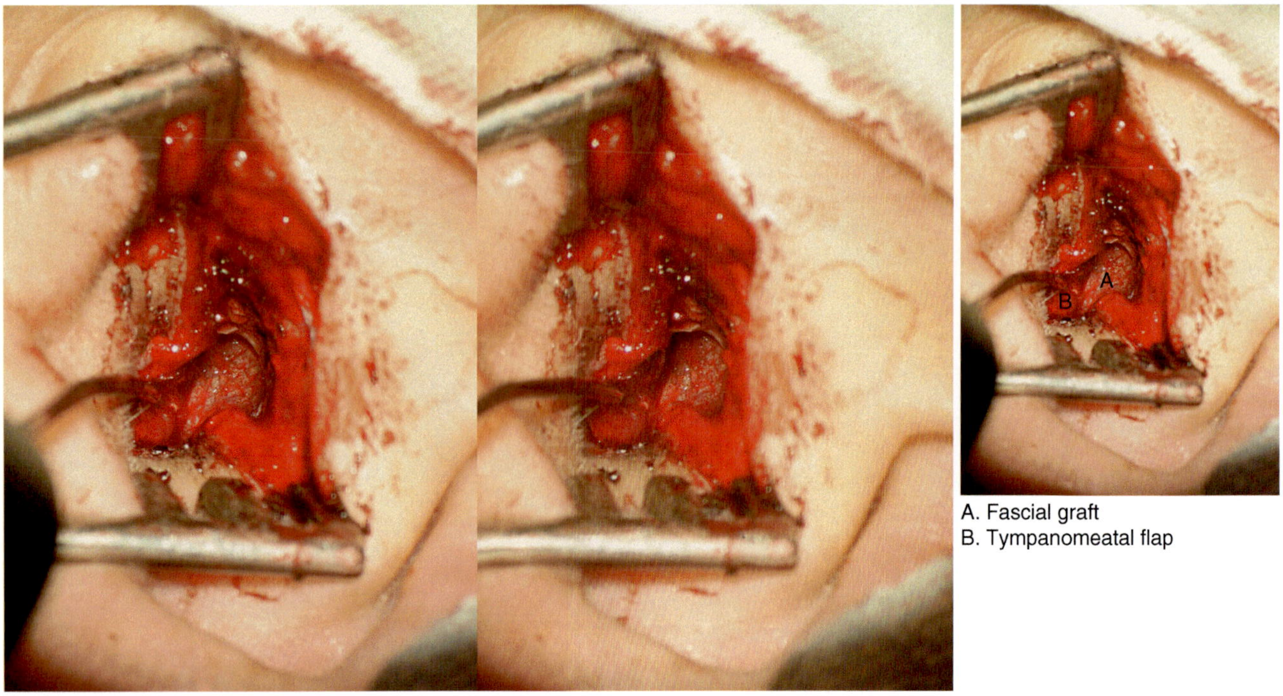

Fig. 2.29 Introducing the temporal fascia graft
The graft is introduced between the fibrous layer of the tympanic membrane and the epithelial tympanomeatal flap

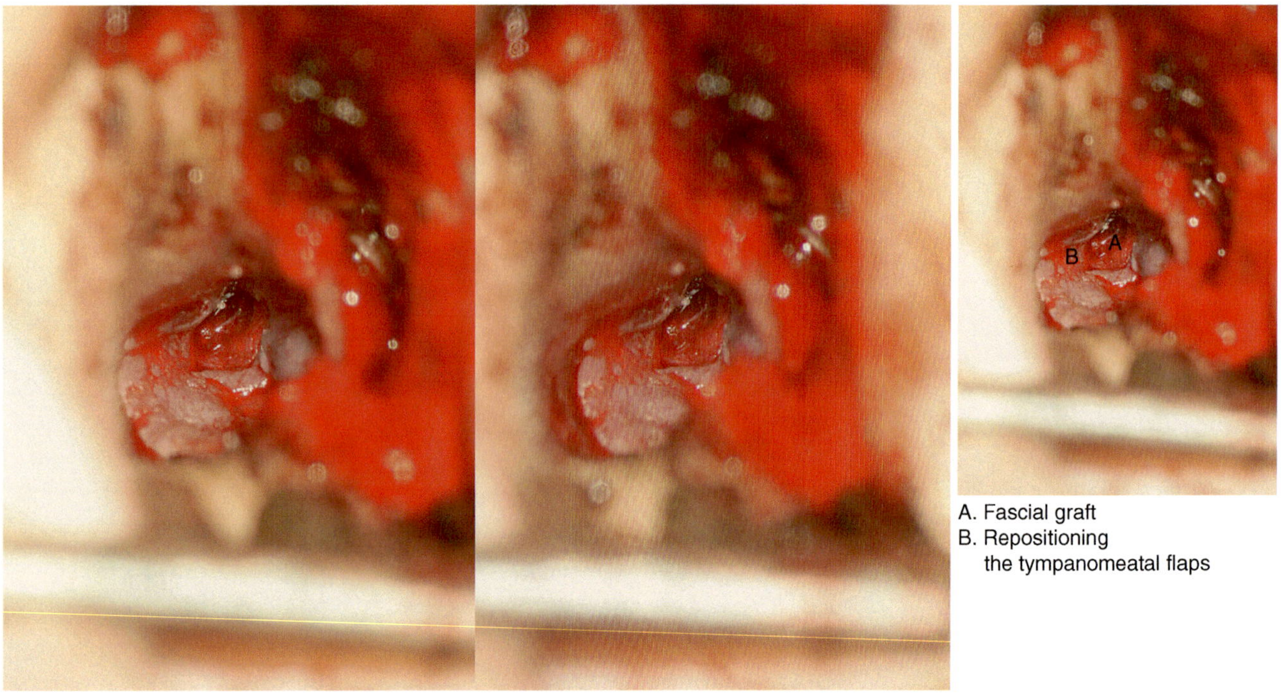

Fig. 2.30 Repositioning the tympanic membrane
The tympanic membrane is placed in its original position. Care is taken to ensure the temporal fascia graft fully covers the perforation

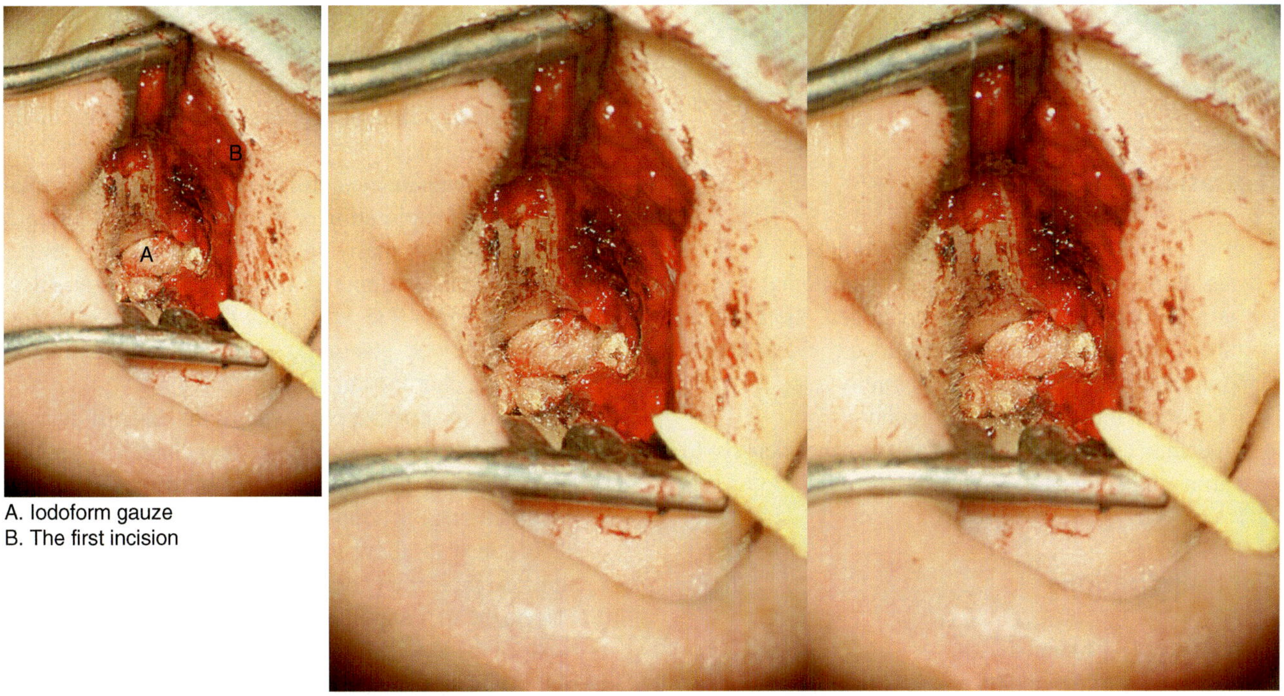

Fig. 2.31 Packing the ear canal
Placing the gelfoam on the surface of the drum, packing the external canal with a strip of iodoform gauze, and closing the incision

Tympanoplasty

Yi Sun and Yue-shuai Song

Indications

1. Tympanoplasty can be used in Chronic otitis media and mastoiditis patients (including cholesteatoma), but only when middle ear infection is controlled, the Eustachian tube is not obstructed and there is good cochlear function.
2. Traumatic ossicular chain discontinuity
3. Congenital middle ear malformation
4. Ossicular erosion or fixation or tympanosclerosis from chronic otitis media

Contraindications

1. Poor cochlear function
2. Malignancy of the middle or external ear (combined with radiation therapy)
3. Pseudomonal infection in diabetic patients
4. Otogenic intracranial complications
5. Patient unfit for surgery

Operative Procedures

1. Anesthesia: Local anesthesia can be used in adults. General anesthesia is used for children. Local anesthetic solution is injected into the skin of the wall of the external auditory canal. Cotton wool soaked with 2 % decicaine is placed on the surface of the tympanic membrane around the perforation for additional surface anesthesia.
2. Graft preparation: Temporalis fascia is harvested. A 2.5 cm long horizontal skin incision is made parallel to the hairline at the top of ear. After division of the subcutaneous tissue the white and tough fascia can be identified over the temporalis muscle. A circular fascial graft of 1.5–2.0 cm in diameter is taken. The graft is cleaned of muscle and loose connective tissue. It is placed in 75 % alcohol solution until use.
3. The first incision: A longitudinal incision is made at the top of EAC, with a 1.0 cm lateral extension along anterior border of crus of helix.
4. The second incision: Make a semicircular incision at bony part of auditory canal, which extends from 6 o'clock up to the inner end of first incision along the posterior wall 0.5 cm away from the tympanic annulus.
5. Elevation of the EAC skin flaps: Elevate the skin and periosteum of EAC towards the tympanic annulus. Curette away the spine of Henle if is prominent.
6. The epithelial layer of the tympanic membrane is separated from the fibrous layer in an anterior direction to form the bed for the graft in the inlay technique.

   The drum remnant is elevated as one layer in the underlay technique.
7. Once the tympanomeatal flap is prepared for the inlay technique, if exploration of the middle ear and ossicular chain is needed, the tympanic annulus can be elevated from the postero-superior part of the tympanic sulcus (right side from 9 to 12 o'clock position, left side from 12 to 3 o'clock position), whilst paying attention to protect the chorda tympani nerve.
8. Part of the postero-superior wall of the external auditory canal can be removed with a curette or chisel to expose the long process of the incus and the incudostapedial joint.
9. After entering the tympanic cavity, blood and any debris is suctioned to allow inspection of the ossicular chain and clearance of any disease associated with it.
10. Placement of temporalis fascia: the fascia is inserted between the outer epithelial layer and fibrous inner layer of the tympanic membrane (inlay technique), or inserted under the drum and between the tympanomeatal flap and auditory canal bony wall. If there is no residual rim of the tympanic membrane anteriorly, the fascia is placed right to the anterior wall of the middle ear and a small extension is placed over the annulus to anchor the graft. The anterior and inferior middle ear space is well packed with gelfoam to ensure it stays in contact with the under surface of the drum remnant.
11. If ossicular chain reconstruction is needed, the temporalis fascial graft is reflected forward with the tympanic membrane remnant to expose the middle ear space. Suitable materials and methods for reconstruction are selected depending on the status of ossicular chain.
12. Repositioning the EAC skin flap: Replace the tympanomeatal flap with the graft that has been inserted. Ensure that the graft covers the perforation and does not extend laterally beyond the edge of the skin flap.
13. Fill the EAC with gelatin sponge and then iodoform gauze.
14. Suture the incision.

Special Comments

1. Inject local anesthetic solution under the skin to cause blanching but avoid excessive swelling, bruising or disruption of the canal skin.
2. Carefully dissect the tympanic membrane and handle of malleus, to avoid injury. The incudostapedial joint can be separated temporarily if necessary to prevent injury to the inner ear with consequent tinnitus, or even irreversible sensorineural hearing loss.

3. Ensure the gelfoam placed in the middle ear is only lightly moistened with normal saline
4. If an autograft incus is used to reconstruct the ossicular chain, ensure that it is healthy and does not contain cholesteatoma.
5. Make sure the attic lateral wall is intact at the end of the procedure, with any defect repaired

Complications

1. Perforation of ear drum: this may happen if the fascial graft is too small and does not cover the perforation completely, or if it is too large and does not lie correctly to make good contact with the recipient bed and develop a good blood supply.
2. Lateral healing of the tympanic membrane: this is mostly caused by inappropriate graft placement and packing, either by excessive separation of anterior edge skin of the recipient bed or loss of and blunting of the acute angle between the tympanic membrane and the anterior EAC wall.
3. Cholesteatoma: a small cholesteatoma or epidermoid can be seen frequently on the surface of tympanic membrane, or on the EAC recipient bed due to implantation of squamous epithelium. When this occurs, it can be removed simply in the clinic without harmful effects. This should be done early to avoid ingrowth of Cholesteatoma to the middle ear.
4. Inner ear injury: dissection of disease or tympanosclerosis from the ossicular chain may cause inner ear damage if it is not done delicately. The stapes can even be dislocated, leading to inner ear injury and creating a pathway for infection to spread to the inner ear. Inner ear damage is seen more frequently in the aged and those with poor inner ear function.
5. EAC stenosis: excessive trauma to the skin of the EAC, infection and proliferation of granulation can cause EAC stenosis.

   Widening of the bony ear canal and repair of any areas skin loss with full-thick skin grafts will help prevent this.
6. Tympanic membrane retraction pocket: when extensive removal of the postero-superior bony canal wall is required, a retraction pocket can occur even in the presence of normal Eustachian tube function. Bone defects in this area should be repaired with a cartilage composite graft to prevent formation of a retraction pocket which may progress to cholesteatoma.
7. Facial palsy: facial nerve damage mostly occurs at the second genu, in the postero-superior region of the tympanic cavity, where dissection may be blind and the bony facial nerve canal is likely to be deficient leaving the nerve exposed and possibly herniating.

   Chemicals (such as acetaldehyde and peroxyacetic acid) contained in the gelatin sponge used to pack the tympanic cavity may cause facial nerve protein denaturation.

Surgery 1: Tympanoplasty, ossiculoplasty

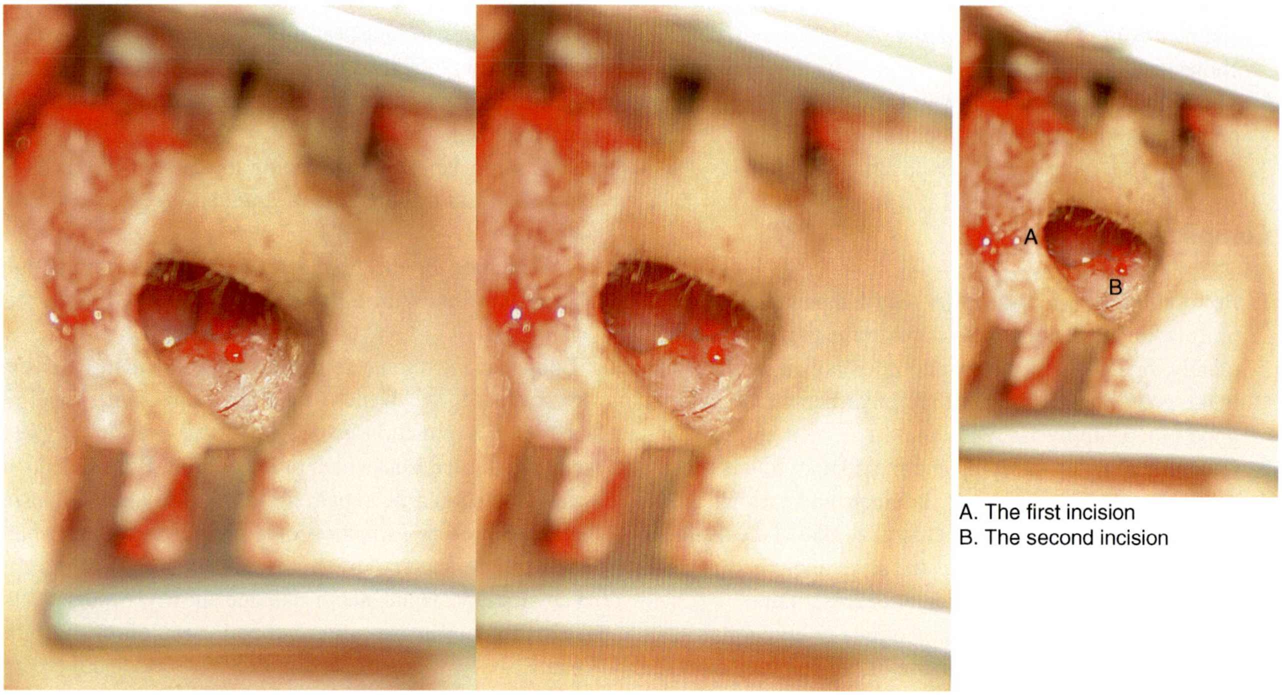

Fig. 2.32 Endaural incision
A longitudinal incision is made at the top of EAC, and extended about 1.0 cm along anterior border of the crus of helix. The inner end of the incision stops 0.8–1.0 cm lateral to the pars flaccida of the tympanic membrane. The second incision is circumferential and made 0.5 cm behind the tympanic annulus. It extends from the 6 o'clock position, over the posterior EAC wall to meet the inner end of the first incision

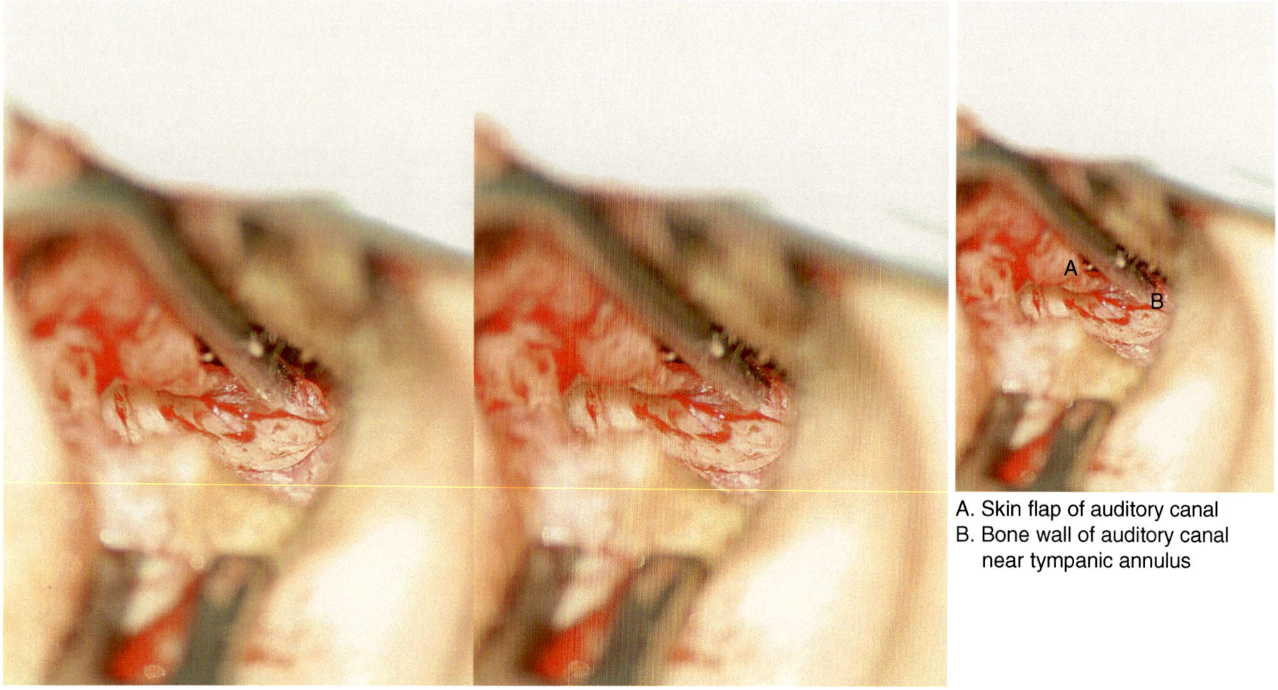

Fig. 2.33 Elevation of EAC Skin flap
The skin and periosteum of the EAC is elevated from the second incision inwards to the tympanic annulus. The dissection is carried out over a broad front avoid too much elevation in one area alone. The dissector is kept tightly on the bone and a fine bore sucker is used to avoid trauma to the flap which is often quite thin

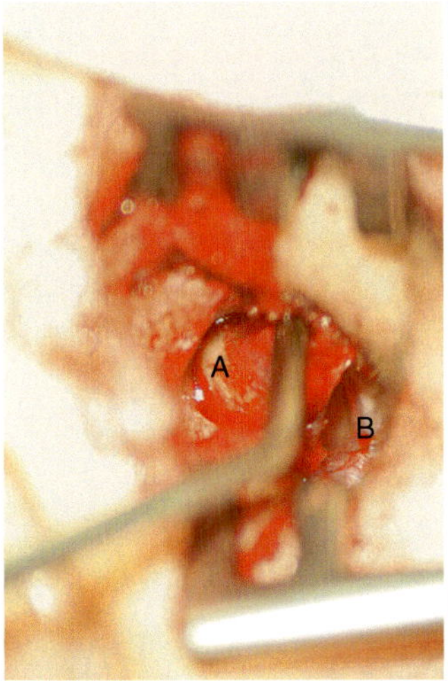

A. Skin flap of EAC with a yellow-white color resulting from inflammation
B. Tympanic membrane residual anterior rim

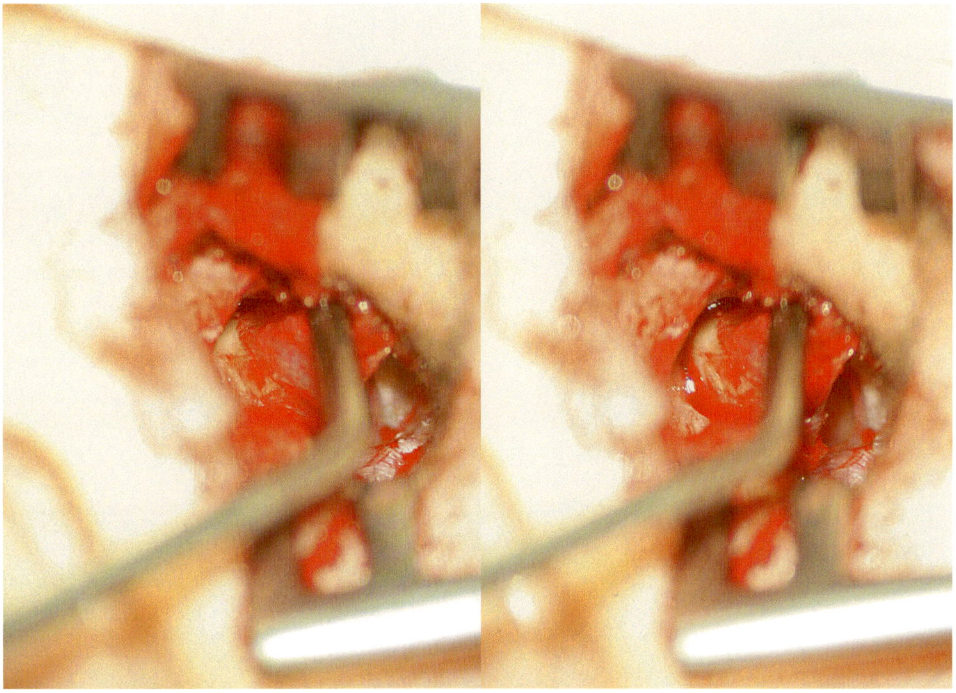

Fig. 2.34 Elevation of superior EAC skin flap
The posterior and inferior skin flap of the EAC is elevated, then the superior skin flap is reflected to the anterior wall. The anterior superior spine of bone is exposed and removed if it is too prominent.
This picture shows the bony part of superior wall of EAC to be eroded leading to expansion of the EAC. The inner end of the EAC skin has turned a yellow-white color due to inflammation

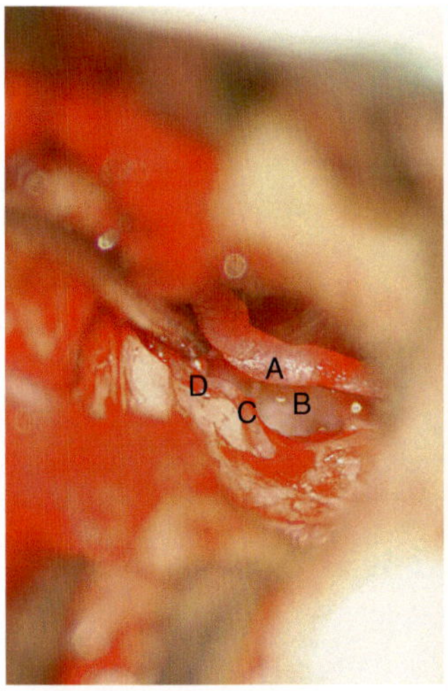

A. Elevated tympanomeatal flap
B. Promontory
C. Chorda tympani nerve
D. Granulation surrounding ossicles

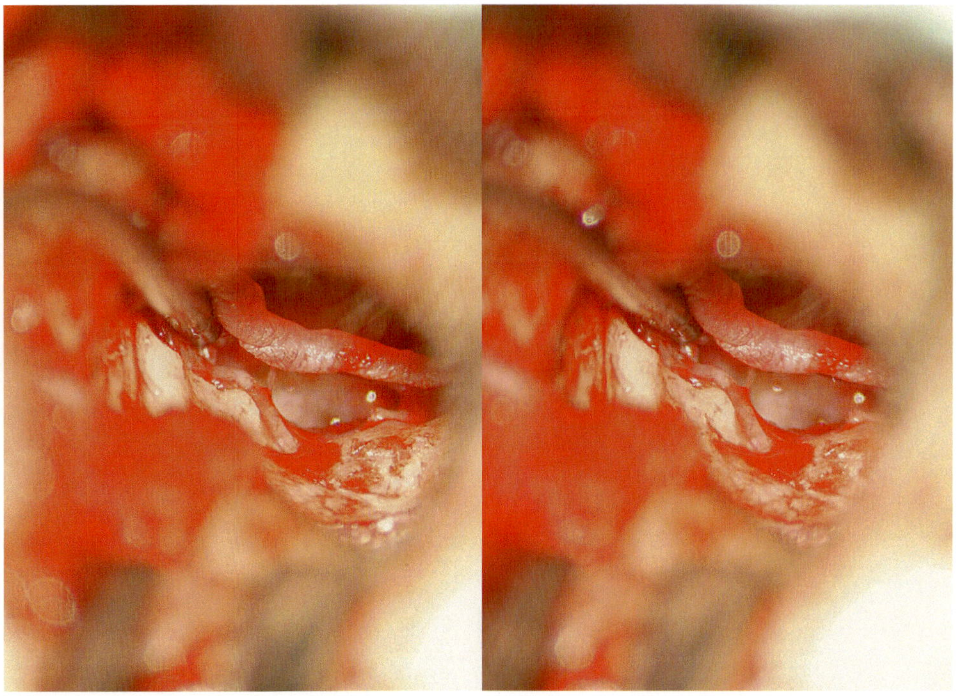

Fig. 2.35 The tympanic membrane is elevated to expose the tympanic cavity.
After the skin flap of the EAC was elevated to the tympanic annulus, a large tympanic membrane perforation could be seen with no posterior residual rim. Part of the postero-superior bony EAC wall, between the 9 o'clock and 12 o'clock positions, was eroded, exposing the chorda tympani nerve. Part of the lateral attic wall is also missing and the ossicles were surrounded by granulation tissue. The pars flaccida was carefully elevated

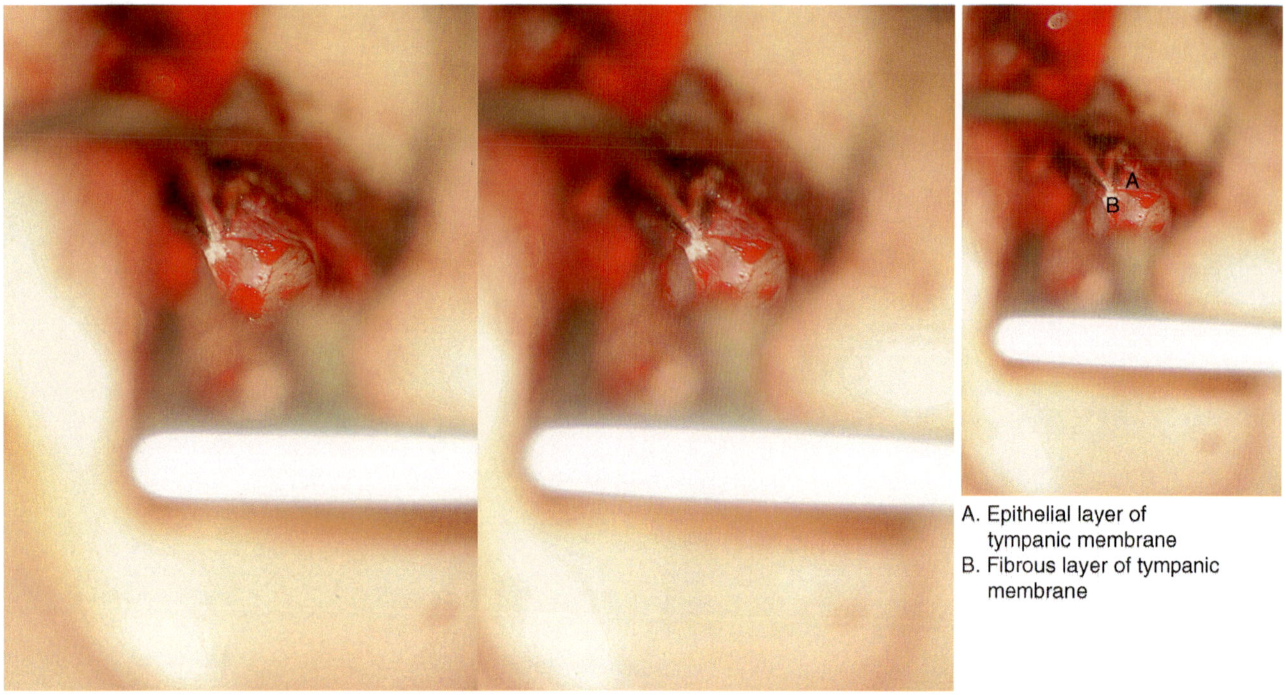

Fig. 2.36 The residual epithelial and fibrous layers of the tympanic membrane were separated from the lamina propria
In this case, there was no postero-superior residual rim of the tympanic membrane. The residual posterior and inferior epithelial layer of the tympanic membrane was separated from the fibrous layer. A calcified plaque can be seen on the surface of the inferior fibrous layer of the tympanic membrane

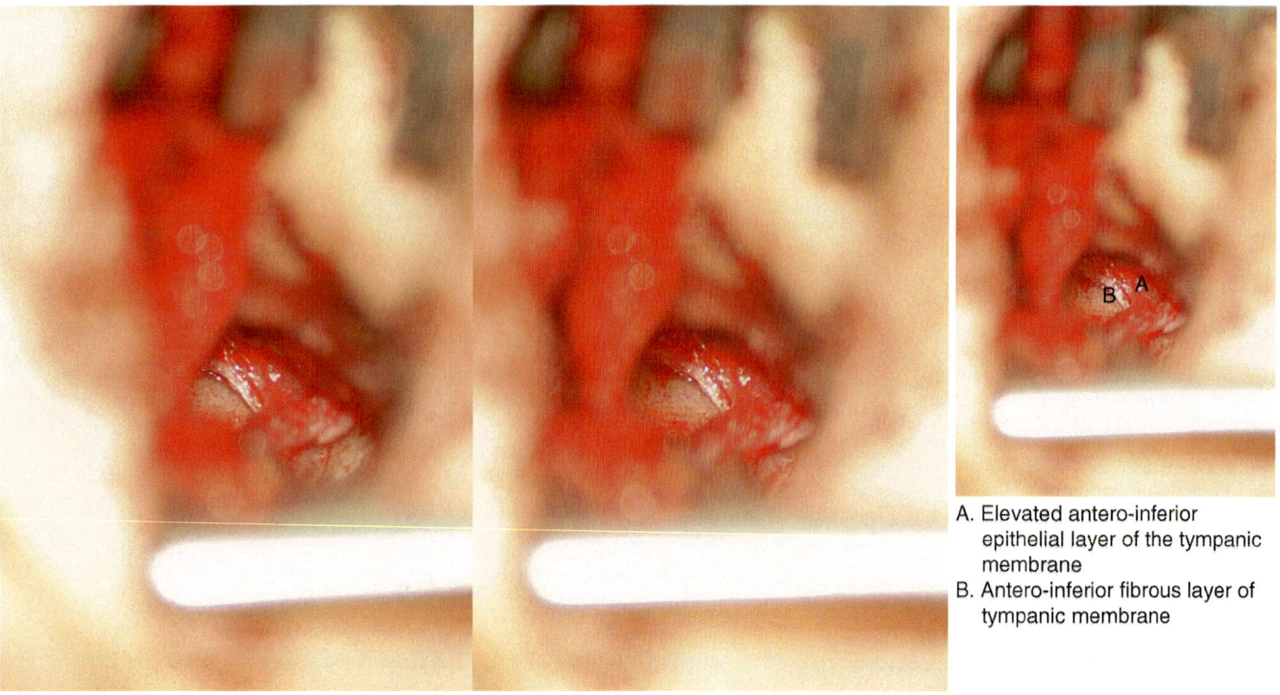

Fig. 2.37 The recipient bed for repairing the tympanic membrane is prepared
The residual epithelial layer of the anterior tympanic membrane is elevated. Dissection should advance evenly from the antero-superior and antero – inferior walls of the EAC and converge on the incisions. The epithelial layer of the tympanic membrane is then replaced to check its integrity. It must be separated completely from the fibrous layer in the area where the fascial graft is to be placed

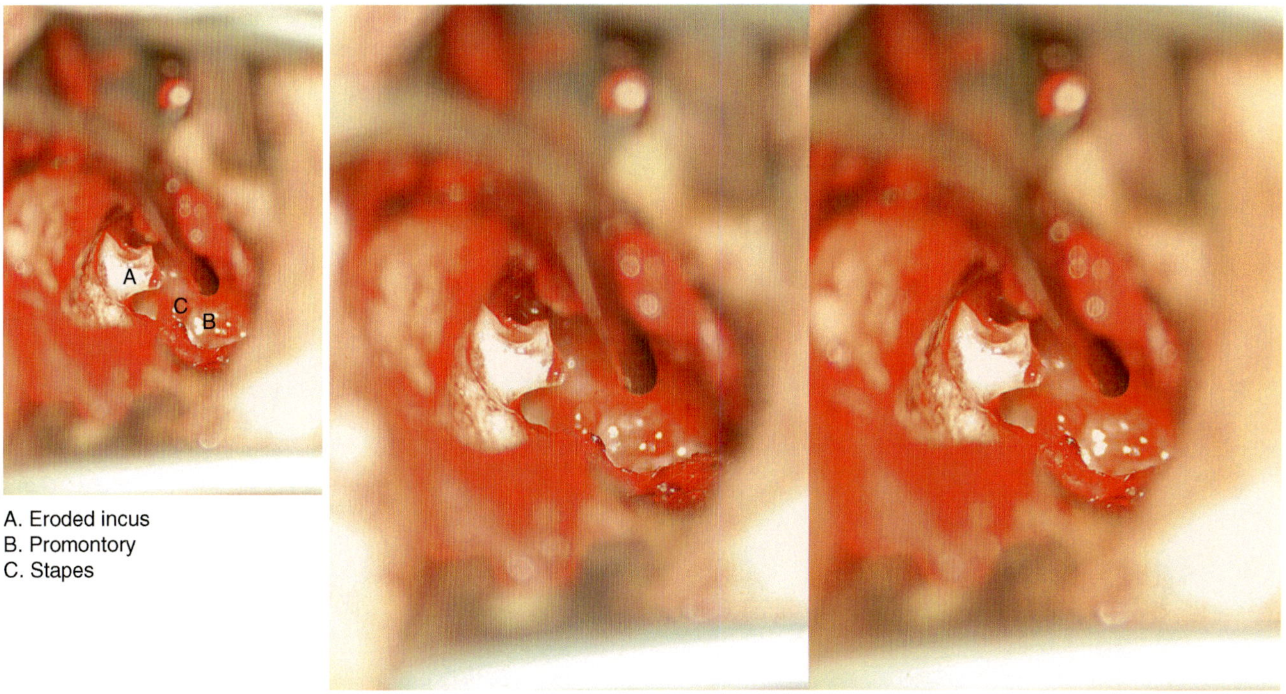

Fig. 2.38 Exposure of the ossicles
The microscope is adjusted to look superiorly. The attic was partly open due to erosion of its lateral wall. Granulation tissue surrounding the ossicular chain was cleaned up. The malleus was absent and the incus long process was mostly missing. The stapes is surrounded by swollen mucous membrane binding it to the surface of the promontory. This picture shows the incus in the process of being removed

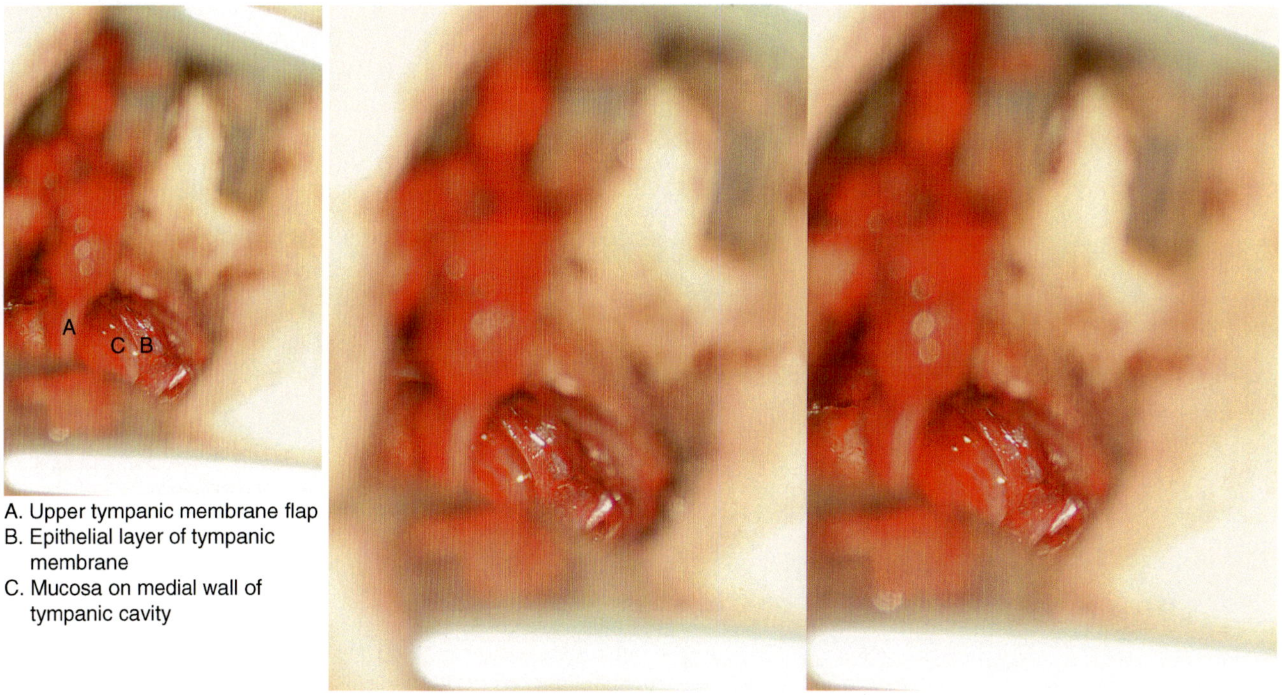

Fig. 2.39 Tympanic membrane is replaced
EAC tympanic membrane flap is replaced. The tympanomeatal flap is totally separated from the bony wall and the residual fibrous layer of the tympanic membrane, making the recipient bed for repairing the tympanic membrane

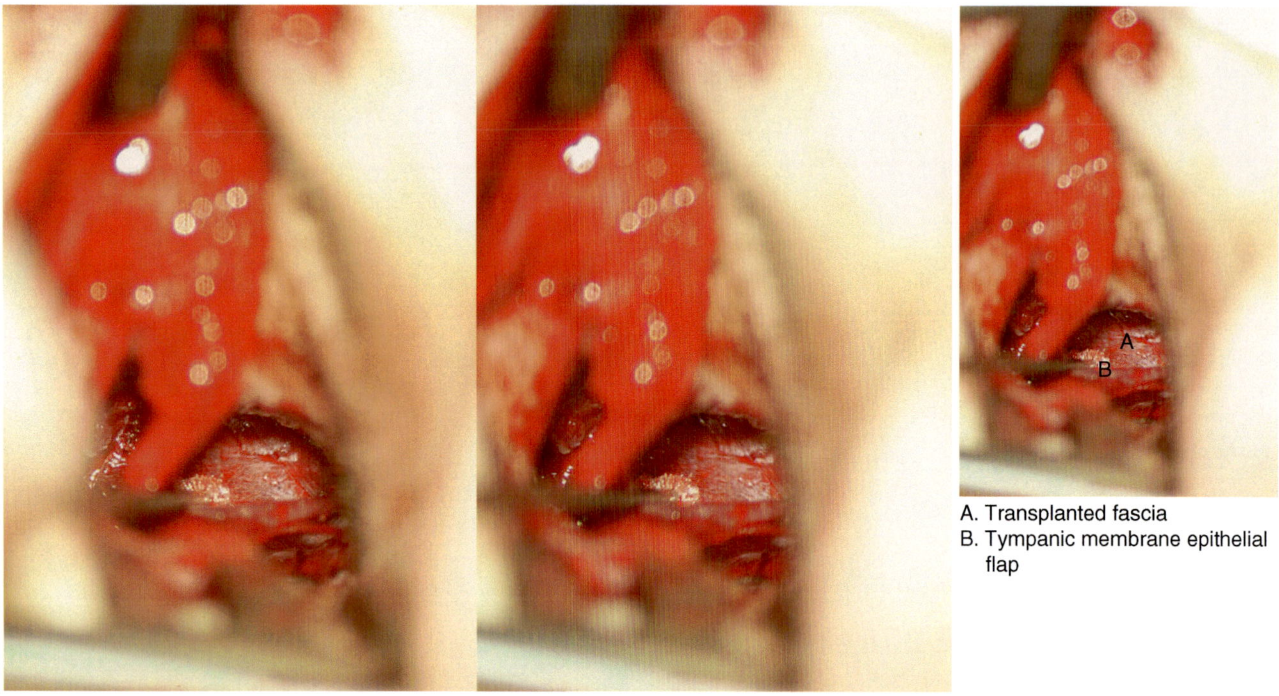

A. Transplanted fascia
B. Tympanic membrane epithelial flap

Fig. 2.40 Transplanted temporalis fascia is positioned for repair of the tympanic membrane
The temporalis fascia is inserted between the epithelial and fibrous layers of the tympanic membrane. The size of fascia is important and should not be folded over, but in direct contact with the residual fibrous layer of tympanic membrane and bony wall near the tympanic sulcus. The graft should cover the perforation completely to prevent a recurrent membrane defect

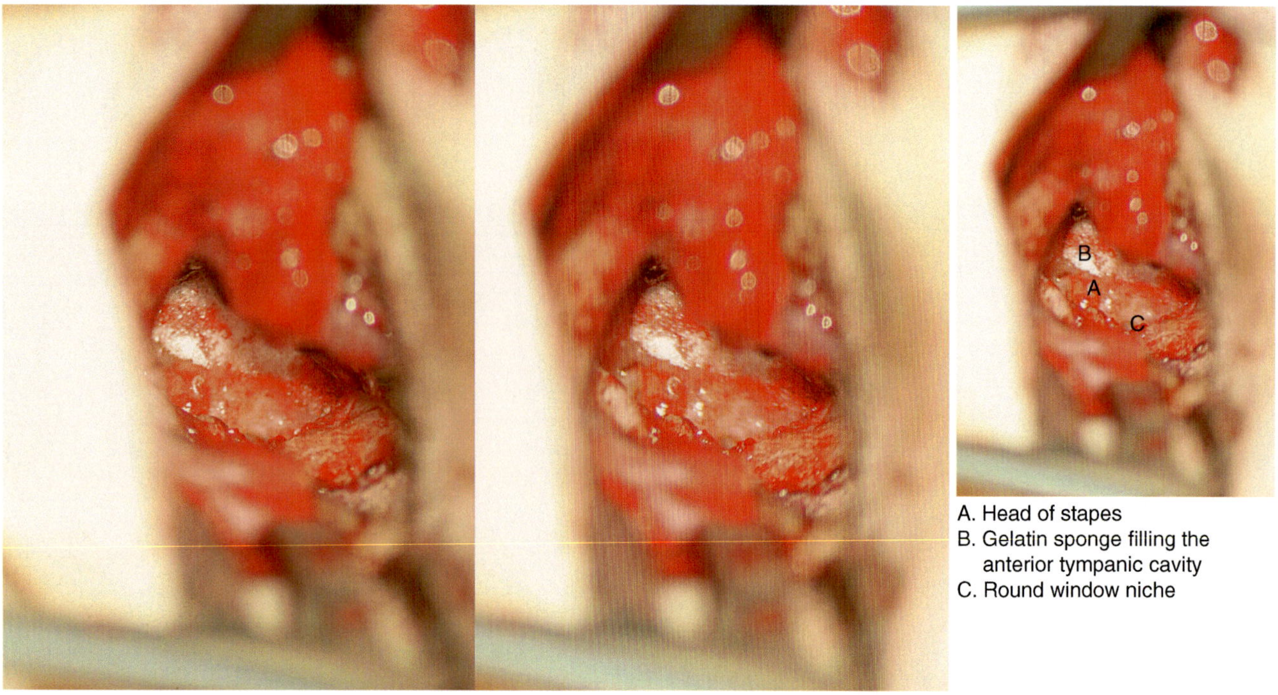

A. Head of stapes
B. Gelatin sponge filling the anterior tympanic cavity
C. Round window niche

Fig. 2.41 The incus has been removed and the stapes superstructure is seen
The tympanomeatal flap with the embedded temporalis fascia is reflected forwards to expose the tympanic cavity. After the incus is taken out, the stapes superstructure is seen to be intact. The anterior and inferior tympanic cavity is filled with erythromycin soaked gelatin sponge to support the temporalis fascial graft

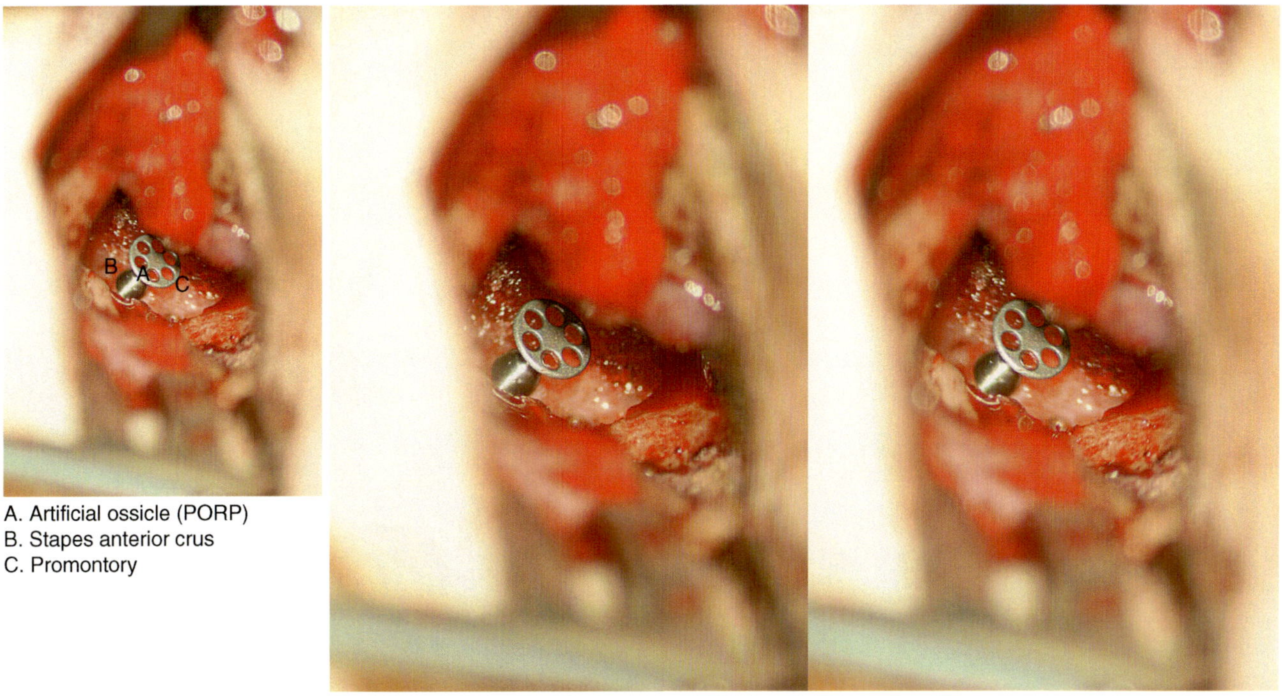

Fig. 2.42 Artificial ossicle (PORP) is positioned
After cleaning the disease from around the stapes, its mobility was checked and seen to be good. The ossicular prosthesis (PORP) was positioned on the stapes head. As there was a good fit between the cup of the prosthesis and the stapes head, no additional support was necessary to hold it in correct position

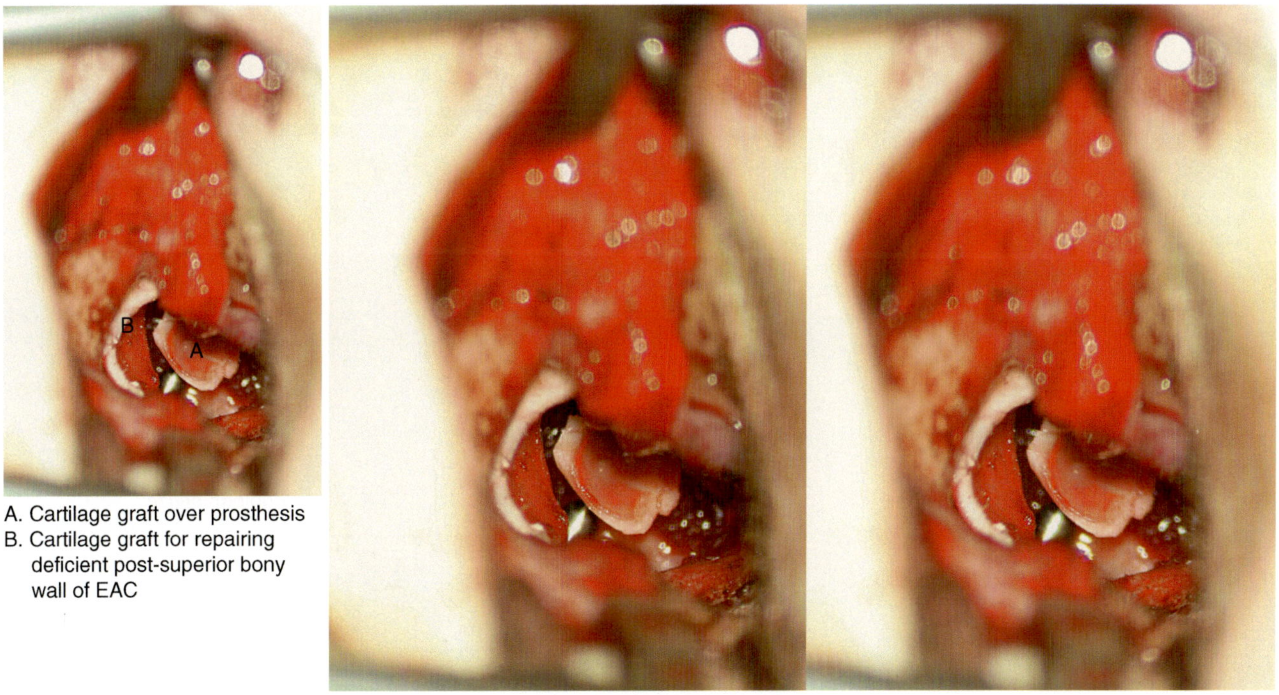

Fig. 2.43 A cartilage graft was inserted between the lateral face of the prosthesis and the temporalis fascia
In order to prevent extrusion of the prosthesis a cartilage graft is taken from the crus of helix and inserted between the lateral face of the prosthesis and the temporalis fascia. A rectangular curved cartilage graft is also used to repair the deficient postero-superior bony EAC wall in the 9–12 o'clock position to prevent retraction of the repaired tympanic membrane

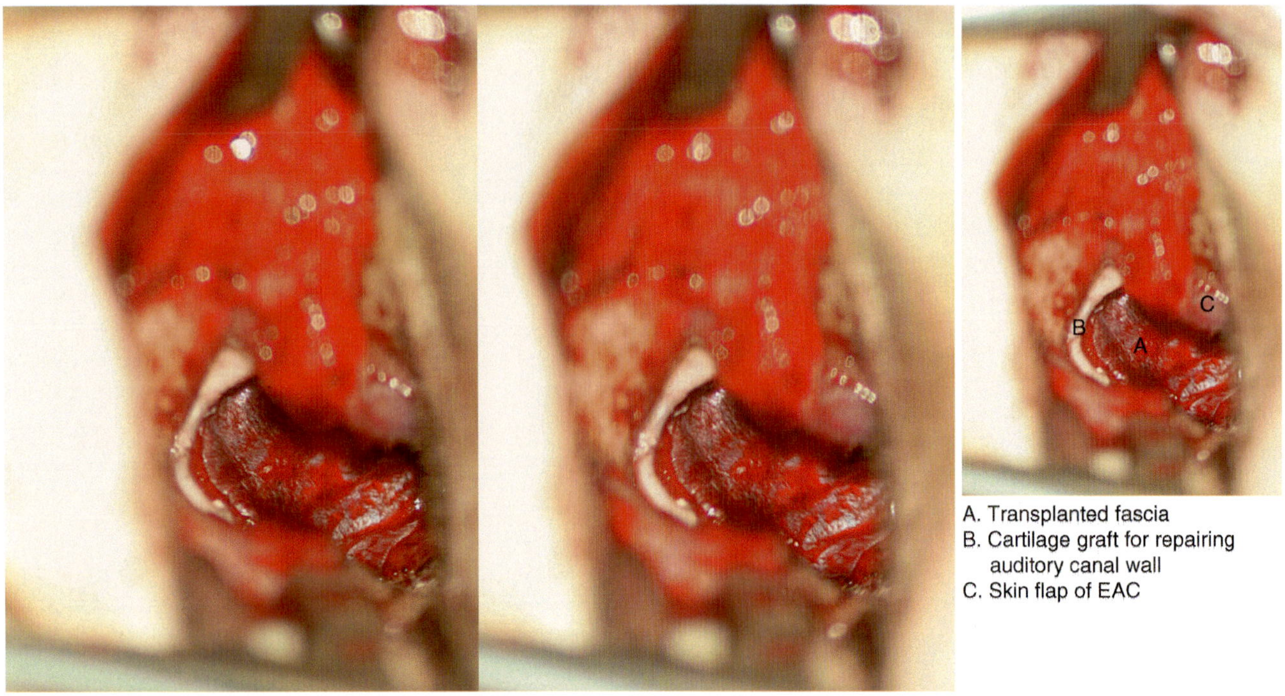

Fig. 2.44 Transplanted fascia
The fascial graft is used to cover the surface of the ossicular prosthesis and the two cartilage grafts, making sure they remain in their correct position

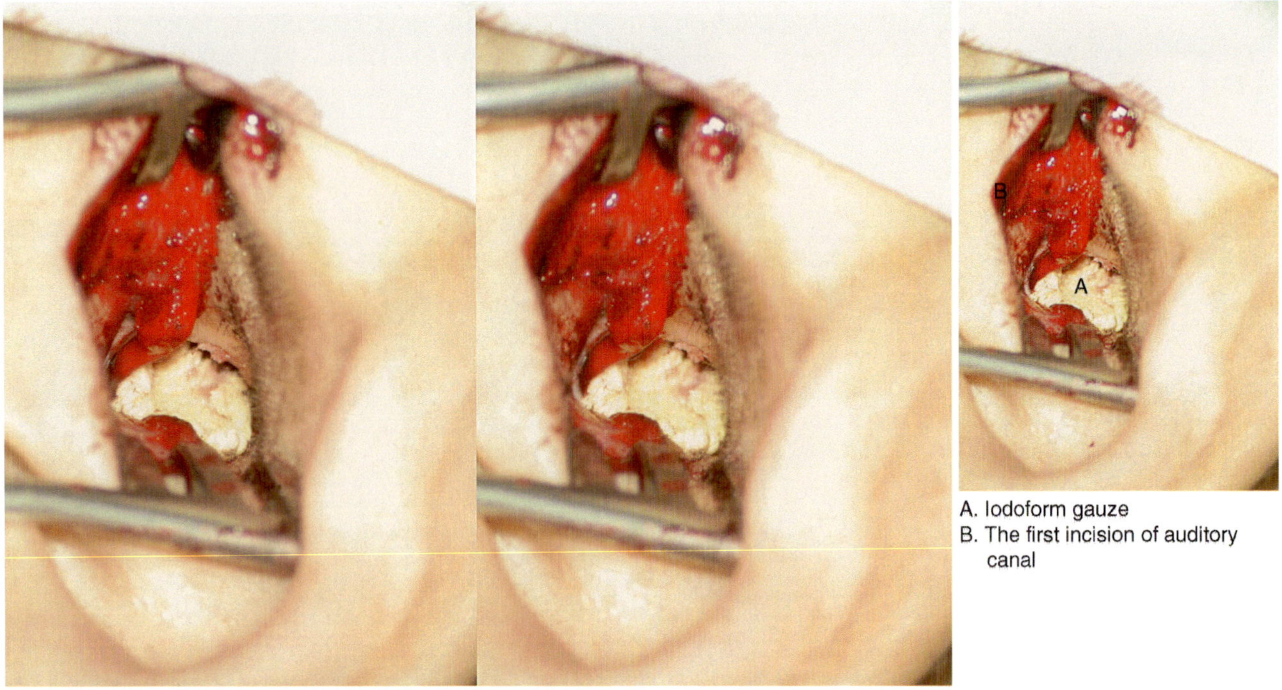

Fig. 2.45 Iodoform gauze is used to pack the EAC
The tympanomeatal flap is replaced and positioned with a dissector
Care is taken to ensure the fascia covers the perforation and does not extend beyond the lateral end of the skin flap. Gelatin sponge is used to cover the lateral surface of the drum and iodoform gauze pieces are placed to pack the EAC

Surgery 2: Tympanoplasty

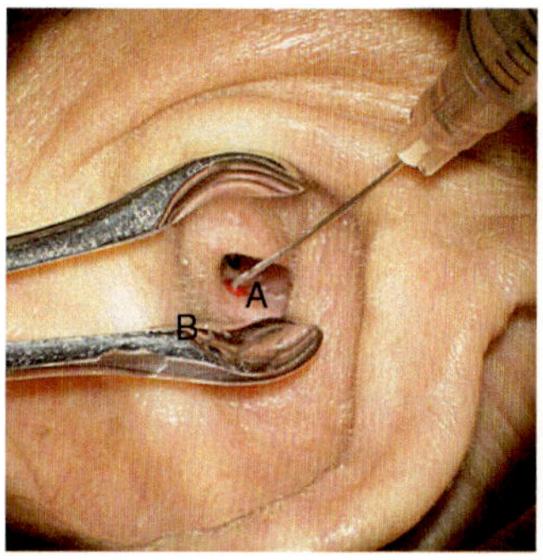

A. Junction of cartilage and bony part of EAC
B. Expand the external meatus with a nasal speculum

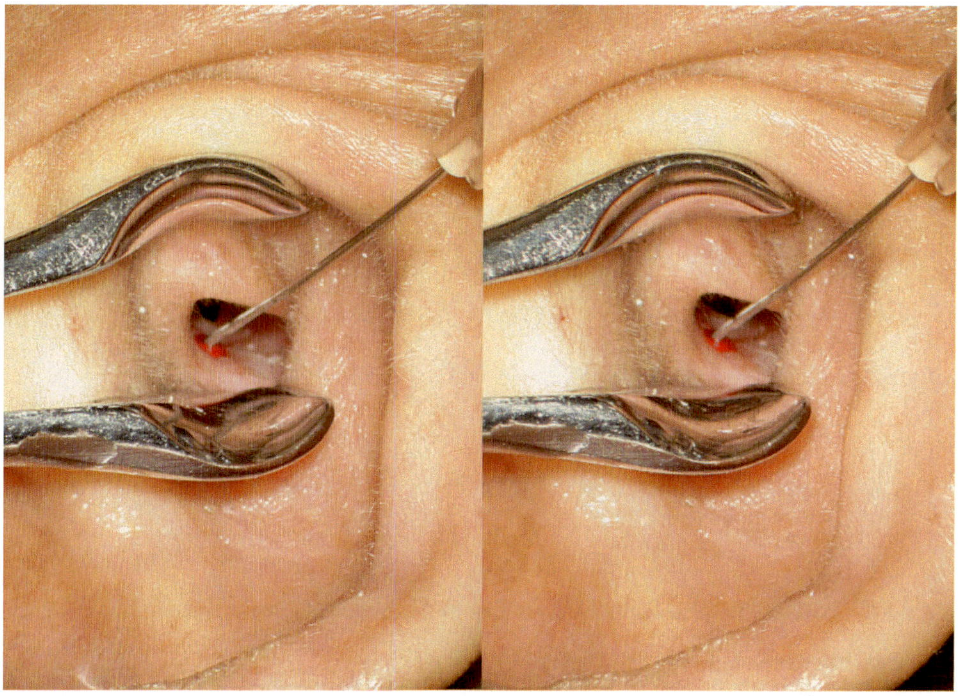

Fig. 2.46 Local anesthetic is injected
10 ml of local anesthetic solution in normal saline is mixed with 10 drops of 0.1 % epinephrine and injected as local infiltration anesthesia. The injection is performed at three to four points along the junction of the cartilage and bony parts of the EAC. The needle is inserted through the lateral skin on to the EAC bone and the infiltration is performed slowly to blanch the skin and anesthetize the skin

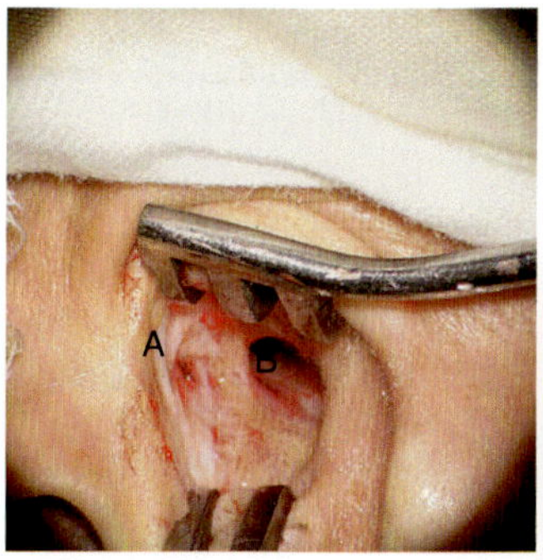

A. The first incision
B. Posterior edge of perforation of ear drum

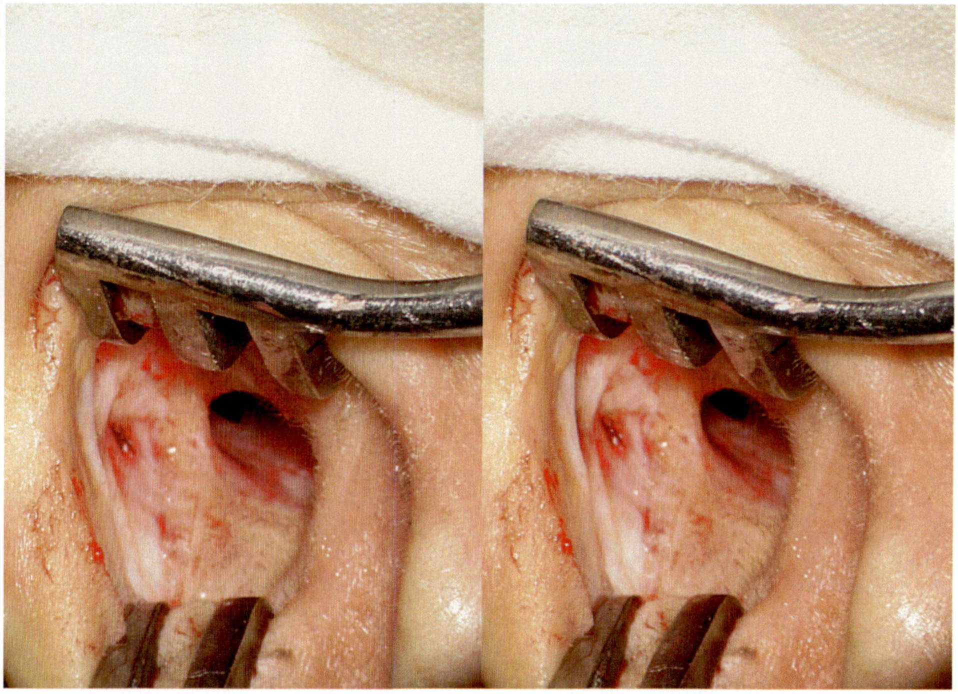

Fig. 2.47 The first incision
A longitudinal incision is made at the top of EAC, and extended about 1.0 cm along anterior border of the crus of helix. Any bleeding vessels are coagulated with bipolar diathermy. The inner end of the incision stops 0.8–1.0 cm lateral to the pars flaccida of the tympanic membrane. The second incision is circumferential and made 0.5 cm behind the tympanic annulus. It extends from the from the 6 o'clock position, over the posterior EAC wall to meet the medial end of the first incision

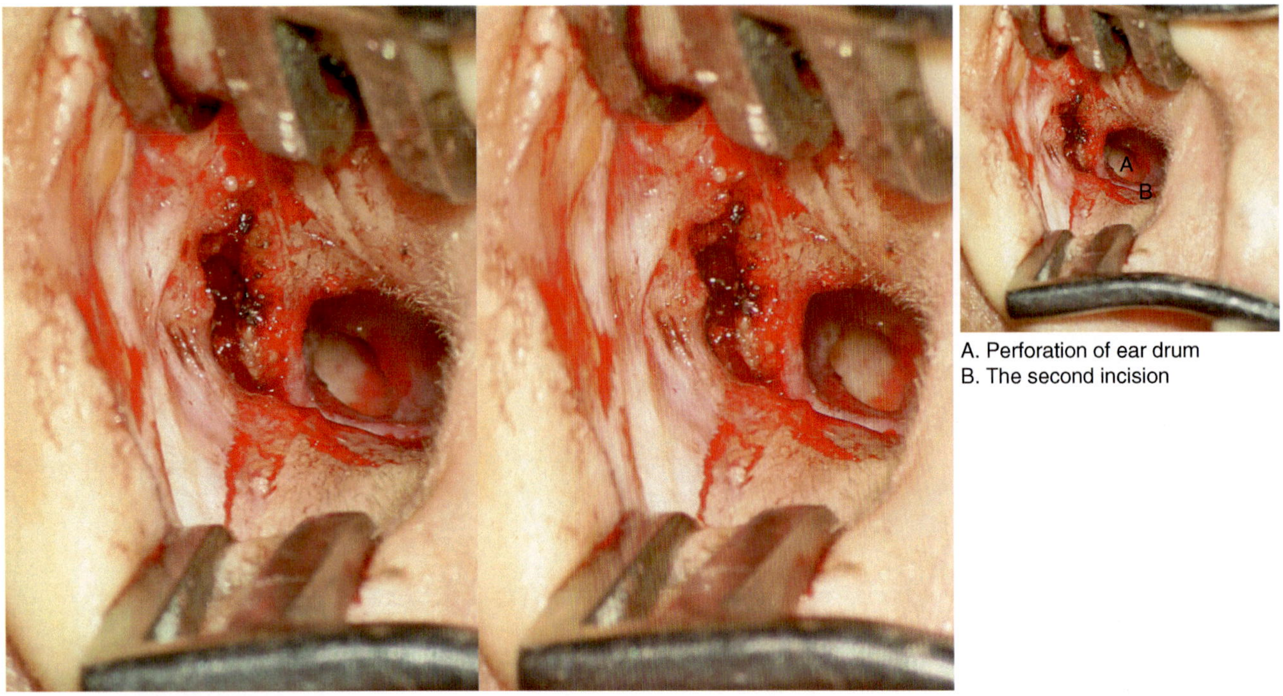

A. Perforation of ear drum
B. The second incision

Fig. 2.48 The second incision
The second incision is made over the posterior bony auditory canal wall from the 6 o'clock position, 0.5 cm away from the tympanic annulus, to join the inner end of the first incision. The large perforation at the center of the pars tensa and the residual tympanic membrane can be seen

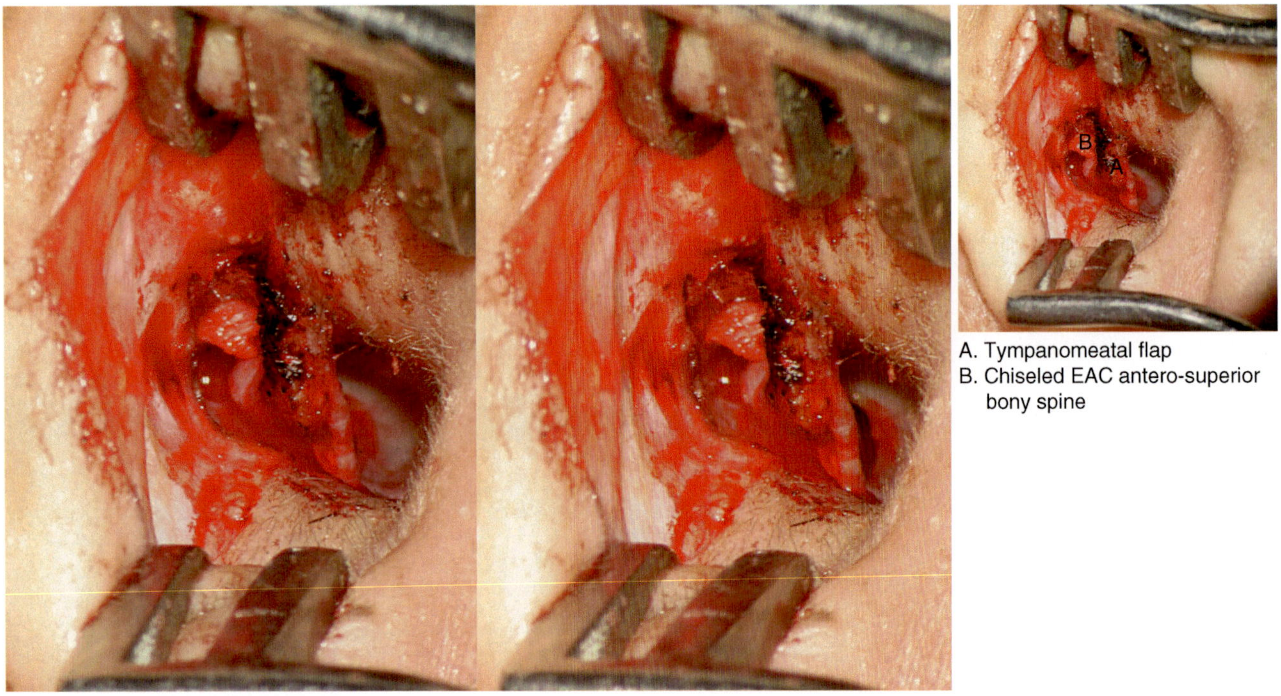

A. Tympanomeatal flap
B. Chiseled EAC antero-superior bony spine

Fig. 2.49 Elevation of EAC skin flaps
The skin and periosteum of the EAC are elevated from the bony wall along incisional margin to the tympanic annulus. The anterior skin flap is elevated and the anterior superior spine is exposed with sharp and blunt dissection. Any prominent anterior superior spine is removed. This is an important part of the procedure to expose the anterior part of the tympanic membrane and of the middle ear

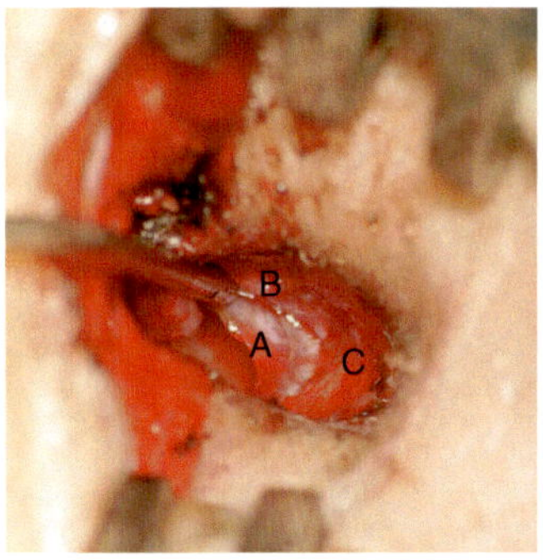

A. Lamina propria
B. Epithelial layer of tympanic membrane
C. EAC inferior wall

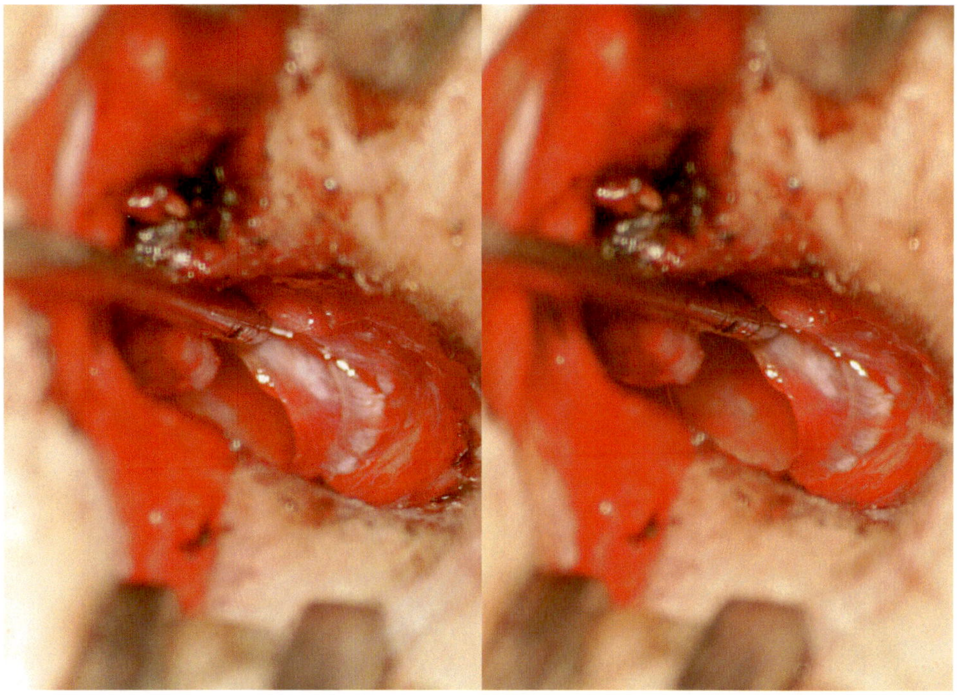

Fig. 2.50 Remnant epithelial layer and fibrous layer of the tympanic membrane are separated
The skin flap of the EAC is elevated to the tympanic annulus and whole remnant epithelial layer of the tympanic membrane is separated carefully upwards, forwards and downwards. The fibrous layer of the tympanic membrane is left in situ

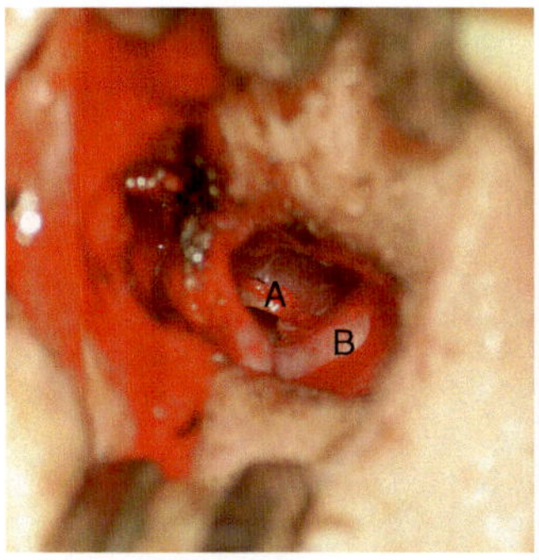

A. Epithelial layer of tympanic membrane
B. Tympanomeatal flap

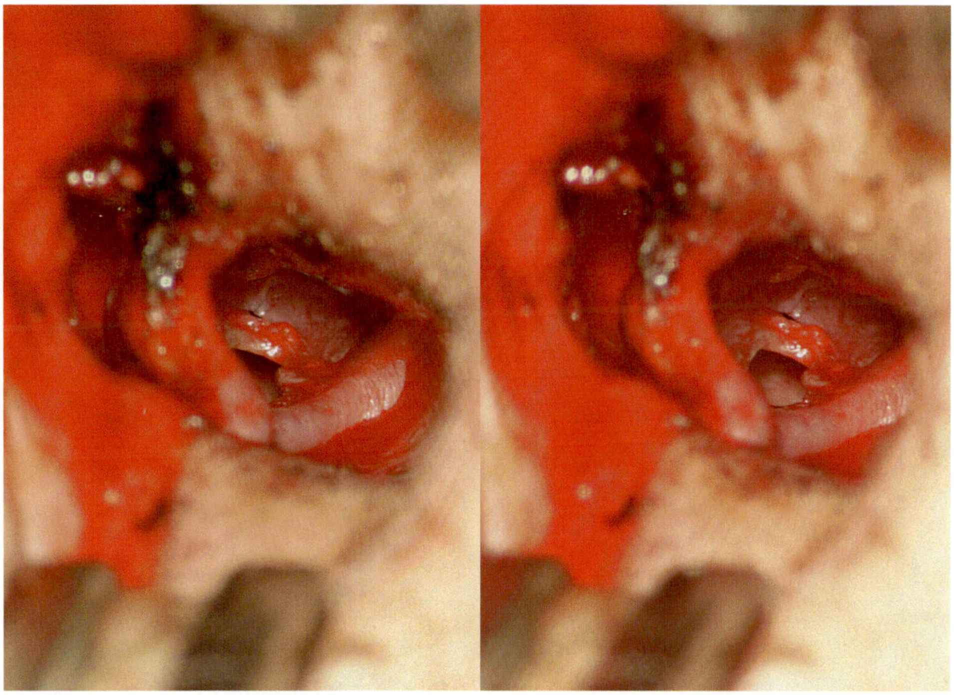

Fig. 2.51 Repositioning of EAC skin flap
After replacing the tympanomeatal flap, the integrity of the epithelial layer of tympanic membrane is checked to ensure that it is completely separated from the lamina propria. Any areas of adhesion are identified and separated. The site and size of the ear drum perforation are also assessed. The epithelial layer of the tympanic membrane is preserved as far as possible

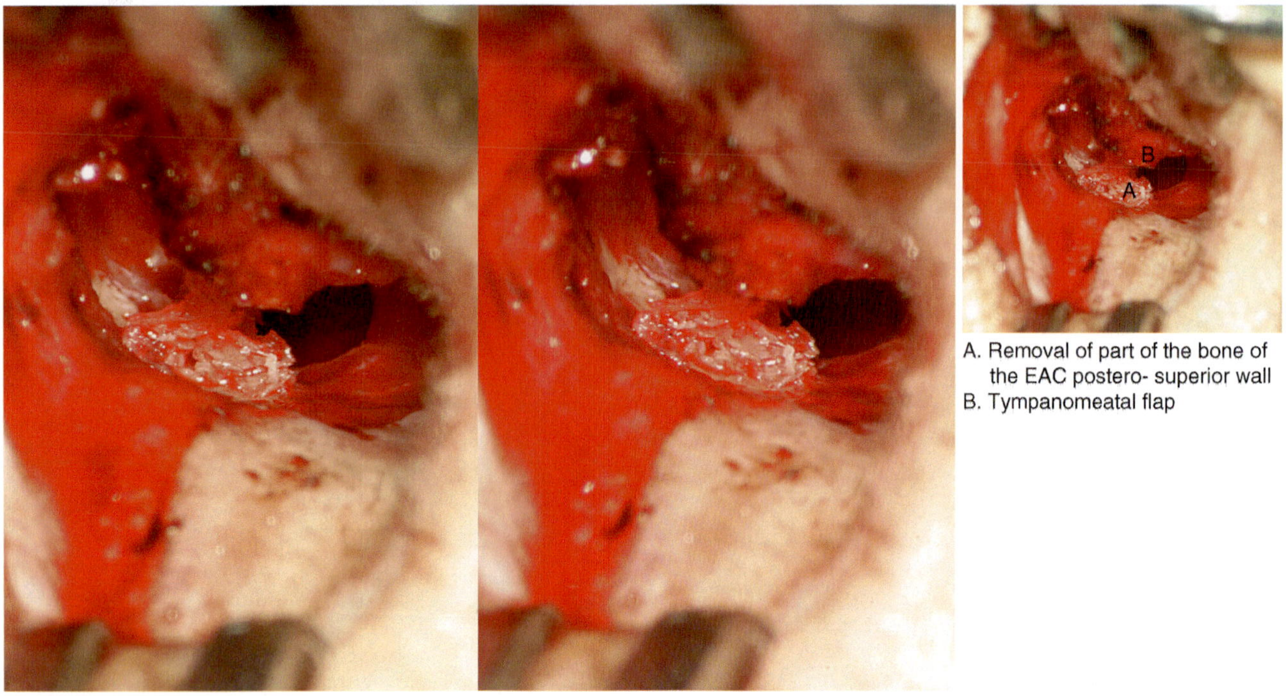

Fig. 2.52 A segment of the lateral bony wall of postero-superior tympanic cavity is chiseled off
If exploration of the ossicular chain or attic is required, the remaining base layer of the tympanic membrane (right side from 9 to 11 o'clock) is elevated from the tympanic sulcus. Bone can be removed delicately in small pieces to extend the exposure as required, avoiding injury to the chorda tympani and the ossicular chain

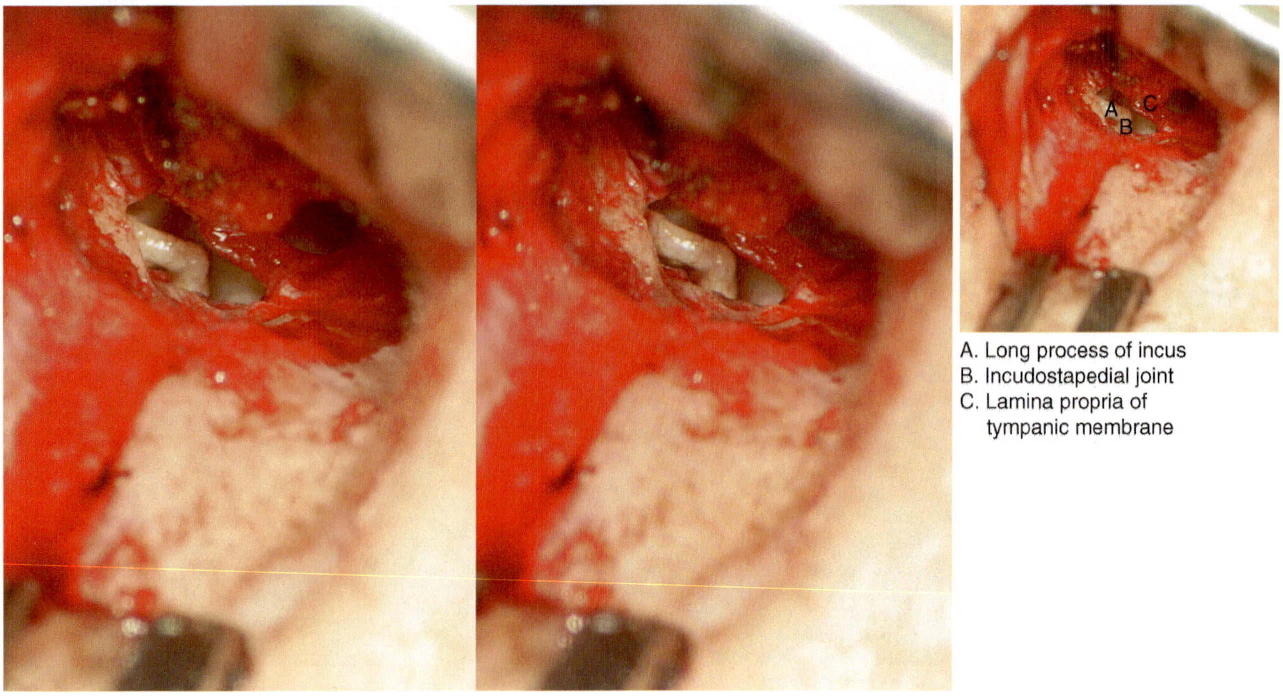

Fig. 2.53 The long process of incus and incudostapedial joint are exposed
In order to explore the integrity and mobility of the ossicular chain, bone of the postero-superior EAC wall can be removed to expand the field of vision. This picture shows the lamina propria, chorda tympani nerve, long process of incus and stapes. The ossicular chain is seen to be intact and mobile

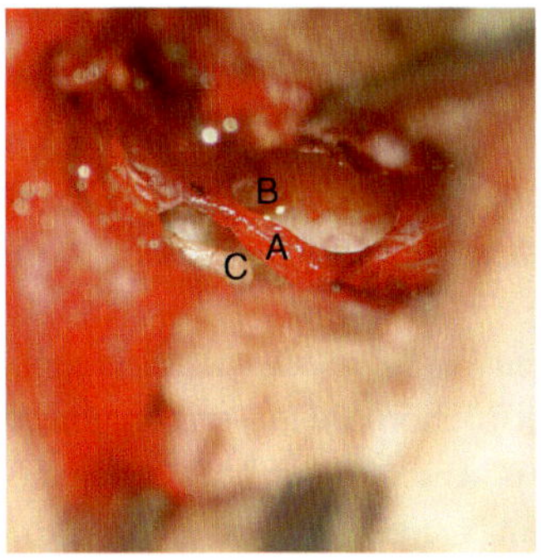

A. Chorda tympani nerve and lamina propria
B. Handle of malleus
C. Long process of incus

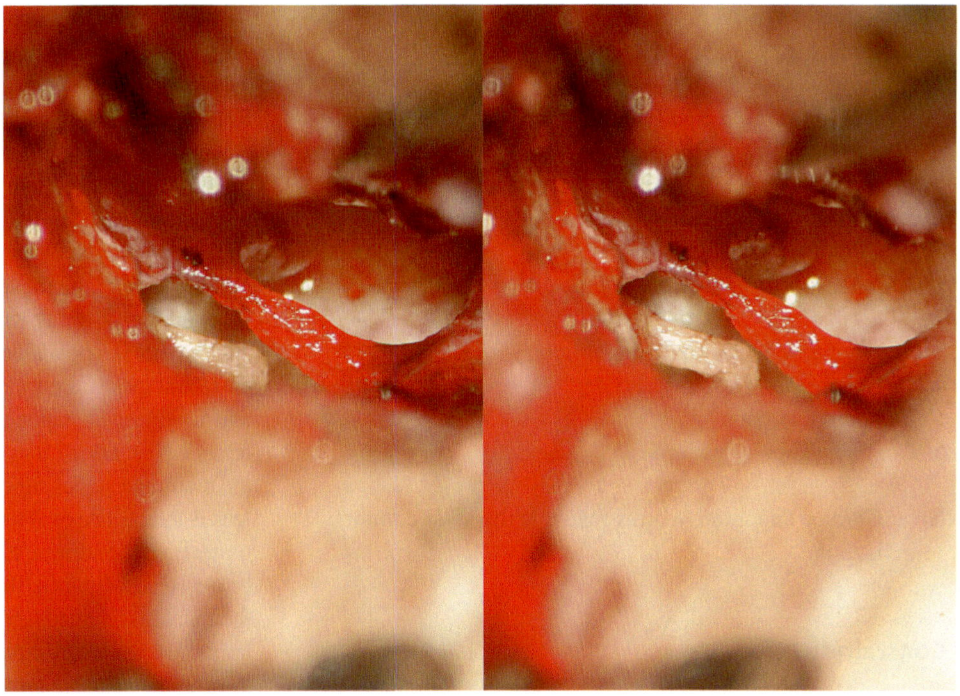

Fig. 2.54 Relation between chorda tympani nerve and lamina propria
Zoom in with the microscope; identify the lamina propria extending from the tympanic sulcus. The chorda tympani nerve sits under the lamina propria lateral to the long process of the incus. The handle of the malleus and remaining lamina propria surrounding it are seen in the front of the field of vision

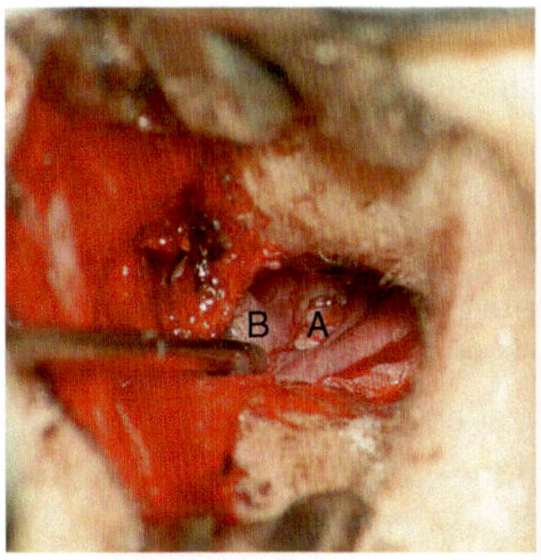

A. Transplanted fascia
B. Lateral tympanomeatal flap

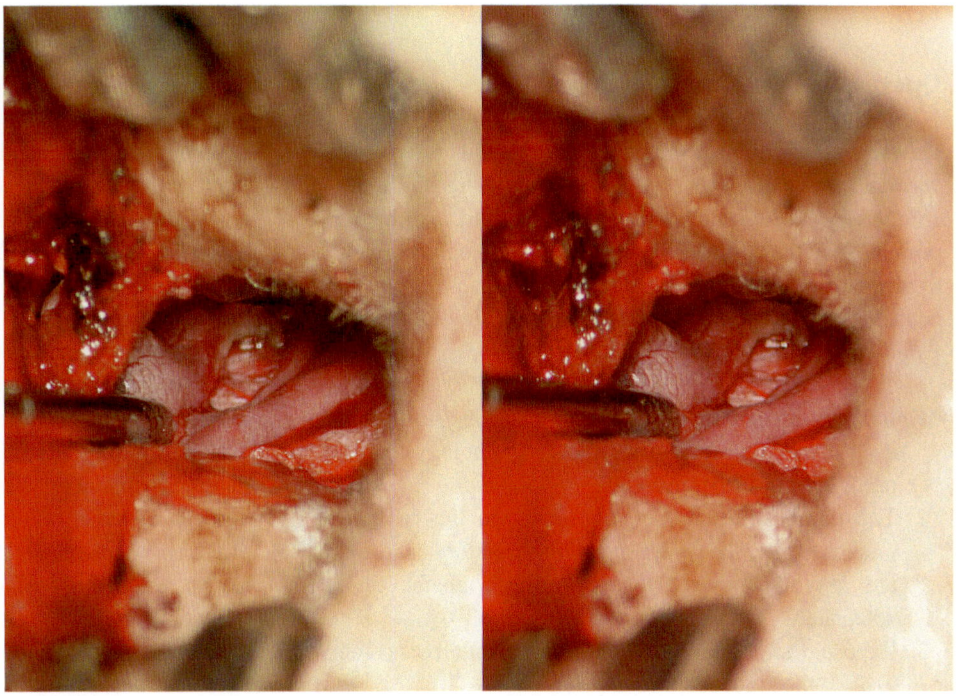

Fig. 2.55 Repair of tympanic membrane; replacement of tympanomeatal flap.
Harvest the temporalis fascia at the beginning of the operation and stiffen it in 75 % alcohol solution. Lay it between the epithelial layer of tympanic membrane and the lamina propria, covering the perforation completely. Replace the lateral and tympanomeatal flaps, ensuring the fascia is well seated and fully covers the perforation, and does not extend lateral to the end of the tympanomeatal flap

Reconstruction of Ossicular Chain/ Ossiculoplasty

Yu-hua Zhu, Xue Gao, and Pu Dai

Indications

1. Chronic suppurative otitis media
2. Abnormality of ossicular chain
3. Traumatic ossicular chain disruption
4. Otospongiosis (Otosclerosis)
5. Tympanosclerosis
6. Congenital cholesteatoma

Note: Chronic suppurative otitis media is the most common indication.

Contraindications

1. Patients unfit for the operation
2. Dysfunction of Eustachian tube
3. Residual cholesteatoma in the tympanic cavity
4. Perforation of ear drum with persistent discharge
5. Acute otitis externa and otitis media

Operative Procedures

Different reconstructive methods and materials are used in various approaches to ossiculoplasty depending on the disease status and ossicular status (continuity and mobility). If possible, it is the best to make full use of autologous ossicles to reconstruct hearing. Maintaining the tympanic cavity and continuity and stability of the ossicular chain are two key points in ossiculoplasty.

1. Incision: an endaural or a postauricular incision can be used, depending on the middle ear pathology and the preference of the surgeon
2. The tympanomeatal flap, consisting of the tympanic membrane and the posterior external auditory canal skin are carefully elevated to expose the tympanic cavity adequately.
3. Expose the lateral wall of epitympanic recess and explore the malleus.
4. Open the epitympanic recess to completely remove cholesteatoma, and explore the incus and malleus.
5. The antrum and mastoid should be opened until normal air cells and mucosa are reached.
6. Evaluate the status and mobility of the residual ossicles and prepare available autologous ossicle(s) for further use.
7. Select the type of ossicle to be transplanted, measure the length required, shape the ossicle for ossicular reconstruction.
8. Reconstruction of ossicular chain: there are different types of reconstruction according to the status of the residual ossicular chain.

   A. Manubrium of malleus -Head of stapes: this is applicable for ossicular chain disruption due to a missing incus, attic fixation of the malleus head or incus body, tympanosclerosis and so on. B. Manubrium of malleus-Footplate of stapes: this is applicable for the lesions where the incus and the stapes superstructure are damaged and the malleus and footplate of stapes are intact. C. Manubrium of malleus-Oval window: it is applicable for the lesions where the incus and stapes superstructure are absent and the malleus is intact. The oval window may need to be sealed with tissue (perichondrium, fascia or vein). D. Tympanic membrane-Head of stapes: this is applicable for lesions where the incus and malleus are absent and the stapes is intact. A partial ossicular substitute (PORP) can be used to bridge the gap between the tympanic membrane and head of stapes. E. Tympanic membrane- Footplate of stapes: this is applicable for lesions including absence of the malleus, incus and superstructure of stapes, but the footplate of stapes present and mobile. A total ossicular substitute (TORP) may be used to connect the tympanic membrane and footplate of stapes.
9. The stabilization of reconstructed ossicular chain: there are a number of techniques used for stabilizing the ossicular chain, including residual manubrium of malleus, homogenous cartilage/perichondrium tissue and chorda tympani nerve, either used alone or in combination according to the actual situation. The chorda tympani nerve should be preserved for ossicular stabilization as far as possible.
10. Reconstruction and packing of the external auditory canal.

    Note: Many materials may be used for reconstruction of the ossicular chain: A. Autologous grafts: including residual ossicles, cortical bone and cartilage. B. Allogeneic grafts: including auditory ossicles, and nasal septum cartilage. C. Artificial ossicles: They are more commonly used and can be made of Teflon, silicone, ceramics, titanium, etc. Transplanted materials must meet the following criteria: no residual tissue antigen, no inflammatory or foreign body response in the middle ear, easy to shape, conducive to establishing a stable connection.

Special Comments

1. Remove all disease and promote good ventilation of the new tympanic cavity.
2. Assess the residual ossicular chain thoroughly.

3. Retain or re-use healthy autologous materials as far as possible, such as ossicles and the tympanic membrane remnant.
4. Various tissues and materials can be used to stabilize the reconstructed ossicular, such as manubrium of malleus, homogenous cartilage, chorda tympani nerve, fibrin glue, gelatin sponge and so on.
5. Confirm the structural integrity and mobility of the stapes: a mobile footplate is required for successful ossicular reconstruction. Stapedectomy or stapedotomy may be considered at a second stage if the footplate is fixed. If the stapes arch is missing or disconnected, a direct connection to the footplate may be considered.
6. Care should be taken not to damage the chorda tympani nerve or the tendon of the tensor tympani muscle when severing the neck of the malleus and removing the incus. The chorda tympani and the tensor tympani tendon can be used for fixing implanted ossicles or prostheses. (Disease processes often exist in the epitympanic recess, necessitating removal of the malleus. This favours ventilation and drainage of the epitympanic recess).
7. Carefully measure the length of transplanted ossicles to prevent displacement or protrusion of ossicle, and to prevent fracture of the stapes arch or footplate.
8. The external auditory canal should be carefully packed after myringoplasty and ossicular chain reconstruction, taking care not to deform the tympanic membrane or the reconstructed chain.

Complications

1. Fixation of ossicles: Both residual lesions in the tympanic cavity or improper position of ossicles can lead to fixation of ossicles. The implanted ossicle or prostheses should be positioned in the center of the stapes footplate in order to acheive maximum hearing gain and avoid poor conduction.
2. Displacement of ossicles: Implanted ossicles or prostheses that are too short can often result in displacement of ossicles. The best part of the tympanic membrane to connect with the reconstructed chain is the posterosuperior quadrant.
3. Ossicles protruding: A small disc of cartilage should be laid between the tympanic membrane and ossicular prosthesis in order to prevent it extruding. Re-perforation of the tympanic membrane may occur when implanted ossicles or prostheses are too long and apply excessive pressure to the repaired tympanic membrane.
4. Fracture of stapes arch or footplate: This may occur when the implanted ossicles or prostheses are too long or too heavy.
5. Transplanted ossicles may be absorbed.

Surgery 1: Mastoidectomy with reconstruction of external auditory canal and ossicular chain

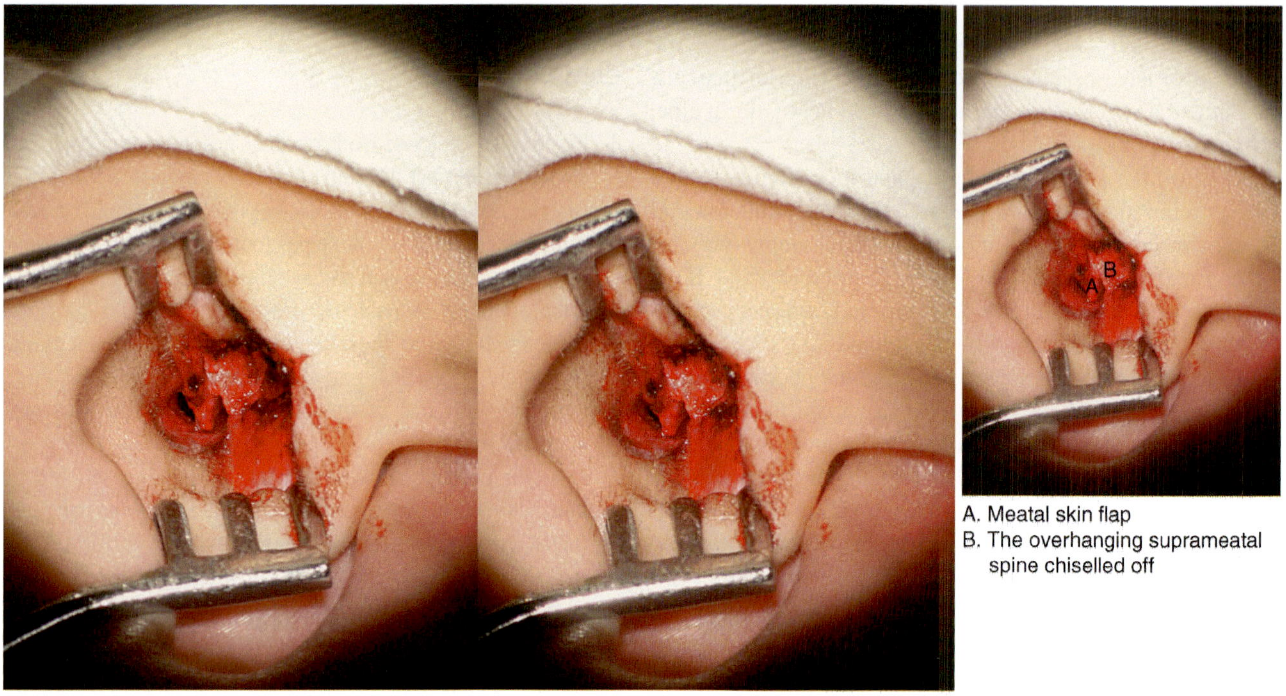

Fig. 2.56 Endaural incision and removal of the overhanging suprameatal spine
The first skin incision is made at the 12 o'clock position of EAC just lateral to the bony-cartilaginous junction and carried down to the bone, and then under the operating microscope the first incision is extended inward to a point about 0.8–1.0 cm lateral to the tympanic annulus. The second incision starts from the 6 o'clock position of EAC, and remains 6–8 mm lateral to the tympanic annulus along the posterior meatal wall in an ascending spiral (or curved) fashion to meet the first incision. The overhanging suprameatal spine can be removed by a small burr or chisel for good exposure

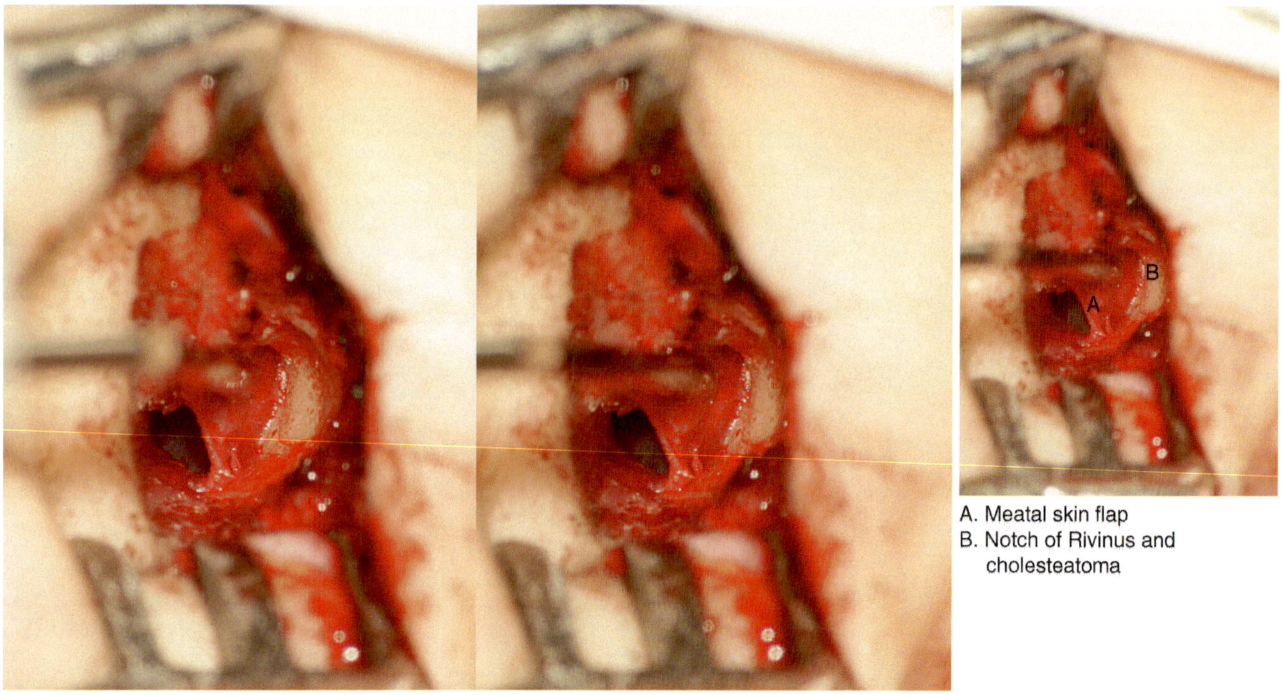

Fig. 2.57 Elevation of the meatal skin flap
The meatal skin flap of posterio-superior part of the external auditory canal is elevated and cholesteatoma is seen in the notch of Rivinus in this case

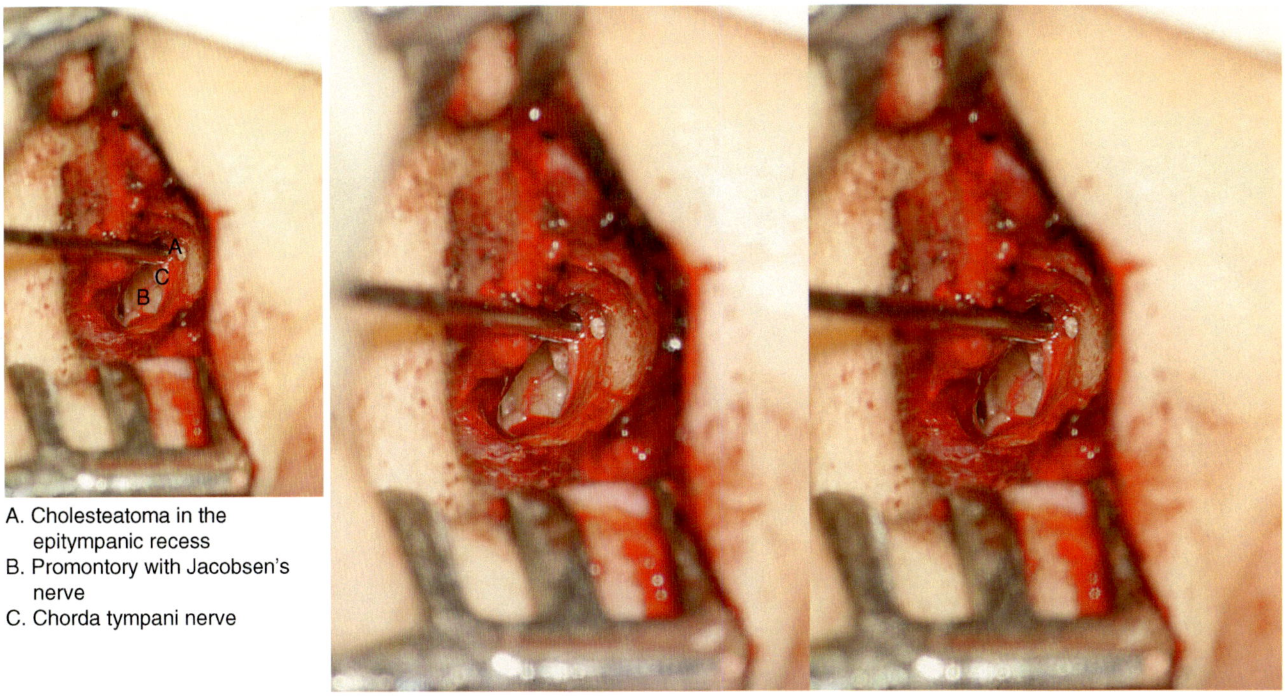

A. Cholesteatoma in the epitympanic recess
B. Promontory with Jacobsen's nerve
C. Chorda tympani nerve

Fig. 2.58 Expose the tympanic cavity and the lateral wall of the epitympanic recess
The fibrous annulus of the tympanic membrane is dissected and separated from the posterior tympanic sulcus. The meatal skin flap and tympanic membrane are raised anteriorly to the level of short process of malleus. The tympanic cavity is thus exposed and the cholesteatoma in the postero-superior part of tympanic cavity can be seen. Care should be taken not to injure the chorda tympani nerve during the procedure

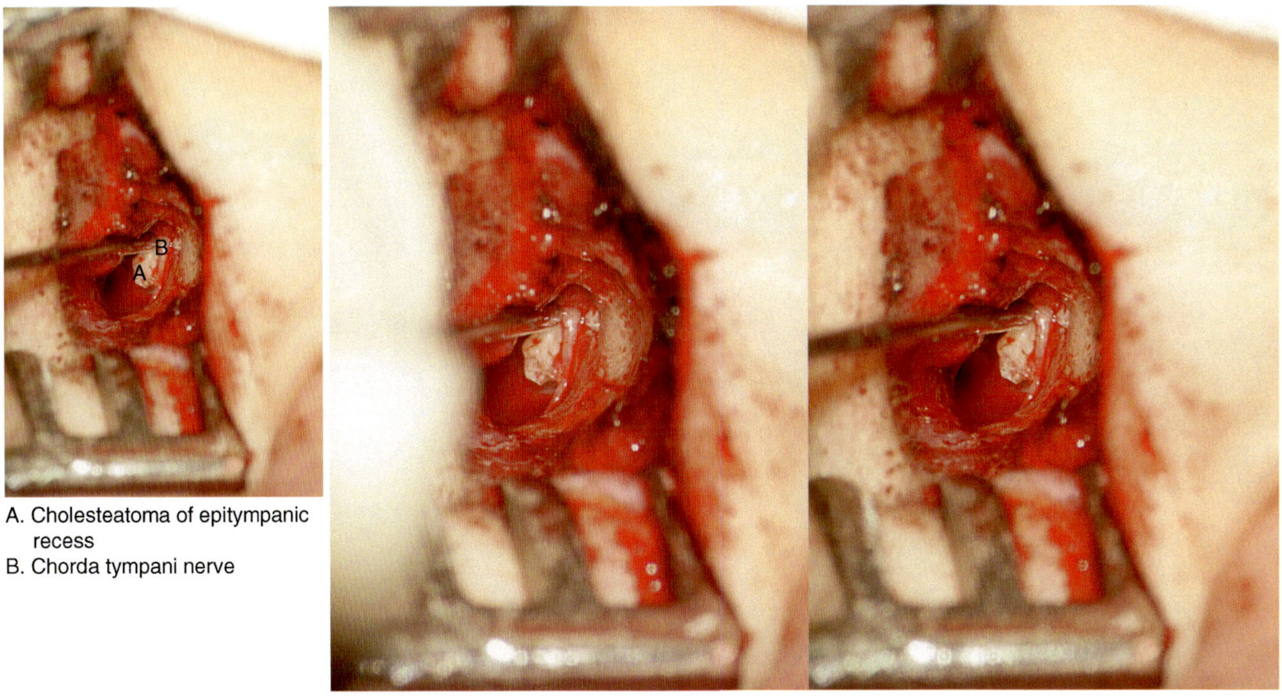

A. Cholesteatoma of epitympanic recess
B. Chorda tympani nerve

Fig. 2.59 Remove cholesteatoma from the tympanic cavity
Remove part of the lateral wall of epitympanic recess. The chorda tympani nerve and cholesteatoma in the epitympanic recess are clearly exposed

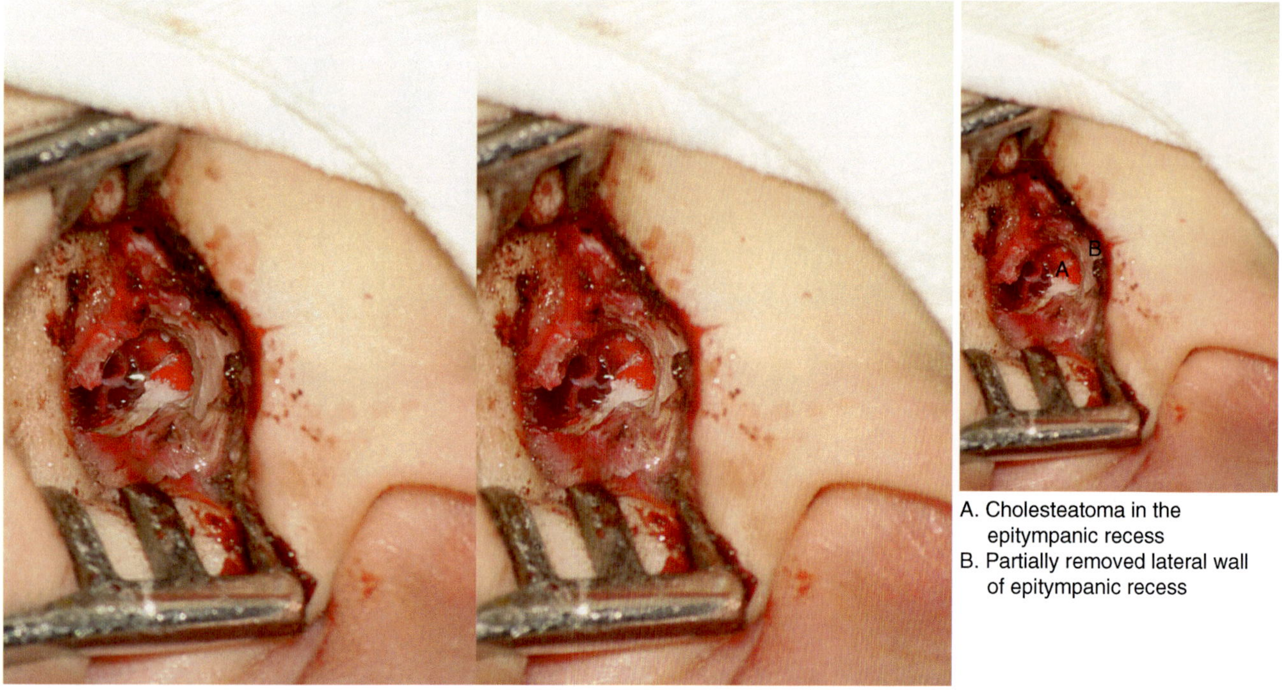

Fig. 2.60 Open the epitympanic recess
The attic is opened with an electric drill to expose the anterior border of attic to the same level as the anterior wall of external auditory canal. When the attic is partially opened, the extent of the cholesteatoma in the attic cavity can be determined, including any extension to the mastoid antrum

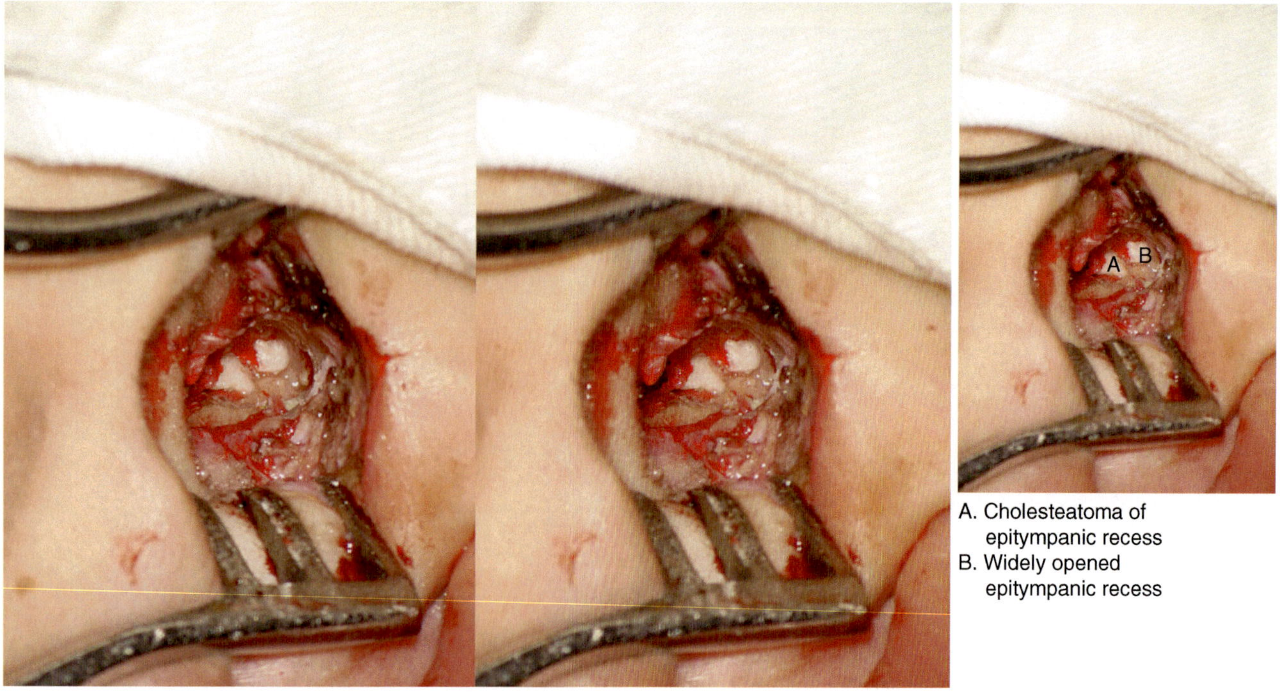

Fig. 2.61 Expose the cholesteatoma of epitympanic recess completely
Continue to remove the lateral wall of epitympanic recess with a drill to expose epitympanic recess adequately. The epitympanic recess is filled with the cholesteatoma, which is seen extending to the aditus ad antrum

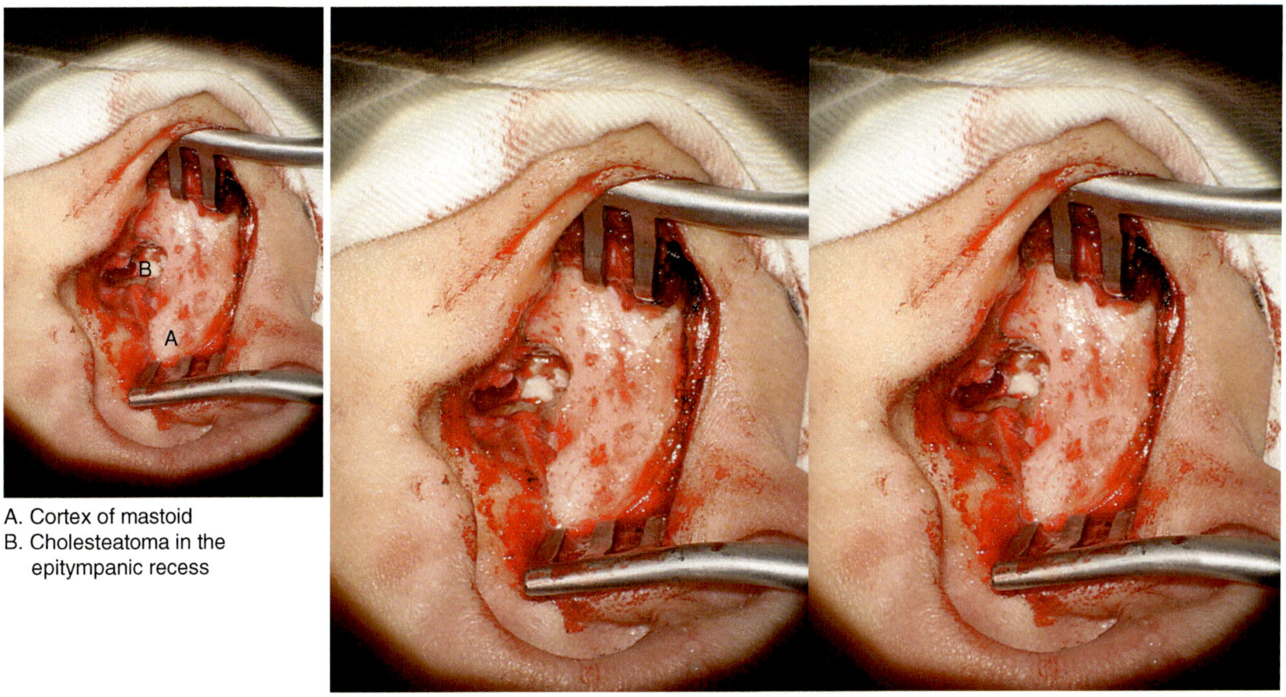

Fig. 2.62 Expose the cortex of mastoid
Make an outward prolongation of the original incision and separate the periosteum from the mastoid surface. Replace the self-retaining retractor to adequately expose the upper part of mastoid cortex

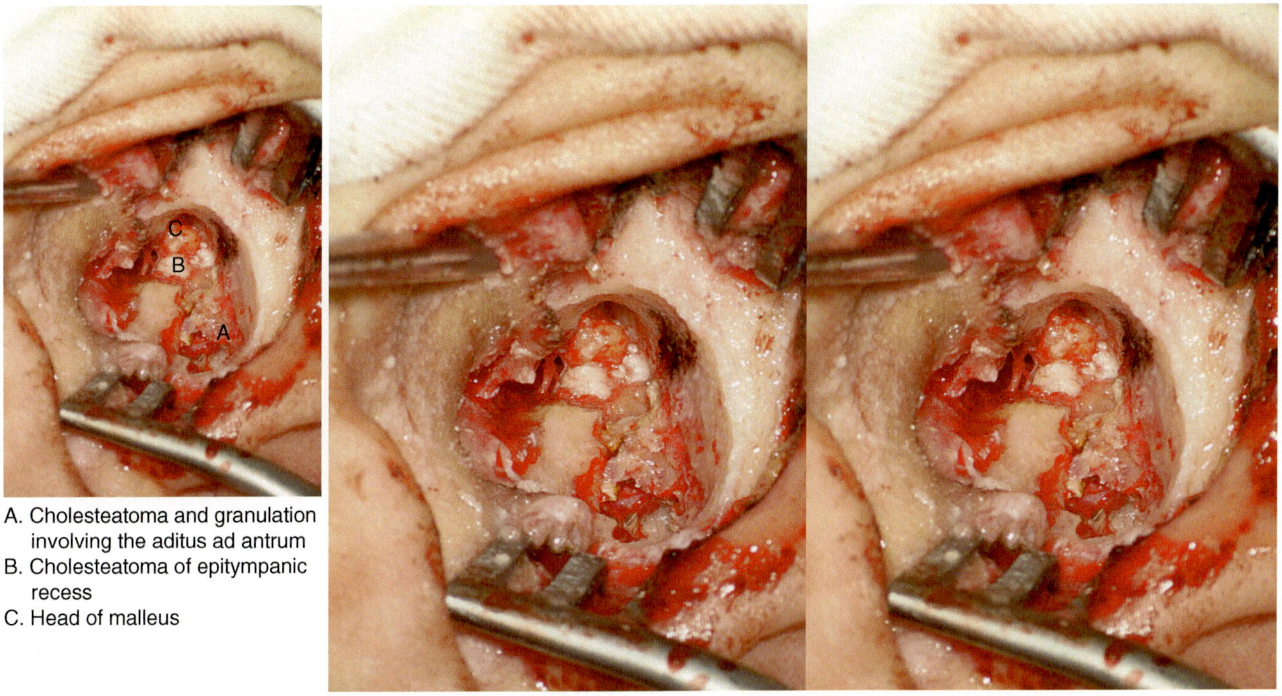

Fig. 2.63 Expose the disease in the tympanic antrum and mastoid cavity
An electric drill is used to open the antrum and mastoid to fully expose the cholesteatoma. Inflammatory granulation is seen in the aditus ad antrum after removal of cholesteatoma at this site. Surgical exposure should extended beyond the disease to see normal air cells and mucosa

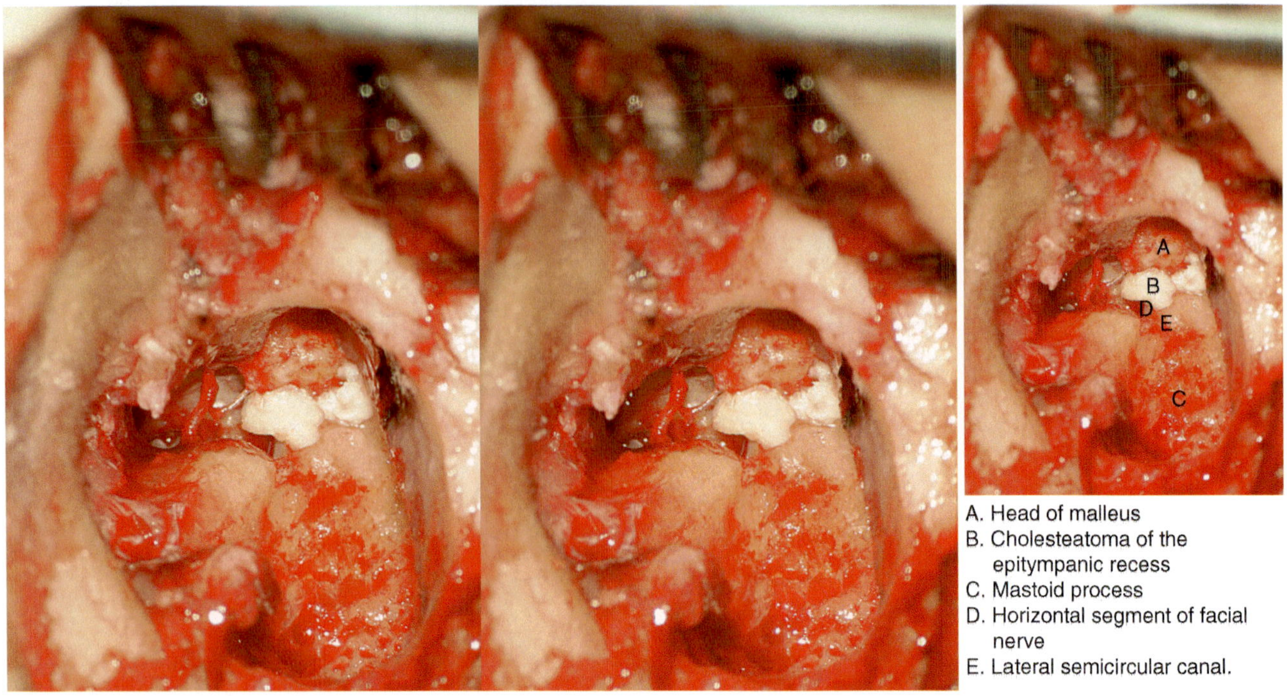

A. Head of malleus
B. Cholesteatoma of the epitympanic recess
C. Mastoid process
D. Horizontal segment of facial nerve
E. Lateral semicircular canal.

Fig. 2.64 Eradicate all disease from the mastoid
Disease in the antrum and mastoid cavity is removed totally and the walls of mastoid cavity are polished with a diamond burr. The upper wall of surgical cavity is the thin bony plate of the middle fossa. The lateral semicircular canal and facial nerve which are partially covered by the cholesteatoma can be seen at this point

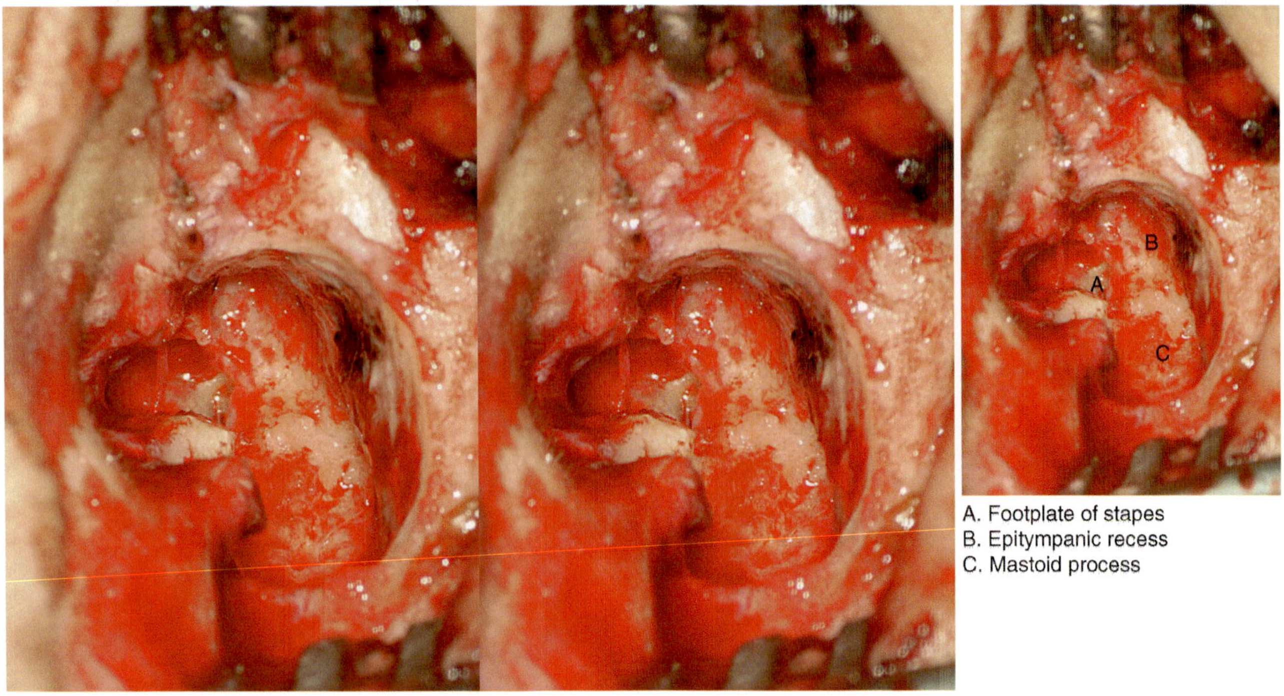

A. Footplate of stapes
B. Epitympanic recess
C. Mastoid process

Fig. 2.65 Remove the head of malleus and cholesteatoma from the epitympanic recess
The cholesteatoma can also be hidden medial to the head of malleus. In order to eradicate all cholesteatoma, the head of malleus is removed. The superstructure of stapes is absent, but the footplate of the stapes is present and mobile

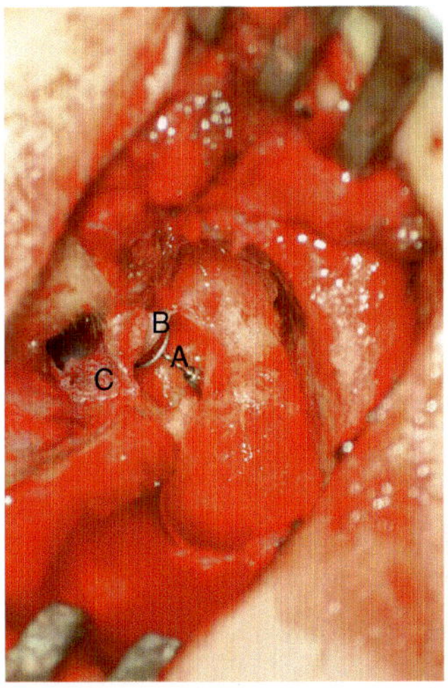

A. Ossicular prosthesis
B. Cartilage
C. Tympanomeatal flap

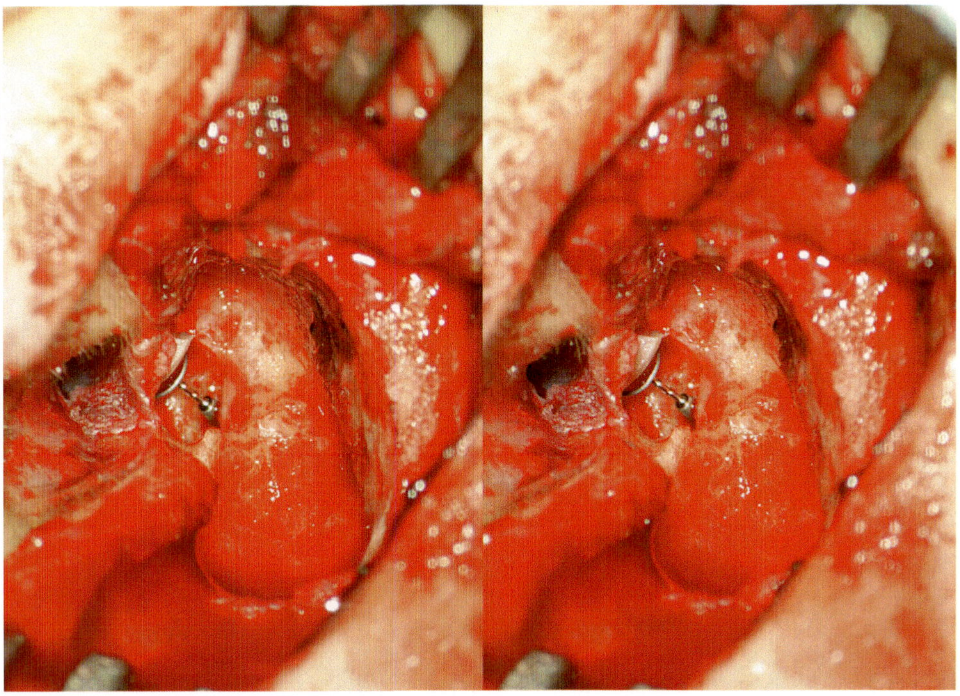

Fig. 2.66 Reconstruction of the ossicular chain
A groove is drilled in the bone of the anterior and posterior arch of the epitympanic recess and opened mastoid cavity. The tympanic membrane was intact and the ossicular prosthesis (TORP, Spiggle & Theis, total titanium ossicle replacement prosthesis) is positioned to connect the tympanic membrane and footplate of stapes. It is important to place a small piece of cartilage between the tympanic membrane and the prosthesis to prevent later extrusion through the tympanic membrane

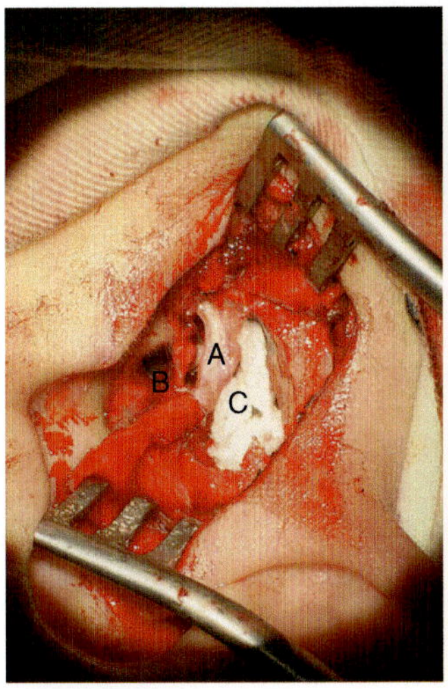

A. Cartilage
B. Tympanomeatal flap
C. Gelatin sponge

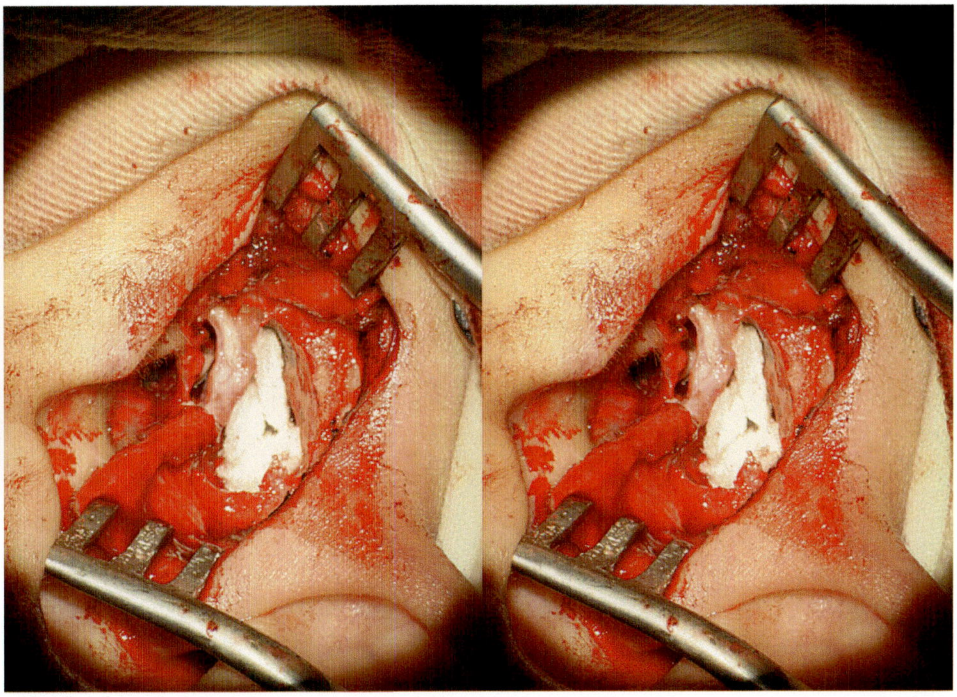

Fig. 2.67 Reconstruction of external auditory canal and obliteration of operation cavity
The superior and partial posterior walls of external auditory canal are repaired with tragal cartilage and the mastoid cavity is closed off. After the reconstruction of the ossicular chain and the repair of tympanic membrane, the surgical cavity should be carefully filled by small pieces of absorbable gelatin sponge to prevent adhesion and displacement of reconstructed ossicles and transplanted cartilage

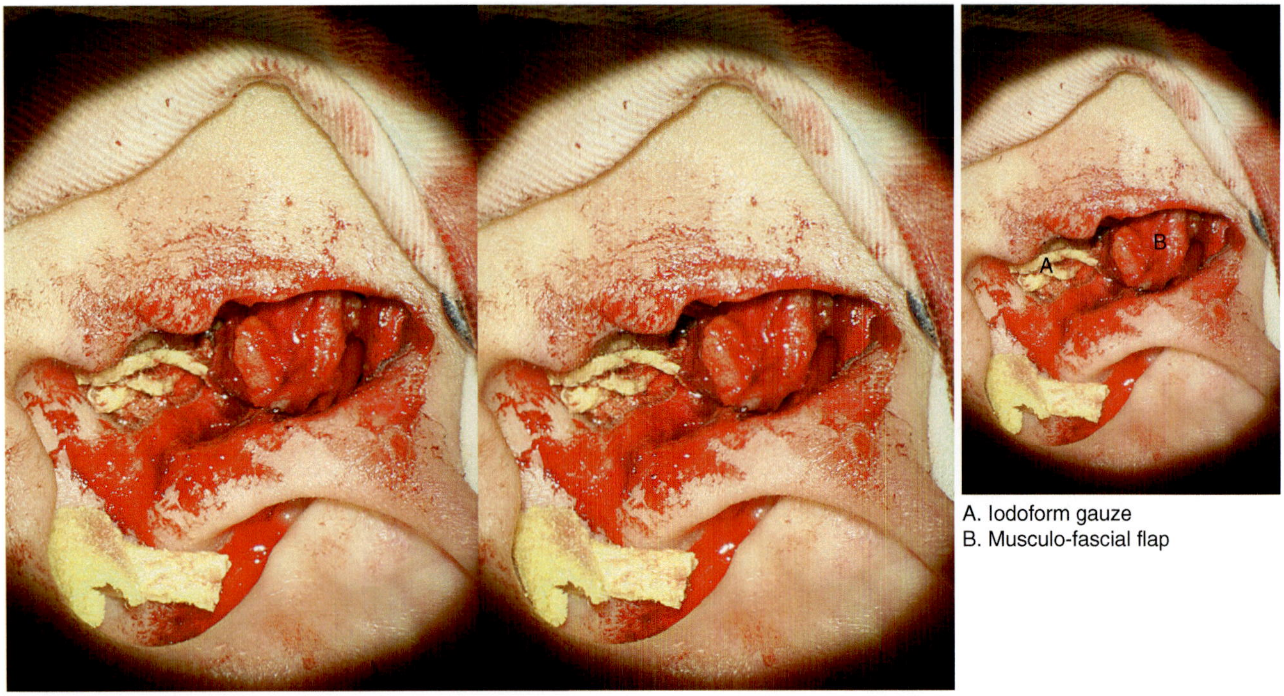

Fig. 2.68 Packing of external auditory canal
The pedicled temporalis muscle is put in the defect of mastoid to support the reconstructed external canal wall. It is important to pack the external auditory canal carefully with the iodoform gauze to prevent canal stenosis and displacement of reconstructed ossicular chain

Surgery 2: The tympanoplasty and ossiculoplasty

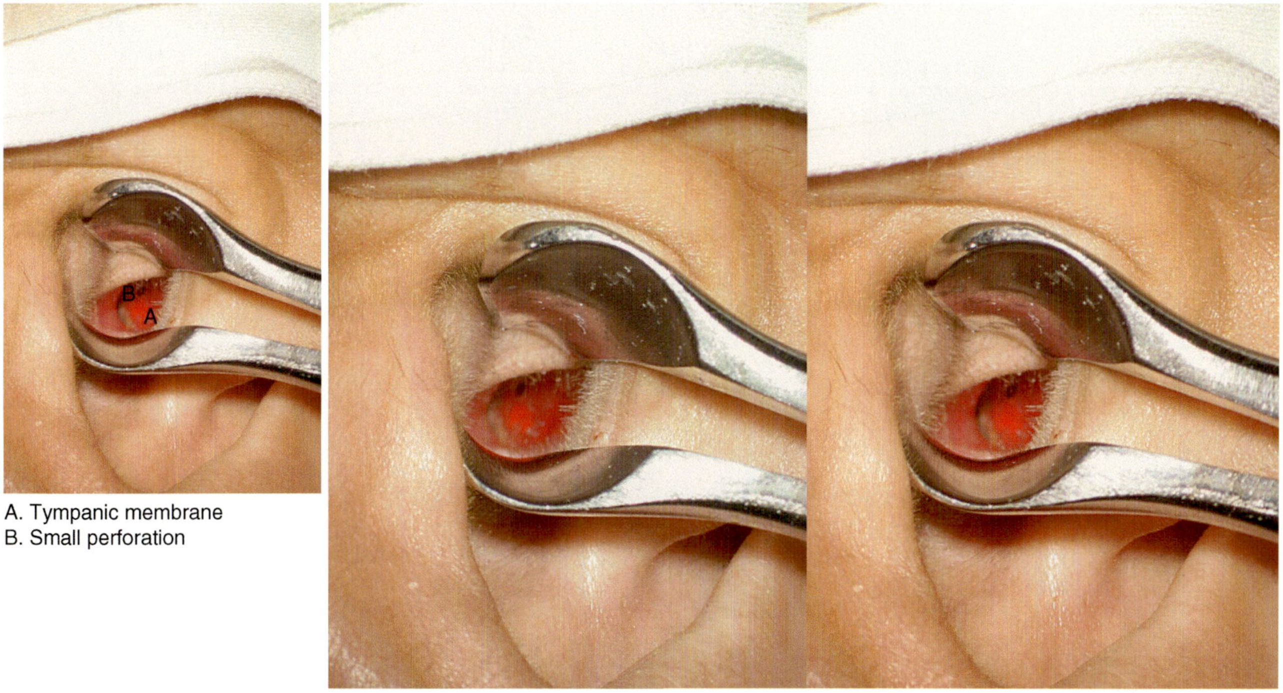

A. Tympanic membrane
B. Small perforation

Fig. 2.69 Examine the tympanic membrane
The external auditory canal and tympanic membrane are carefully examined under the microscope. In this case, there is a small perforation in the pars tensa of the tympanic membrane, with a calcified plaque in the residual tympanic membrane

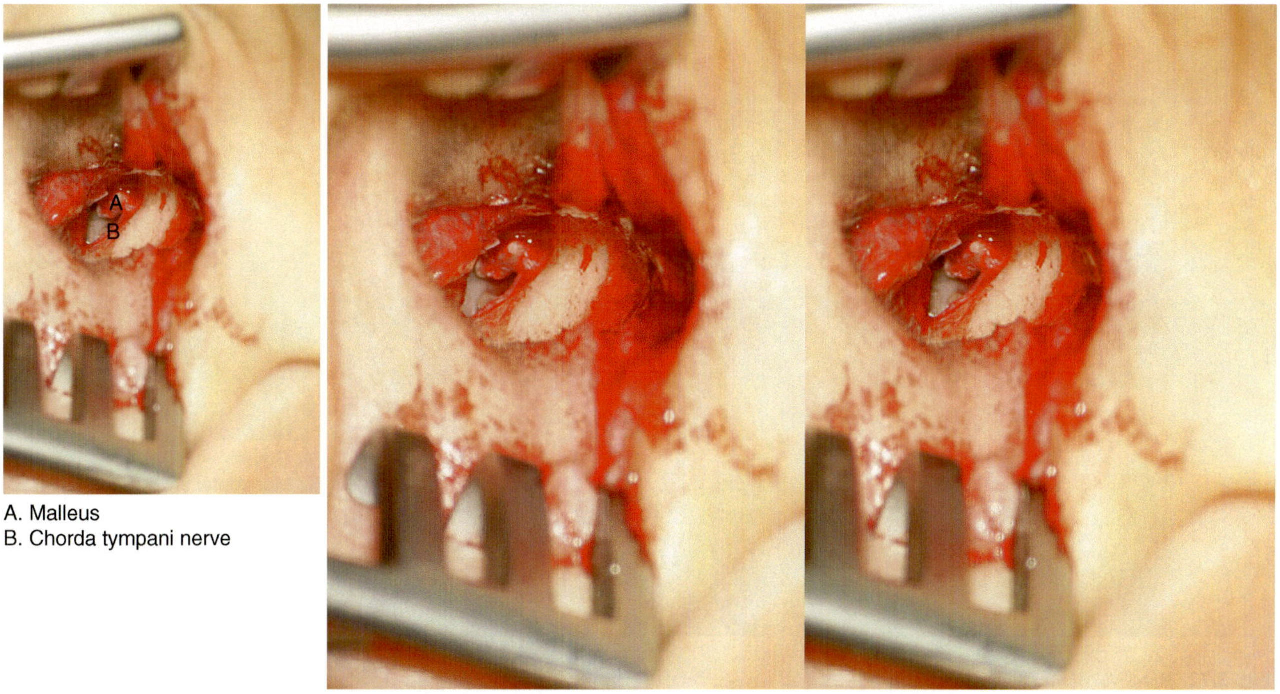

A. Malleus
B. Chorda tympani nerve

Fig. 2.70 Elevate the tympanic membrane to enter the tympanic cavity
The underlay grafting technique is used for tympanoplasty in this case. The skin incision is made between the tragus and the root of helix, and an inward extension is made to a point about 1.0 cm lateral to the tympanic annulus. The second incision starts from the 6 o'clock position of the EAC, and remains 6–8 mm lateral to the tympanic annulus along the posterior meatal wall in an ascending spiral fashion to meet the inner part of the first incision. The tympanomeatal flap is elevated anteriorly to expose the tympanic cavity

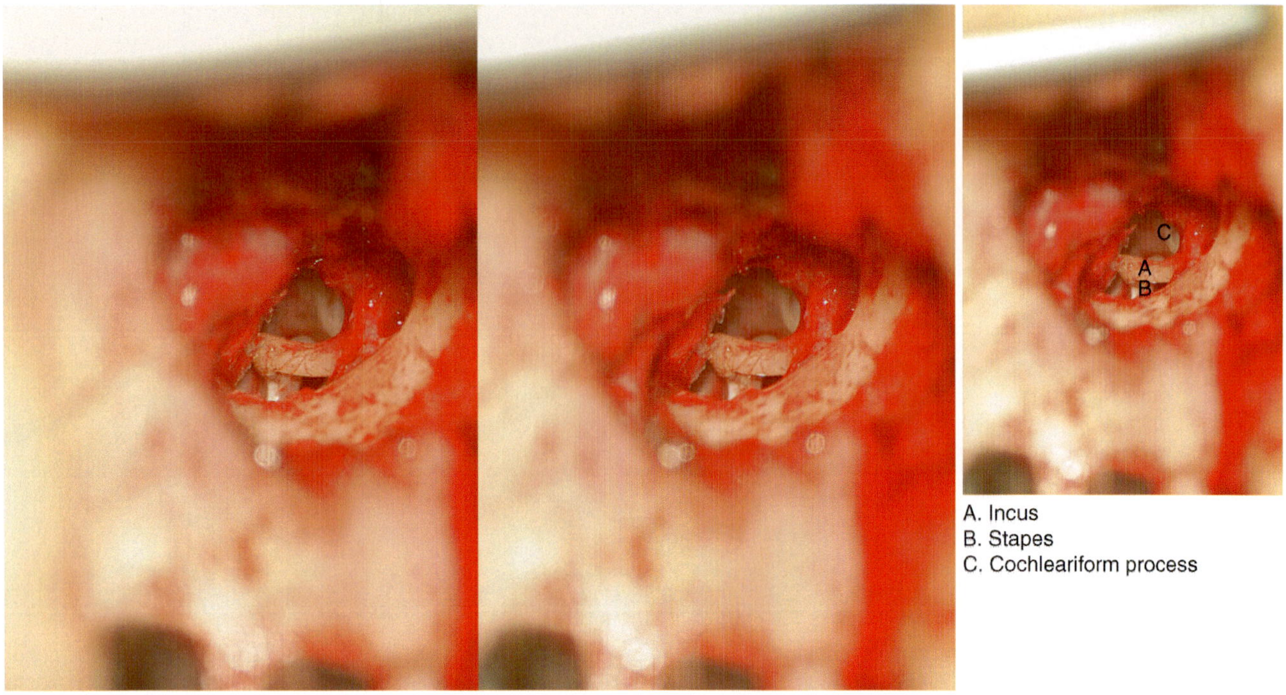

Fig. 2.71 Examine the incus and stapes
The excess bone of the postero-superior canal is removed. The incus and stapes are visible. There is hyperplastic fibrous tissue between the malleus and the incus. The cochleariform process is whitish, which is a sign of tympanosclerosis

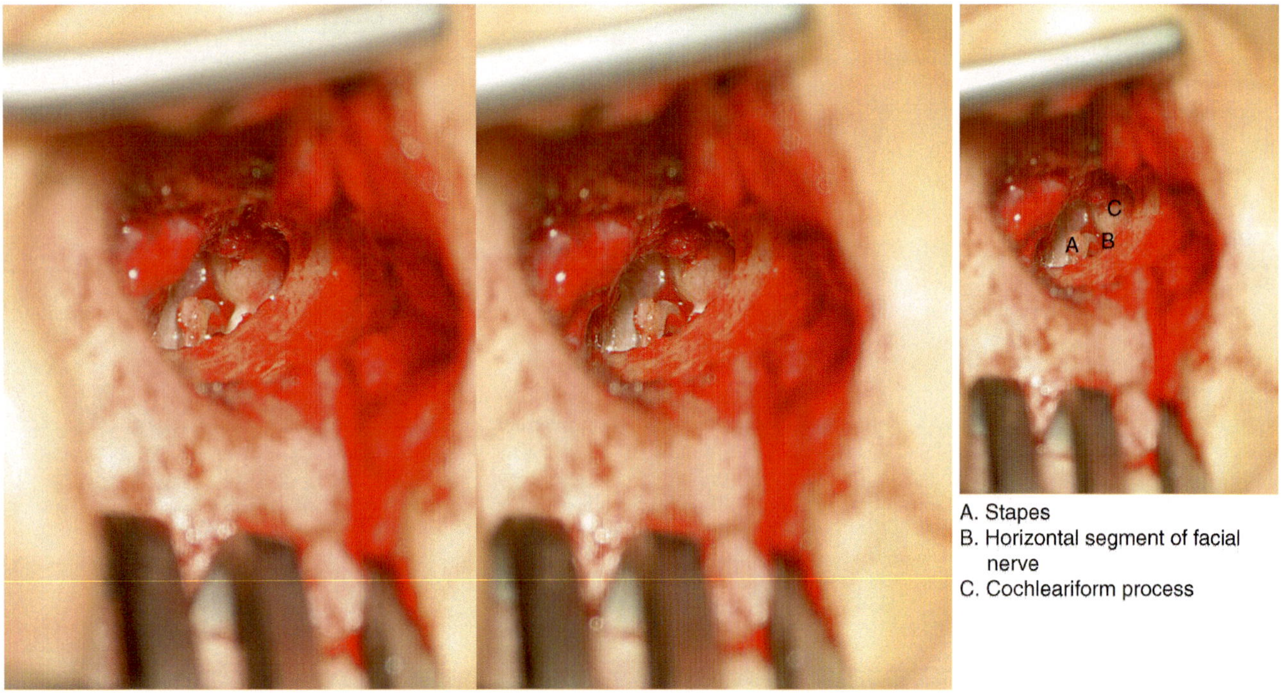

Fig. 2.72 Removal of the incus
The incus is taken out due to its fixation. The epitympanic recess is exposed sufficiently and the mobility of the stapes is evaluated carefully. The stapes and malleus are seen to have good mobility after removal of the incus

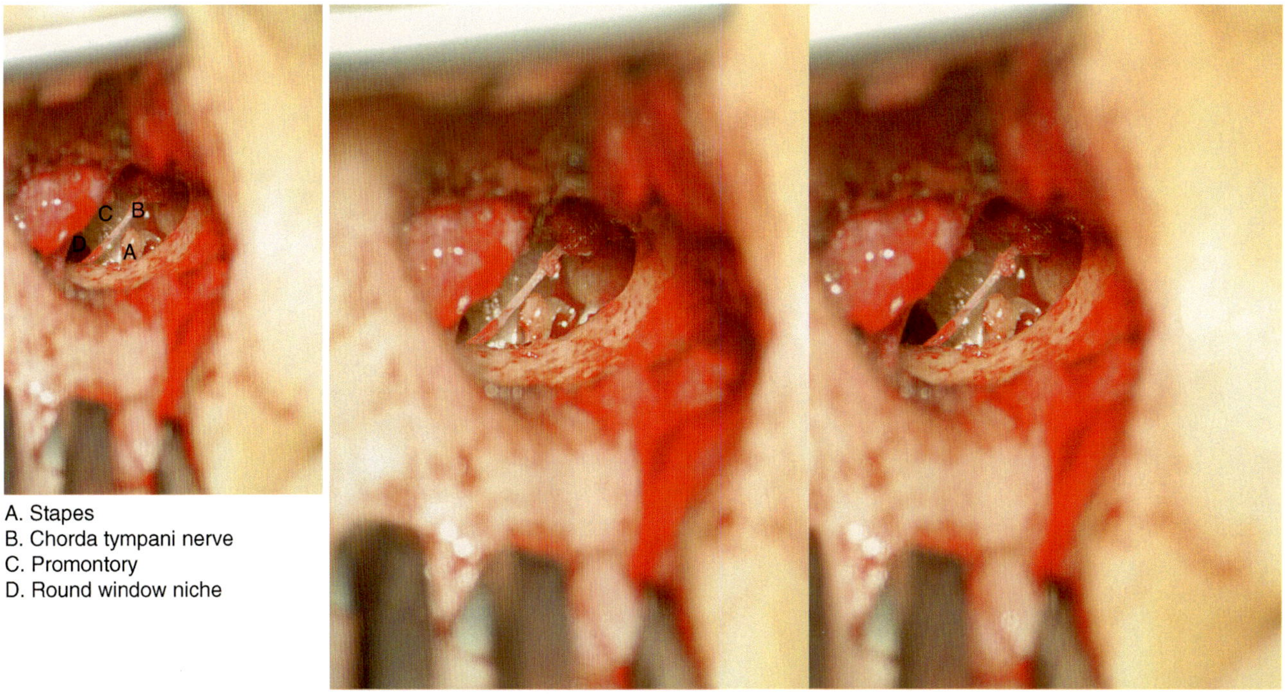

Fig. 2.73 Dissect the chorda tympani nerve
Dissect the chorda tympani nerve from the tympanic sulcus and expose the mesotympanum and hypotympanum. The mucosa of the tympanic cavity is normal and smooth, and there is no obstructive lesion in the round window niche

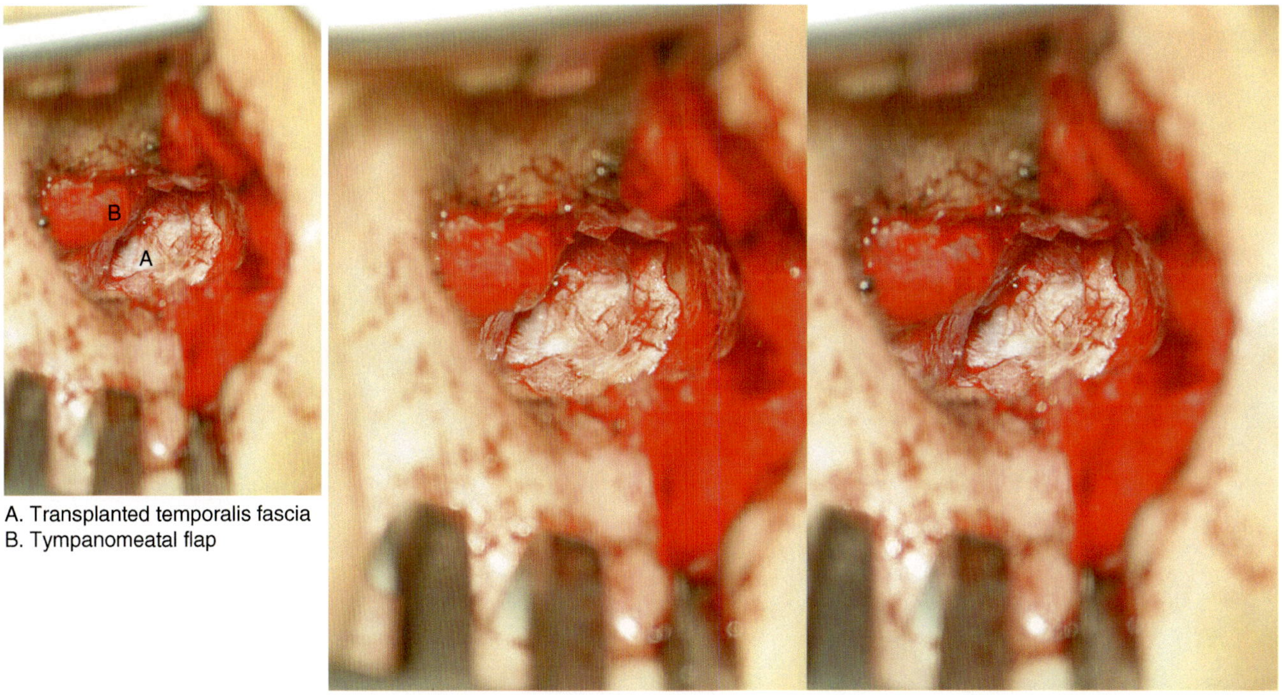

Fig. 2.74 Repair of the tympanic membrane
The temporalis fascia was fixed in 75 % alcohol and trimmed to a suitable size, then placed under the internal surface of the residual tympanic membrane

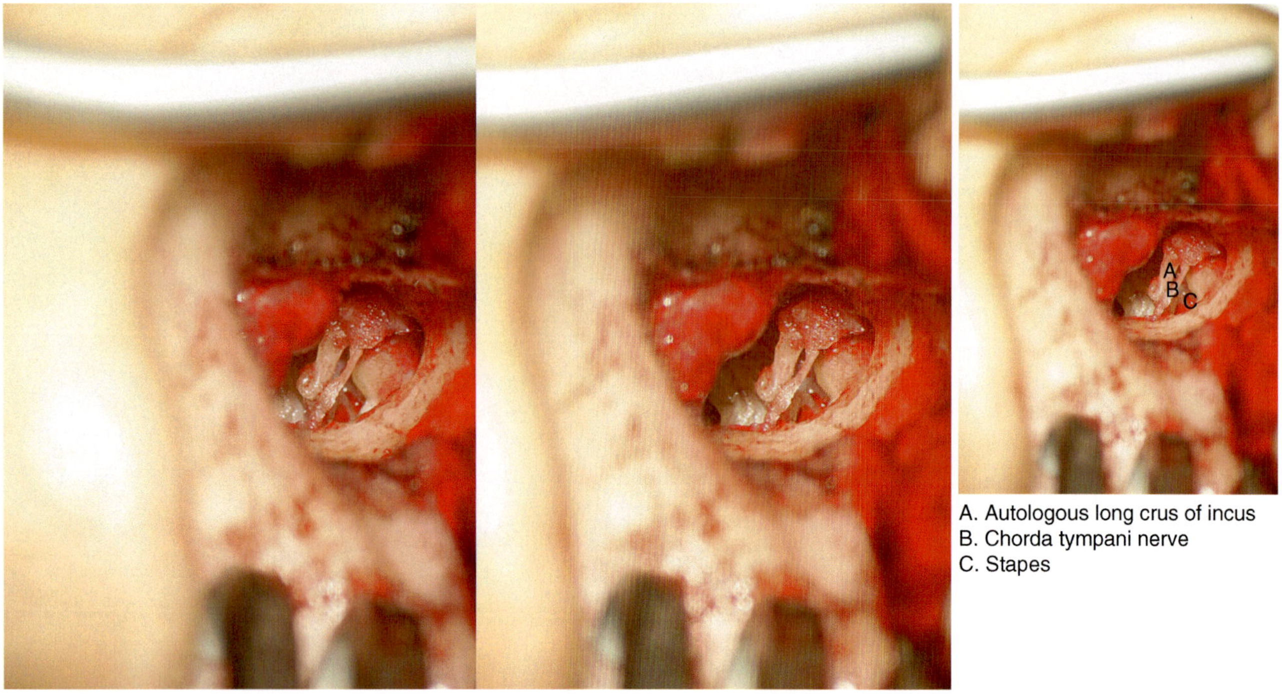

A. Autologous long crus of incus
B. Chorda tympani nerve
C. Stapes

Fig. 2.75 Reconstruction of the ossicular chain with autologous incus
Raise the temporalis fascia again. The sculptured autologous incus long process is implanted to connect the head of stapes and manubrium of malleus. Fibrinogen glue can be used to support the connections of the reconstructed ossicular chain. The preserved chorda tympani nerve is also helpful in stabilization of the reconstructed ossicles

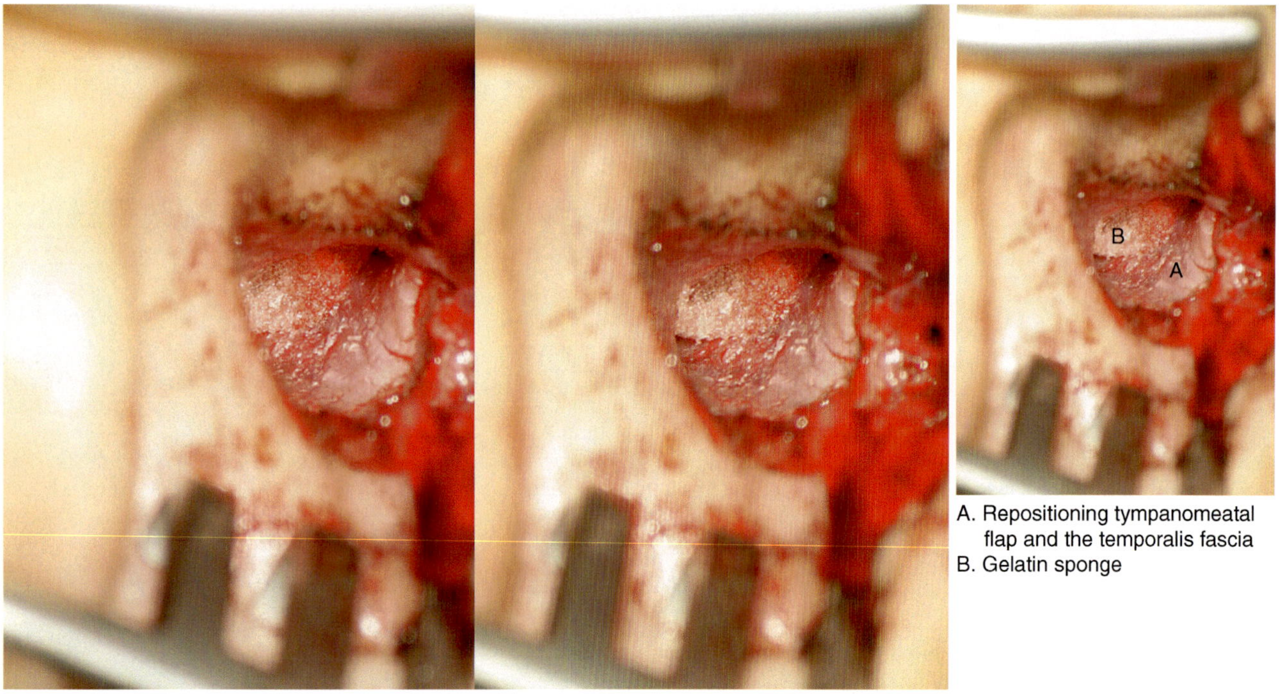

A. Repositioning tympanomeatal flap and the temporalis fascia
B. Gelatin sponge

Fig. 2.76 Repositioning the tympanomeatal flap and the temporalis fascia
At the end of the procedure, the temporalis fascia and the tympanomeatal flap with tympanic membrane remnant are returned to its natural position. Several pieces of gelatin sponge are placed in the anteroinferior part of tympanic cavity to support the implanted fascia. Then pack the external auditory canal with gelatin sponge and iodoform gauze

Mastoidectomy (Open Cavity)

Zhao-hui Hou, Xue Gao, and Pu Dai

Indications

1. When there is no ability of reconstructing the ossicular chain due to extensive erosion by cholesteatoma or severe bone erosion in chronic purulent mastoiditis.
2. Uncertainty of complete removal of cholesteatoma, or patients who have a completely squamous epithelial lined medial wall of the middle ear with permanent loss of Eustachian tube function.
3. Chronic suppurative otitis media with intracranial complications, petrous bone inflammation, suppurative labyrinthitis, facial paralysis, etc., that are not suitable for hearing reconstruction.
4. Tuberculous otitis media with bone destruction or sequestrum formation.
5. Benign tumor, such as facial never neurinoma, glomus tumor.

Contraindications

1. Simple chronic suppurative otitis media.
2. Allergic otitis media.
3. Secretory otitis media.
4. Acute purulent otitis media.
5. Tuberculosis of the middle ear or mastoid without destruction of bone or sequestrum.

Operative Procedures

1. Incision: usually endaural but may be postauricular incision. Postauricular incision is used in cases of otogenic complications, middle ear and mastoid tuberculosis, middle ear tumors etc.
2. Mastoid cortex exposure, show the landmarks: suprameatal spine, suprameatal triangle and temporal line.
3. Suprameatal triangle is used as a guide to the mastoid antrum, remove disease in the mastoid, then drill out the mastoid cavity.
4. Remove posterior wall of EAC and the bone bridge, lower the facial ridge as much as possible for unobstructed drainage.
5. Open anterior attic fully, remove all disease and remnants of the malleus and incus, leaving only the stapes.
6. Scarify the mucosa of tympanic opening of Eustachian tube and fill the entrance with muscle.
7. EAC skin flap is used to cover mastoid cavity. A meatoplasty is fashioned later.
8. Fill operating cavity with iodoform gauze, then close the skin incision and apply a dressing.

Special Comments

1. Fully open and clean the anterior attic to ensure complete removal of cholesteatoma.
2. Lower the facial nerve ridge as much as possible to improve drainage: no higher than lateral semicircular canal superiorly and at level of the EAC inferiorly.

   Pay particular attention to the vertical segment of the facial nerve.
3. When dealing with middle ear disease, take care to avoid injury to the horizontal segment of facial nerve which is exposed.
4. It is also important to remove all the deceased tissue from posterior tympanic cavity.
5. A wide open external auditory meatus is important to ensure a long term dry ear.

Complications

1. Facial paralysis.
2. Sensorineural hearing loss, due to inner ear injury caused by stapes or lateral semicircular canal injury at operation.
3. Sigmoid sinus or dural laceration.
4. Wet ear with persistent suppuration postoperatively.
5. EAC stenosis or auricular perichondritis.

Surgery1: Mastoidectomy (Open Cavity)

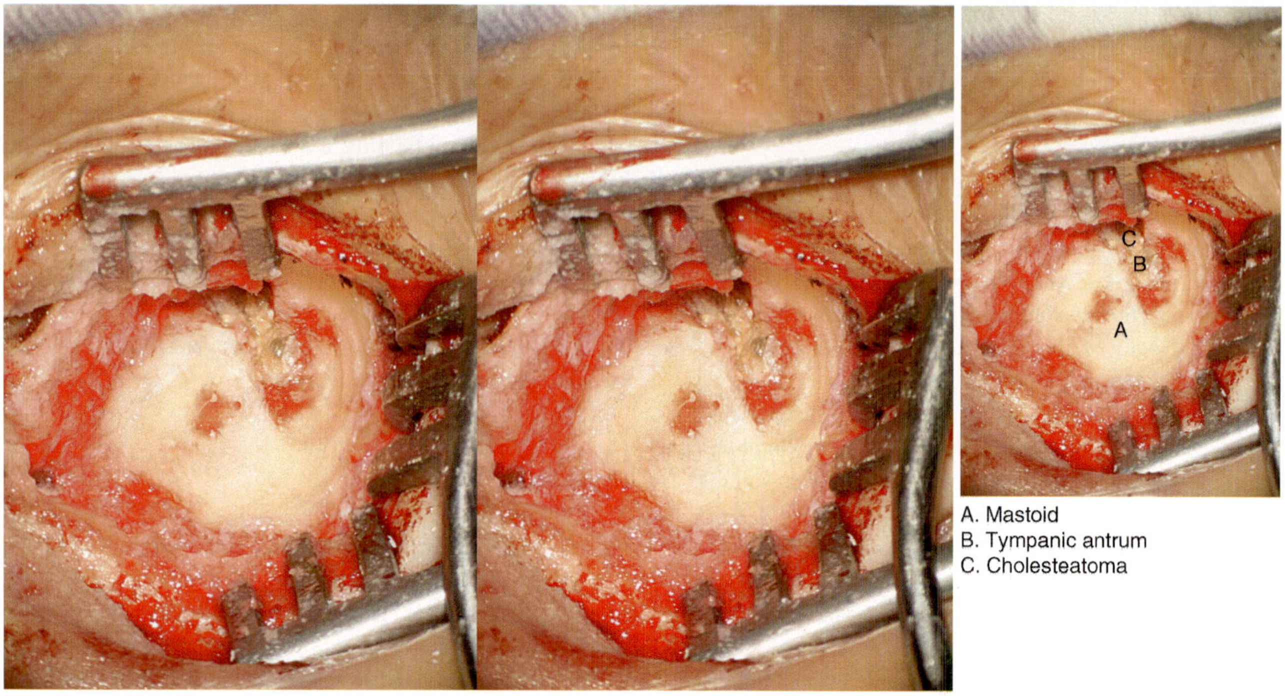

Fig. 2.77 Open mastoid antrum through Macewen's triangle.
Lempert endaural incision has been made and the tympanomeatal flap prepared, then exposure of the mastoid cortex, using Macewen's triangle as a landmark to the antrum, then opening antrum tympani and mastoid cavity. Cholesteatoma can be seen

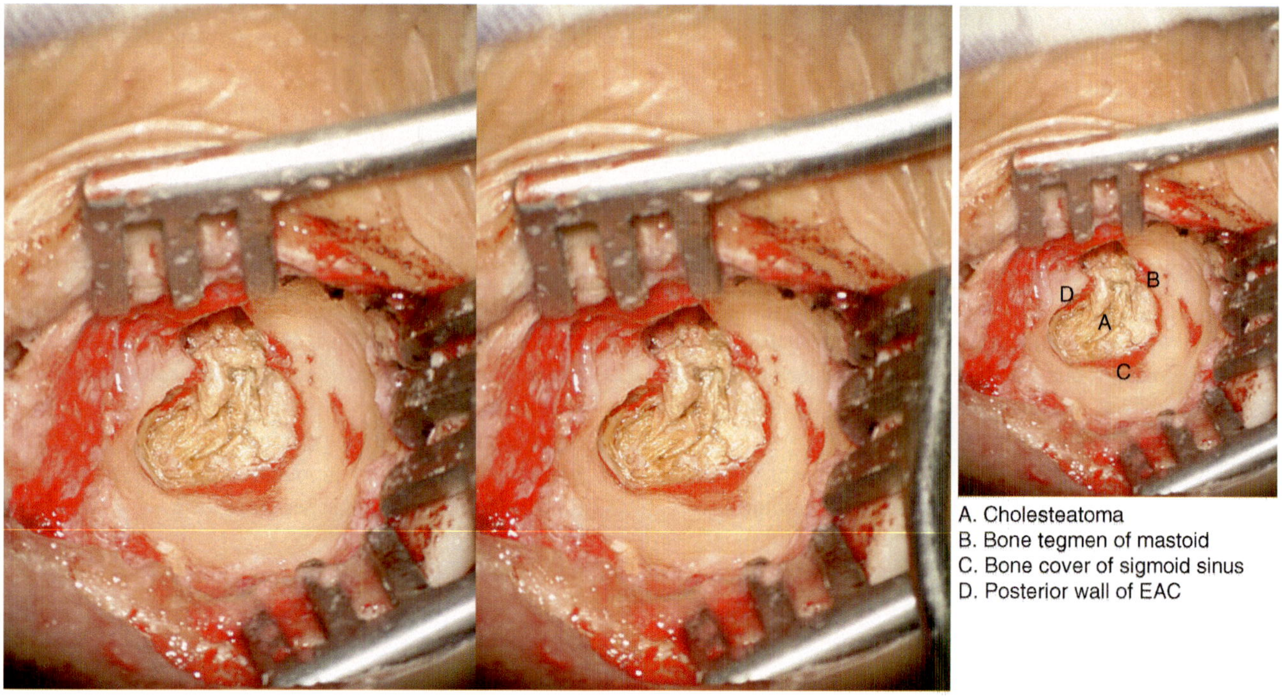

Fig. 2.78 Part of the attic is exposed
An extensive cholesteatoma is shown. It was necessary to enlarge the mastoid cavity from the open antrum and to the attic, to expose the cholesteatoma which was filling it

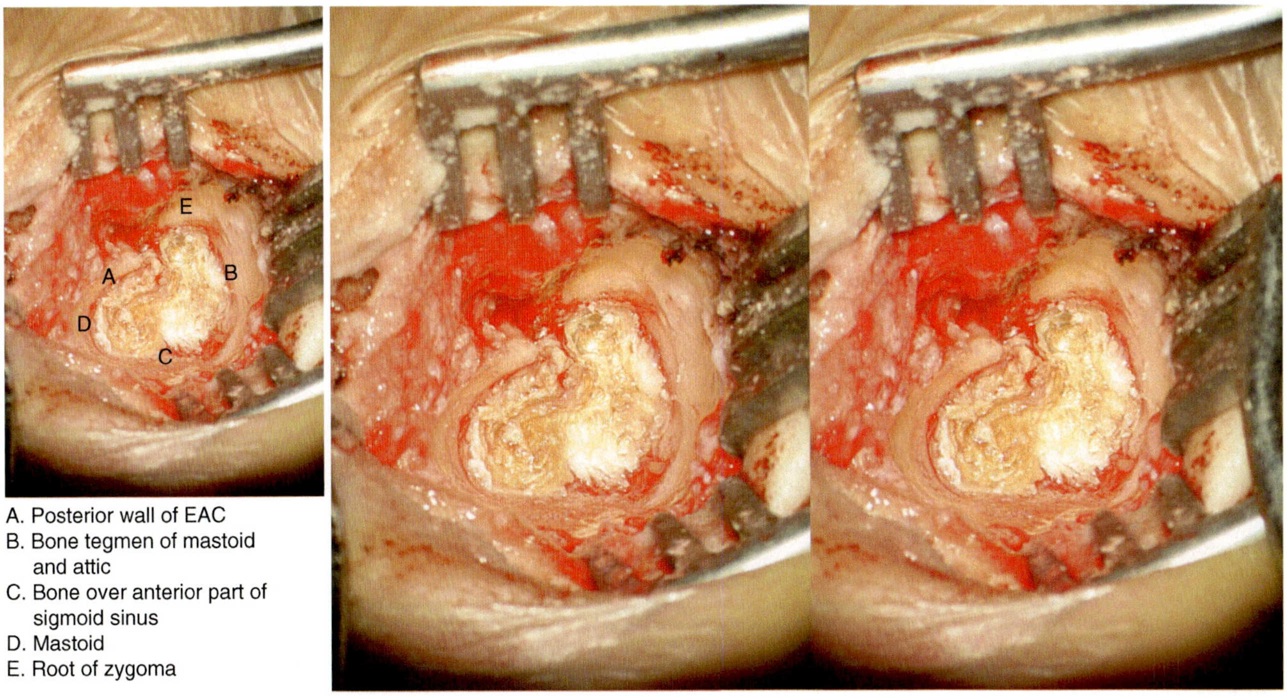

A. Posterior wall of EAC
B. Bone tegmen of mastoid and attic
C. Bone over anterior part of sigmoid sinus
D. Mastoid
E. Root of zygoma

Fig. 2.79 Opening of the attic
Enlarge the cavity, open the air cells forward into the root of zygoma, skeletonize bone tegmen of mastoid and attic superiorly. At the same time, drill bone cover of the sigmoid sinus posteriorly as thin as possible, and open the mastoid inferiorly. Gradually remove the posterior wall of EAC

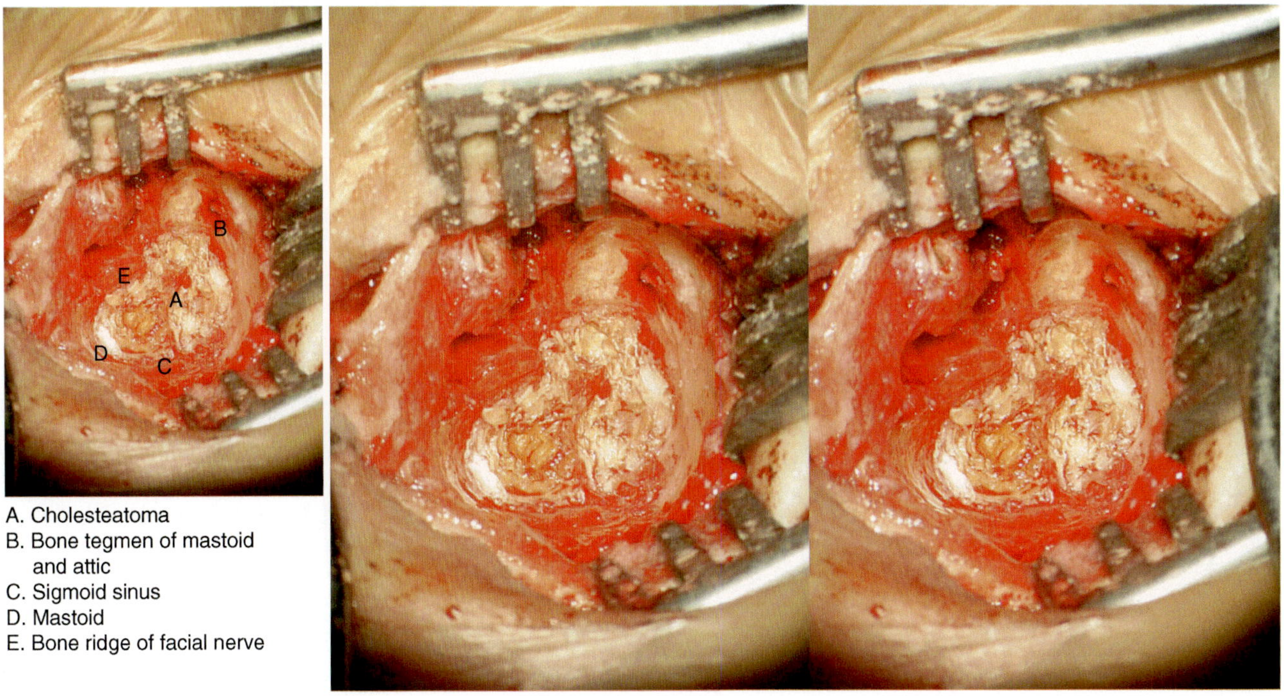

A. Cholesteatoma
B. Bone tegmen of mastoid and attic
C. Sigmoid sinus
D. Mastoid
E. Bone ridge of facial nerve

Fig. 2.80 Surgical cavity skeletonization
Continue the cavity skeletonization until attic, antrum and mastoid form a single cavity

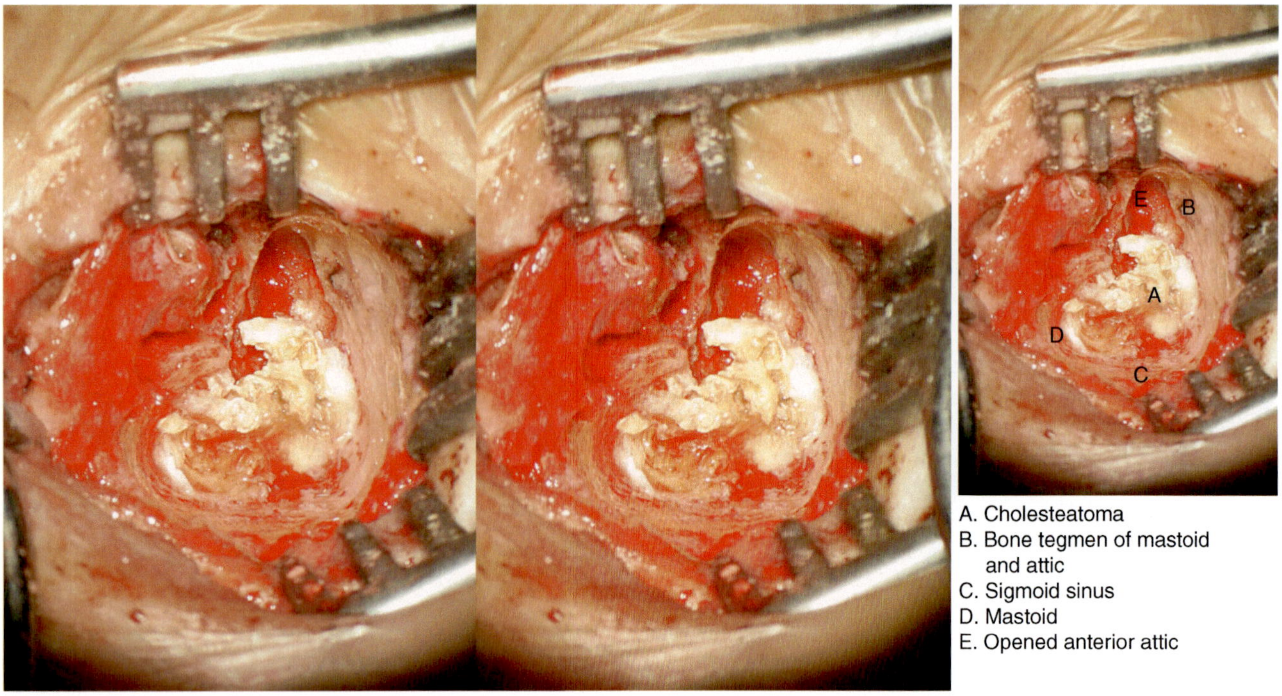

Fig. 2.81 Remove disease completely
Open the attic until it is flush with anterior wall of EAC, expose the anterior attic fully. An almost completely skeletonized cavity can be seen. Next, remove the cholesteatoma matrix in continuity from front to back

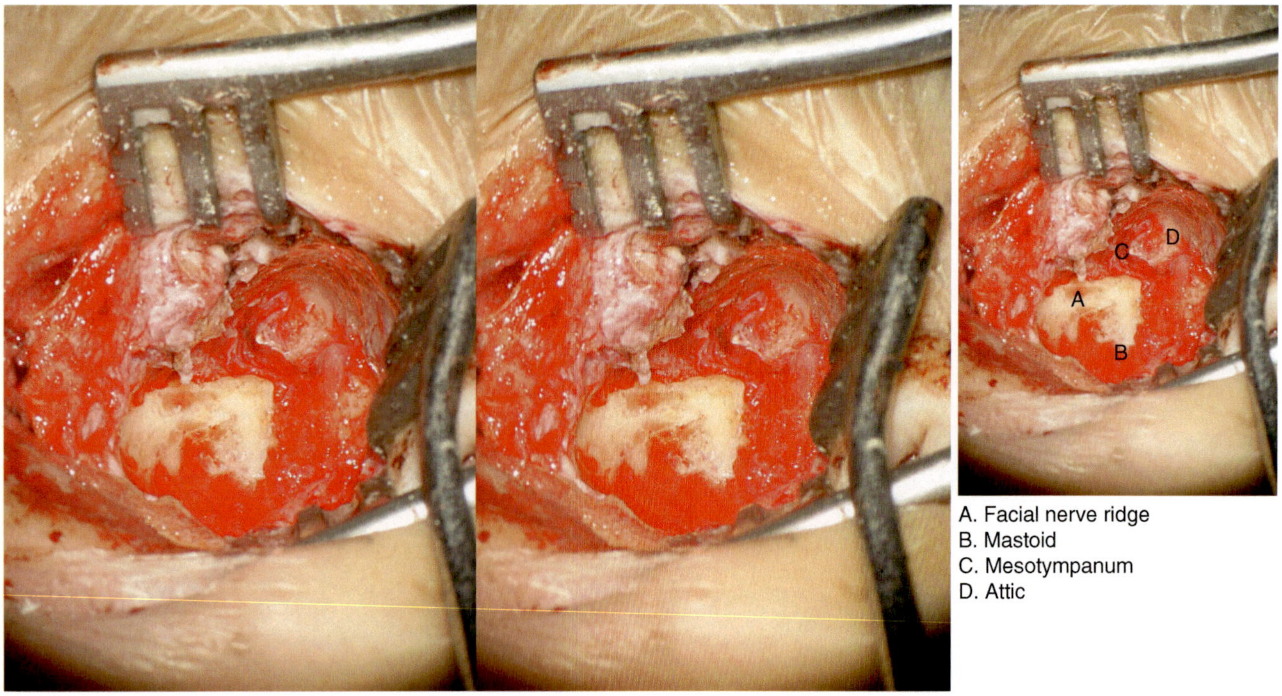

Fig. 2.82 Remove the bony bridge
Further medial bone erosion can be seen after most of the cholesteatoma was removed. Remove the bridge, expose the middle ear, lower the posterior buttress and facial nerve ridge as much as possible: no higher than lateral semicircular canal superiorly, and about the same height as the EAC floor inferiorly. Complete skeletonization of the cavity

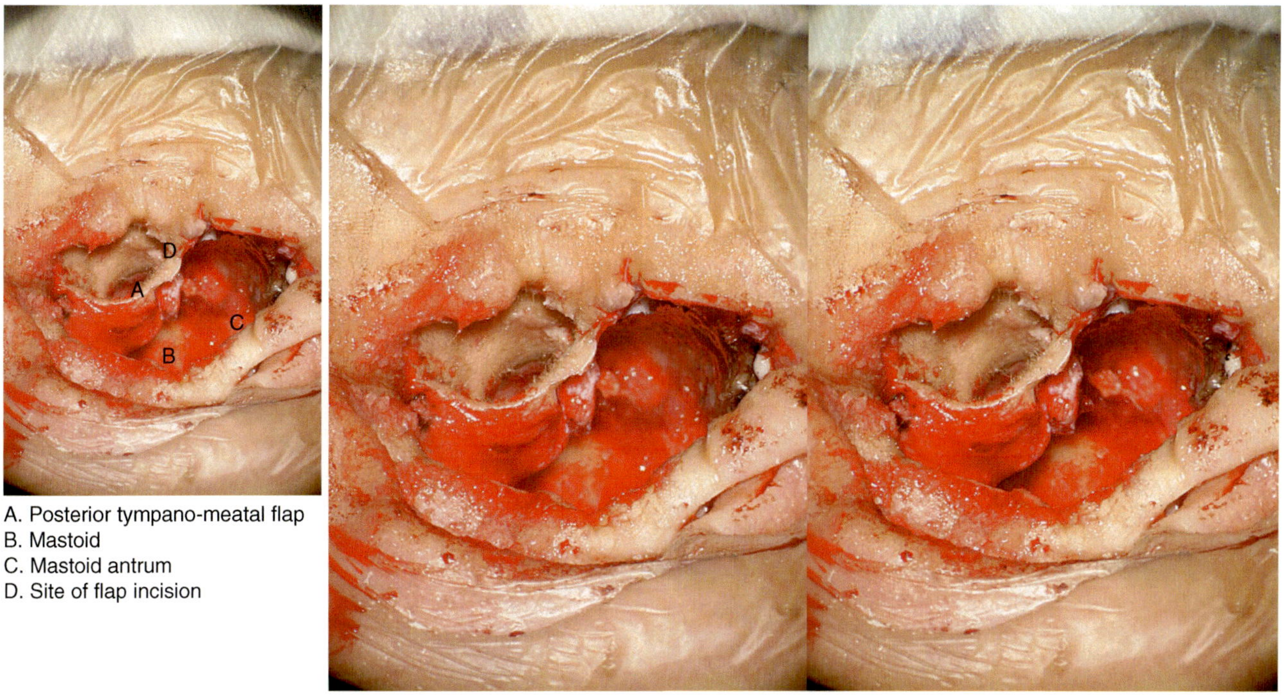

A. Posterior tympano-meatal flap
B. Mastoid
C. Mastoid antrum
D. Site of flap incision

Fig. 2.83 Posterior EAC flap incision
Incise tympano-meatal flap at 12 o'clock, ensure the flap can cover the mastoid cavity posteriorly

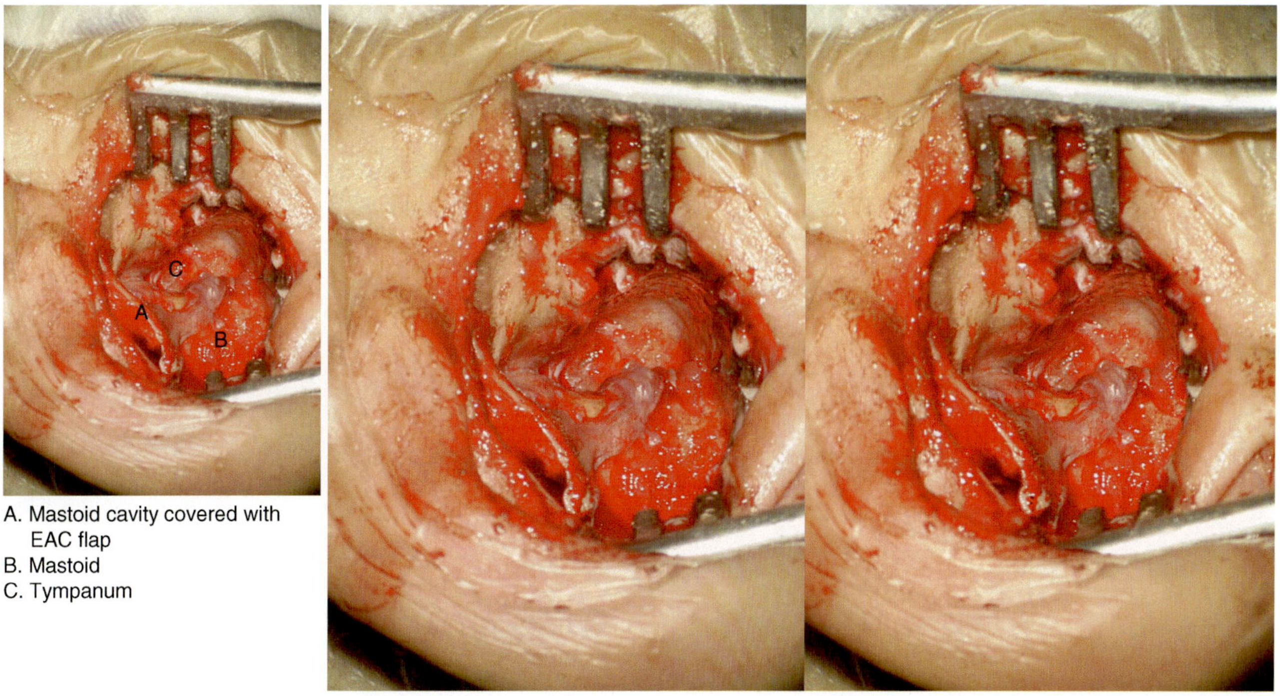

A. Mastoid cavity covered with EAC flap
B. Mastoid
C. Tympanum

Fig. 2.84 Mastoid cavity covered with flap
Turn the flap back into mastoid cavity, pars tensa perforation and tympanic membrane remnant can be seen, tympanic mucous membrane was partly epithelized

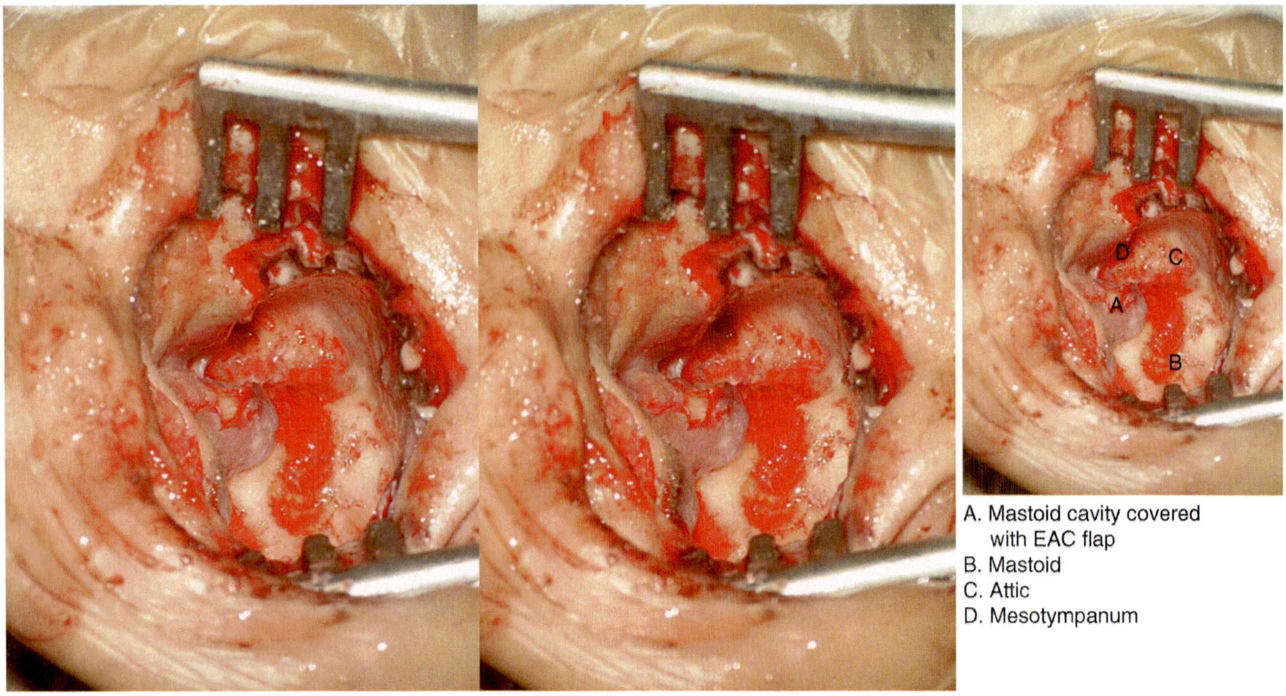

A. Mastoid cavity covered with EAC flap
B. Mastoid
C. Attic
D. Mesotympanum

Fig. 2.85 Removal of cholesteatoma and cavity skeletonization
Remove all cholesteatoma and granulation tissue, polish all cavity walls with diamond or finishing bur to smooth them out, leaving no covered space or bone ridge which can block drainage. At completion, the bony ear canal, middle ear, attic and mastoid form a single open space

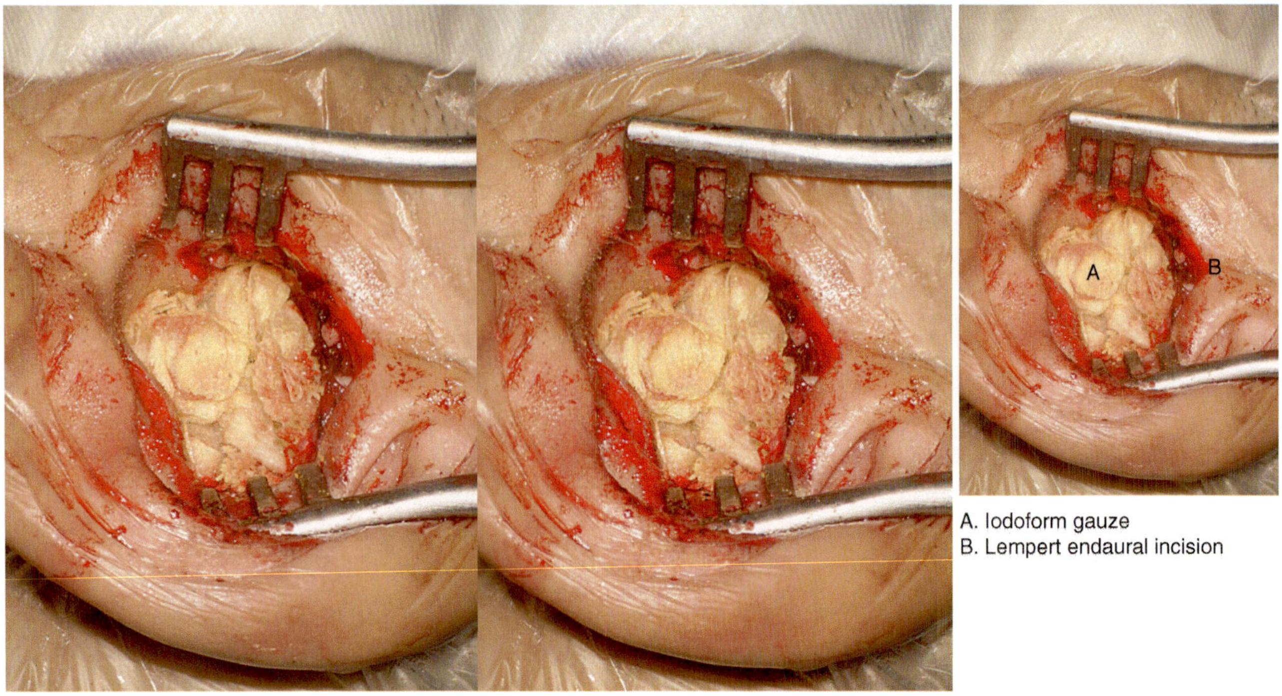

A. Iodoform gauze
B. Lempert endaural incision

Fig. 2.86 Meatoplasty and cavity closure
Excise conchae cartilage to enlarge the EAC opening, fill the surgical cavity with iodoform gauze in layers. Note: the EAC flap should be placed on to the surface of the bone. Close the wound with three to four stiches

Surgery 2: Mastoidectomy (Open Cavity)

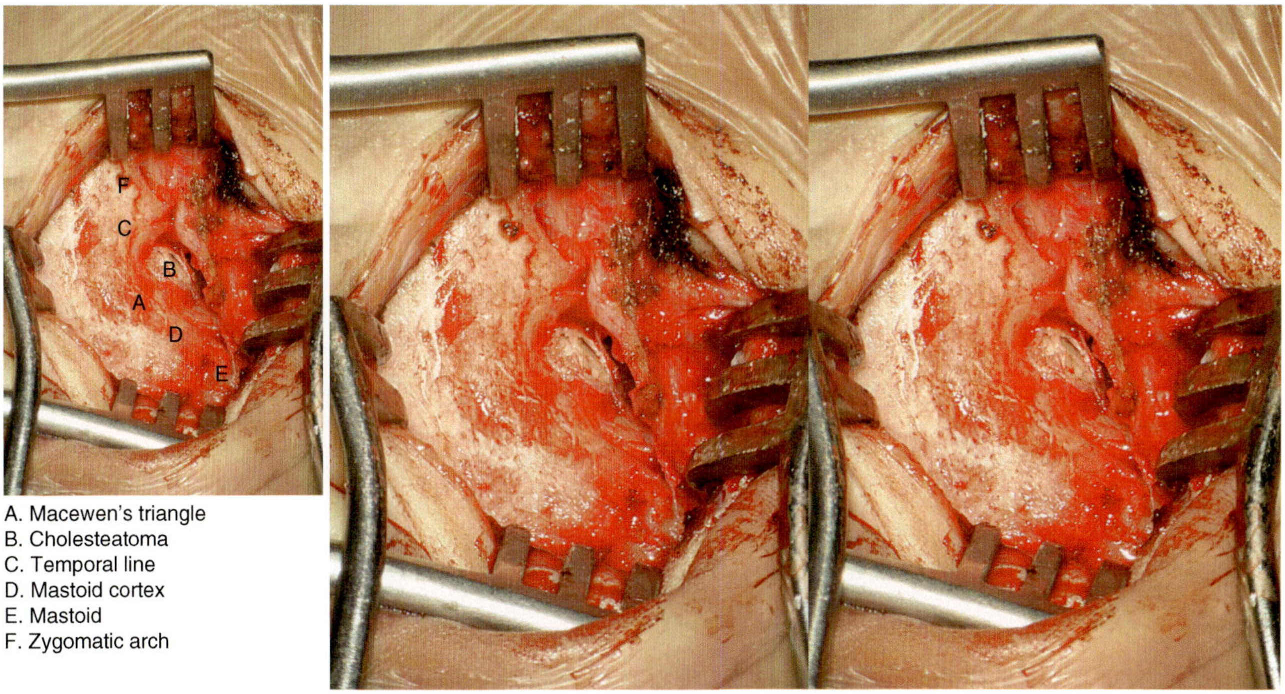

A. Macewen's triangle
B. Cholesteatoma
C. Temporal line
D. Mastoid cortex
E. Mastoid
F. Zygomatic arch

Fig. 2.87 Make lempert endaural incision and enlarge surgical field by displacing the EAC flap forward
Make Lempert endaural incision, elevate the EAC flap to widen the surgical field. The area should expose the zygomatic arch and temporal line superiorly, most of mastoid posteriorly, the anterior wall of EAC and temporomandibular joint in front. In this case, bone medial to the spine of Henle has been eroded by cholesteatoma

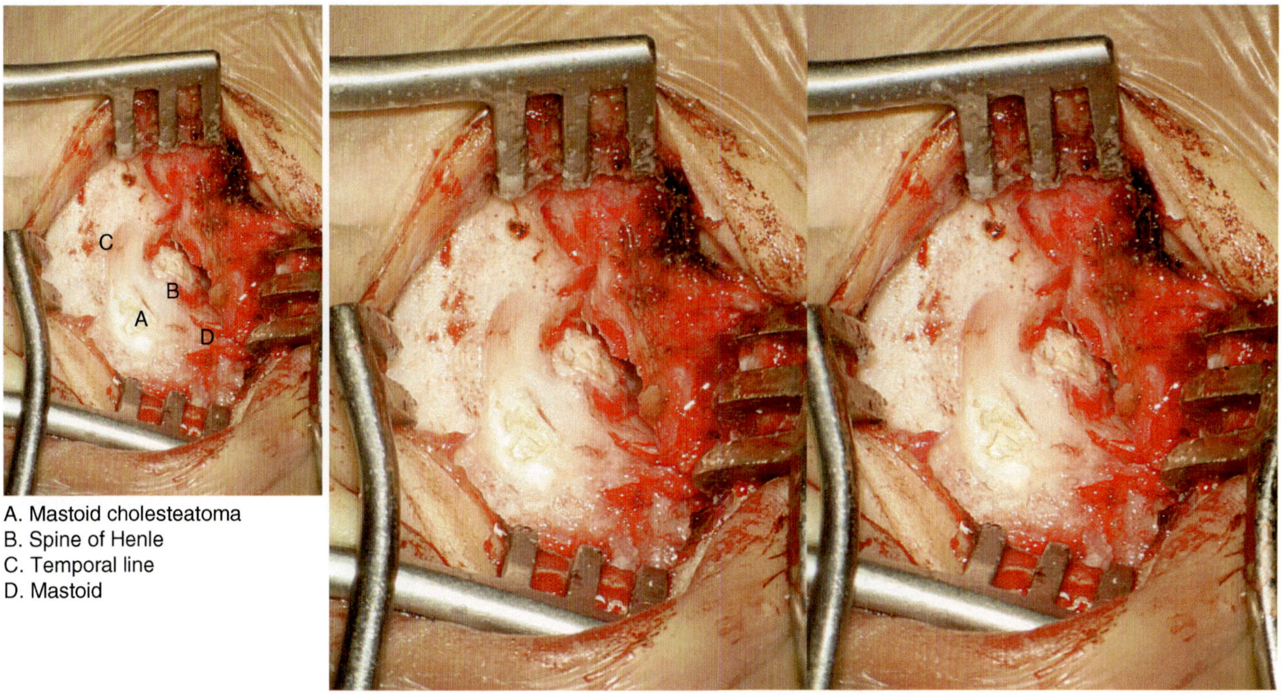

A. Mastoid cholesteatoma
B. Spine of Henle
C. Temporal line
D. Mastoid

Fig. 2.88 Tympanic antrum opening
Drill marker lines along temporal line and posterior wall of EAC. Drill the mastoid cortex of this triangle to expose the antrum, then proceed to locate the tympanic attic and mastoid. In this case, cholesteatoma can be seen when drilling the mastoid

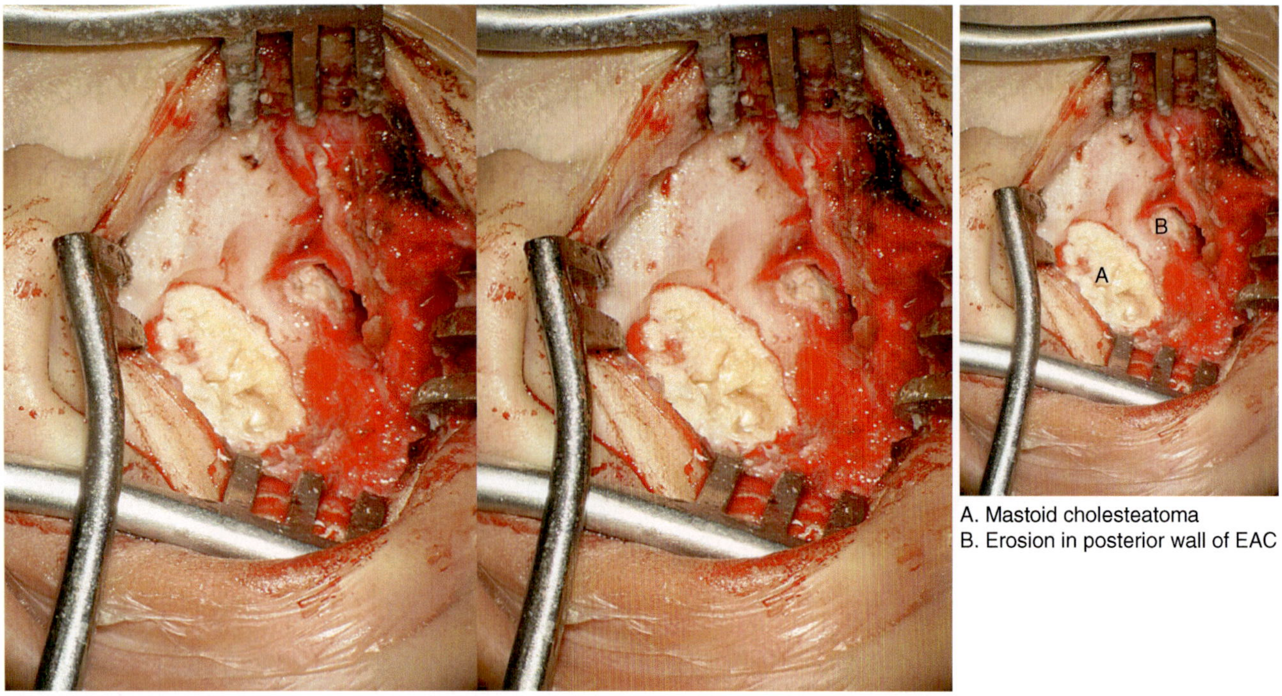

Fig. 2.89 Stepwise opening of the mastoid cavity
Progressively open the mastoid cavity around the exposed cholesteatoma. The cortex of mastoid in this case was markedly thinned by the large cholesteatoma

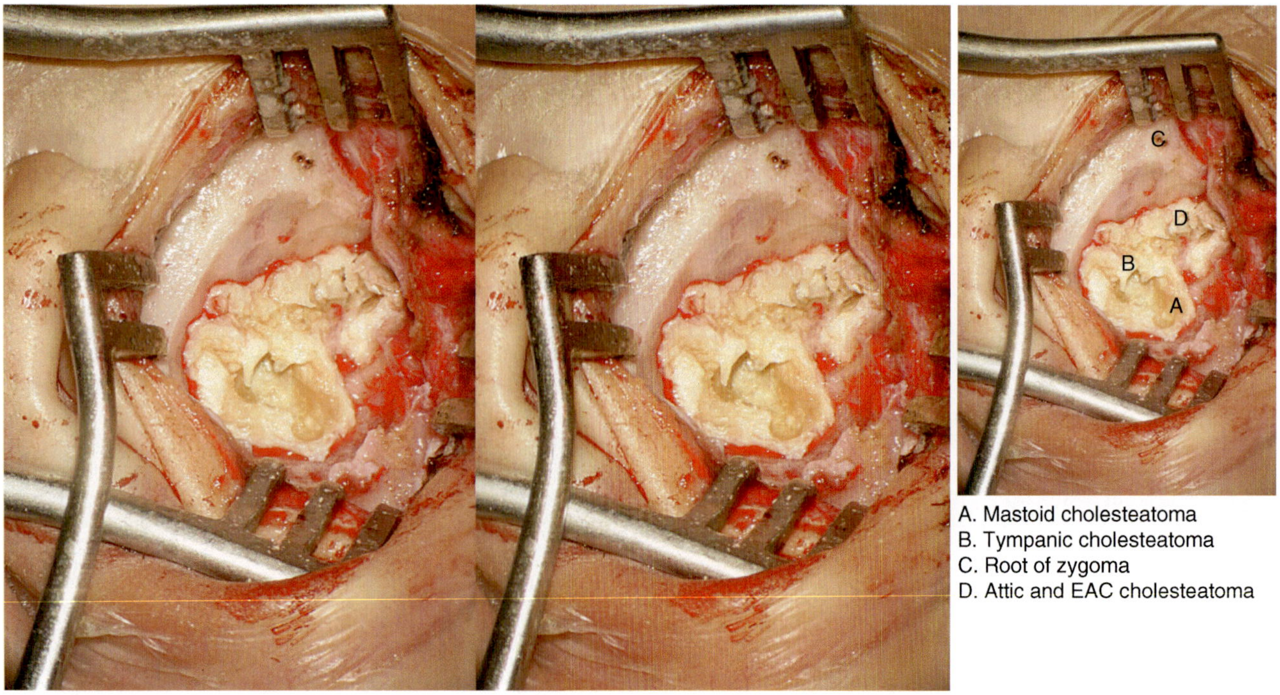

Fig. 2.90 Removal of the bony bridge
Enlarge surgical cavity around the cholesteatoma which can be seen filling the middle ear and attic. Remove the posterior wall of EAC (bone bridge) which can be seen to be eroded by disease in this case

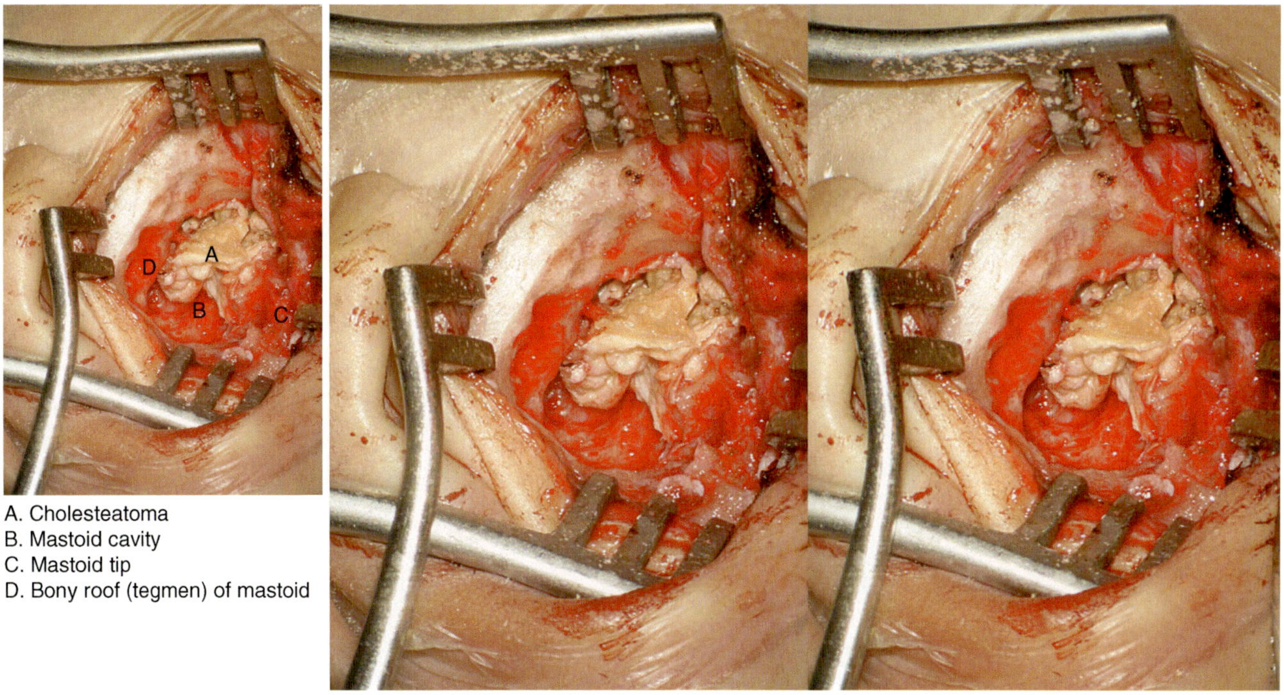

A. Cholesteatoma
B. Mastoid cavity
C. Mastoid tip
D. Bony roof (tegmen) of mastoid

Fig. 2.91 Cholesteatoma removal
Completely elevate the cholesteatoma along its upper and lower borders. Take care in removal of disease form the facial ridge. Risk to the facial nerve can be reduced with use of a facial nerve monitor, particularly by less experienced surgeons. Always work along the long axis of the nerve to minimize trauma

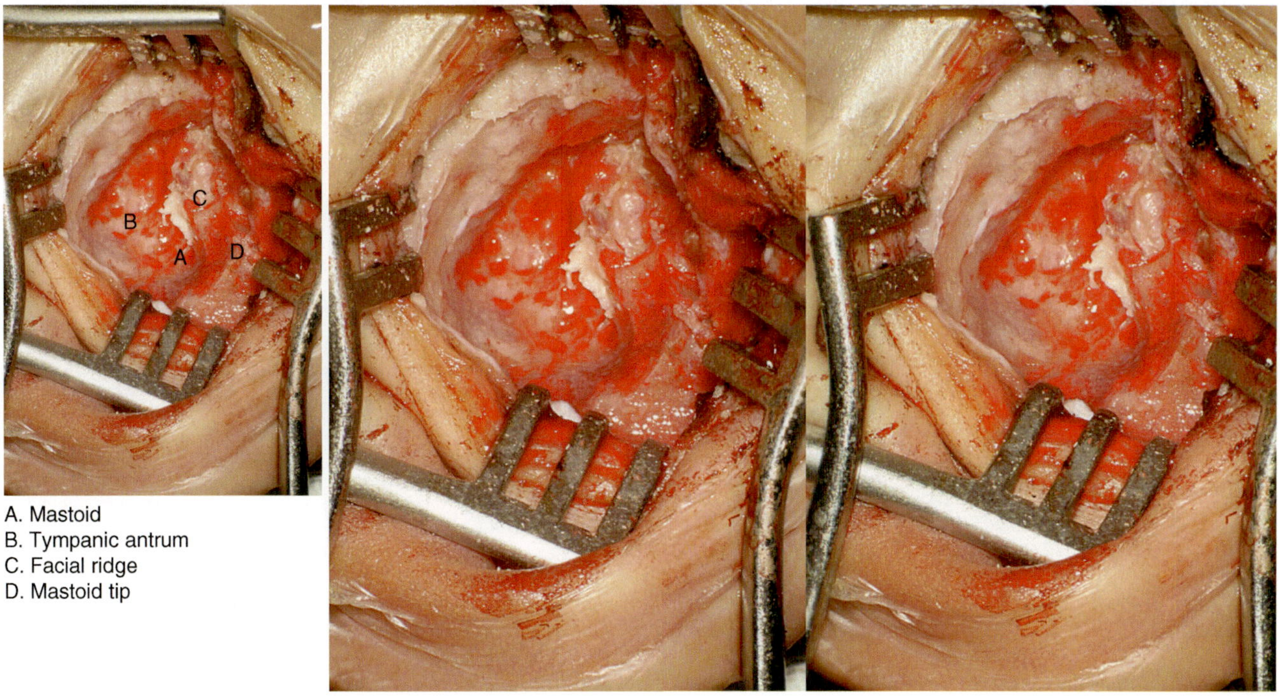

A. Mastoid
B. Tympanic antrum
C. Facial ridge
D. Mastoid tip

Fig. 2.92 Facial ridge exposure
After removal of cholesteatoma the facial ridge is exposed. In this case, an abnormal facial ridge can be seen due to bone erosion

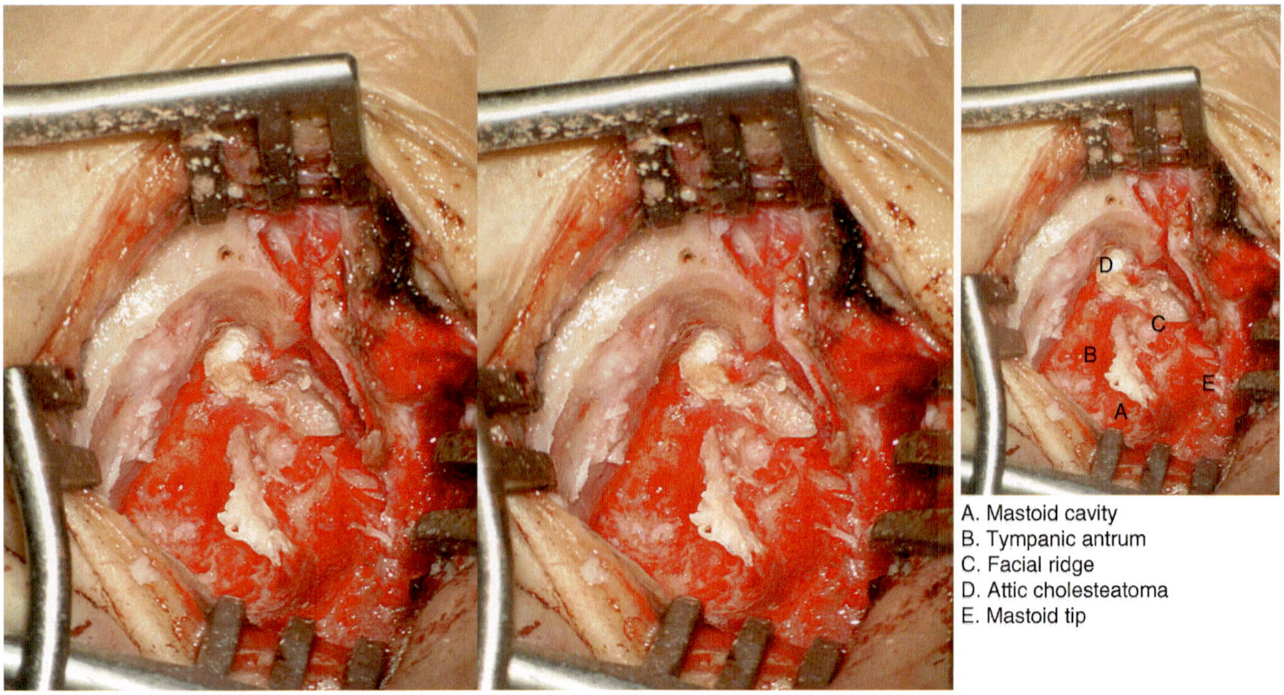

Fig. 2.93 Open attic fully
Continue drilling until the anterior wall of attic is flush with the anterior wall of EAC, in order to ensure complete removal of cholesteatoma in this region

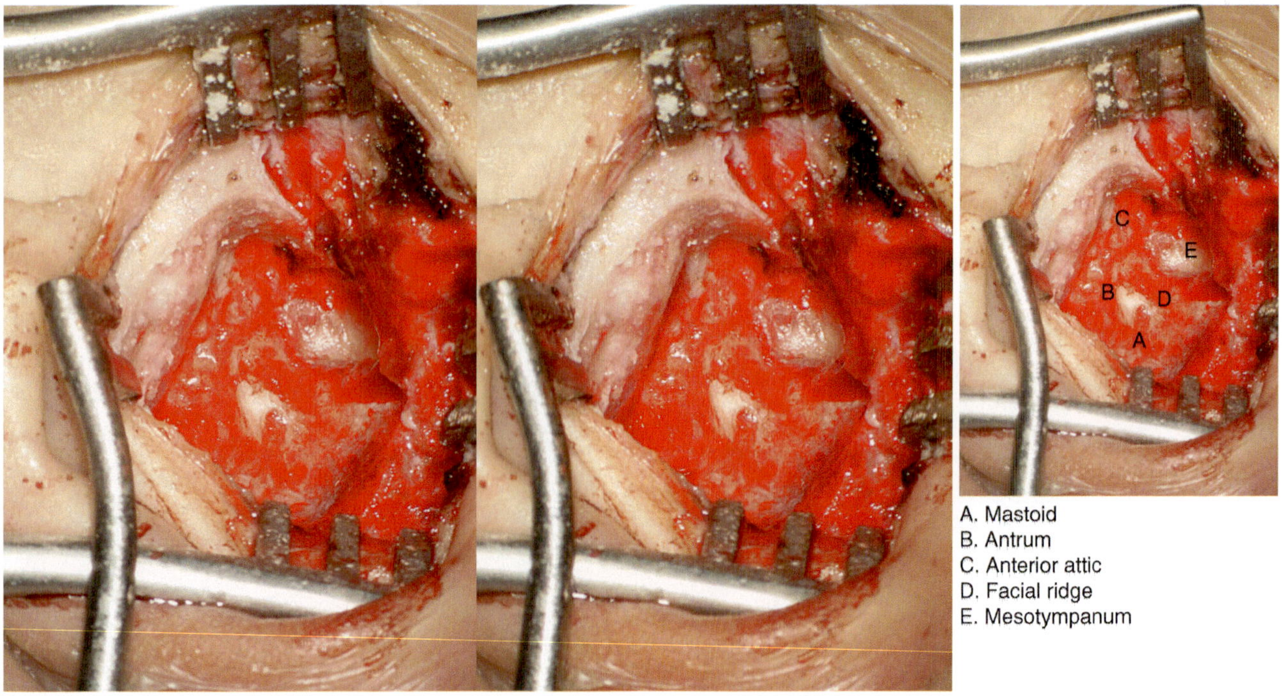

Fig. 2.94 Complete the surgical cavity
Clear disease from anterior attic, lower the facial ridge, and skeletonize the middle and posterior fossa dural plates until mastoid cavity, antrum and middle ear form a single cavity, which will drain well. Ensure the mastoid cavity walls are drilled smooth without any bony overhangs

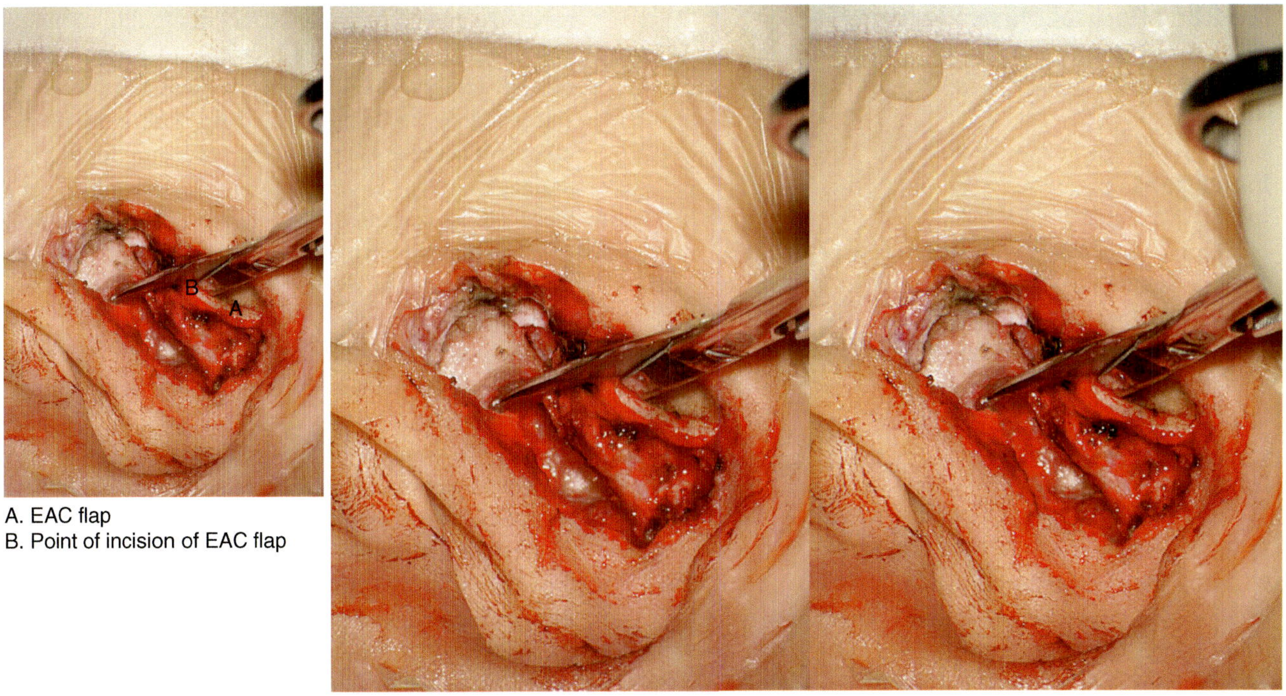

Fig. 2.95 Incise the canal wall flap
Incise the EAC flap at 12 o'clock, and complete the flap

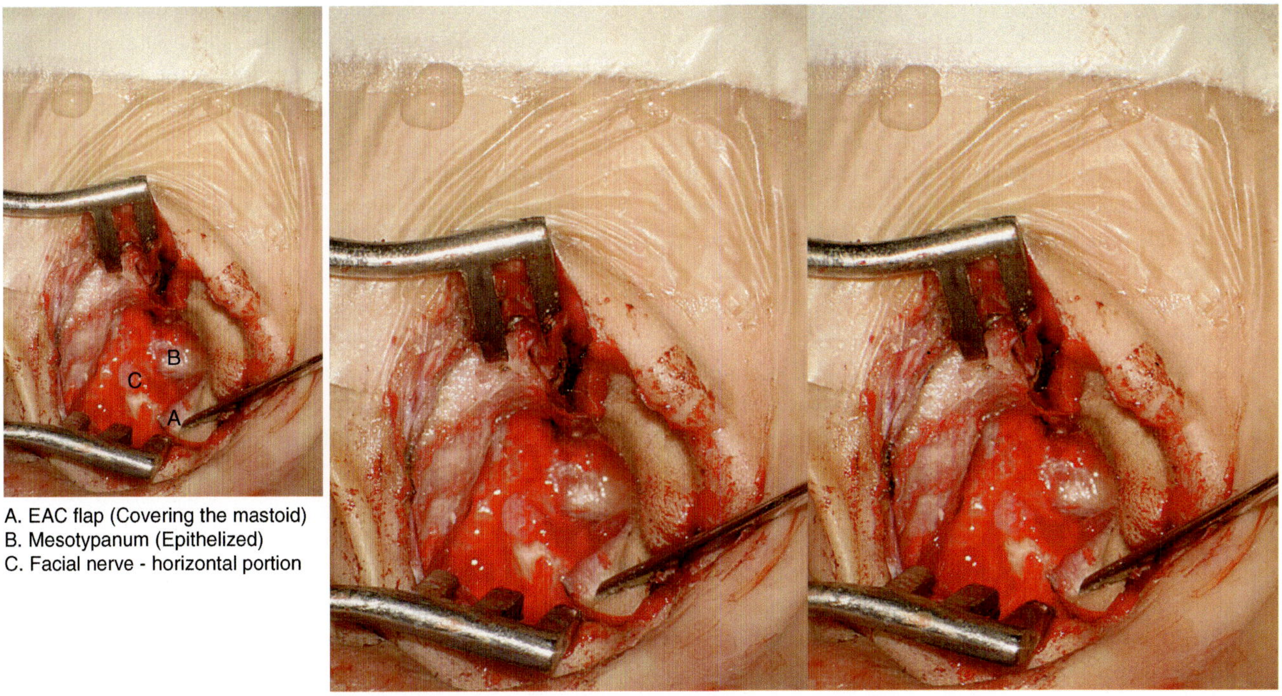

Fig. 2.96 Meatoplasty
Turn the flap back into mastoid cavity and fashion the meatoplasty

Modified Radical Mastoidectomy

Fei Yu, Pu Dai

Indications

1. Chronic otitis media with cholesteatoma
2. Persistent purulent secretion, unsuitable for tympanoplasty.
3. Provide easy access for long term follow-up
4. No surgical contraindication

Contraindications

1. Poor systemic condition
2. Acute upper respiratory infection
3. Unable to resect cholesteatoma thoroughly with this technique
4. Atresia of oval window and round window, mucosa of tympanic cavity is epithelized entirely
5. Hearing aid is important postoperative
6. Women in menstrual phase

Operative Procedures

1. Terminal sulcus (endaural) incision or postauricular incision. By using terminal sulcus incision, the meatoplasty with removal of conchal cartilage must be performed at the same time, and meatal stenosis can be prevented. The meatoplasty also facilitates drainage, ventilation and epithelization of the operative cavity. The better exposure ensures easy cleaning and care of the cavity.

   Alternatively, the operative field is well exposed by a postauricular incision, and the meatoplasty should be performed at the end of the operation to prevent meatal stenosis.
2. Incise the skin, subcutaneous tissue and periosteum. Expose the mastoid cortex, the posterior and superior wall of external auditory meatus, tympanic notch, tympanic ring, temporal line and suprameatal spine.
3. Drill the mastoid cortex and cells from cribriform area and open the mastoid antrum.
4. Open the attic, find the short process of the incus.
5. Saucerize the mastoid cavity. The cavity is bound by the posterior wall of the external acoustic meatus, perpendicular part of facial nerve, sigmoid sinus, tegmen mastoideum, sinodural angle, and mastoid tip. Thin the bone of the posterior wall of the external auditory meatus, preserve the facial nerve canal and protect the sigmoid sinus. Fill the mastoid tip with bone dust or other soft tissue at the end of the procedure for easier to drainage.
6. Open the attic, expose the anterior and superior walls and drill down the lateral wall.
7. Resect the bridge by removing the bony postero-superior wall and clear the mesotympanum.
8. Separate the incudo-stapedial joint. Shear the superior ligament of the malleus. Take out of the defective malleus and incus.
9. Identify the position of the cochleariform process, the horizontal part of the facial nerve and the prominence of the lateral semicircular canal. Remove the lateral and posterior-inferior walls. Lower the facial ridge. Smooth the cavity walls to assist with easy drainage.
10. Implant the ossicular prosthesis to rebuild the ossicular chain. Use a PORP if the stapes superstructure is intact, or a TORP if the superstructure is missing.
11. Fashion the plastic meatal flaps, making a flap with an inferior pedicle. Incise the subcutaneous tissue and cartilage of the external acoustic meatus. Fold the flap inferiorly to cover the mastoid cavity. With the postauricular incision, make a circumferential incision along the terminal sulcus, extend the incision to the point between root of the helix and tragus, then make plastic meatal flaps.
12. Fashioning the meatoplasty. Excise a semilunar segment of conchal cartilage without perichondrium from the endaural incision, cut the skin flaps transversely into two to three small ones along the free edge of cavity of concha skin, and use these at the end of the procedure to cover the mastoid cavity.
13. Repair the tympanic membrane with air dried temporalis fascia.
14. Reflect the fascia, fill the cavity with absorbable hemostatic gauze or erythromycin-soaked gelatin sponge.
15. Place a cartilage disc with periosteum between the ossicular prosthesis and the fascia. Reset the temporalis fascia and skin flap to cover the facial ridge.
16. Place erythromycin-soaked gelatin sponge or absorbable hemostatic gauze over the tympanic membrane, pack the external auditory meatus by using iodoform gauze to secure the flap.
17. Suture the incision using an interrupted silk suture, cover the incision with a sterile dressing.

Special Comments

1. Clear the mastoid cavity, aditus ad antrum and attic thoroughly to avoid recurrent disease.
2. Preserve the structure of mesotympanum and hypotympanum to give the best possibility of tympanoplasty and ossicular chain reconstruction.
3. Protect the integrity of ossicular chain as far as possible.
4. Protect the facial nerve and semicircular canal to prevent facial palsy and perilymph leak.
5. Preserve the mucosa of the tympanic cavity as far as possible.

Complications

1. Hemorrhage and infection. Use aseptic operative technique, good hemostasis and postoperative antibiotics. Avoid injury to the sigmoid sinus and jugular bulb.
2. Deafness or severe hearing loss. Avoid excessive stapes manipulation and injury to the inner ear.
3. Facial paralysis. Pay attention to facial nerve position and the state of its bony canal. Decompress the facial nerve immediately if it is injured during surgery or peripheral facial paralysis is apparent immediately after the operation.
4. Leakage of cerebrospinal fluid. Avoid injury to the dura and repair it immediately if it is injured during operation.
5. Perilymph leak. Avoid opening the horizontal semicircular canal. Dissect cholesteatoma carefully.
6. Persistent purulent secretion post operation. Resect disease thoroughly and drill the facial ridge as low as possible. Ensure adequate drainage of the attic and mastoid cavity.

Surgery 1: Modified radical mastoidectomy and Tympanoplasty

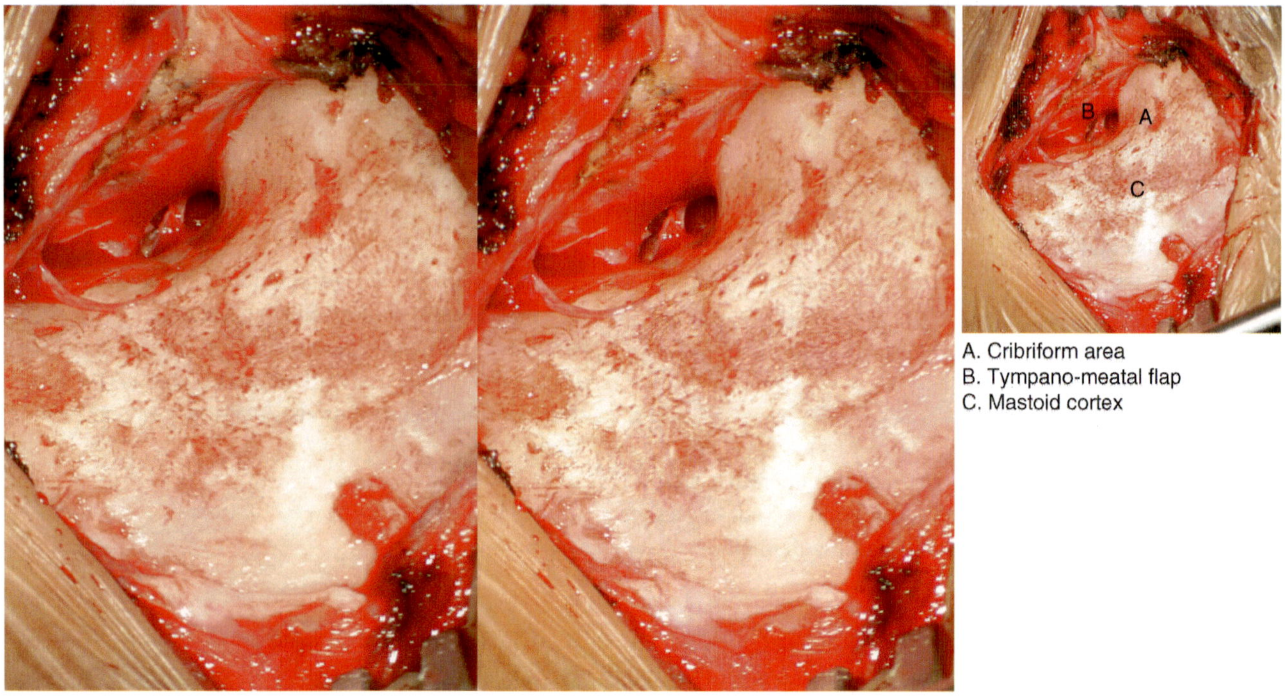

A. Cribriform area
B. Tympano-meatal flap
C. Mastoid cortex

Fig. 2.97 Postauricular incision, exposure of the mastoid cortex
A sterile operation towel is spread over the skin after the external auditory canal and the skin around the ear is sterilized. The incision of the skin, the subcutaneous tissue and the periosteum is made behind the ear, the mastoid cortex is then exposed. Separate the meatal flaps from the subcutaneous tissue

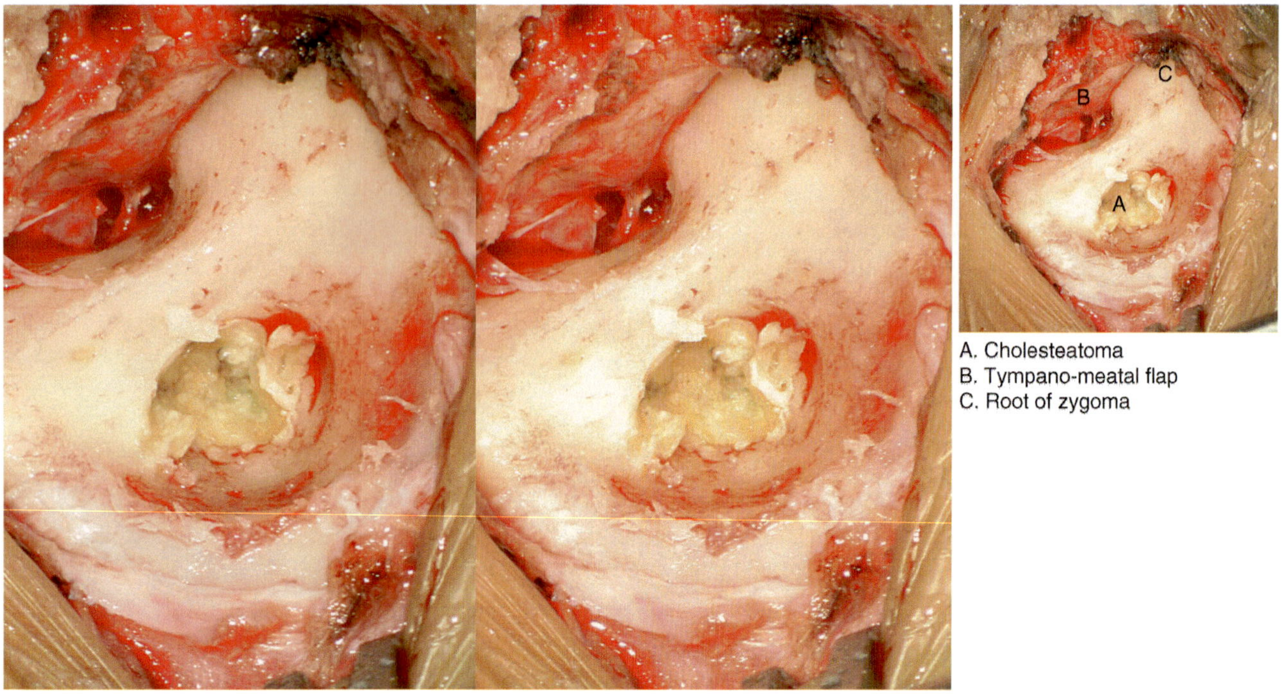

A. Cholesteatoma
B. Tympano-meatal flap
C. Root of zygoma

Fig. 2.98 Cholesteatoma exposure though cribriform area approach
After exposing the posterior wall of the external auditory canal, the mastoid cavity is contoured though a cribriform area approach to the mastoid antrum. The cholesteatoma is then exposed

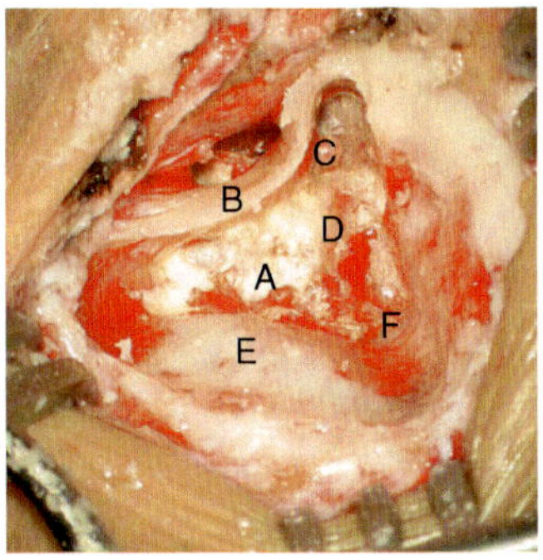

A. Mastoid
B. Posterior wall of external auditory canal
C. Residual ossicles
D. Prominence of lateral semicircular canal
E. Sigmoid sinus
F. Sinodural angle

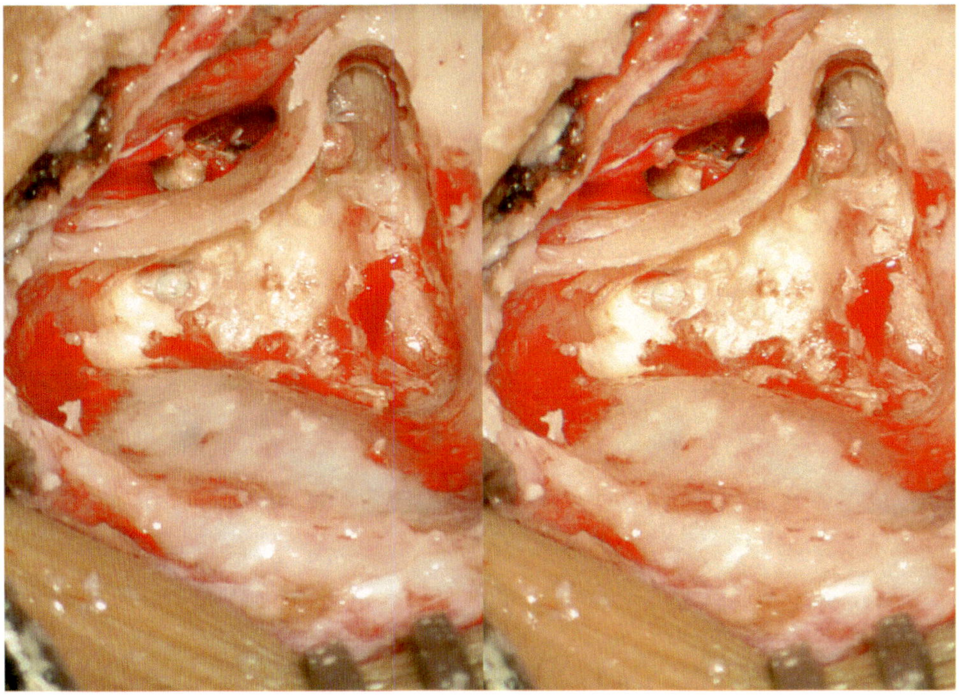

Fig. 2.99 Shaping of mastoid cavity
After the mastoid cavity is fashioned, the cholesteatoma is exposed in the mastoid antrum and attic, and then the mastoid tip and the sinodural angle are exposed thoroughly. The exposure includes the posterior wall of external auditory meatus, perpendicular part of facial nerve, sigmoid sinus, tegmen mastoideum, sinodural angle, and mastoid tip. Open the attic and expose the anterior and superior walls

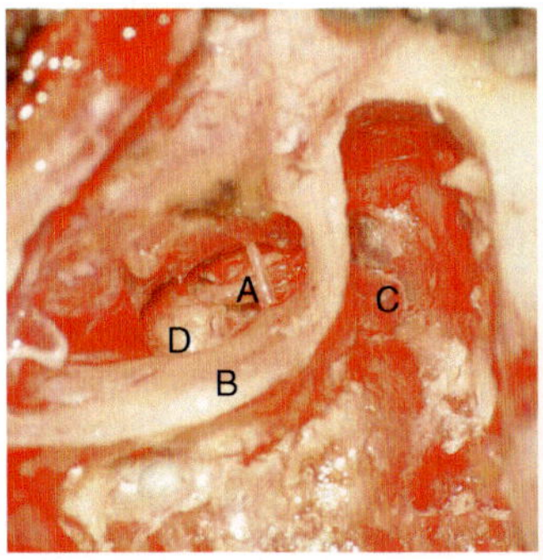

A. Handle of malleus
B. Posterior wall of external auditory canal
C. Head of malleus
D. Cholesteatoma in middle & posterior tympanum

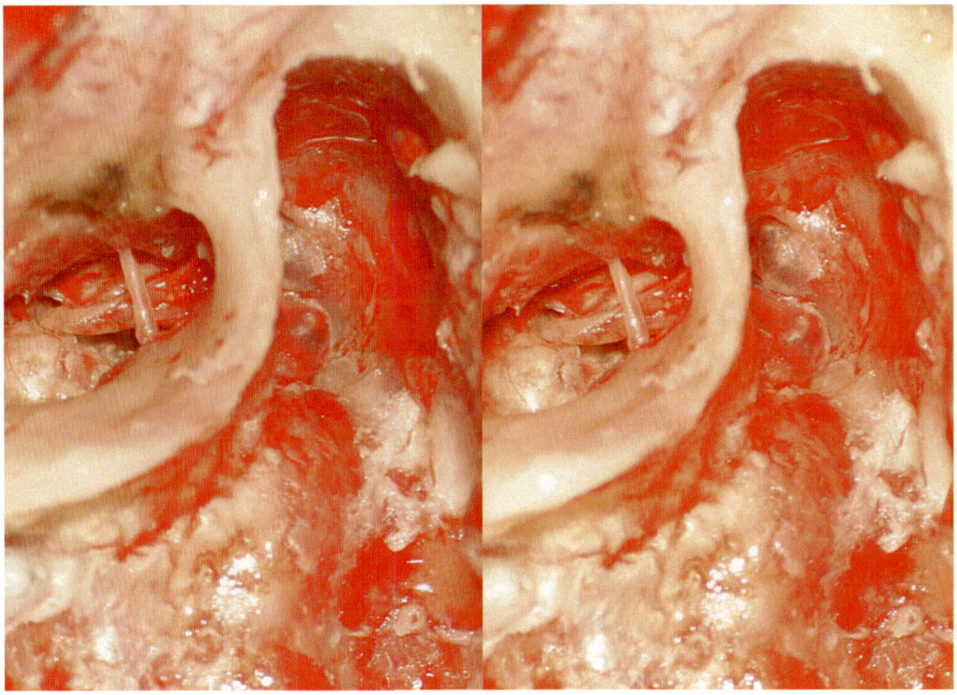

Fig. 2.100 Disease in mastoid and tympanic cavity are exposed via a combined approach
After adjusting the amplification of the microscope, the tympano-meatal flap is elevated to expose the tympanic cavity containing cholesteatoma. The residual tympanic membrane is also visible

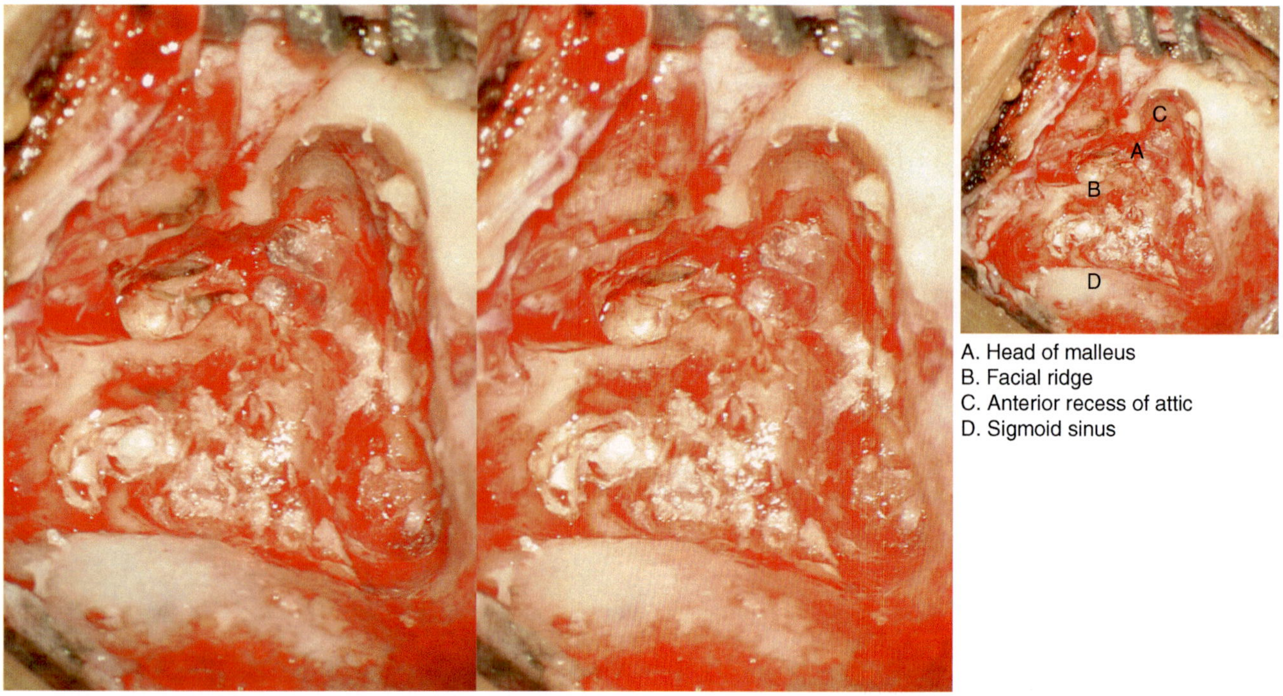

A. Head of malleus
B. Facial ridge
C. Anterior recess of attic
D. Sigmoid sinus

Fig. 2.101 Removal of the bridge
The surgical bridge is taken down because of extensive cholesteatoma. The cholesteatoma which is surrounding the head of malleus and covering the medial wall of the tympanic cavity is removed carefully

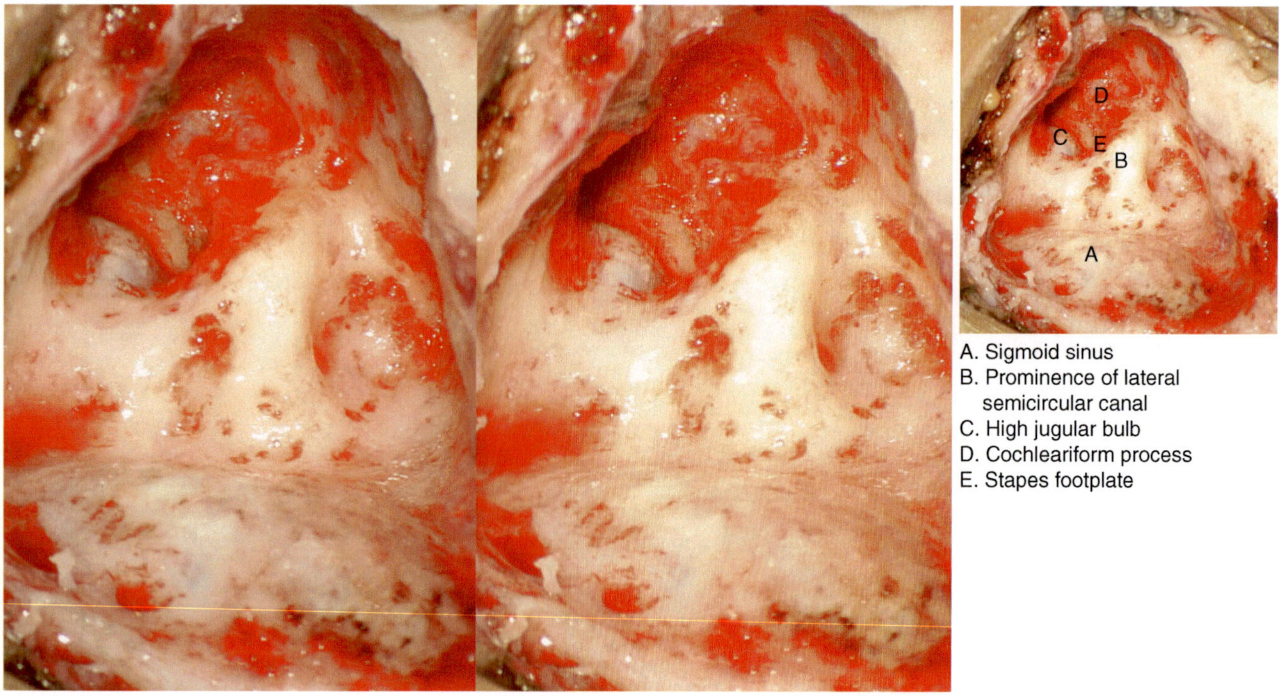

A. Sigmoid sinus
B. Prominence of lateral semicircular canal
C. High jugular bulb
D. Cochleariform process
E. Stapes footplate

Fig. 2.102 Full view of operation cavity
The full view of operation cavity is shown clearly. The attic is opened fully. Its anterior wall is further forward than that of the external auditory canal. The tegmen mastoideum is drilled as thin as possible. The sinodural angle is exposed thoroughly. The facial ridge is made lower than the lateral semicircular canal. Contouring of the sigmoid sinus, mastoid tip and high riding jugular bulb region is completed. The mesotympanic cholesteatoma is cleaned and the mucous membrane of medial wall of tympanic cavity is left intact

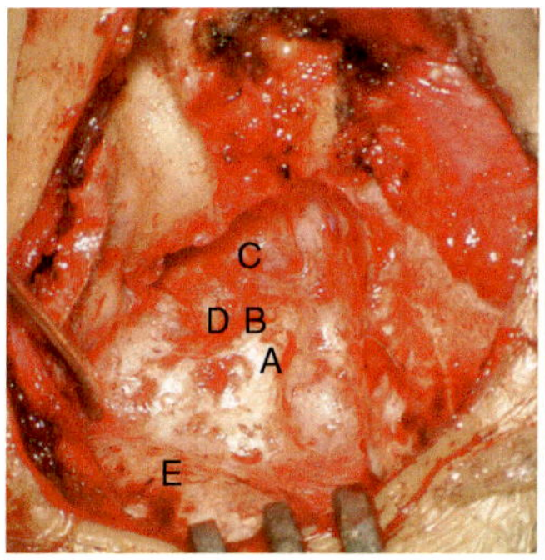

A. Prominence of lateral semicircular duct
B. Bone canal of facial nerve
C. Cochleariform process
D. Stapes footplate
E. Sigmoid sinus

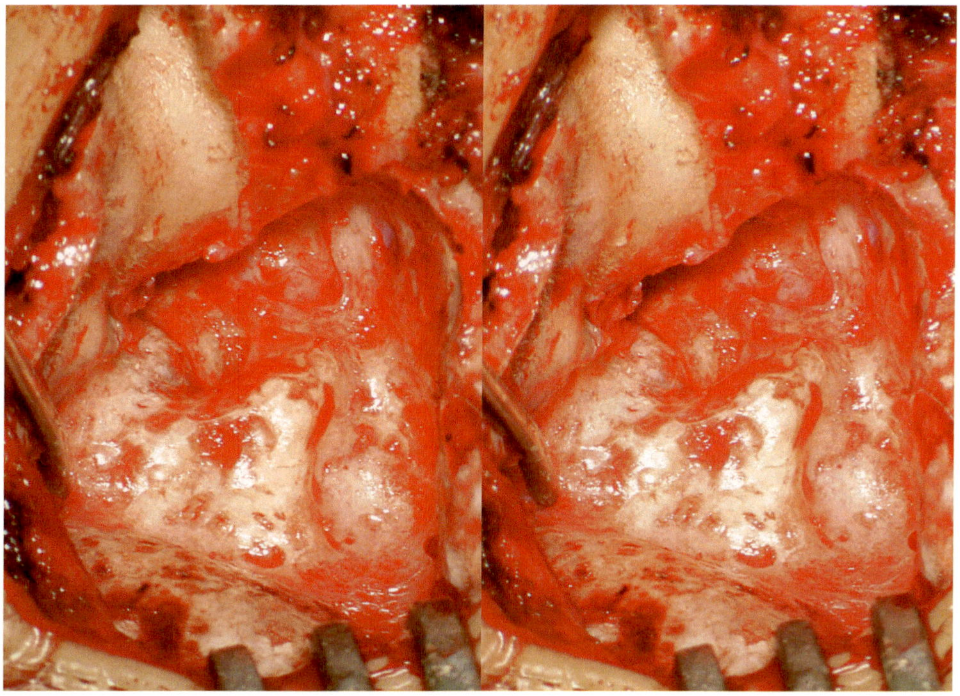

Fig. 2.103 Lower the facial ridge and remove the disease
After the facial ridge is lowered, the cholesteatoma over horizontal part of facial nerve and oval window is removed thoroughly. The stapes superstructure is absent, the stapes footplate is mobile and the mucosa is healthy. The horizontal part of facial nerve, the prominence of the lateral semicircular canal and the cochleariform process are exposed after the cholesteatoma is cleared

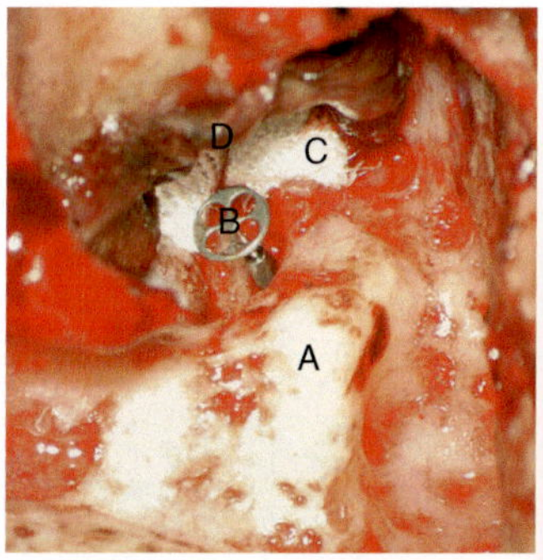

A. Lateral semicircular canal
B. Ossicular prosthesis (TORP)
C. Absorbable non-adhesive gauze
D. Temporalis fascial graft

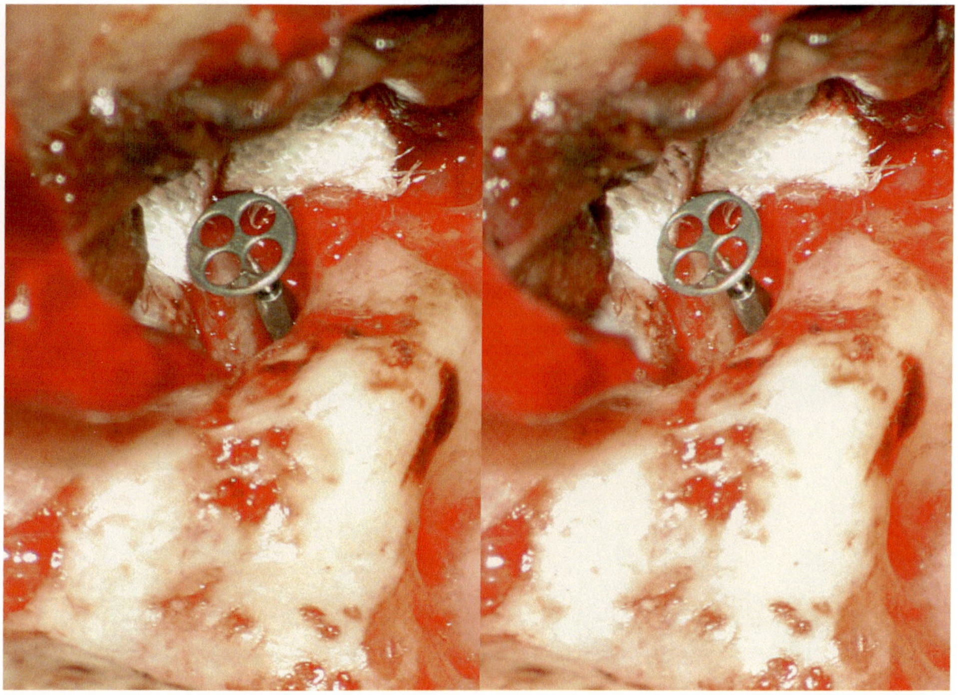

Fig. 2.104 Ossicular prosthesis implantation
Underlay the tympanic membrane with temporalis fascia that has previous been air dried. Turn the fascia back and fill the tympanic cavity with absorbable non-adhesive gauze to support the graft and prevent post-operative adhesions. The prosthesis (TORP) is cut to the appropriate length and placed on the stapes footplate

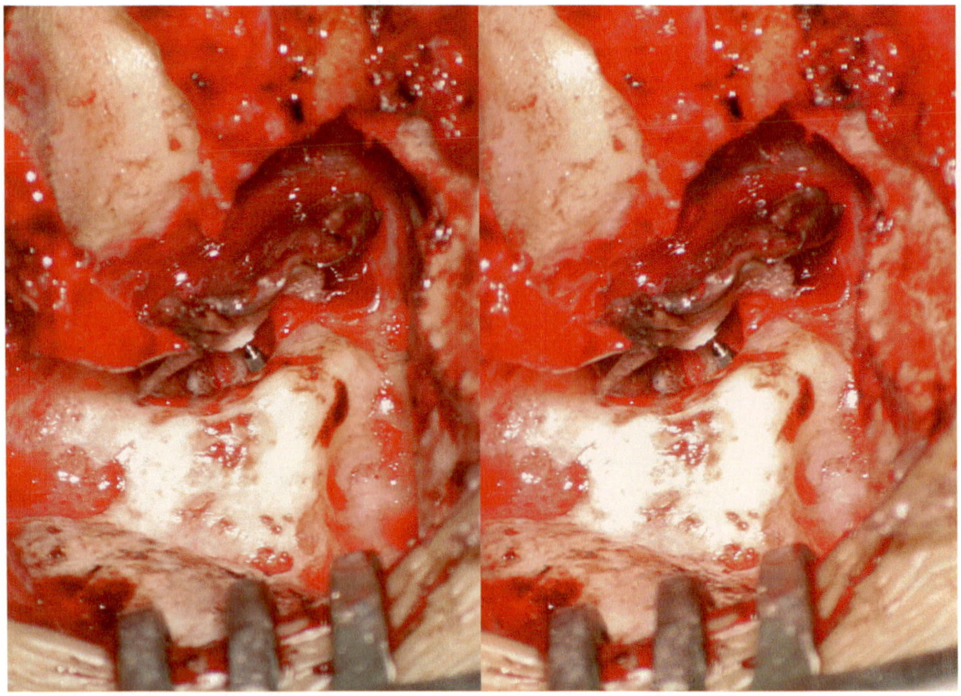

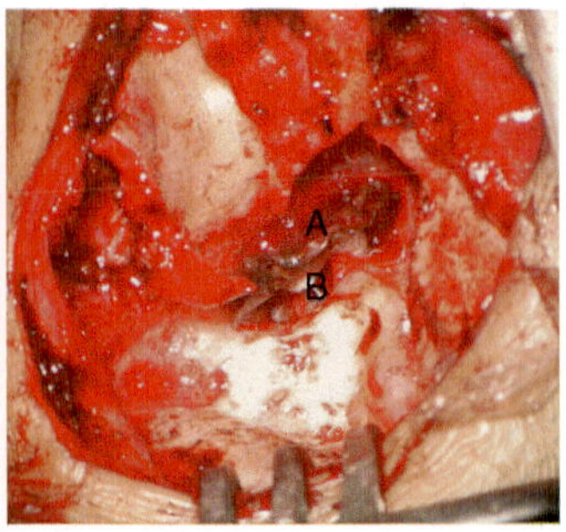

A. Transplanted fascia
B. Cartilage disc

Fig. 2.105 Place the cartilage disc
A cartilage disc with attached perichondrium is taken from the auricle and inserted over the TORP. The temporalis fascia graft is placed over this under the tympano-meatal flap

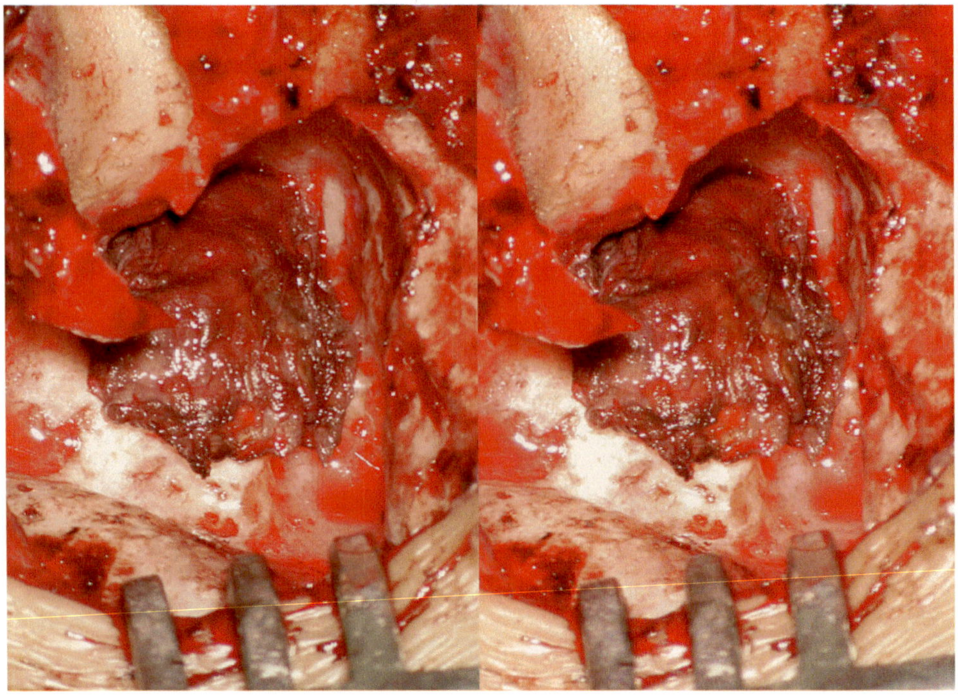

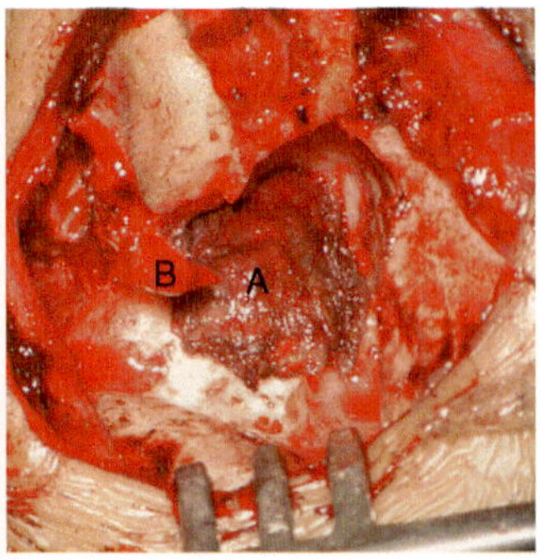

A. Fascial graft
B. Tympano-meatal flap

Fig. 2.106 Placement of fascia
Reposition the temporalis fascia and skin flap over the facial ridge, TORP and tympanic cavity

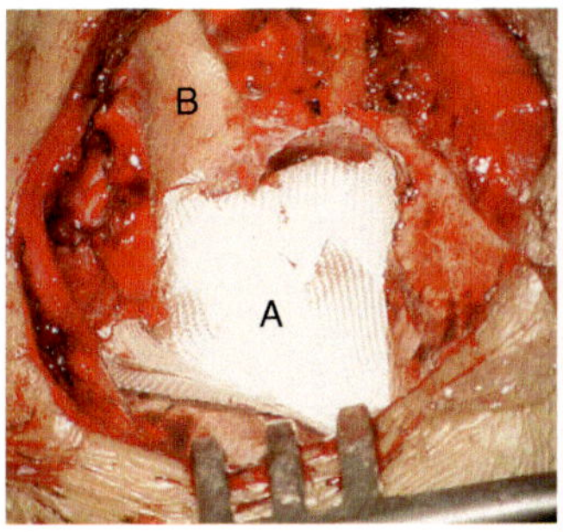

A. Absorbable non-adhesive gauze
B. External auditory canal skin

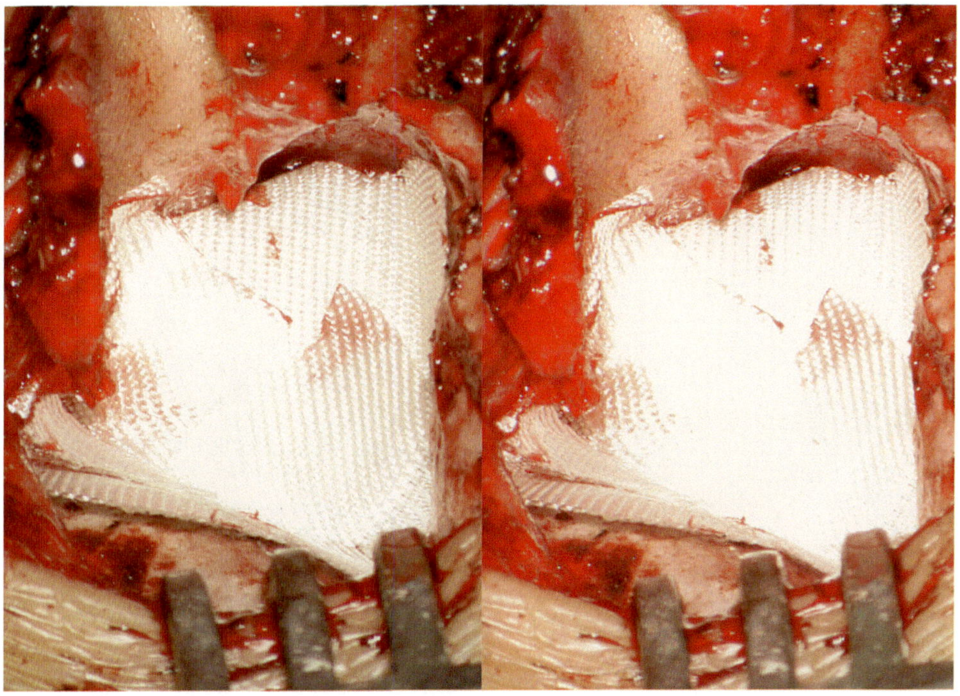

Fig. 2.107 Mastoid cavity packing
The absorbable non-adhesive gauze is placed over the tympanic membrane

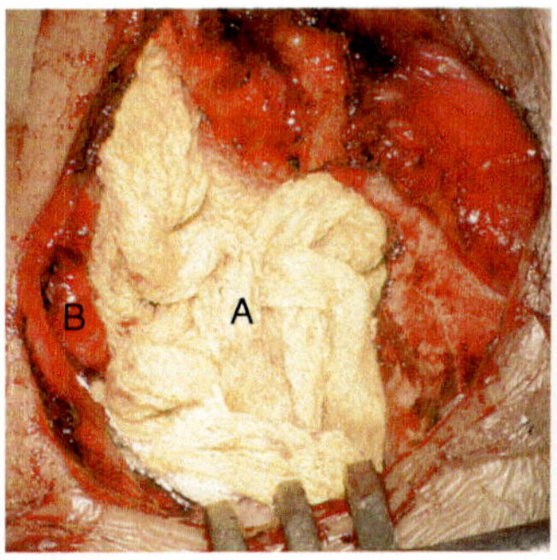

A. Iodoform gauze
B. Tympano-meatal flap

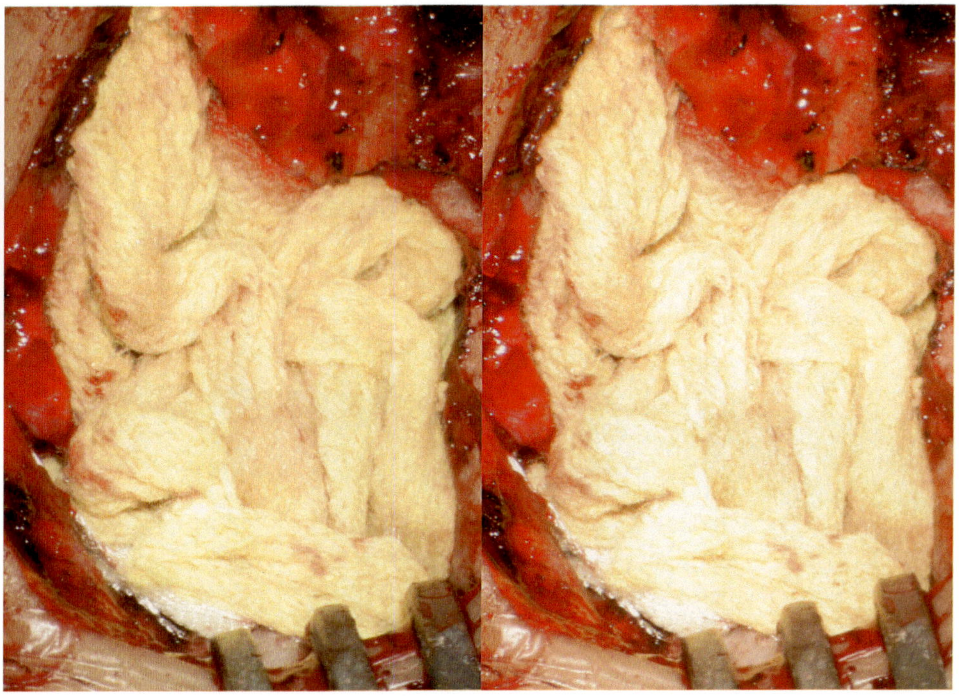

Fig. 2.108 Mastoid cavity packing
The iodoform gauze is packed into the external auditory meatus to hold the flap

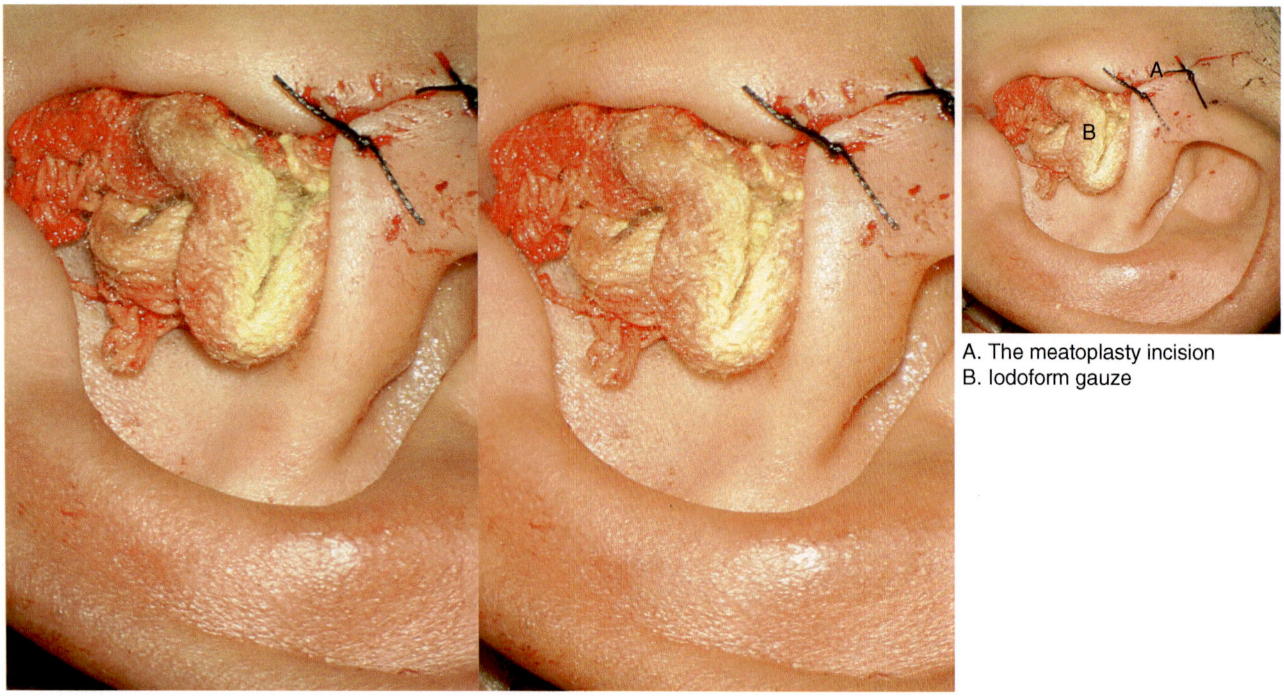

Fig. 2.109 Wound closure
The incision and the meatoplasty of auricular concha is performed to enlarge the external auditory meatus. Close the wound with interrupted silk sutures. Cover the wound with a sterile dressing to complete the operation

Surgery 2: Modified radical mastoidectomy and Tympanoplasty

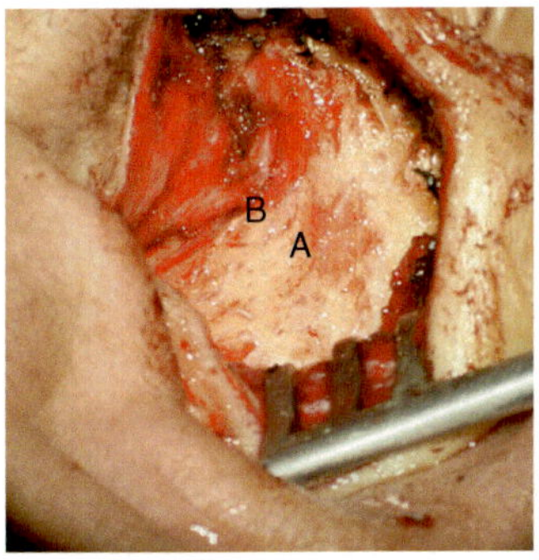

A. Cribriform area
B. Suprameatal spine of external auditory canal

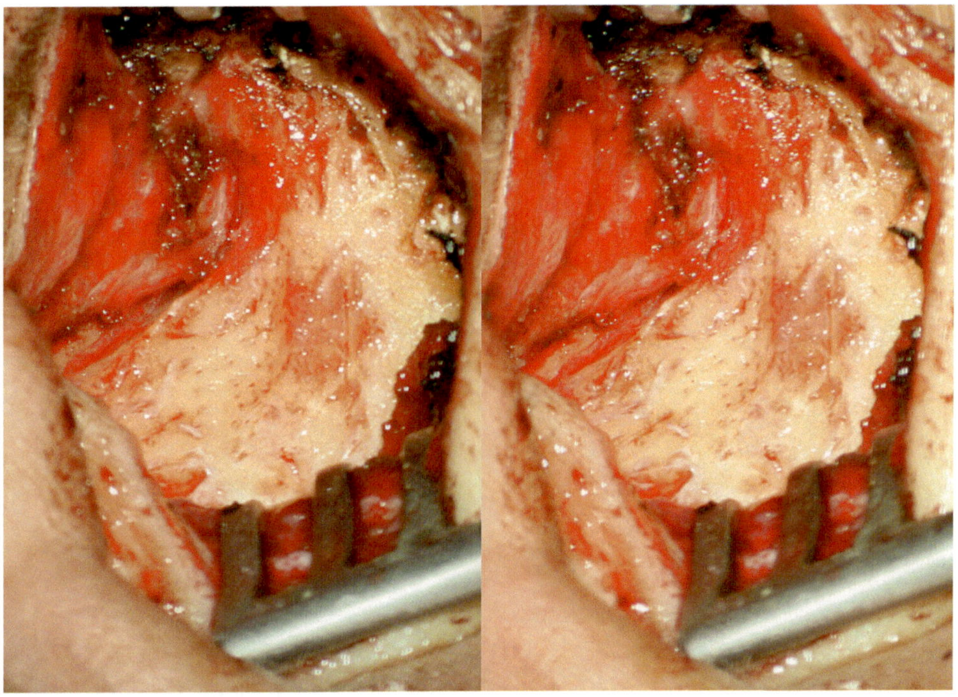

Fig. 2.110 Make Lempert endaural incision
A sterile operation towel is spread over the skin after the external auditory canal and the skin around the ear is sterilized. Make Lempert endaural incision, the mastoid cortex is then exposed. Perform a mastoidectomy via a cribriform area approach

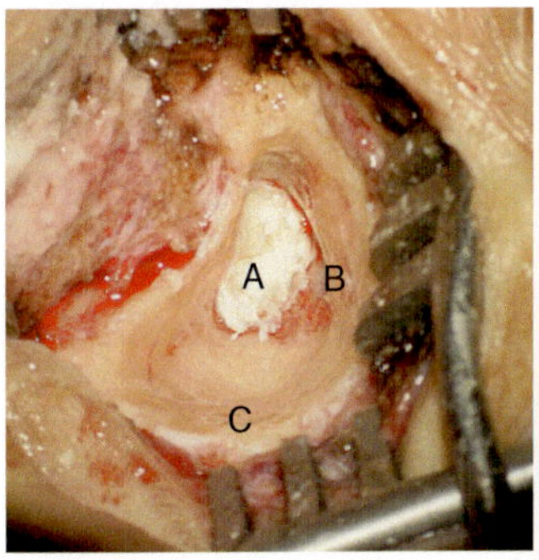

A. Cholesteatoma
B. Tegmen mastoideum
C. Anterior wall of sigmoid sinus

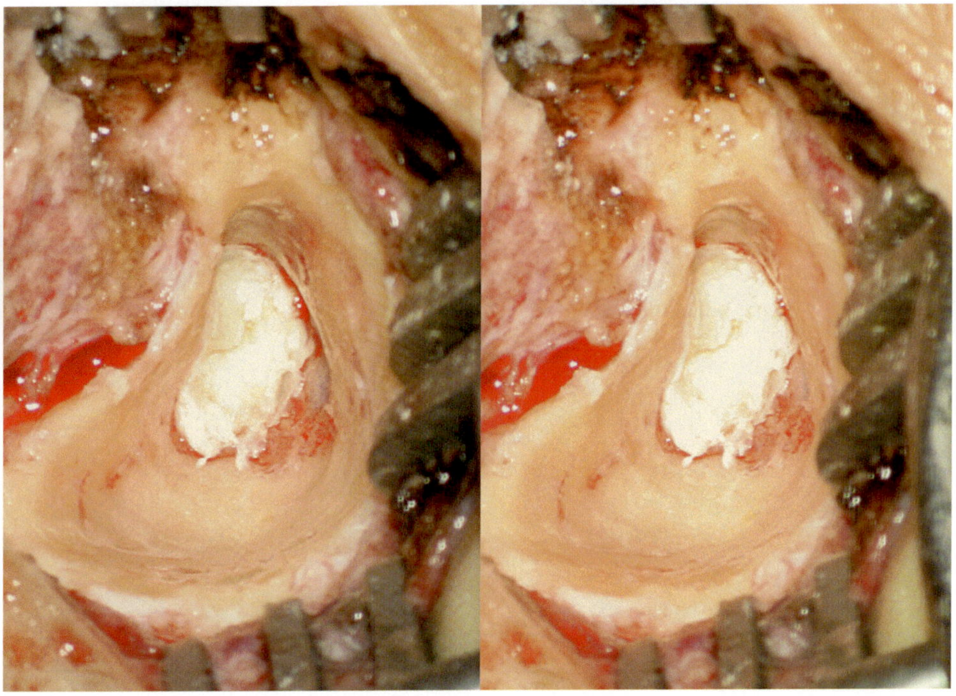

Fig. 2.111 Contour the mastoid cavity
The mastoid cavity is fashioned via a cribriform area approach to expose the sigmoid sinus, the tegmen mastoideum and the cholesteatoma in the antrum and mastoid

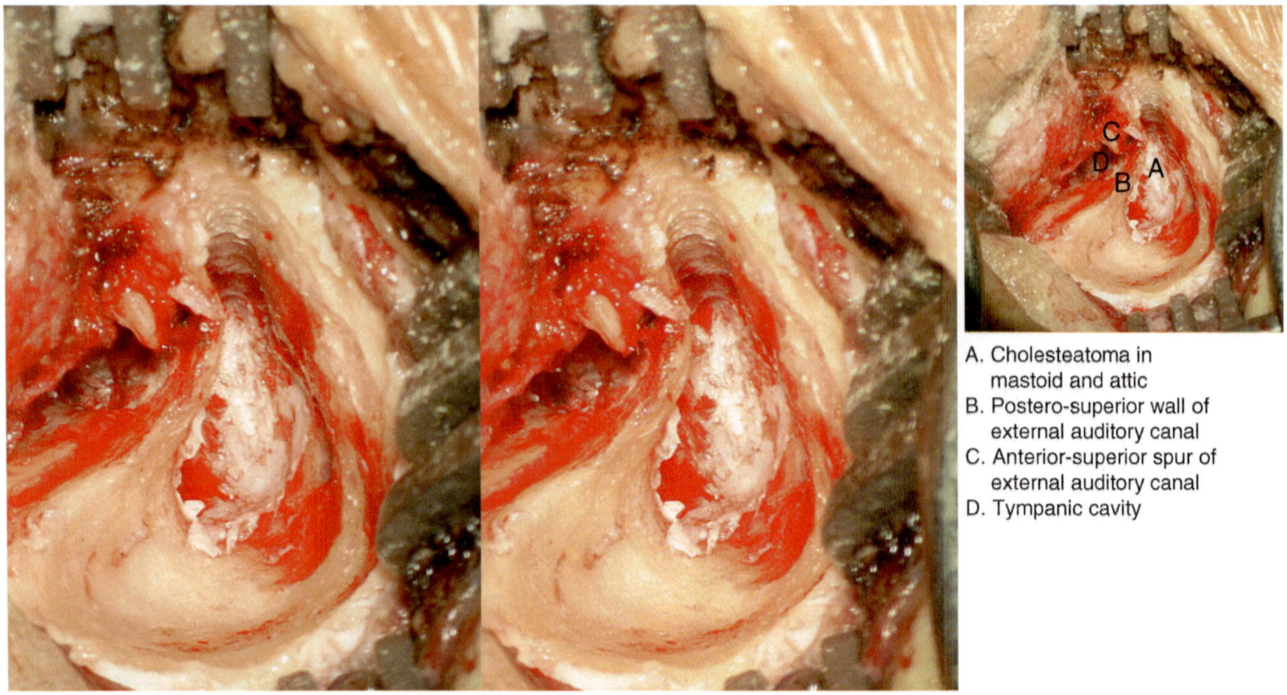

A. Cholesteatoma in mastoid and attic
B. Postero-superior wall of external auditory canal
C. Anterior-superior spur of external auditory canal
D. Tympanic cavity

Fig. 2.112 Open attic
The cholesteatoma in the attic and mesotympanum is exposed after the attic is opened. The middle ear space also contains disease

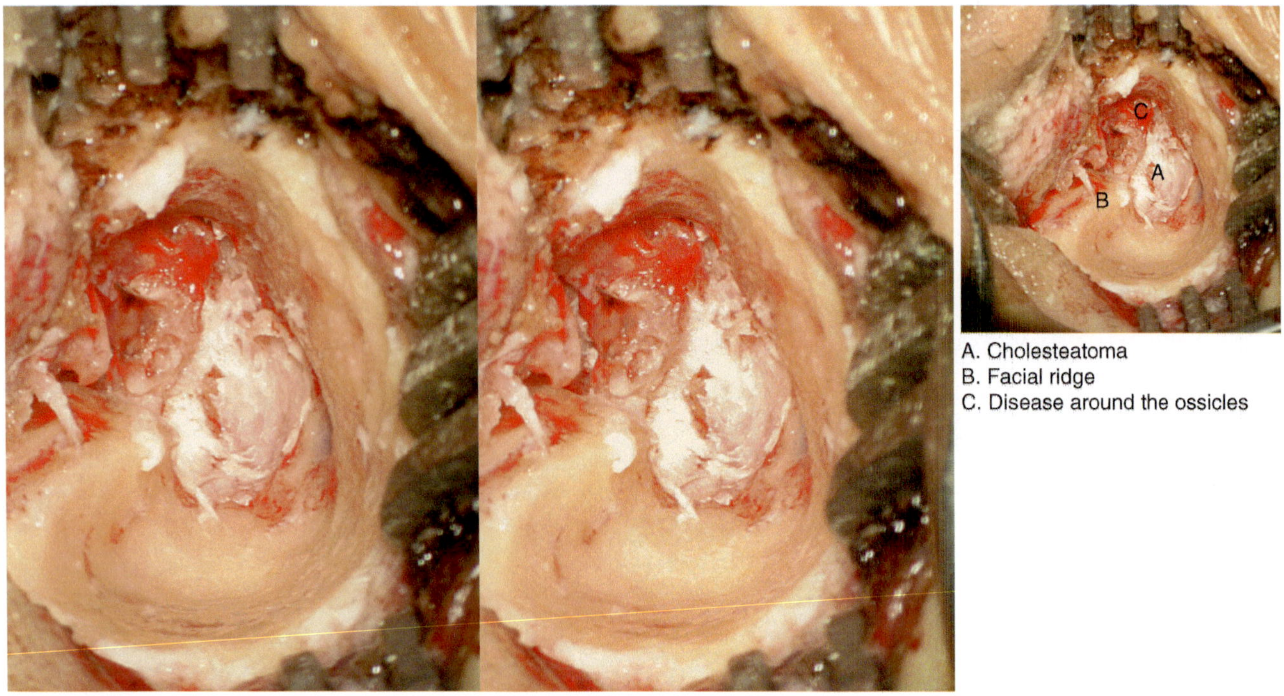

A. Cholesteatoma
B. Facial ridge
C. Disease around the ossicles

Fig. 2.113 Removal of the bridge
The bridge is removed because of the extensive cholesteatoma in the middle ear and around the ossicles which will be difficult to remove otherwise

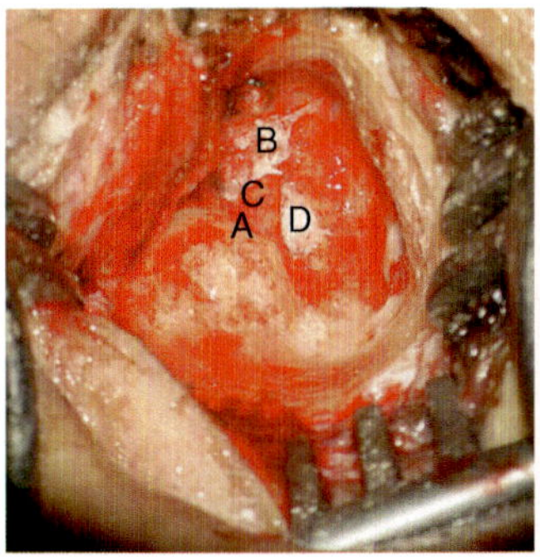

A. Facial ridge
B. Residual cholesteatoma
C. Horizontal part of facial nerve
D. Residual cholesteatoma over the lateral semicircular canal

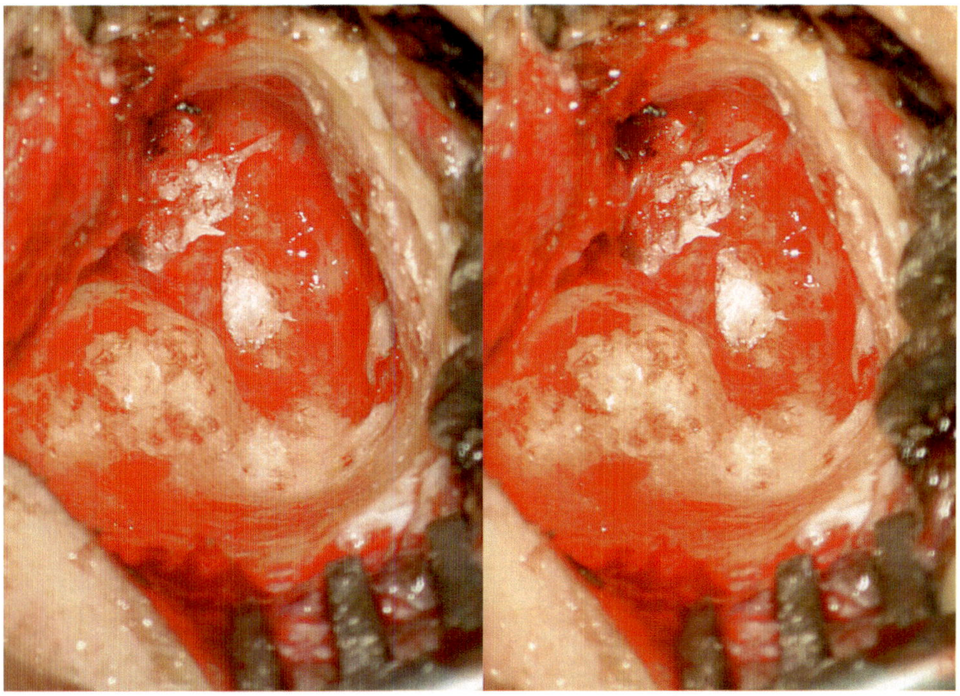

Fig. 2.114 Removal of the facial ridge
The head of malleus is taken out after the bridge is removed. The facial ridge is then lowered to expose the cholesteatoma in the mesotympanum and over the prominence of the lateral semicircular canal. The horizontal part of the facial nerve is also exposed due to erosion of its covering bony canal

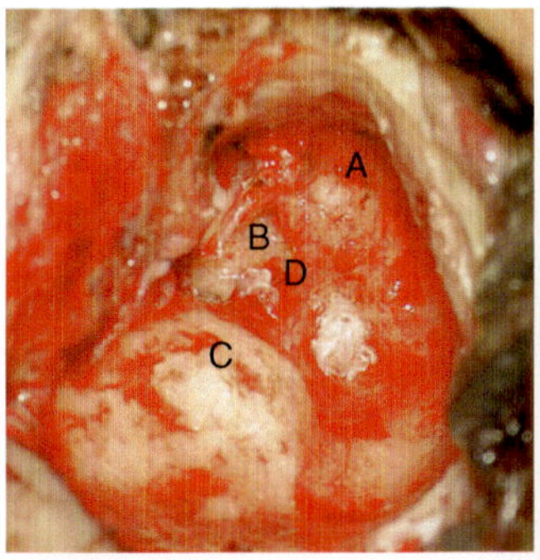

A. Attic
B. Remnant of tympanic membrane
C. Facial ridge
D. Horizontal part of facial nerve

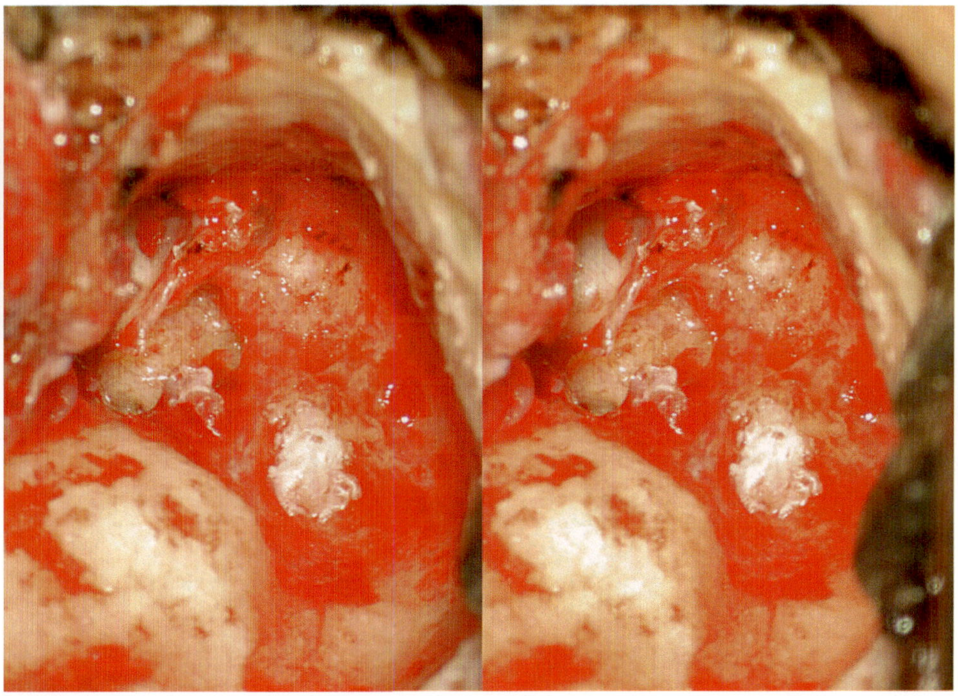

Fig. 2.115 Removal of the cholesteatoma
The cholesteatoma is removed from tympanic cavity, attic and over the lateral semicircular canal leaving the healthy mucosa. The anterior-inferior remnant of the pars tensa and the handle of the malleus are exposed. Fistulization of the lateral semicircular canal is suspected, so removal of any overlying disease should be done with great care

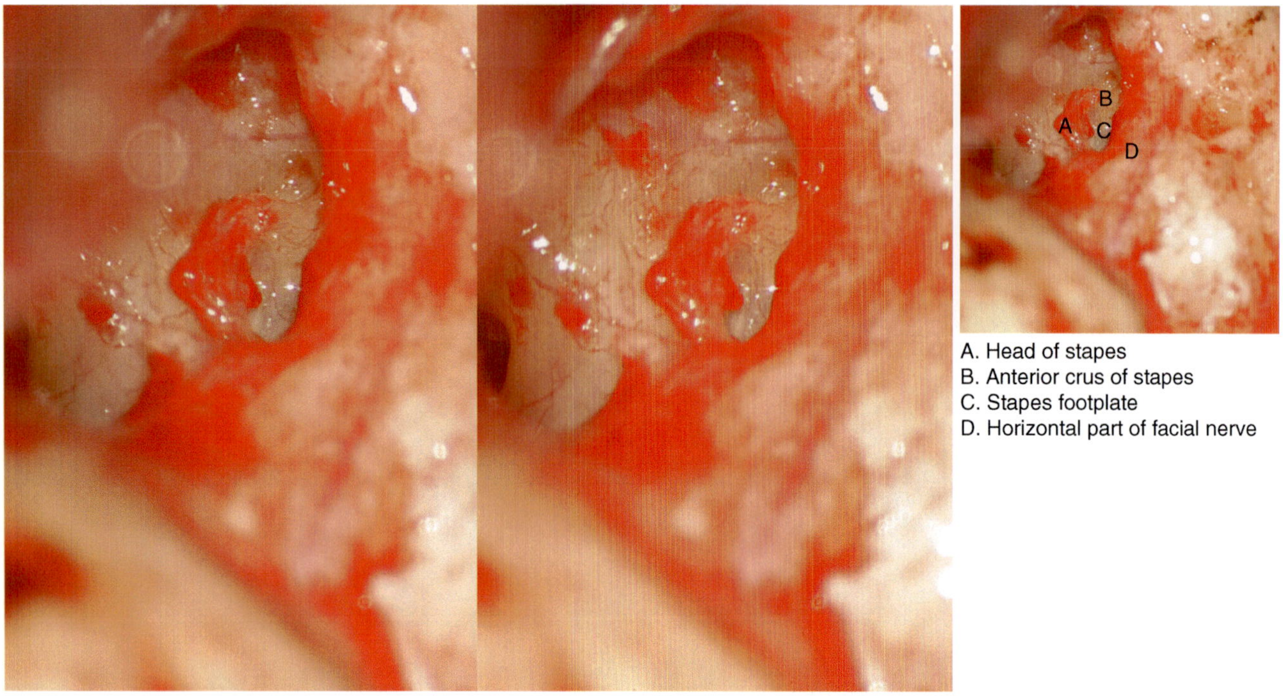

A. Head of stapes
B. Anterior crus of stapes
C. Stapes footplate
D. Horizontal part of facial nerve

Fig. 2.116 Removal of disease
The cholesteatoma over the horizontal part of the facial nerve and oval window is removed thoroughly. The eroded head, crura and footplate of the stapes and the horizontal part of facial nerve are exposed. The stapes is mobile and the covering mucosa is healthy. Part of the head of the stapes is eroded, but the crura and footplate are normal

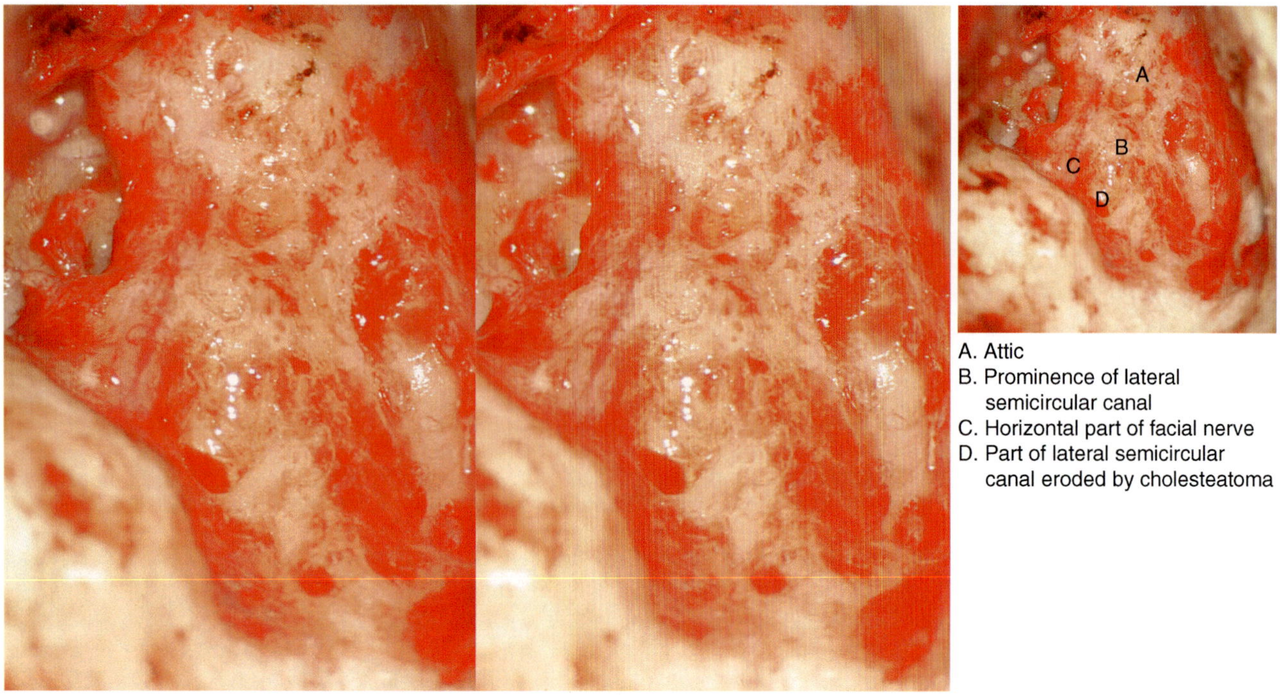

A. Attic
B. Prominence of lateral semicircular canal
C. Horizontal part of facial nerve
D. Part of lateral semicircular canal eroded by cholesteatoma

Fig. 2.117 Removal of the cholesteatoma
The cholesteatoma is removed thoroughly. It can be seen that part of lateral semicircular duct is eroded by cholesteatoma. This is superficial and an osseous fistula has not been created

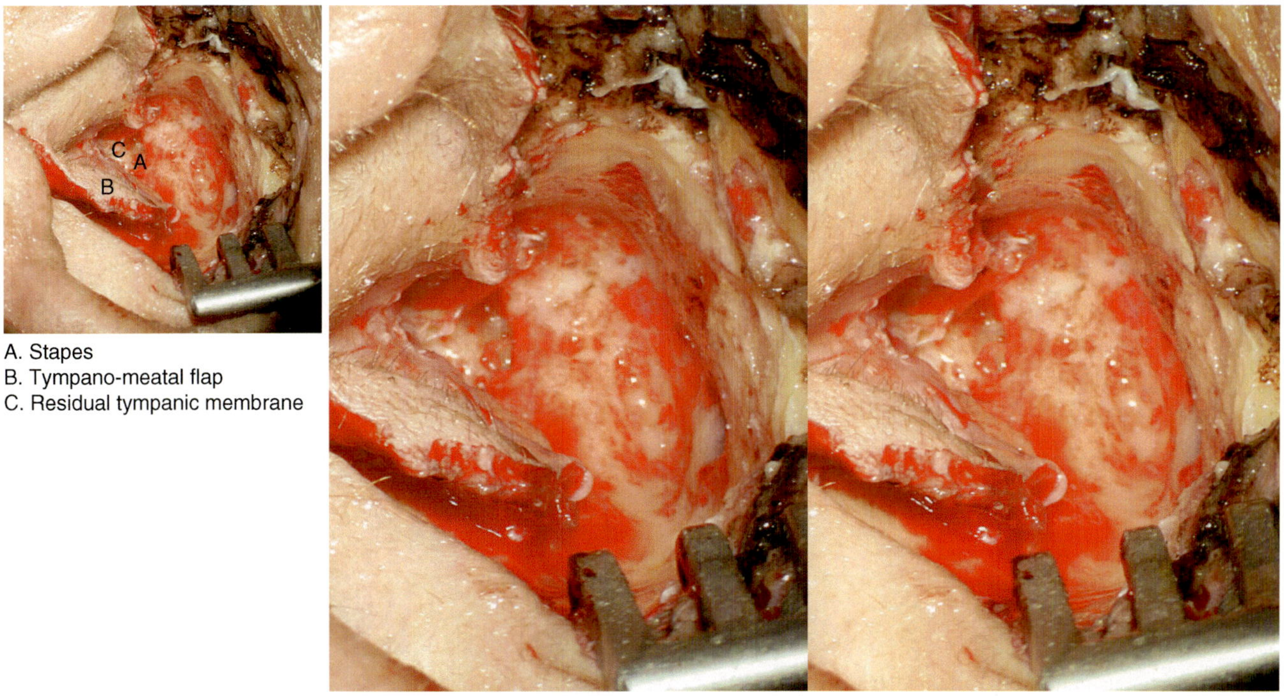

A. Stapes
B. Tympano-meatal flap
C. Residual tympanic membrane

Fig. 2.118 Incise the flap
Cut the flap at the 12 o'clock point, then drape the external part of the cavity and the facial ridge with the flap

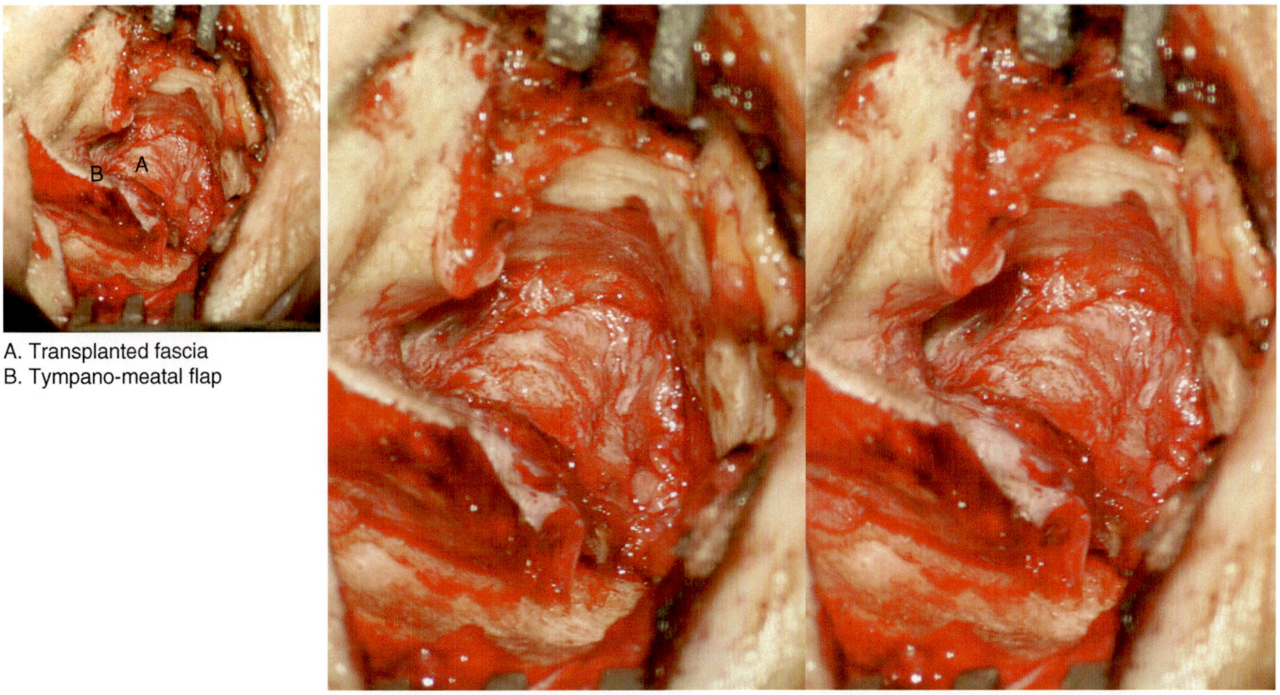

A. Transplanted fascia
B. Tympano-meatal flap

Fig. 2.119 Spread the fascia
Repair the tympanic membrane with temporalis fascia that has been air dried. Spread the fascia on the surface of the mastoid cavity and deep to the flap. Ensure the size of the fascial graft is adequate to repair the drum and cover the bone of the cavity

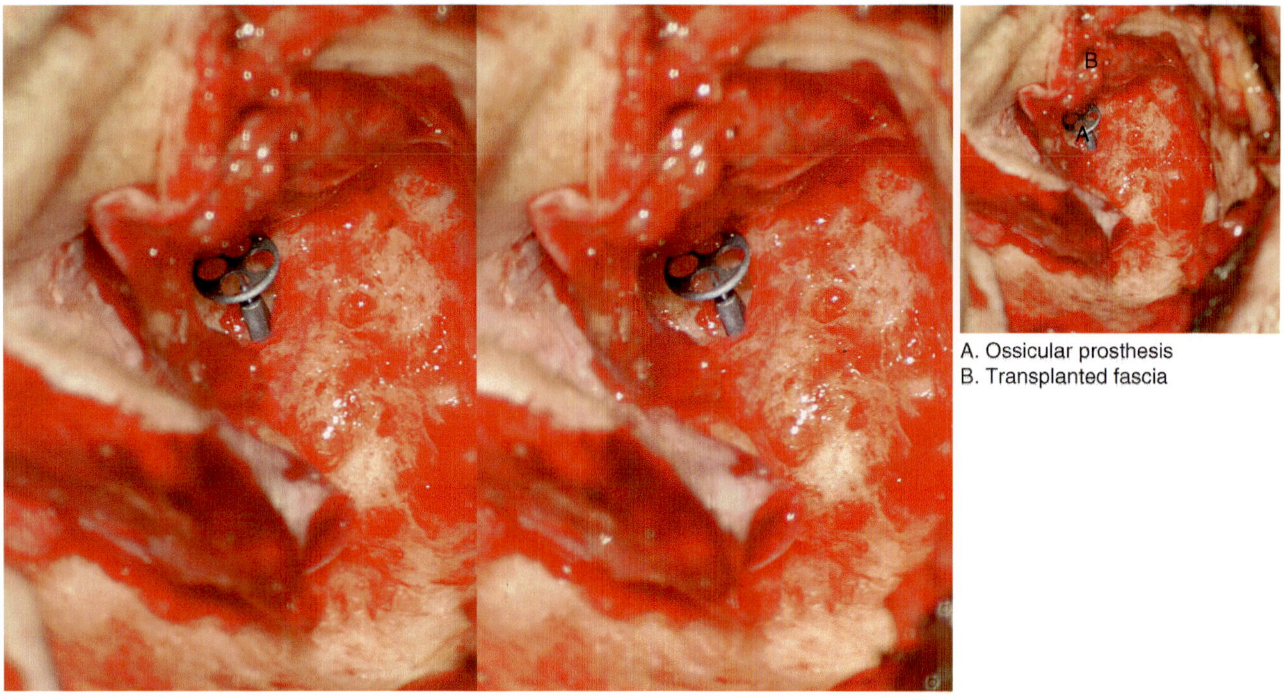

Fig. 2.120 Ossicular prosthesis implantation
The fascia is elevated; the TORP is cut to the appropriate length and implanted on the stapes footplate

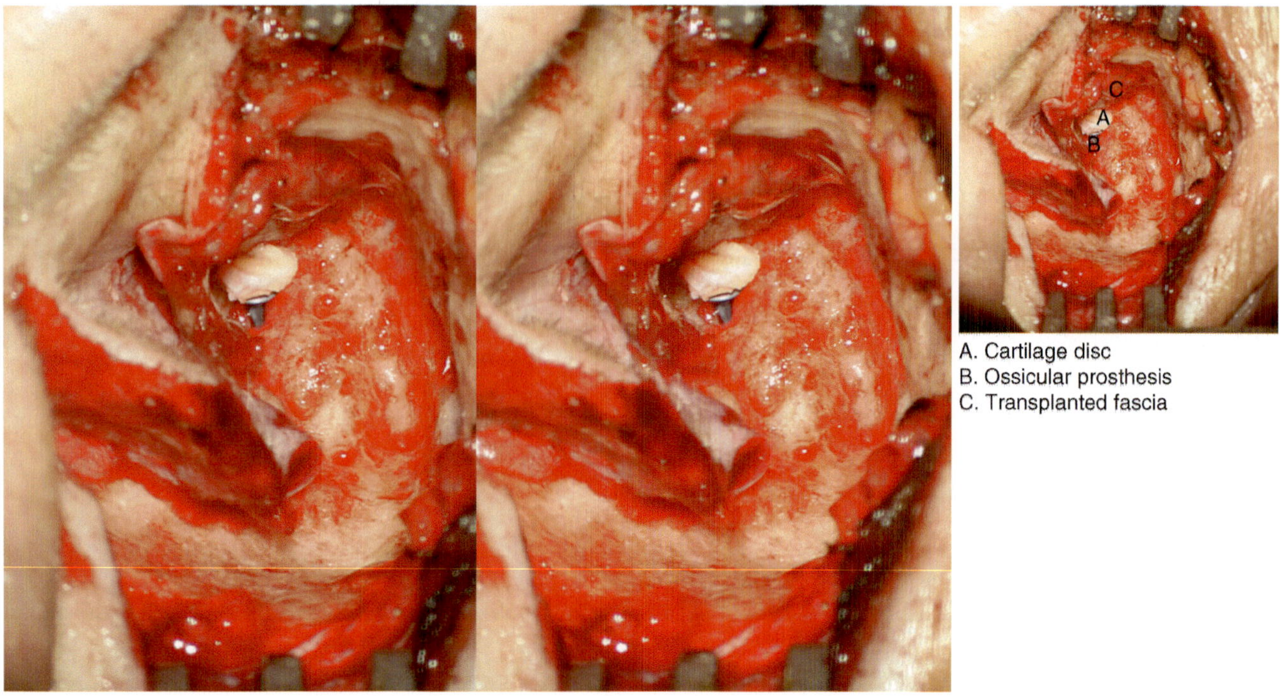

Fig. 2.121 Position the cartilage disc
Place a cartilage disc taken with perichondrium from the auricle between the TORP and the fascia to prevent tympanic membrane erosion and extrusion of the prosthesis

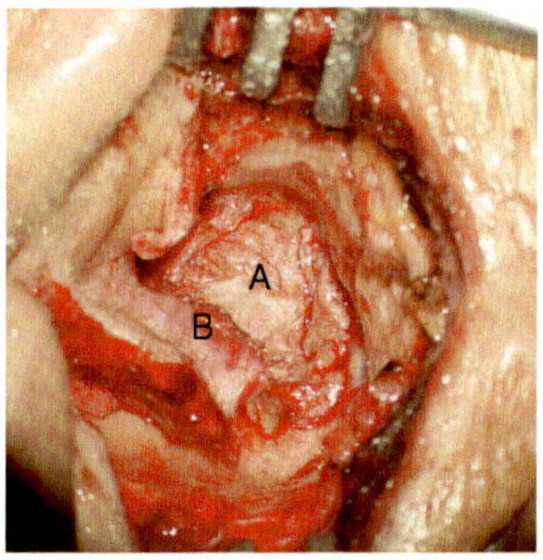

A. Transplanted fascia
B. Tympano-meatal flap

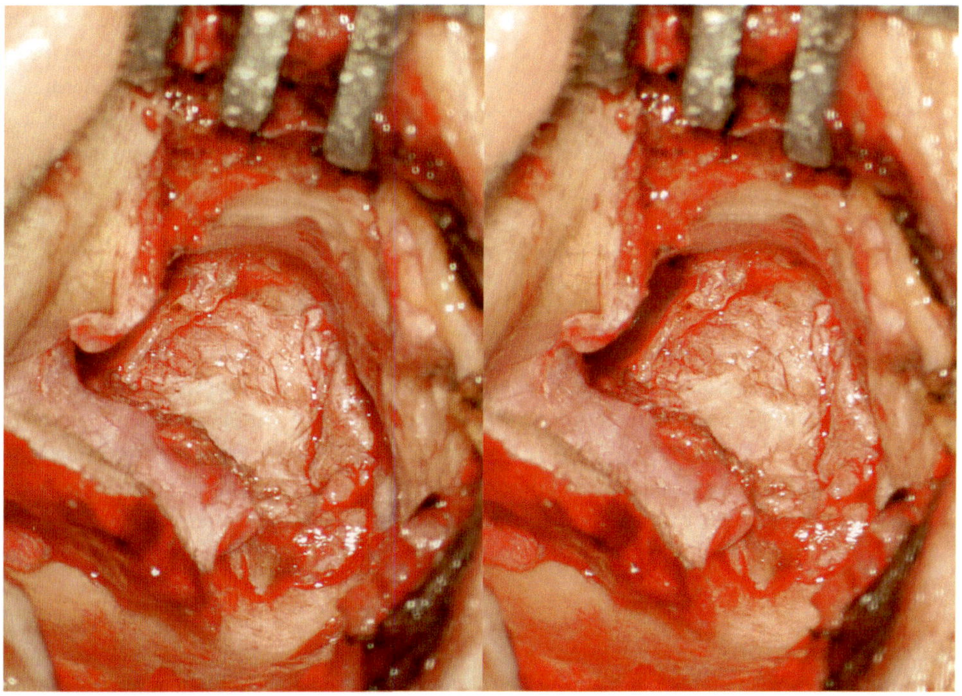

Fig. 2.122 Re-position the fascia
Cover the facial ridge by replacing the temporalis fascia and the skin flap. Place absorbable hemostatic gauze over the tympanic membrane. The external auditory canal and mastoid cavity are packed with iodoform gauze to fix the flap. The incision is closed with interrupted silk sutures. Cover the wound with a sterile dressing to complete the operation

Mastoidectomy (Closed Cavity)

Ming-yu Han, Pu Dai

Indications

1. Chronic otitis media with persistent otorrhea or other symptoms including ear pain and external canal bleeding despite routine medical therapy.
2. Cholesteatoma in middle ear and mastoid, especially involving attic and mastoid antrum; where any disease in the mesotympanum and hypotympanum is able to be controlled.
3. The tumors involving the attic or middle ear.
4. Refractory middle ear effusions unresponsive to conservative measures.

Contraindications

1. Non-functioning Eustachian tube or erosion of the inner ear.
2. Significant erosion of the posterior bony EAC wall.
3. A small sclerotic mastoid, a low-lying middle cranial fossa and an anteriorly positioned sigmoid sinus will limit surgical exposure and may necessitate removal of the canal wall.
4. Irreversible disease in the middle ear.
5. The large area dura mater defects which can lead to cerebrospinal otorrhea or cerebral hernia.
6. Patient unfit for surgery.

Operative Procedures

1. Incision: Under local or general anesthesia, the procedure is usually carried out through a postauricular incision which is 0.5–1.0 cm behind the posterior sulcus. The incision is carried down to the mastoid cortex, and the postauricular flap is elevated anteriorly and inferiorly to expose the mastoid cortex and outer attic wall.
2. Opening the mastoid antrum: The cortex of the mastoid is removed in the cribriform area using a large cutting bur. The mastoid antrum is directly deep to this area. The bone should be widely removed with bevelling of the margins to give adequate exposure of the cavity.

   (PS:If the disease is only limited to the attic and mastoid antrum, atticoantrostomy may be used).

   In this procedure the lateral wall of the attic is exposed by elevating the skin and periosteum of the external auditory canal. Bone is removed progressively from the margin of the tympanic notch to the antrum until all disease is exposed. The short process of incus, incudal fossa and prominence of lateral semicircular canal can be seen with this approach. (In this technique the posterior EAC wall is mostly preserved and the sigmoid sinus is not exposed.)
3. Fashioning of mastoid cavity: The surgical field is expanded from the antrum. The epitympanum is opened to expose the short process of incus by drilling anteriorly. The mastoid is then drilled to identify and skeletonize the sigmoid sinus, the middle cranial fossa dural plate, the digastric ridge, the lateral semicircular canal.
4. Thinning of posterior EAC wall: The bony EAC must be thinned to allow access for the facial recess dissection and eventual visualization of the most posterior mesotympanic structures, such as the round window and the stapedius tendon.
5. Opening the attic: The lateral wall of the attic is removed to expose the incudo-malleal joint drilling from the temporal line to the zygomatic root. The incus may need to be removed depending on the disease. Removal of the ossicles will improve the communication of middle ear and mastoid cavity.
6. Opening the facial recess: Facial recess is a variably pneumatized triangle bounded anteriorly by the chorda tympani, posteriorly by the second genu and descending portion of the facial nerve and superiorly by the bone of the fossa incudis (incus buttress). When opened it forms a posterior tympanotomy exposing the pyramid, the round window and oval window.
7. Eradication of disease: Disease can now be cleared from the attic, the mastoid cavity, the facial recess and the mesotympanum. Cholesteatoma matrix should be completely removed from the mastoid working from posterior to anterior. The malleus head should be removed if it is eroded by cholesteatoma. This will allow exposure of the supratubal recess and assist in eradicating the disease from both anterior attic and upper part of the EAC. Whether an open or closed approach is used, the areas that are most difficult to be seen are the posterior recesses of the middle ear, including the area below the pyramid and tympanic sinus. These areas are located between and behind the oval and round windows, where the cholesteatoma epithelium is easily hidden, especially in cases of marginal tympanic membrane perforations. If the stapes superstructure and stapedial muscle are missing, the pyramid and the surrounding bone should be drilled to assist in eradicating the disease thoroughly.
8. Tympanoplasty: The annulus is elevated via an EAC approach, and tympanoplasty is performed based on the status of ossicular chain.
9. Closing: A drainage tube is placed in the mastoid cavity and the wound is closed in layers.

Special Comments

1. The mastoid cavity should be saucerized to allow better visualization and prevent injury to important structures.
2. Any overhang of the posterior bony EAC wall should be removed in order to fully visualize the drum and middle ear.
3. Care should be taken in clearing disease from the mastoid antrum in order to avoid injury to the facial nerve or lateral and posterior semicircular canals.
4. When removing of lateral wall to the attic, the bone over the incus should be thinned with a diamond bur then gently removed with a curette to avoid injury to the stapes and inner ear.
5. Any defect of the scutum must be identified. These should be repaired. Large defects may be best treated with open cavity surgery. Failure to deal with bony wall defects will allow pars flaccida retraction post operatively leading to recurrent disease.
6. The air cells of the sinodural angle must be removed in order to clear the area behind the semicircular canals.
7. During the careful skeletonization of the facial nerve and chorda tympani a diamond bur is used and liberal irrigation is necessary to avoid thermal injury to the nerve. The tympanic segment of the facial nerve is commonly exposed, either congenitally or by disease. Care needs to be taken to avoid injury to the nerve when dissecting in this area.
8. When working in the region of the anterior part of the lateral semicircular canal, care needs to be taken with the incus and the facial nerve which is covered with only thin bone here. One needs to be certain of clearing all disease from the canal and irrigation will assist with this.
9. Care needs to be taken with the chorda tympani when working at the anterior margin of the facial recess.
10. The facial recess needs to be opened widely for good access and with due care to the facial nerve when working posteriorly.
11. The bone is removed gently in performing the posterior tympanotomy, without undue pressure which may cause accidental injury to the stapes.

Complications

1. Facial paralysis: If the facial nerve is injured, swelling may occur deep to its sheath causing excessive pressure and paralysis. If this occurs, bone should be removed for 5–6 mm from each side of the exposed portion of the facial nerve and the sheath should be incised to relieve the pressure
2. Vertigo: Caused by semicircular canal injury. It is possible to injure the semicircular canals in a sclerosed mastoid or when dealing with inflamed granulation tissue. Any opening in the labyrinth that occurs should be sealed immediately with bone wax and the area covered with temporalis fascia.
3. Sensorineural hearing loss and tinnitus: These can be caused by a direct injury to any of the semicircular canals or cochlea, or indirectly via trauma to the incus or stapes, especially when opening the posterior tympanotomy.
4. Residual and recurrent cholesteatoma: due to incomplete eradication of cholesteatoma, insufficient opening of attic, inflammation, and so on.
5. Hemorrhage: (1) sigmoid sinus injury: It may bleed immediately after being abraded. Bleeding can be suppressed to stop with pieces of cotton for a few minutes. A larger defect can be sutured with 4–0 lines or be repaired with a muscle flap. The packing materials should be sutured with the surrounding tissues in order to avoid embolism caused by displacement in to the vessel. (2) Jugular bulb Bleeding: Bleeding may come from air cells and bone marrow covering the jugular bulb. They are sealed with bone wax, and then use cotton pieces to press bone wax into air cell for more effective hemostasis.

Surgery 1: Intact Canal Wall Mastoidectomy and myringoplasty with maintaining Ossicular Chain intact

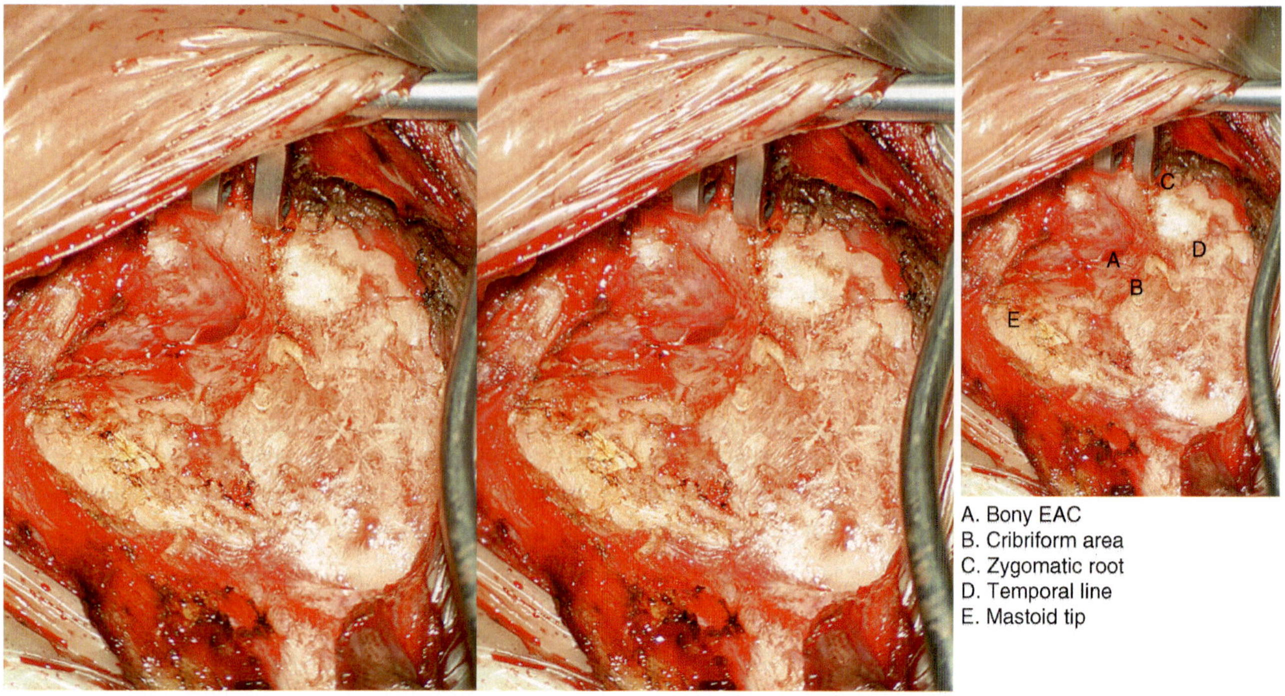

A. Bony EAC
B. Cribriform area
C. Zygomatic root
D. Temporal line
E. Mastoid tip

Fig. 2.123 Post-auricular incision and mastoid exposure
The incision is carried down to the temporalis fascia. The superior periosteal incision was at the level of the temporal line and a second incision extends inferiorly to the mastoid tip over the posterior mastoid. The periosteal flap is elevated in the direction of the EAC

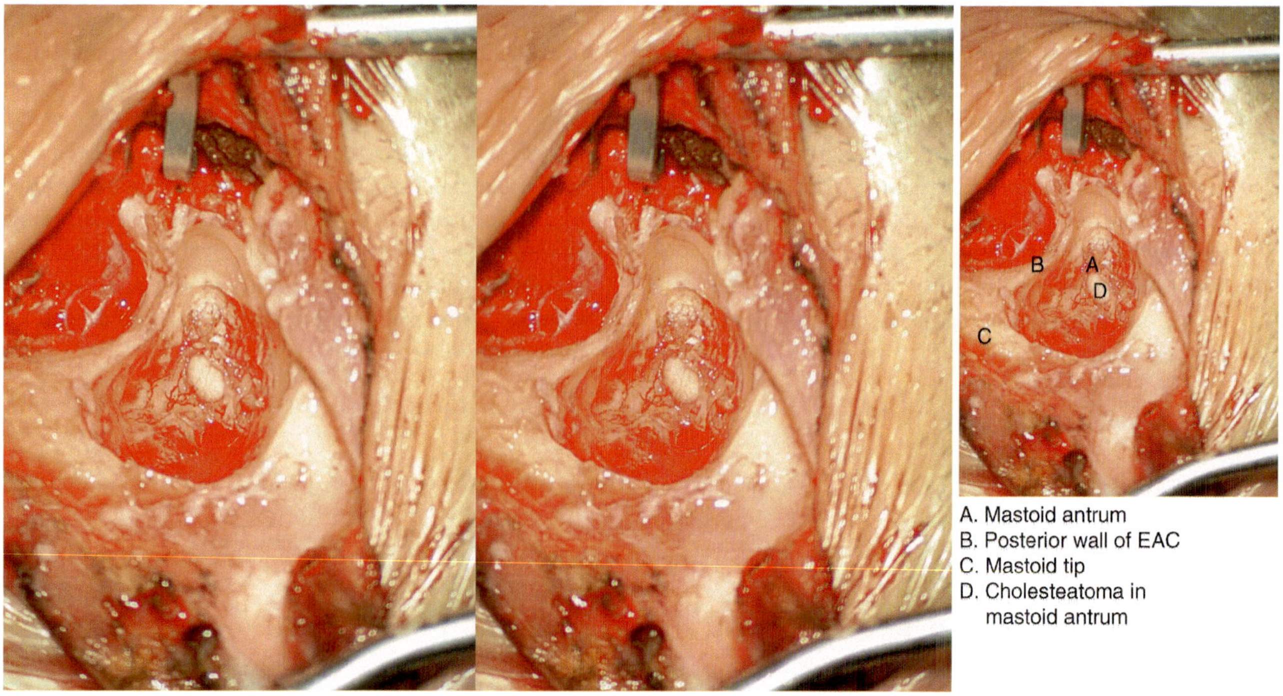

A. Mastoid antrum
B. Posterior wall of EAC
C. Mastoid tip
D. Cholesteatoma in mastoid antrum

Fig. 2.124 Opening the mastoid antrum
The bone is drilled from a triangle made up of the temporal line above, one parallel to the postero-superior EAC wall anteriorly and a vertical line tangential to the posterior curve of the EAC. This bone overlies the mastoid antrum. The bone is "saucerised" to give wide exposure to the antrum and the disease it contains

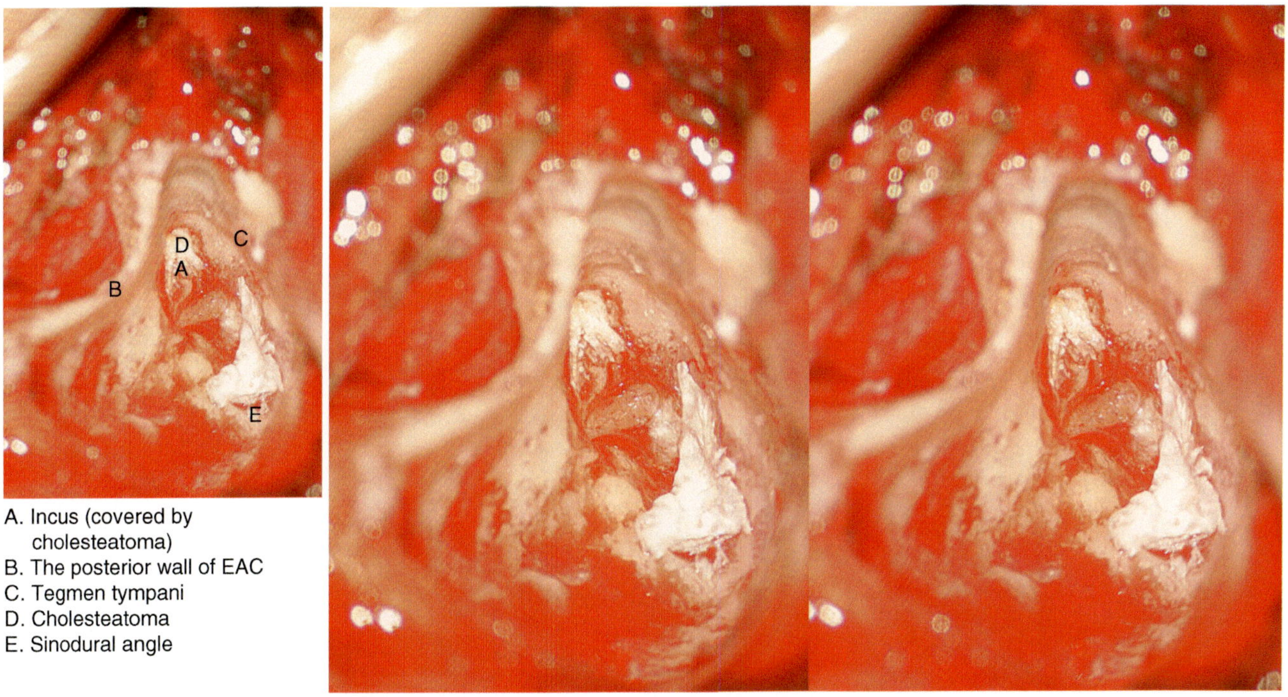

Fig. 2.125 Exposure of the incus and fashioning of mastoid cavity with preservation of the posterior wall of EAC
The attic has been opened antero-superior to the mastoid antrum. Some bone was eroded. The ossicular chain is surrounded by cholesteatoma. After the short process of incus has been exposed, the mastoid cavity is fashioned by drilling posteriorly towards the sigmoid sinus and inferiorly to the mastoid tip. Care needs to be taken with vertical portion of the facial nerve as it runs inferiorly and slightly laterally from the level of the horizontal semi-circular canal

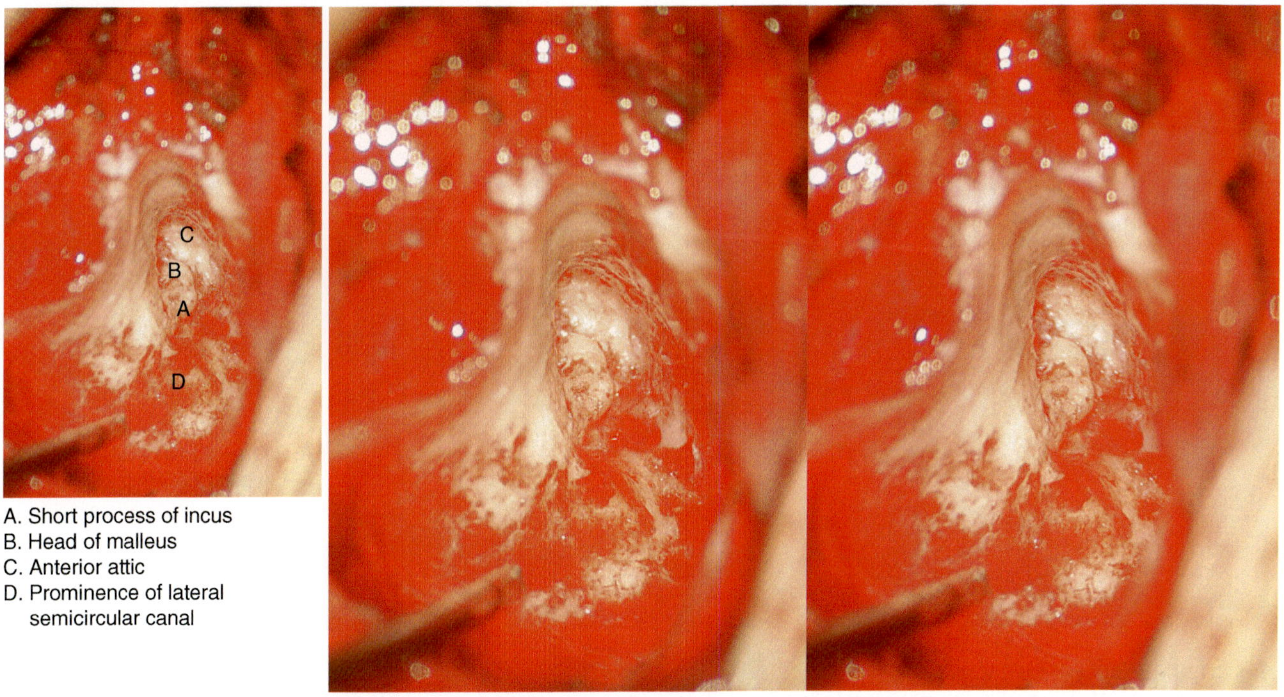

Fig. 2.126 Thinning the posterior EAC wall and opening the attic
The key point of Intact Canal Wall Mastoidectomy is to preserve the posterior wall of EAC, whilst thinning the bony wall as much as possible to expose the operative field
In order to see all disease, the anterior attic should be fully exposed by drilling the anterior and superior walls, leaving a thin postero-superior EAC wall. This figure shows the incudo-malleal joint. Cholesteatoma has been removed from lateral to the ossicles but is still to be cleared from the anterior and medial attic

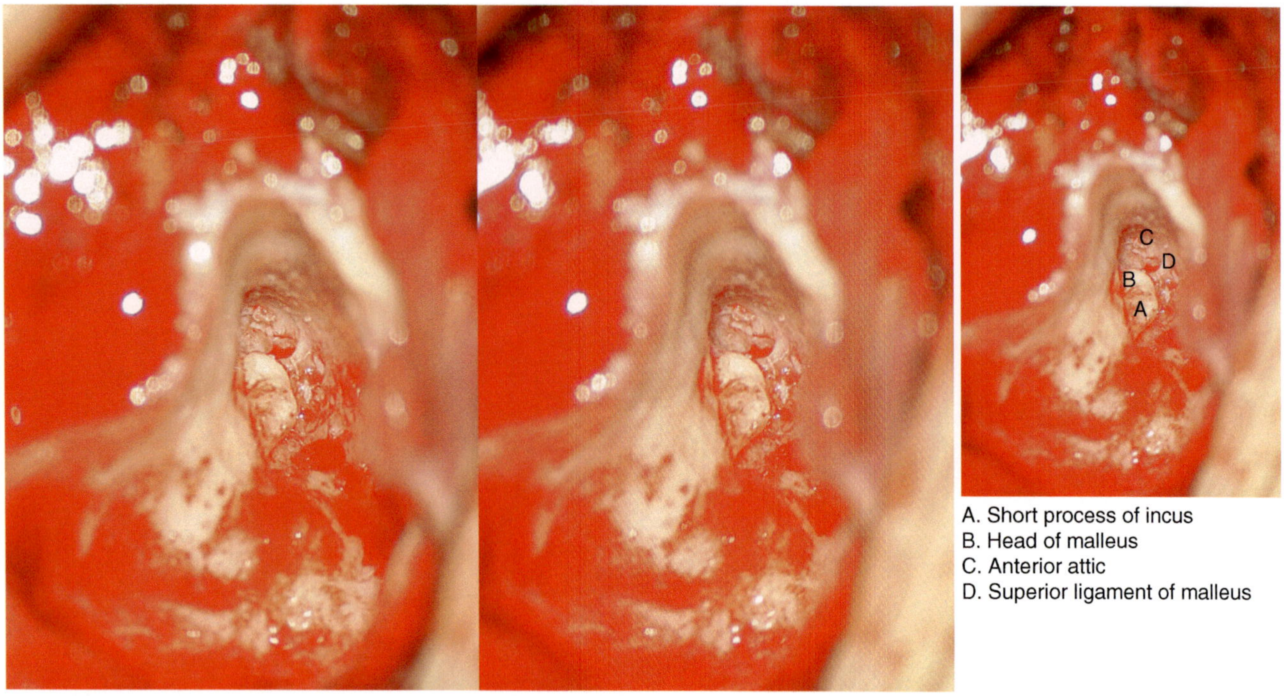

Fig. 2.127 Opening the attic and eradicating the disease
Further opening of the anterior attic allows access to clear the disease. The malleus head and incus body are seen to be intact

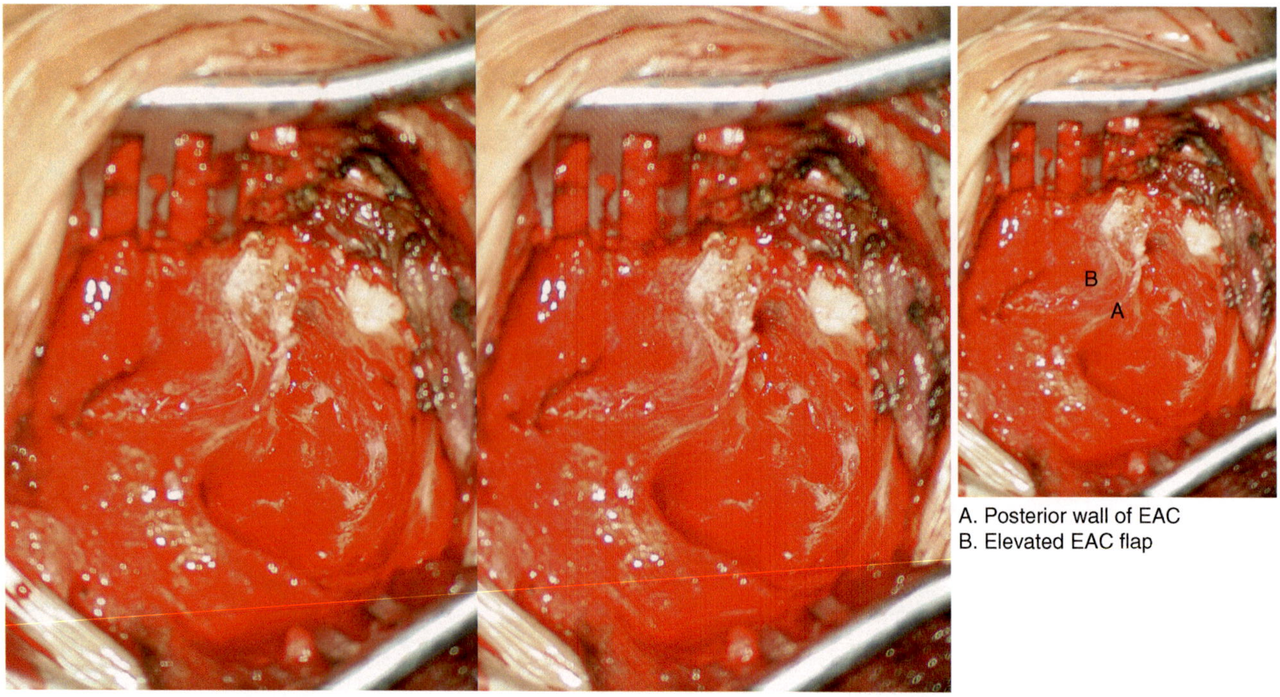

Fig. 2.128 Elevation of the EAC flap
The skin flap of EAC is very thin and care needs to be taken to keep it intact, with gentle dissection along its whole width

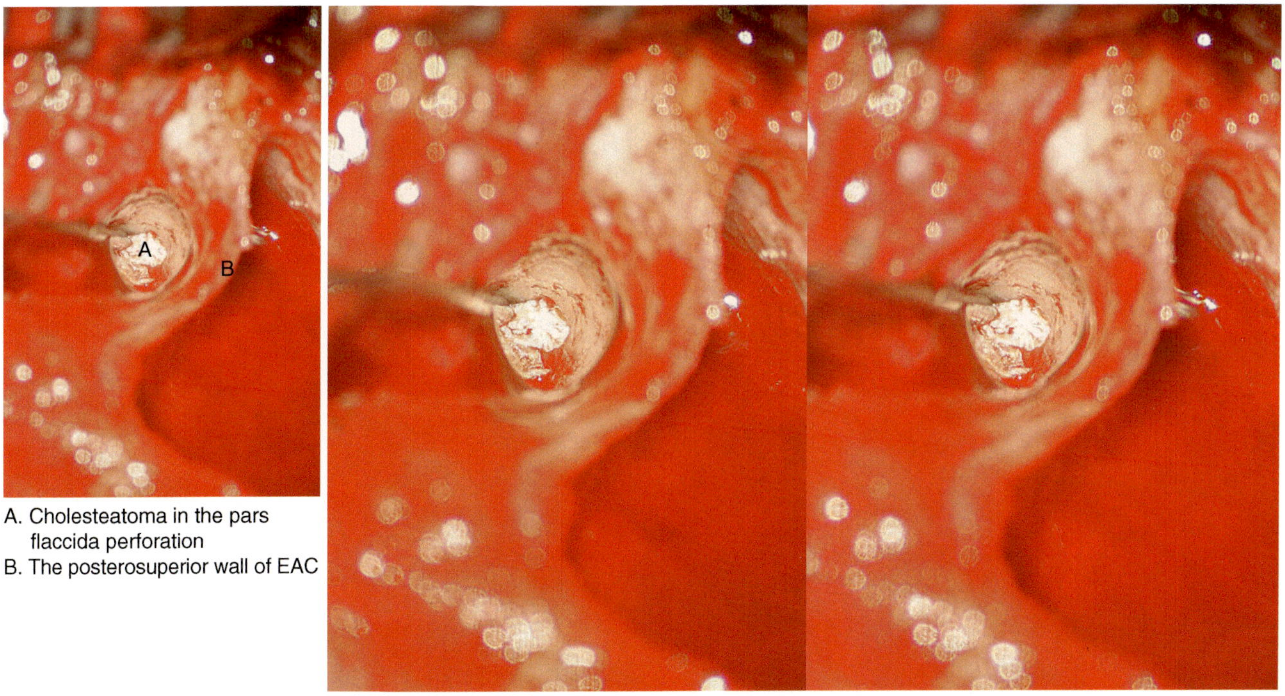

Fig. 2.129 Exploration of the tympanic cavity via a post-auricular approach
Remove the suprameatal spine to enlarge the operative field. Elevate the tympano-meatal flap to enter the middle ear. The cholesteatoma has been partially removed from Prussak's space via the EAC

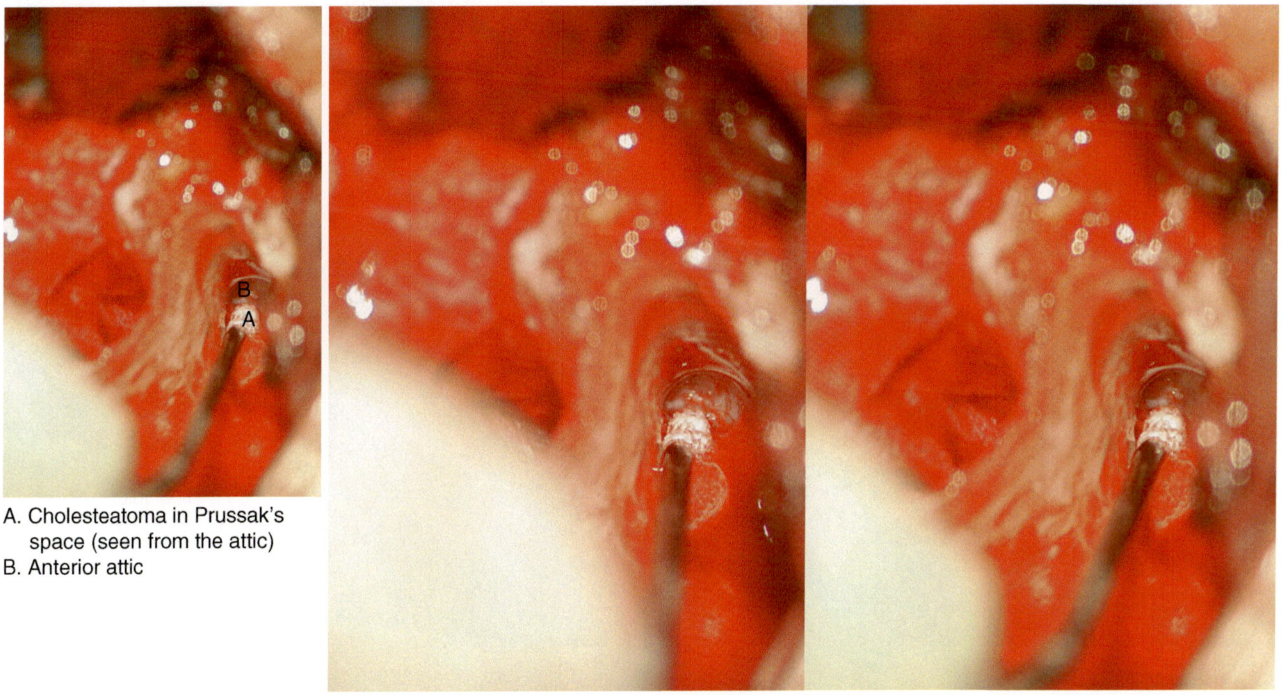

Fig. 2.130 Eradication of attic cholesteatoma
The cholesteatoma has been completely removed from the attic and Prussak's space with combined dissection from the attic above and the EAC below. Ensure no cholesteatoma is left medial to the posterosuperior wall of EAC

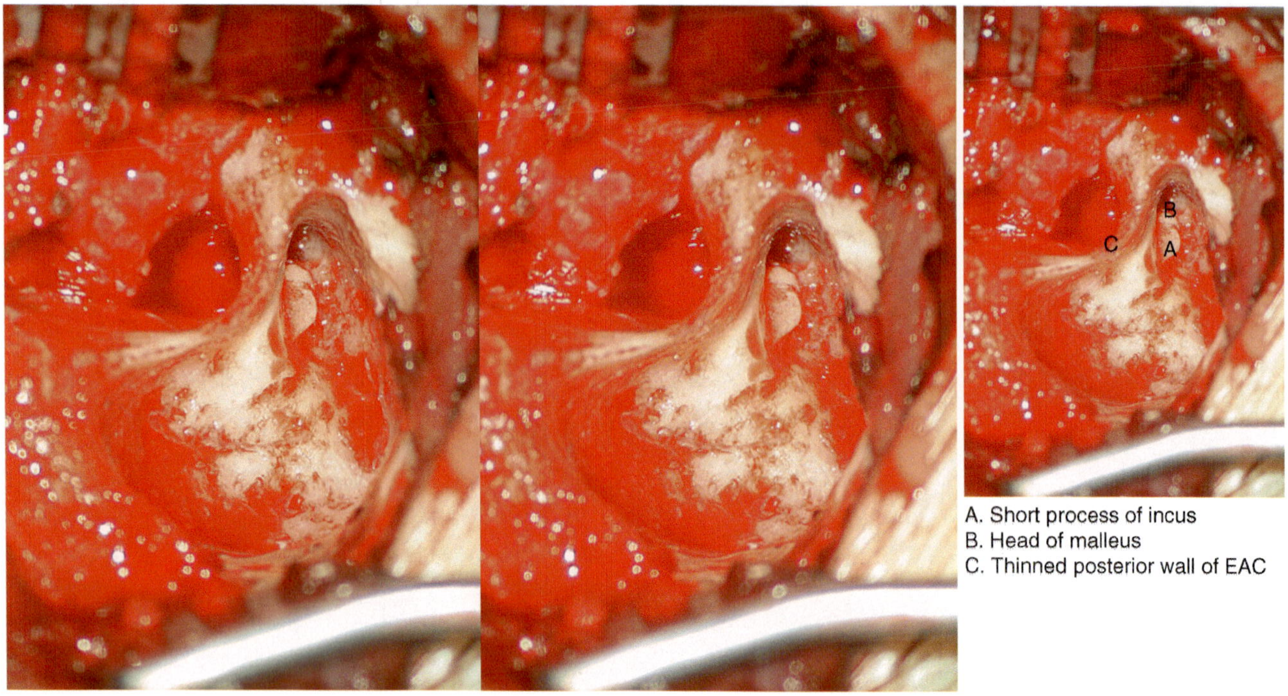

Fig. 2.131 Thinning of the posterior wall of EAC and exposure of the facial recess
A facial recess approach needs to be performed to expose the middle ear and lower part of the ossicular chain and remove any disease present. Firstly, the posterior wall of EAC is further thinned over the facial recess which lies inferior to the incus and lateral semicircular canal

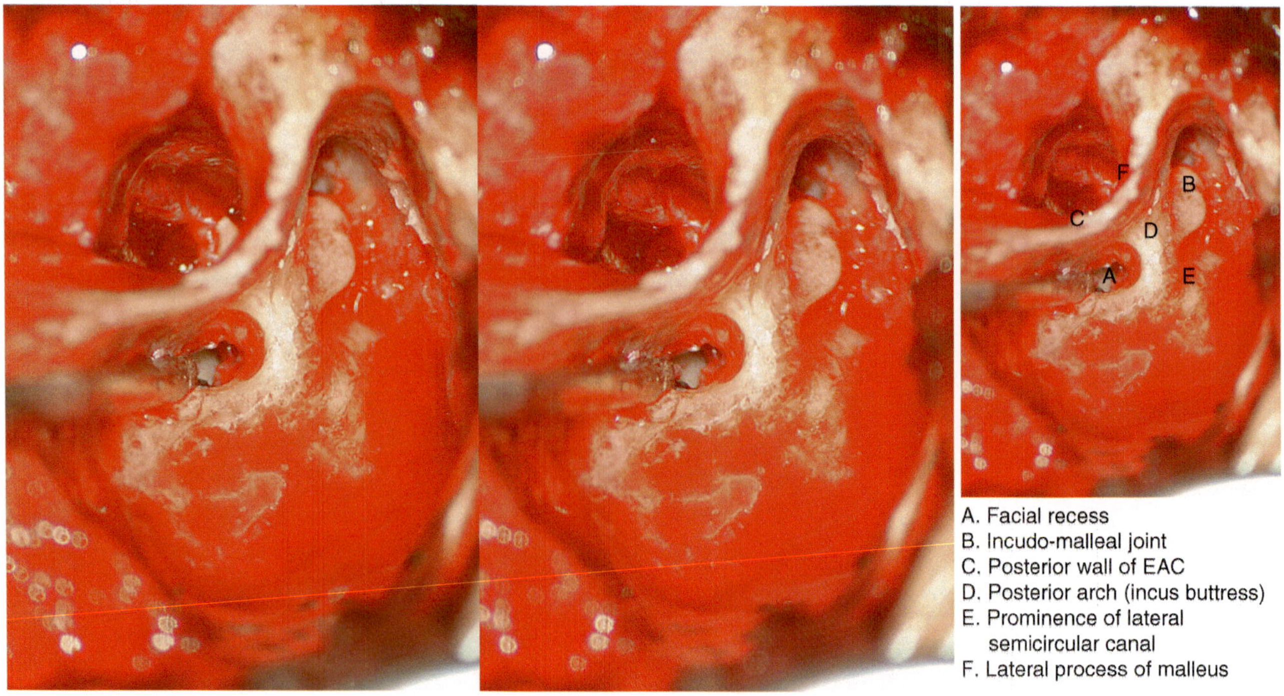

Fig. 2.132 Opening the facial recess
The facial recess is a triangular area bounded superiorly by the bone of incudal fossa, posteriorly by the facial nerve and antero-inferiorly by the chorda tympani. The recess is initially opened superiorly, near to but not touching the incus. This gives the best exposure of the posterior middle ear in intact canal wall mastoidectomy

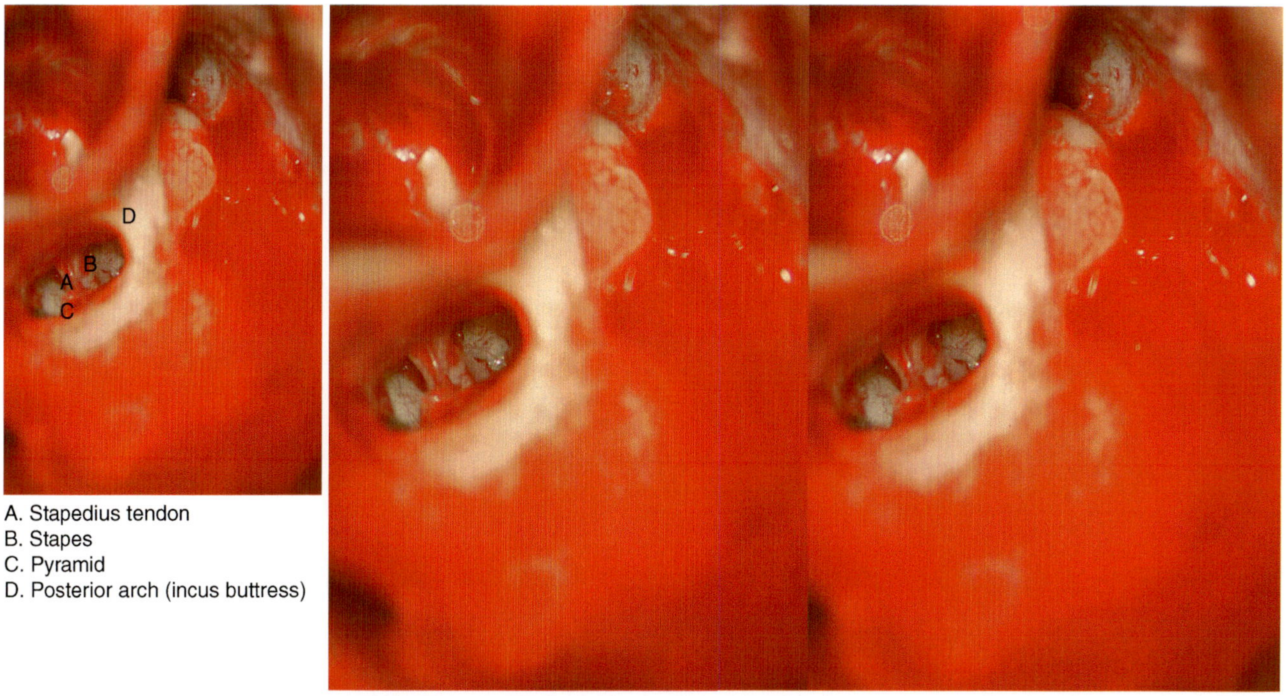

Fig. 2.133 Exploration of the posterior tympanic cavity via the facial recess approach
Exploration via the facial recess revealed mild mucosal edema around the stapes. The incudo-stapedial joint was seen to be intact and the stapes was mobile

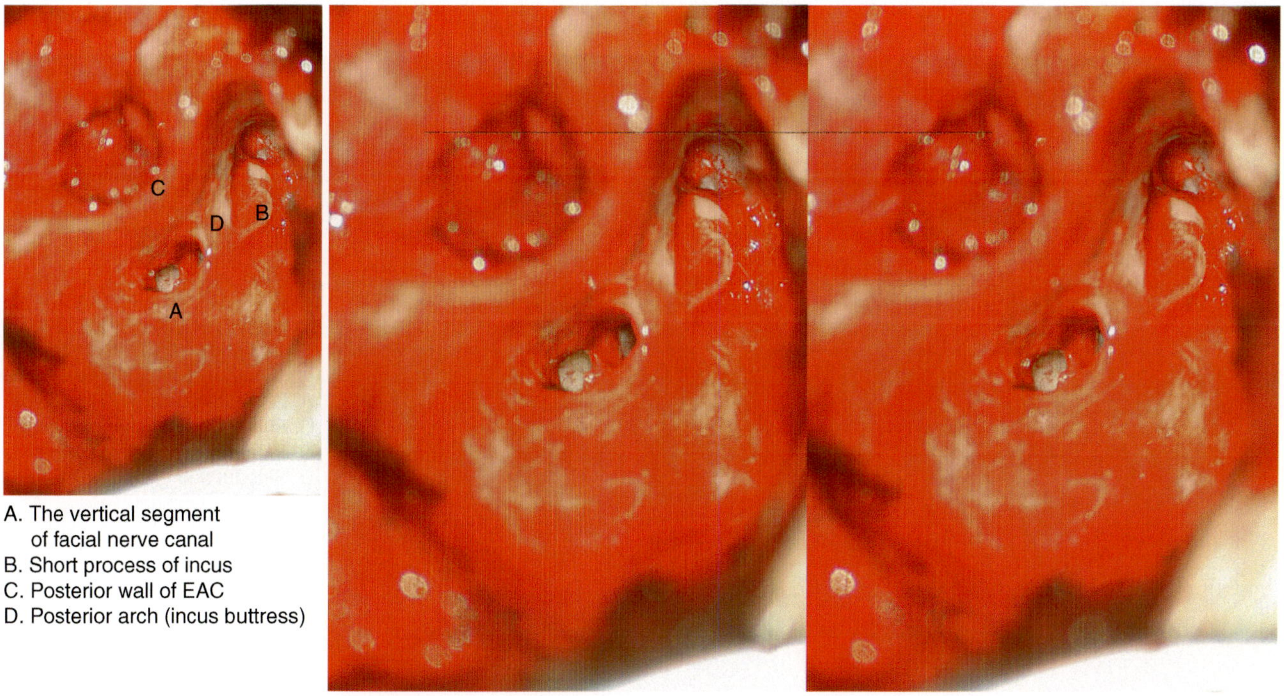

Fig. 2.134 The operative cavity with complete eradication of disease
The operative cavity is seen after complete removal of disease from the attic (both lateral and medial to the ossicles), the antrum and the posterior tympanic cavity (seen via the facial recess approach). The middle ear structures were normal. The pars tensa of the tympanic membrane was intact in this case and the perforation of parts flaccida was repaired with a small piece of fascia

Surgery 2: Intact Canal Wall Mastoidectomy, myringoplasty, and ossiculoplasty with prosthesis

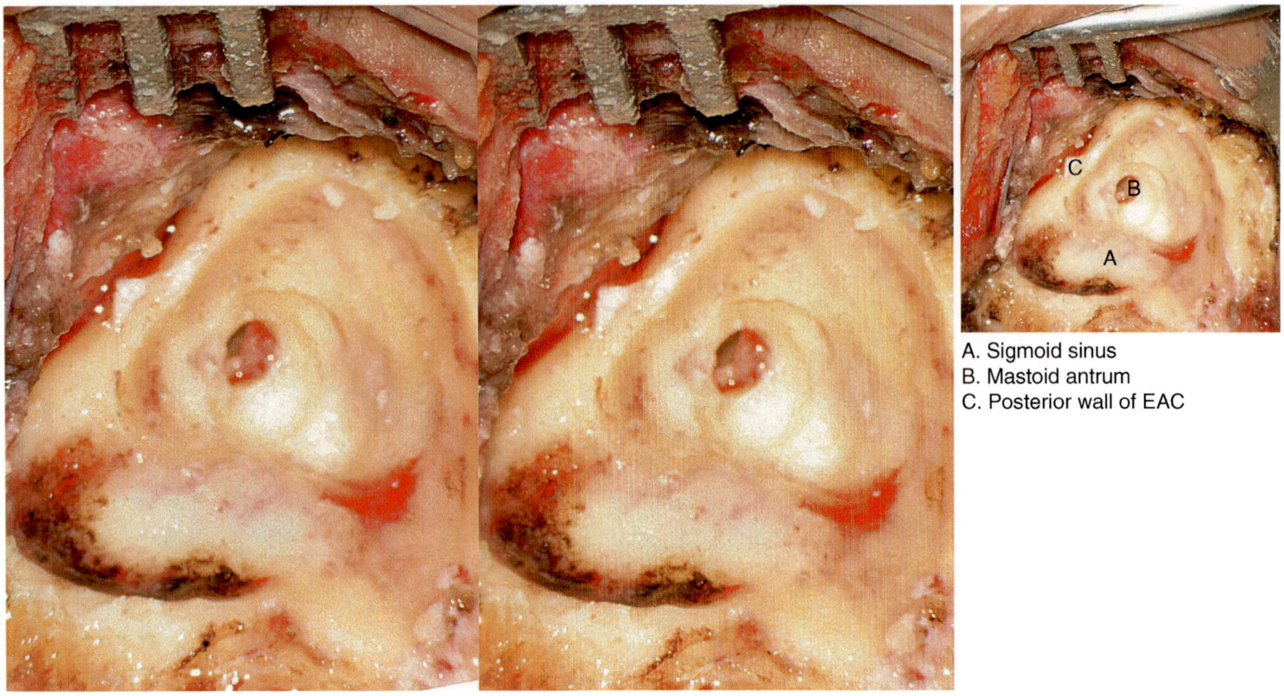

Fig. 2.135 Opening the mastoid antrum
This is a diploic mastoid and a small amount of inflammatory granuloma is seen in the aditus ad antrum

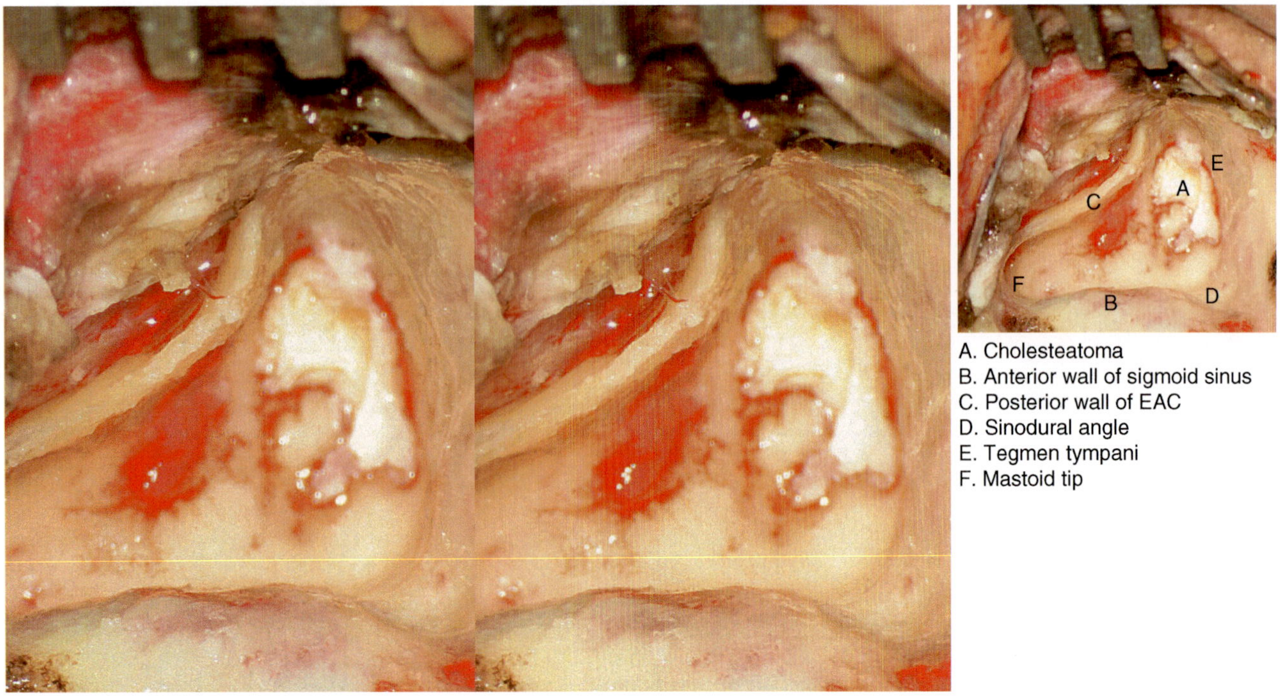

Fig. 2.136 Opening the attic and fashioning the mastoid cavity
In a diploic or poorly developed mastoid the tegmen mastoideum, tegmen tympani and postero-superior wall of EAC all need to be thinned down maximally to obtain the best exposure. The anterior position of the sigmoid sinus and the attic cholesteatoma can be seen

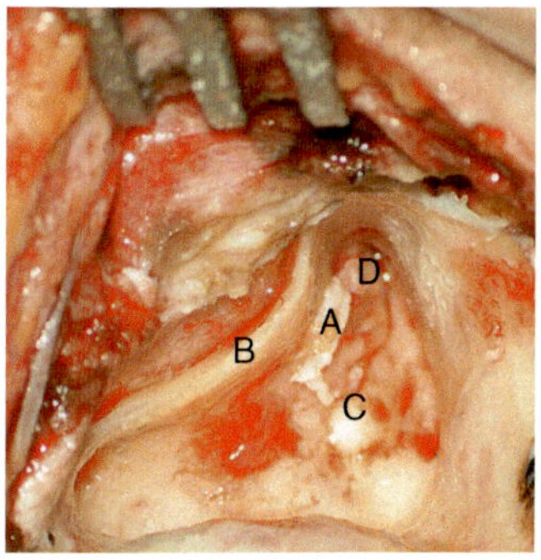

A. Cholesteatoma
B. Posterior wall of EAC
C. Lateral semicircular canal
D. Anterior attic

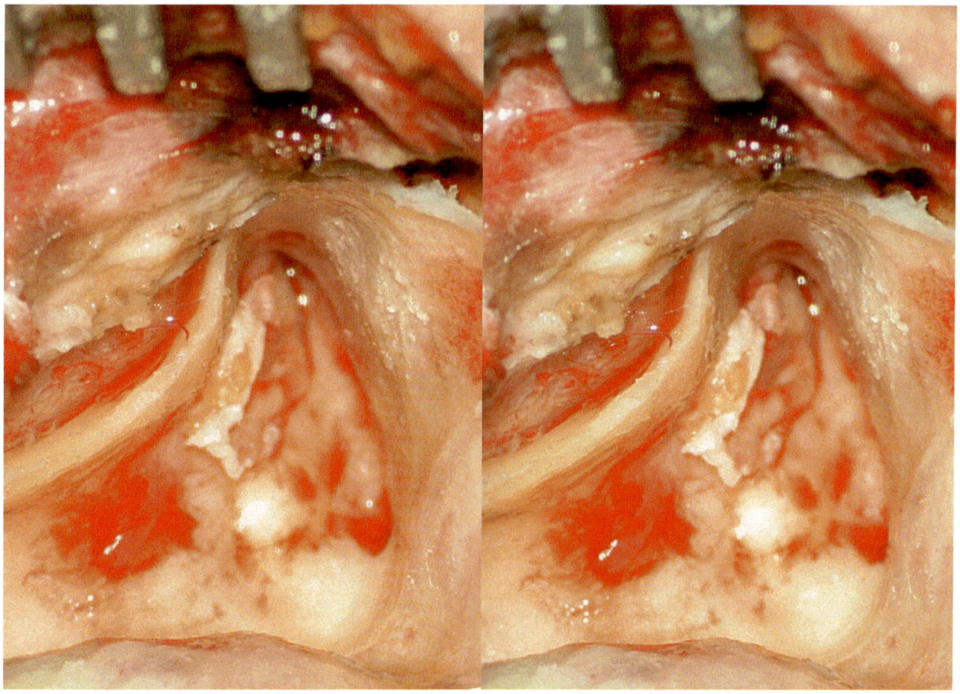

Fig. 2.137 Exploration of the attic
The ossicles are surrounded by cholesteatoma in the attic. This must be completely removed from the ossicles in a posterior and superior direction using a delicate technique to minimize trauma to the ossicular chain

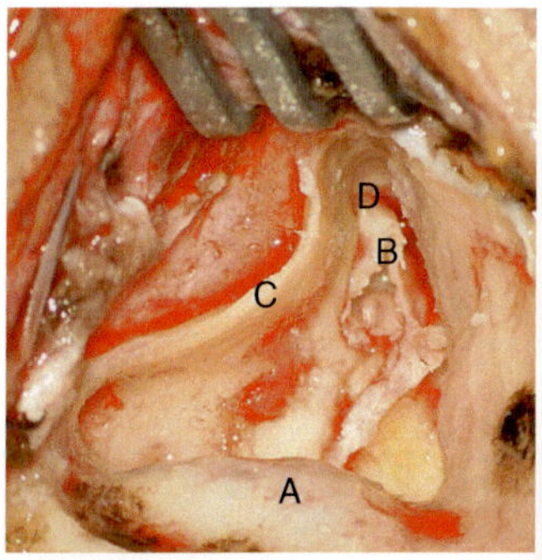

A. Sigmoid sinus
B. Cholesteatoma
C. Posterior wall of EAC
D. Anterior attic

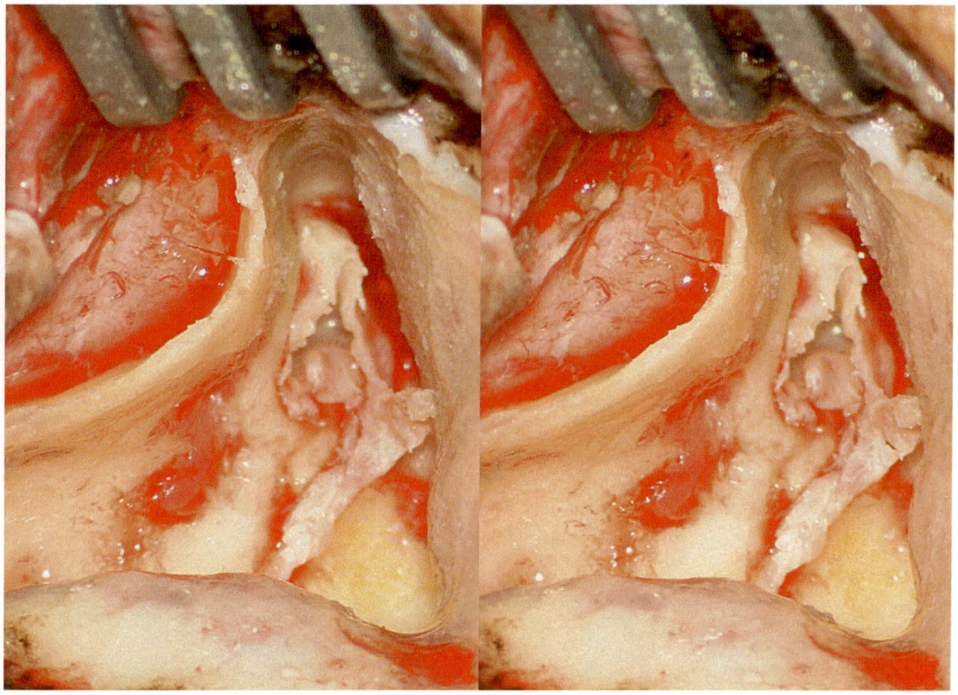

Fig. 2.138 Exploration of the anterior epitympanic recess
After separation of the incudo-stapedial joint, the incus is removed. The neck of the malleus is then cut and the head is removed. This allows removal of cholesteatoma from medial to the malleus in the middle ear and attic

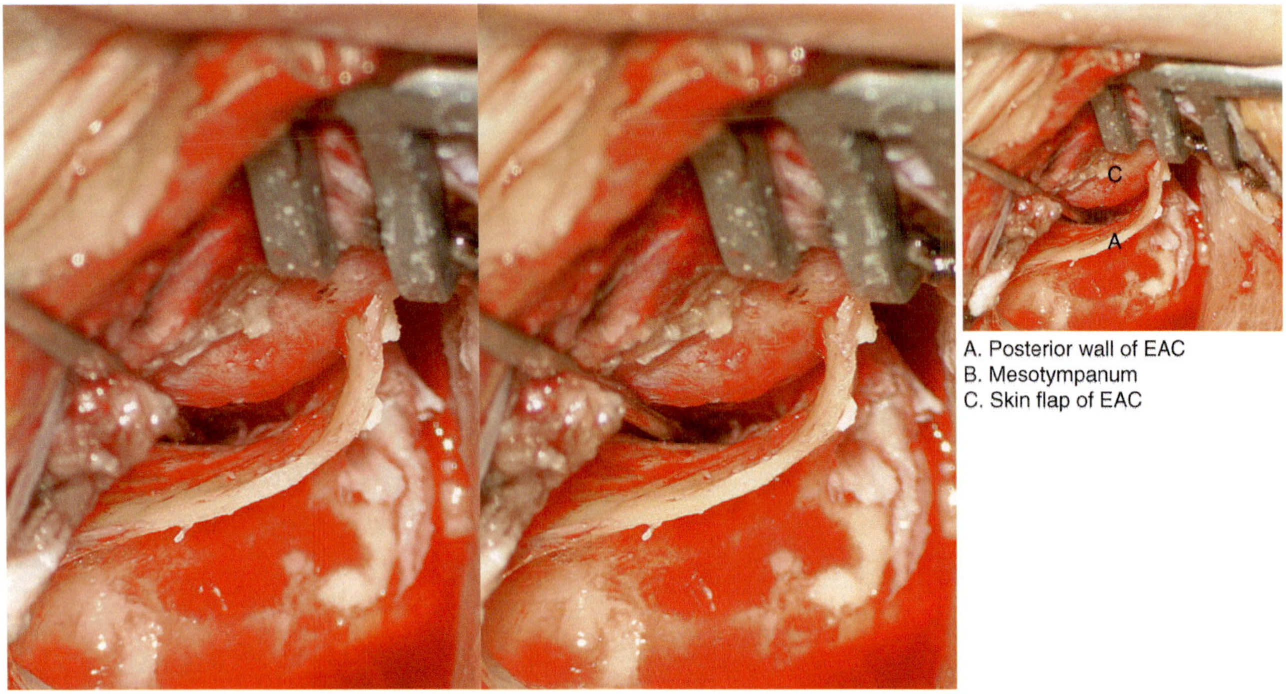

Fig. 2.139 Exploration of the middle ear via EAC.
Elevate the skip flap of EAC to the annulus then elevate the tympanic membrane to enter the mesotympanum. Using this approach, the chorda tympani nerve can be usually preserved and the mesotympanum and hypotympanum can be explored for disease

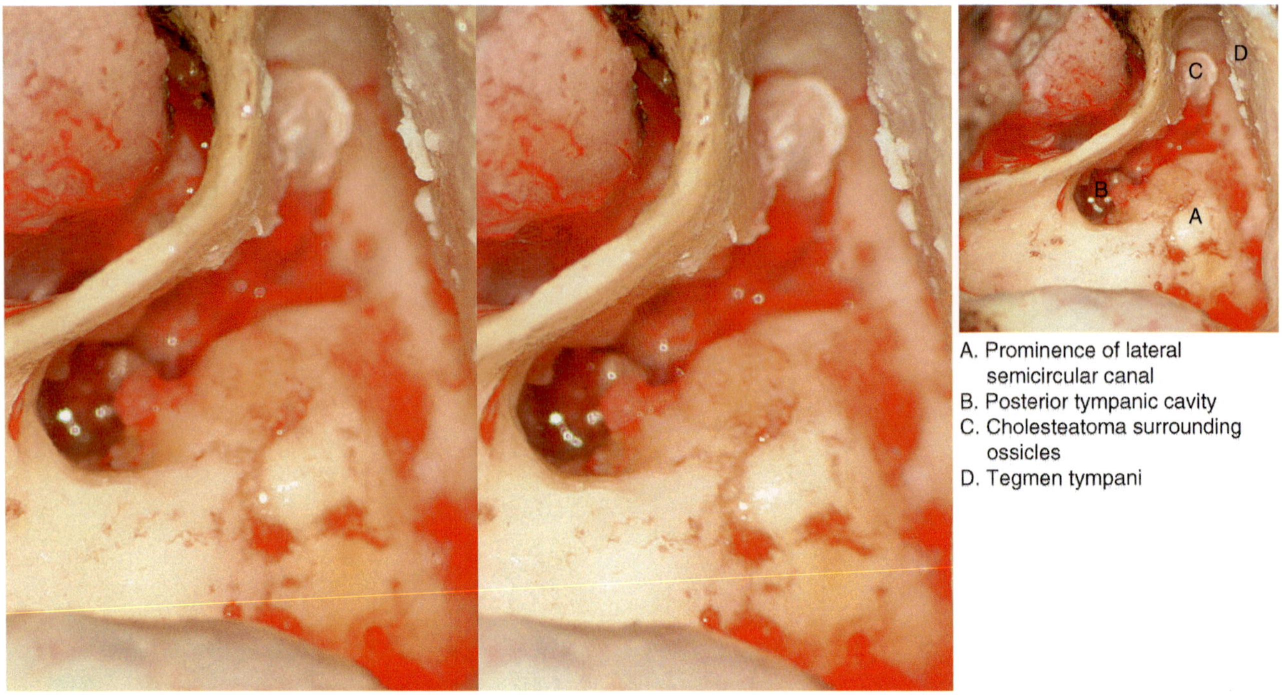

Fig. 2.140 Exposure of the posterior tympanic cavity via a facial recess approach
The posterior tympanic cavity cannot be adequately explored via the EAC. A facial recess approach with removal of the incus buttress was used to widely expose the area. Cholesteatoma and inflammatory granuloma were seen to extend down from the attic

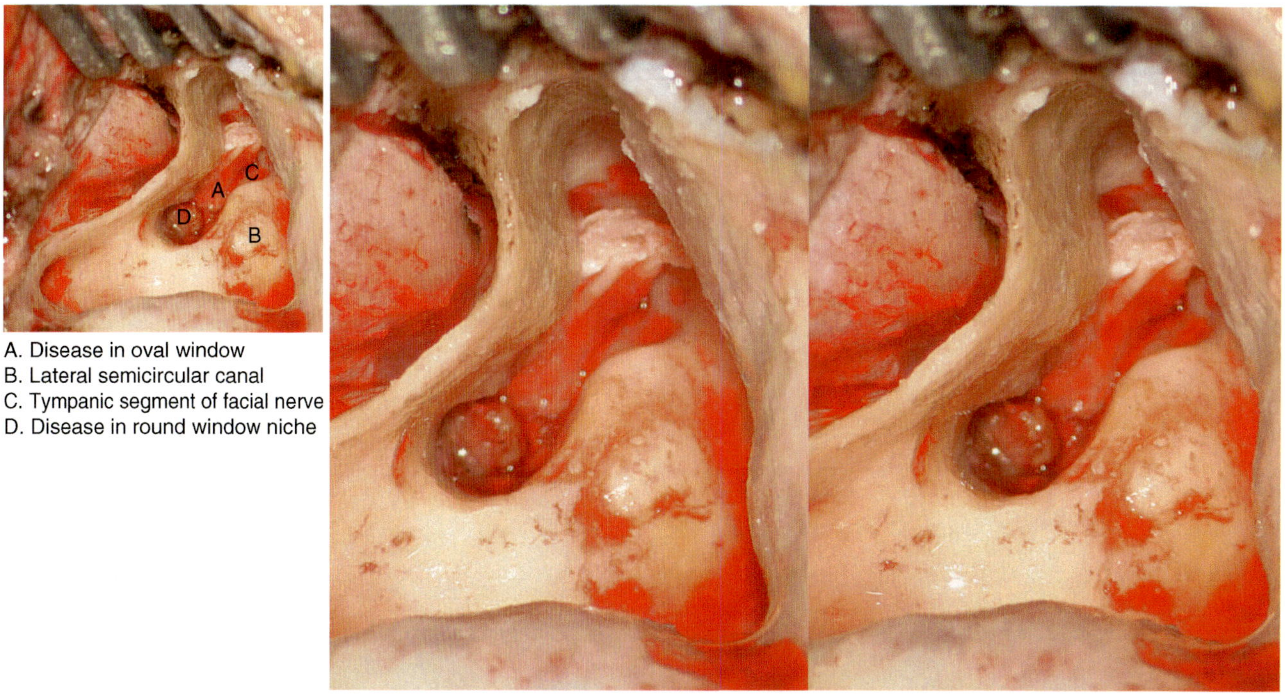

A. Disease in oval window
B. Lateral semicircular canal
C. Tympanic segment of facial nerve
D. Disease in round window niche

Fig. 2.141 Exploration of the posterior tympanic cavity
The posterior arch (incus buttress) has been removed completely to aid visualization of the oval window and posterior tympanic cavity. Bone over the facial nerve has been removed more inferiorly to expose the round window niche and hypotympanum. This allowed removal of cholesteatoma from these areas and exposure of the stapes

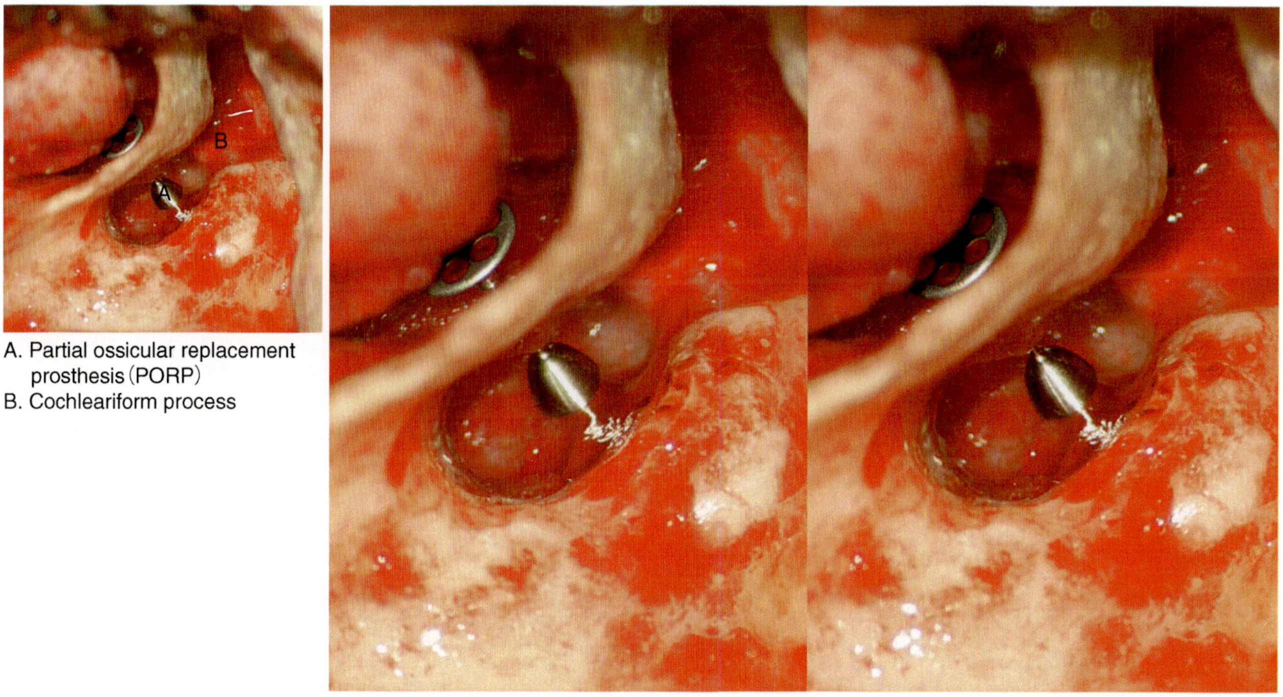

A. Partial ossicular replacement prosthesis (PORP)
B. Cochleariform process

Fig. 2.142 Tympanoplasty
The mucosa on the medial wall of mesotympanum was seen to be intact after removal of all cholesteatoma. The cochleariform process was identified. The stapes was seen to be intact and mobile. The tympanic membrane (TM) defect was then repaired with fascia
Reconstruction of the ossicular chain: The incus and malleus were absent whilst the stapes was intact and mobile. The distance from the head the stapes to the TM was measured. A PORP was trimmed to the correct length and placed on the stapes, with the cup-shaped end on the stapes head and the disc-shaped top under the TM

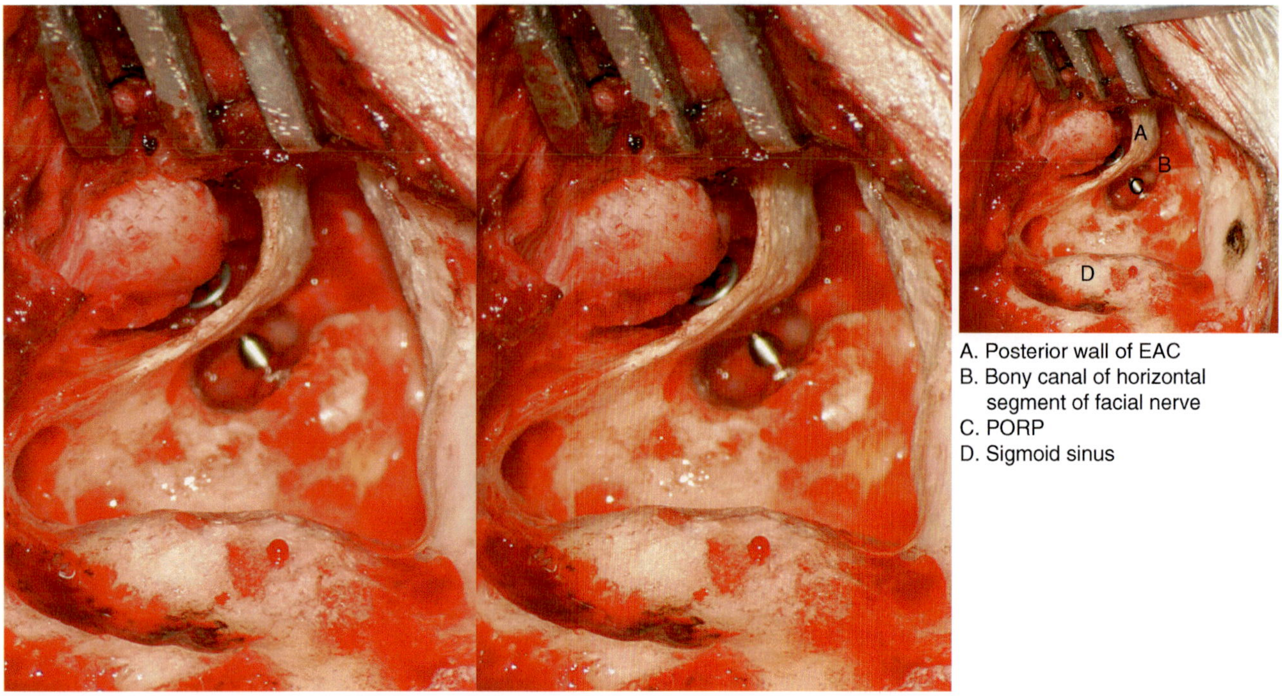

Fig. 2.143 Operative cavity of intact wall mastoidectomy with tympanoplasty
The intact wall mastoidectomy with tympanoplasty is almost complete. The mastoidectomy cavity extends anteriorly to the anterior epitympanic recess, posteriorly to the sinodural angle and inferiorly to the mastoid tip. The eradication of disease and repair of the tympanic membrane and ossicular chain have been accomplished by using the combined-approach through the EAC and facial recess approach via the mastoid

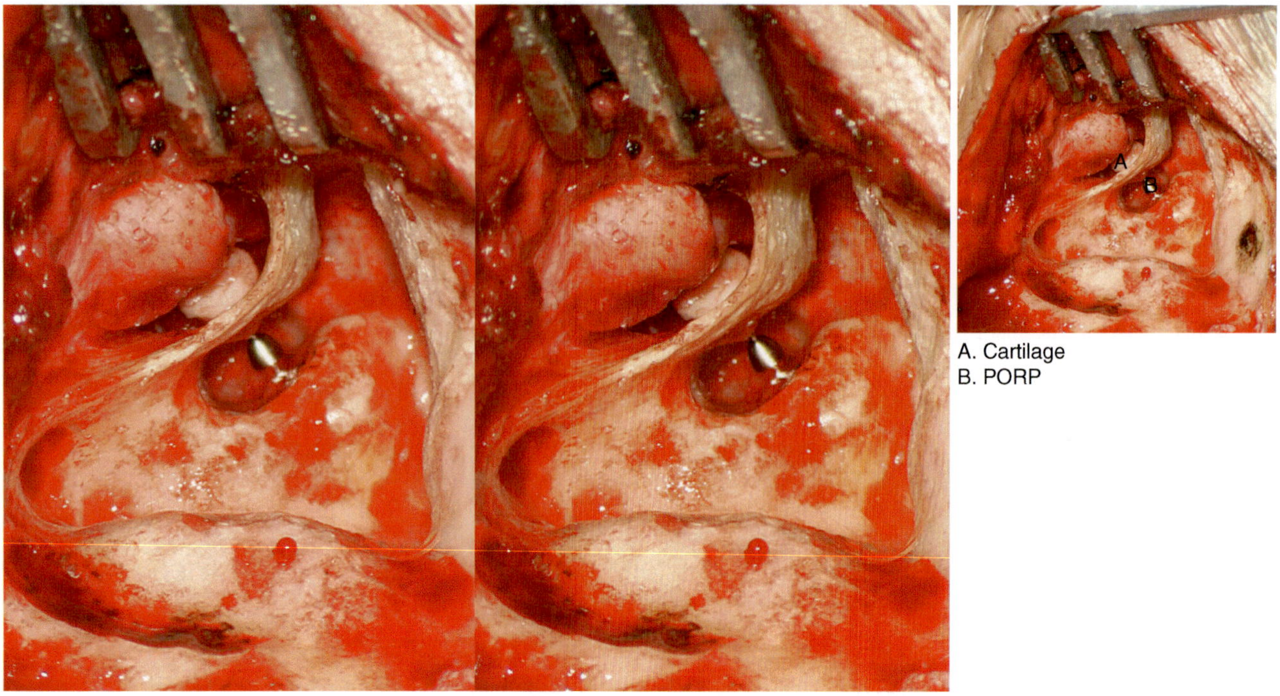

Fig. 2.144 Placement of cartilage disc between TM and prosthesis
A small disc of cartilage has been taken from the tragus. This is placed between the prosthesis and the TM to prevent later extrusion. It also assists in maintaining stability of the PORP

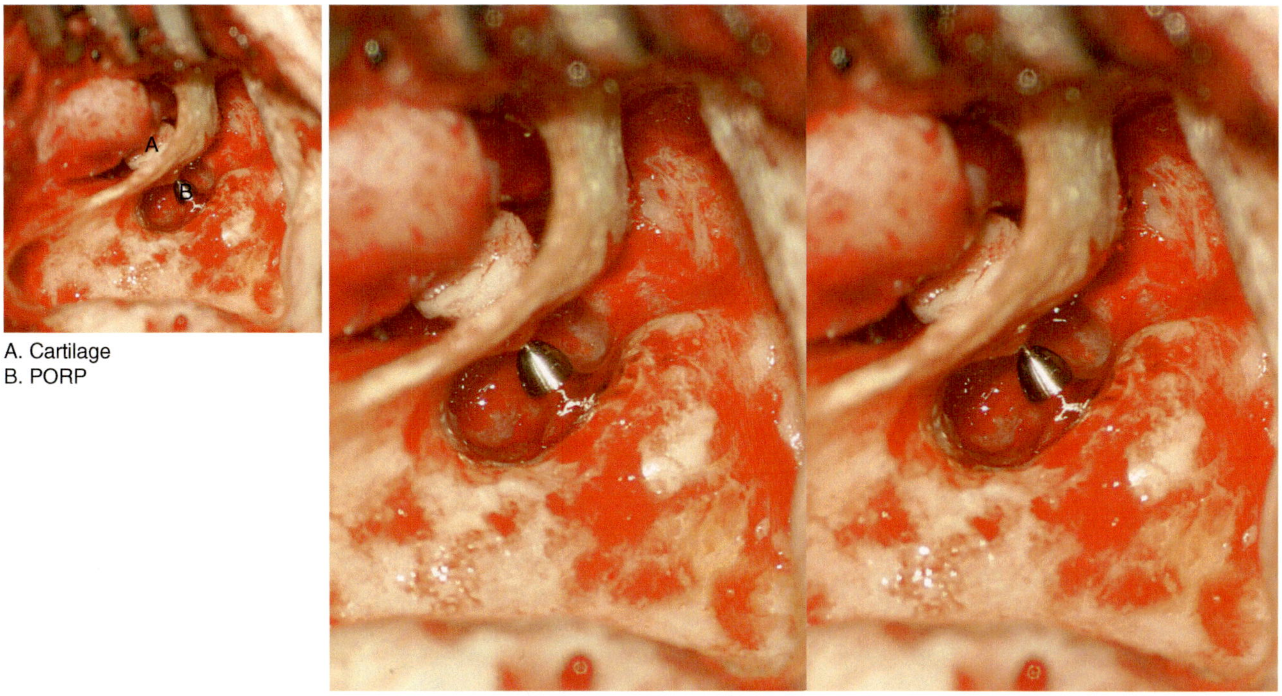

Fig. 2.145 Placement of cartilage disc between TM and prosthesis (High power)
The cartilage should be well-sized and must cover the entire top of the PORP

Surgery 3: Intact Canal Wall Mastoidectomy with preservation of the intact Ossicular Chain

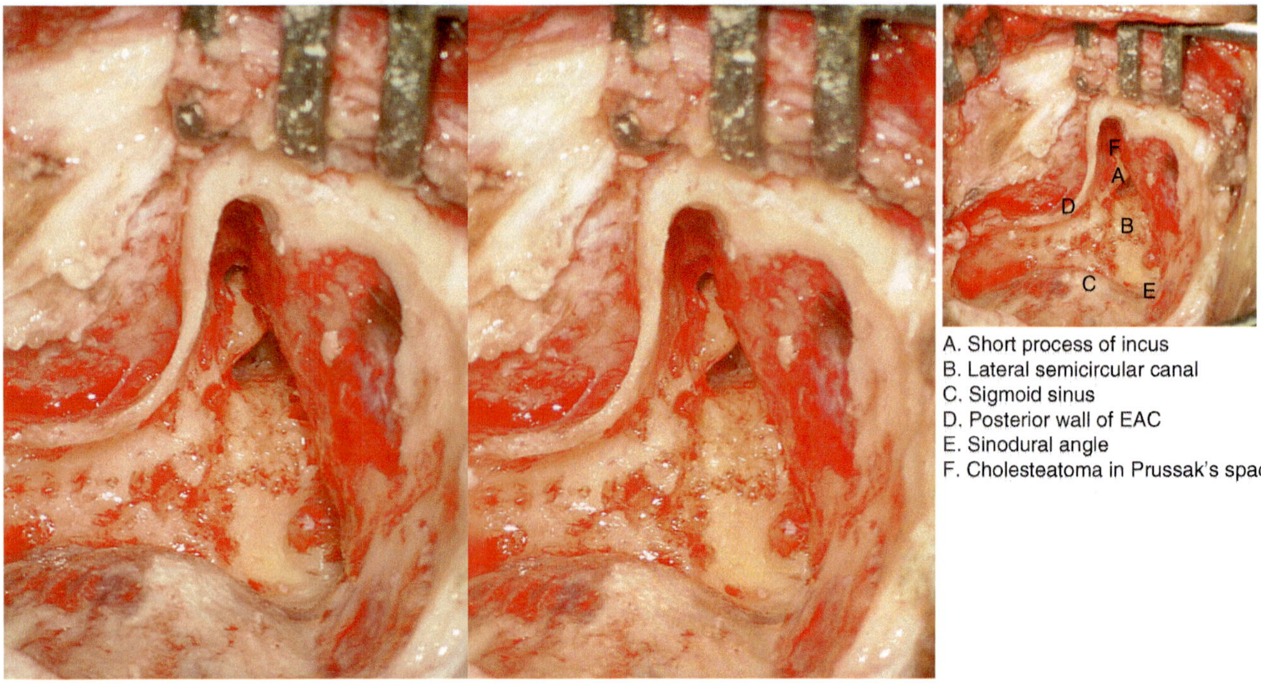

A. Short process of incus
B. Lateral semicircular canal
C. Sigmoid sinus
D. Posterior wall of EAC
E. Sinodural angle
F. Cholesteatoma in Prussak's space

Fig. 2.146 Exposure of the incus and fashioning the mastoid cavity
Intact canal wall mastoidectomy is usually used in cases of limited attic, middle ear or mastoid disease without erosion the ossicular chain. In this case, the attic lesion has been removed while a small amount of cholesteatoma was seen in Prussak's space

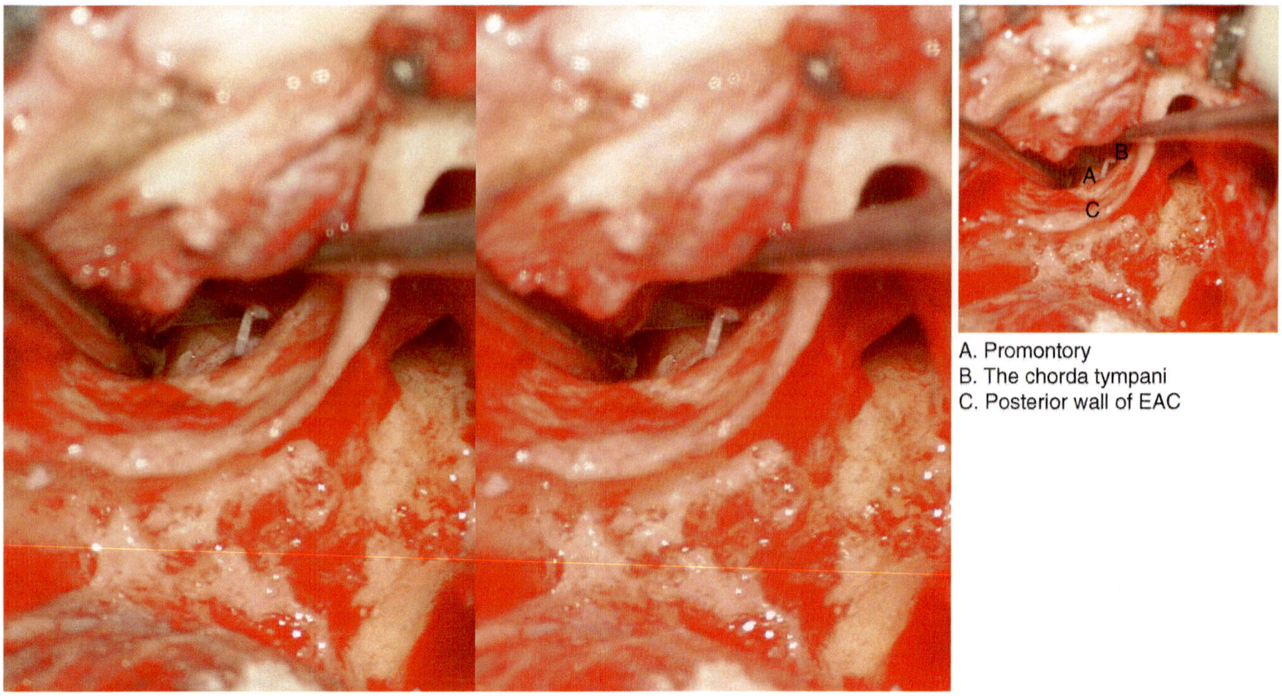

A. Promontory
B. The chorda tympani
C. Posterior wall of EAC

Fig. 2.147 Exploration of the tympanic cavity via a post-auricular approach
This surgery usually requires exploration of the tympanic cavity. The TM has been elevated anteriorly to show the intact pars tensa and separated chorda tympani. The diseases in the pars flaccida and Prussak's space can be eradicated by a combined approach through EAC and attic

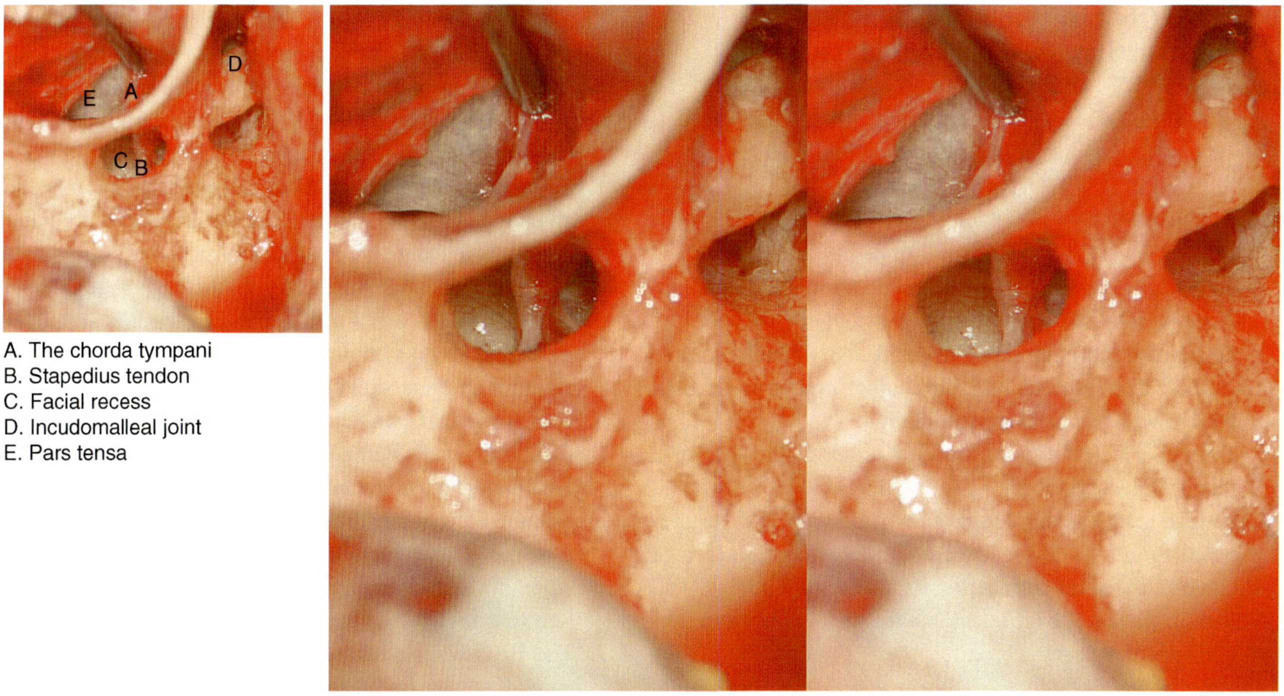

A. The chorda tympani
B. Stapedius tendon
C. Facial recess
D. Incudomalleal joint
E. Pars tensa

Fig. 2.148 Exploration of the posterior tympanic cavity through facial recess
Exploration via the facial recess identified no disease in the posterior tympanic cavity. The ossicular chain was shown to be intact and mobile

Mastoid Obliteration, Canal Wall Reconstruction and Tympanoplasty

Bing Han, Pu Dai

Indications

1. To avoid cholesteatoma recurrence and maintain an adequate middle ear space post-operatively;
2. To avoid the formation of a mastoid cavity which requires regular cleaning and may have other problems such as vertigo with temperature stimulation;
3. To enable hearing reconstruction either at the first or a second stage operation.
4. Patient must undergo long term follow-up and be prepared for a second look operation if there is concern of cholesteatoma recurrence;
5. Patient wishes to expose ear to water. Patient wants a normal appearing ear;

Contraindications

1. Inability to ensure complete clearance of cholesteatoma;
2. Patients are not able to undergo long term follow-up. Patients are not concerned about hearing.
3. Extensive disease or severe complication identified pre-operatively.
4. Patient unable to tolerate multiple procedures.

Operative Procedures

1. Make incision in the hair line, harvest a generous piece of temporalis fascia and place it in alcohol for dehydration. Periosteum from the tragus or conchal cartilage can be used as an alternative;
2. A posterior or endaural incision can be used, with the soft tissues dissected from the surface of the mastoid;
3. Bone can be removed via the antrum or by enlarging the postero-superior part of the EAC. Care must be taken to avoid facial nerve injury;
4. The middle ear cleft is exposed and cholesteatoma is removed thoroughly. The cholesteatoma must be cleared completely from surface of bone or mucous membrane. This is done by dissecting from above down and from below up to the oval window, finally clear disease around the stapes. Care must be taken to avoid opening the inner ear. Healthy mucous membrane is preserved.
5. The lateral wall of the attic is removed to expose the ossicular chain. If the incudo-stapedial joint is intact, it is separated to avoid inner ear injury. The operated cavity should extend from the anterior attic wall, along the tegmen tympani without exposure of the middle cranial fossa (MCF) dura to the mastoid cavity behind.
6. Fashioning the mastoid cavity. Under the microscope, all involved mastoid air cells are exenterated with reducing drills size until all cholesteatoma has been removed. Copious irrigation is used to cool the bone and keep the operative field clear for drilling. The tegmen should be smoothed above without exposure of the MCF dura. The sigmoid sinus is skeletonized posteriorly. The anterior wall is the EAC wall in a closed mastoidectomy, or the EAC if the wall is eroded or needs to be removed. When creating the mastoid cavity one may encounter Koerner's septum before exposing the antrum. The facial nerve and the lateral semicircular canal must be protected when drilling, using a diamond bur and copious irrigation when working near them.
7. The EAC wall is removed if necessary to clear all disease. If it can be preserved, the facial recess must be opened. The upper margin of the recess is the fossa incudis, its anterior border is the chorda tympanic and its posterior border is the vertical segment of the facial nerve. Once the facial recess has been adequately opened, cholesteatoma can be removed from the posterior middle ear cavity
8. Reconstruction of the lateral attic wall or external auditory canal wall: Use free cartilage, pedicled cartilage or artificial material to rebuild the attic lateral wall and/or the external canal wall to keep an adequate middle ear space. Cholesteatoma is thoroughly cleared around the stapes;
9. The temporalis fascia is laid under the tympanic membrane, the ossicular chain is reconstructed as is the external auditory canal wall. Gelfoam is placed in the middle ear and mastoid to support the grafts.
10. The patient's incus or malleus (if present) or a PORP can be used to rebuild the ossicular chain.

    If the stapes footplate is fixed, it is not opened or removed at this stage. A secondary procedure will be necessary.
11. The tympano-meatal flap is re-positioned and supported with gelfoam in the external canal as well. The canal is packed with iodoform gauze. The external meatus can be enlarged if necessary. The incisions are sutured.

Special Comments

1. Cholesteatoma must be cleared thoroughly. The attic and posterior tympanic cavity must be thoroughly checked to avoid recurrence after the operation;

2. Materials used to reconstruct the external auditory canal wall must be stable to avoid cholesteatoma recurrence and to maintain an open middle ear cavity;
3. Any free bone grafts or artificial material must be covered to avoid sequestrum formation or extrusion;
4. Long term regular review is required post-operatively. A temporal bone CT or MRI scan may also be helpful in identifying recurrence. A second operation should be undertaken promptly when a recurrence is found early or a long time after the original surgery;

Complications

1. Facial paralysis: this I more likely if the anatomic landmarks are not clear or when anatomical anomalies are present. The nerve needs to be clearly identified to avoid intra-operative injury;
2. Medial displacement of the reconstructed external auditory canal wall: ensure the transplant material used o reconstruct the wall is firmly fixed to prevent displacement;
3. Cholesteatoma recurrence: this can be due to inadequate initial clearance. Collapse of the reconstructed wall may also allow recurrence of cholesteatoma. Good initial surgery and long term regular follow-up are necessary.

Surgery 1: Closed mastoidectomy with tympanoplasty and reconstruction of the external auditory canal

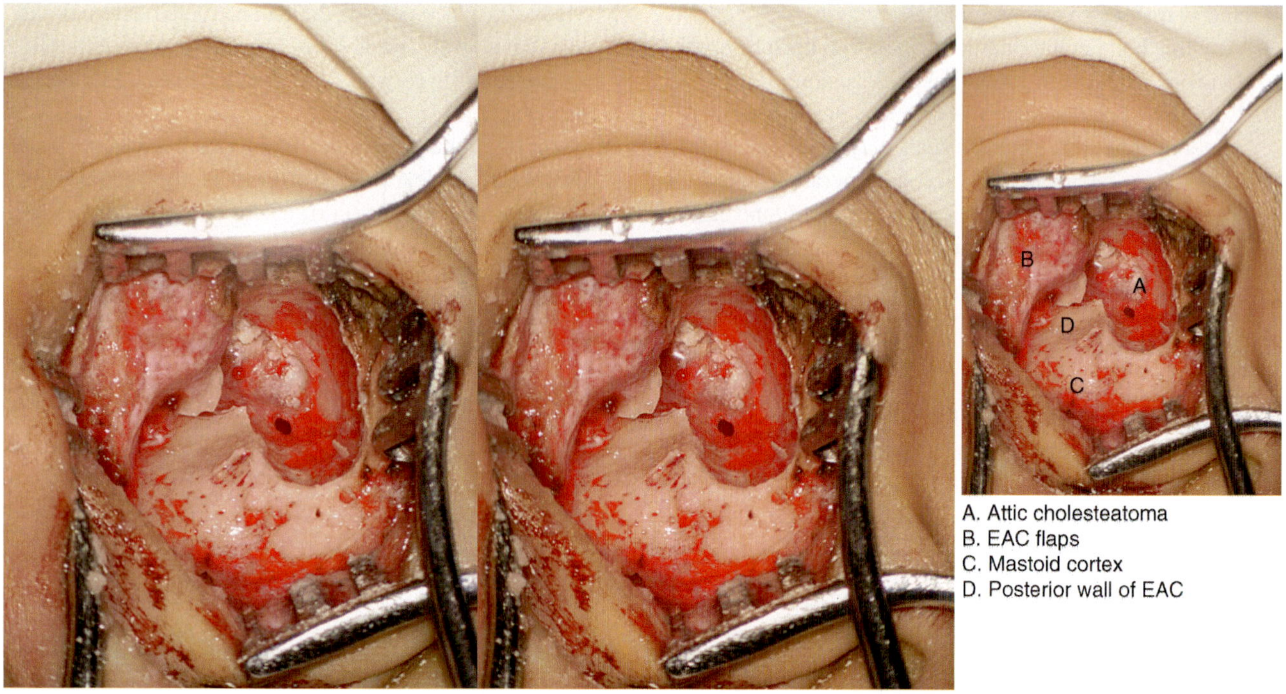

Fig. 2.149 Attic exposure
If cholesteatoma is limited in the attic or the mastoid is diploic, the attic can be opened directly from the external auditory canal. The tympanomeatal flap is elevated. The postero-superior external auditory canal, the cribriform area and mastoid cortex are exposed. The lateral wall of the attic is drilled away to expose the cholesteatoma. The tympanic antrum is also opened out posteriorly

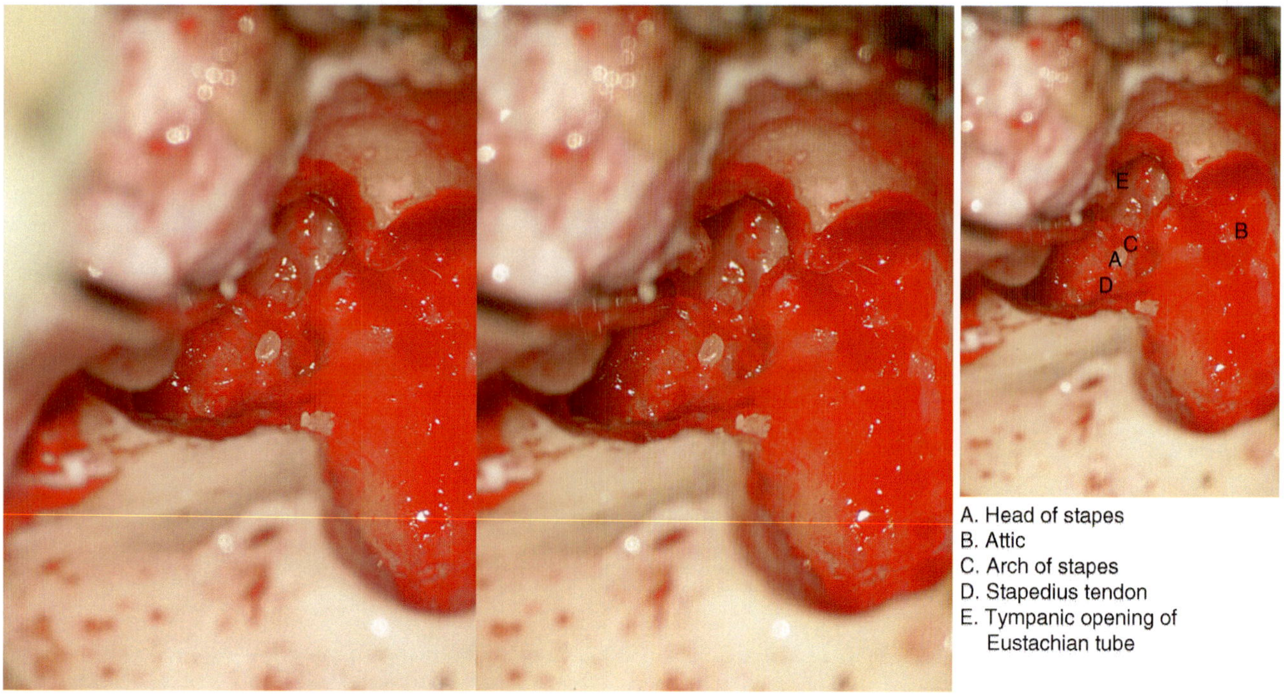

Fig. 2.150 Clearance of attic cholesteatoma and exposure of ossicular chain
Thorough clearance of attic cholesteatoma. The pars tensa is elevated to expose the middle ear contents. The malleus and incus are absent but the stapes is intact and mobile. The middle ear mucosa was normal and the tympanic opening of the Eustachian tube was free of disease

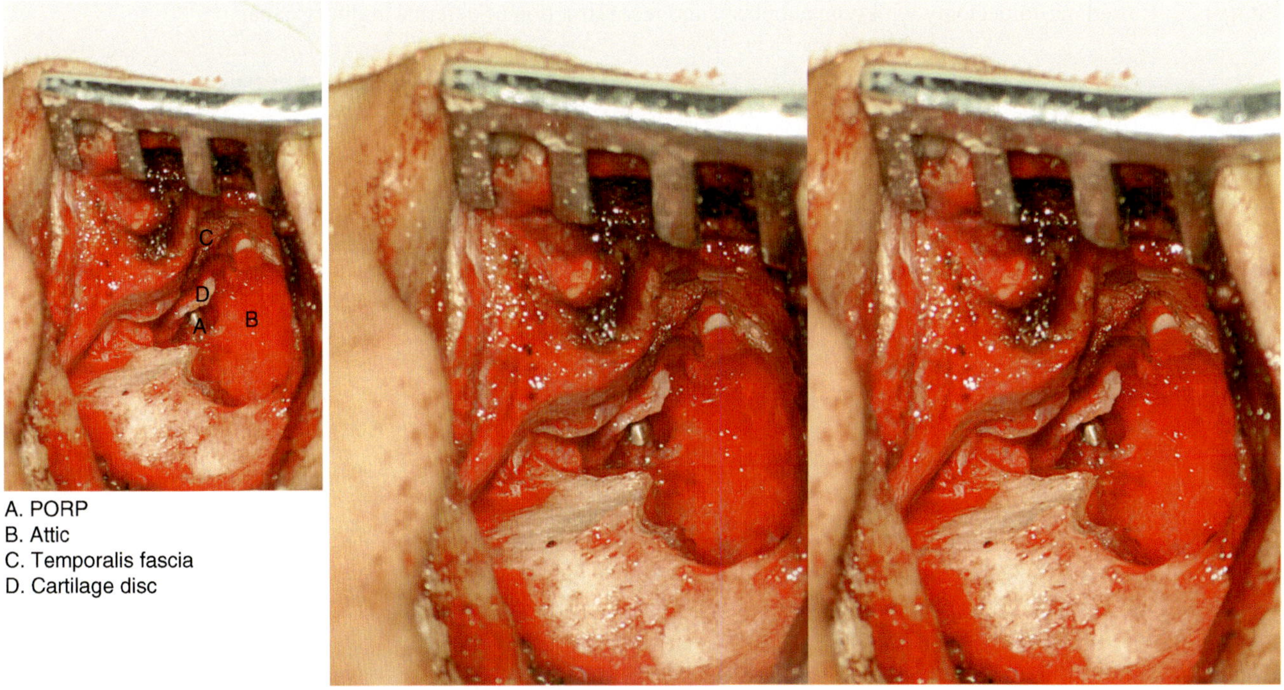

Fig. 2.151 Insertion of PORP and reconstruction of the tympanic membrane
A slot is drilled in the external auditory canal wall to hold the cartilage flap. The PORP is positioned between the head of stapes and temporalis fascial graft. A cartilage disc is placed between the top of the PORP and the fascia

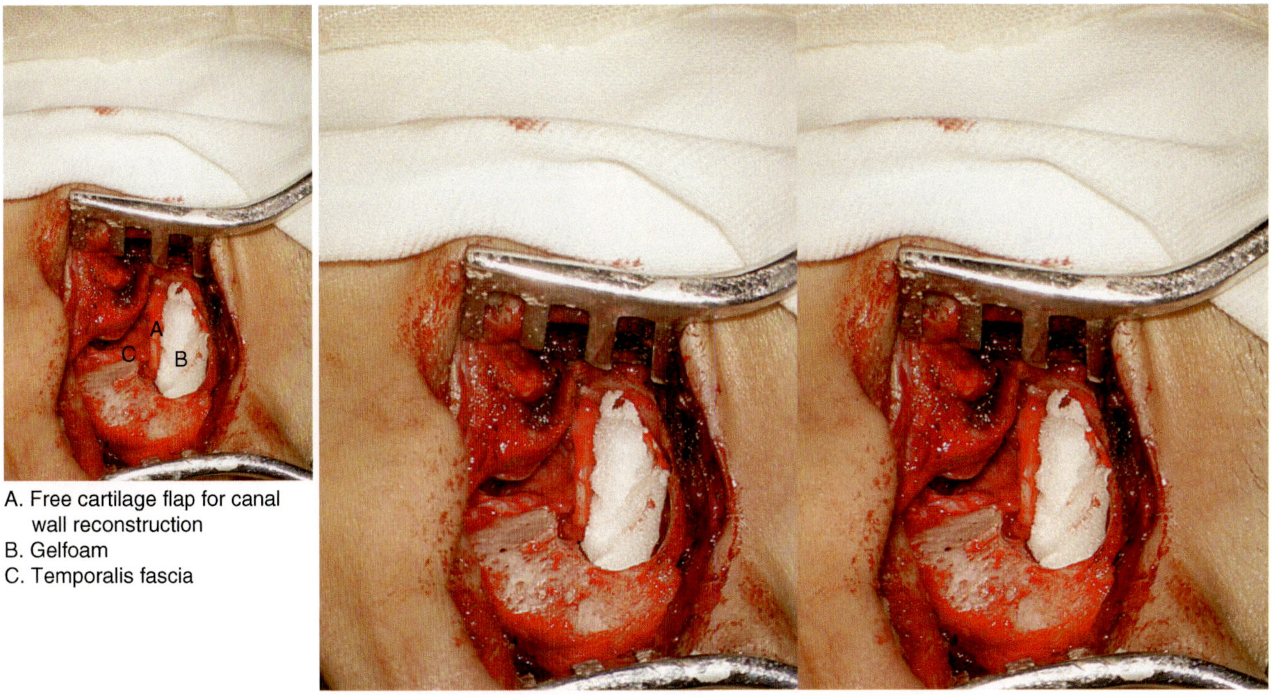

Fig. 2.152 Reconstruct lateral attic and superior external auditory canal walls
The cartilage flap is placed in the bone slot made in external auditory canal and fill the attic with gelfoam. Temporalis fascia covers this and the tympano-meatal flap is re-positioned. The external canal is packed with iodoform gauze. The incision is then sutured

Surgery 2: Closed mastoidectomy with tympanoplasty and reconstruction of external auditory canal

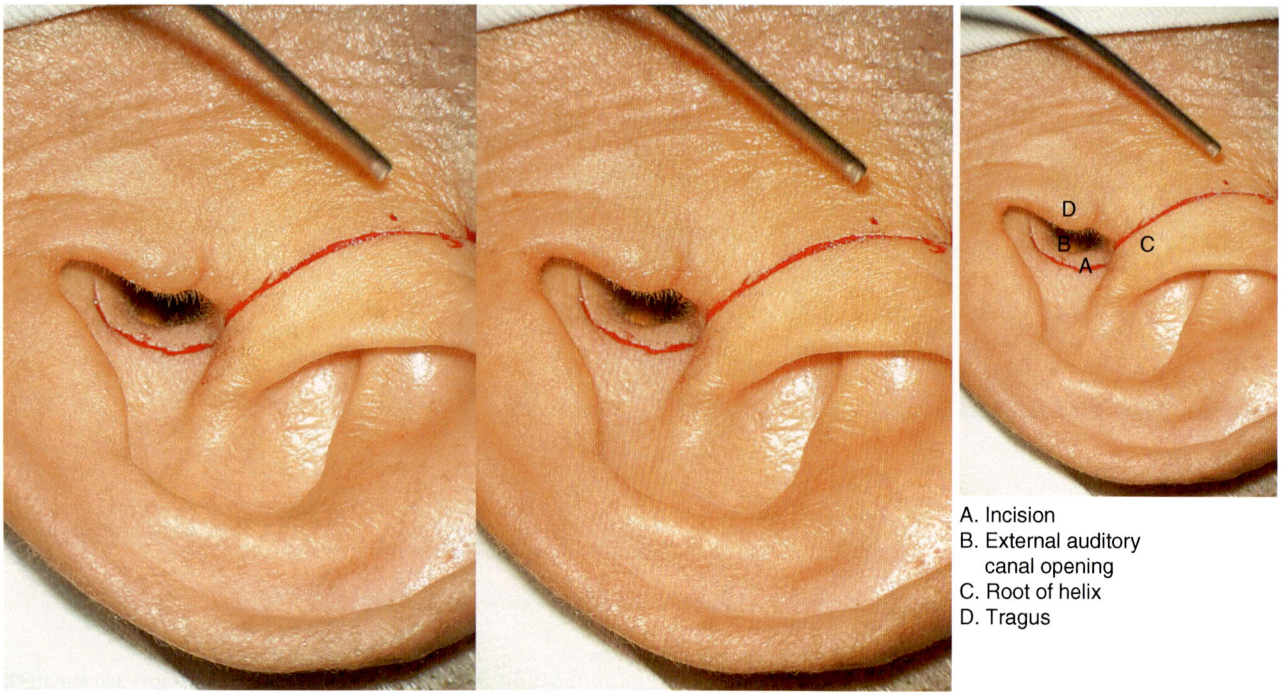

A. Incision
B. External auditory canal opening
C. Root of helix
D. Tragus

Fig. 2.153 Incision
The endaural incision is extended into the external canal. The subcutaneous tissues are extensively removed

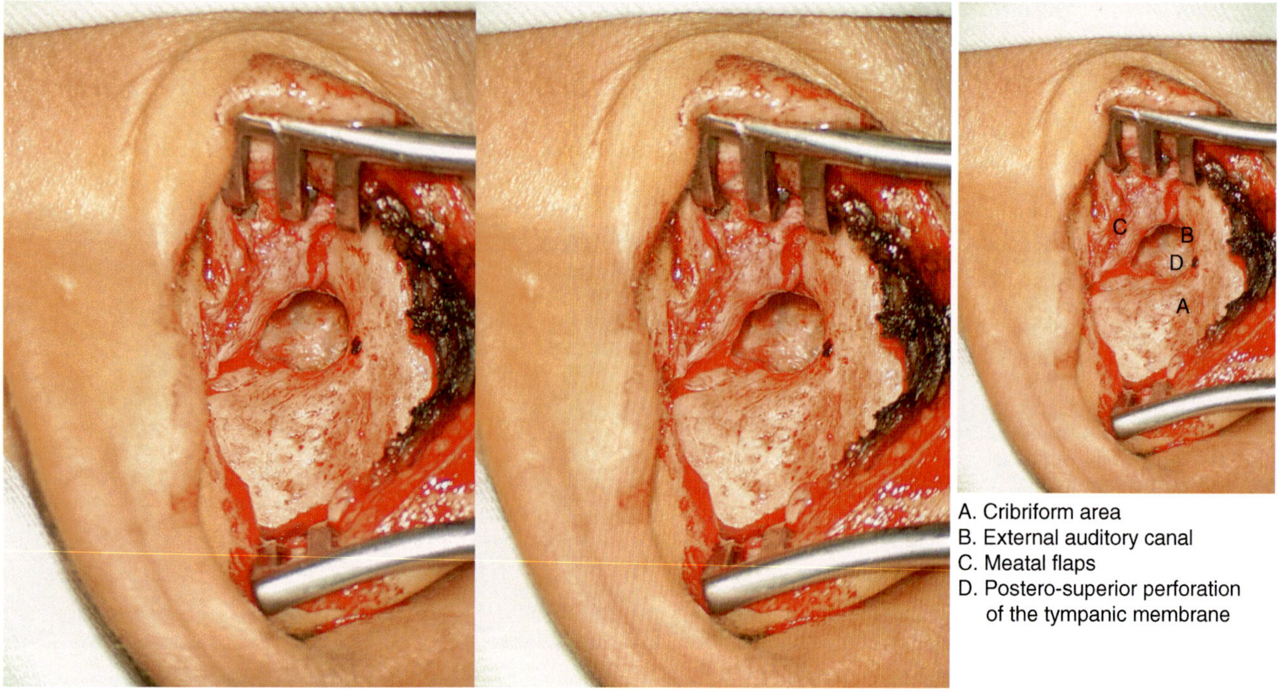

A. Cribriform area
B. External auditory canal
C. Meatal flaps
D. Postero-superior perforation of the tympanic membrane

Fig. 2.154 Exposure of the middle ear cavity
Remove the soft tissues from the back of the meatal flaps, in order to expose mastoid cortex, the root of the zygoma, the cribriform area and mastoid tip clearly. The perforation of tympanic membrane was in the postero-superior quadrant with epithelium extending to the attic and mastoid

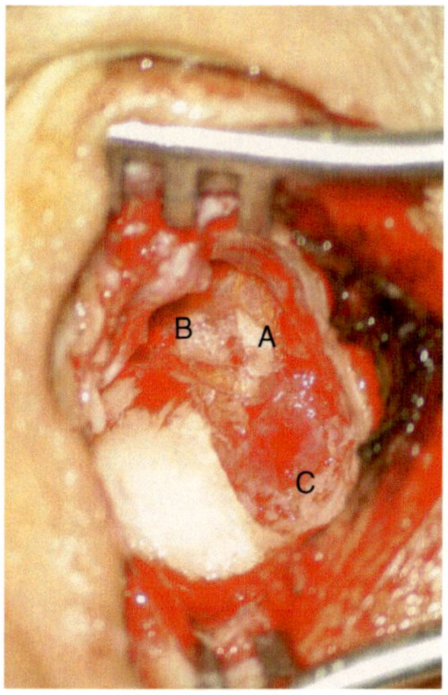

A. Epithelium in attic
B. Residual tympanic membrane
C. Mastoid antrum

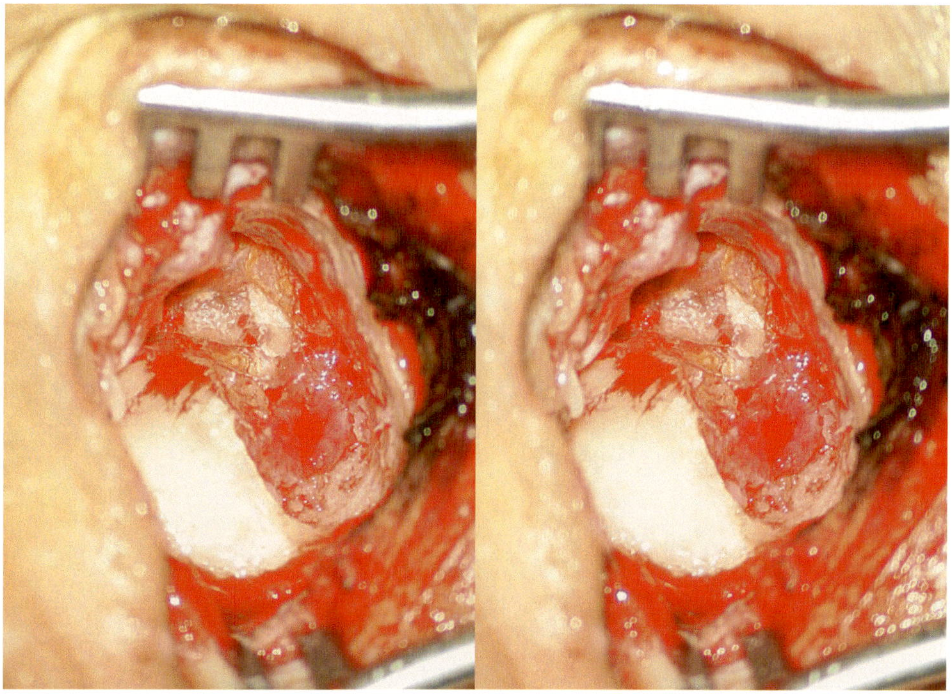

Fig. 2.155 Attic opening
On drilling away the lateral attic wall, cholesteatoma is seen to fill the attic. The mastoid antrum has been opened posteriorly to identify the incus and erosion of the mastoid

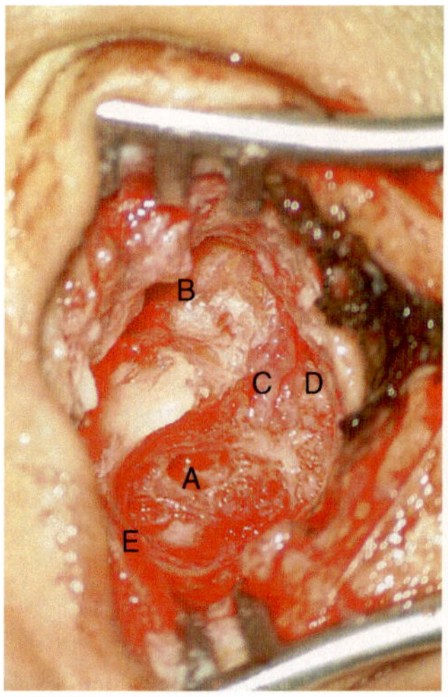

A. Mastoid cavity
B. Residual tympanic membrane
C. Incus
D. Attic
E. Mastoid tip

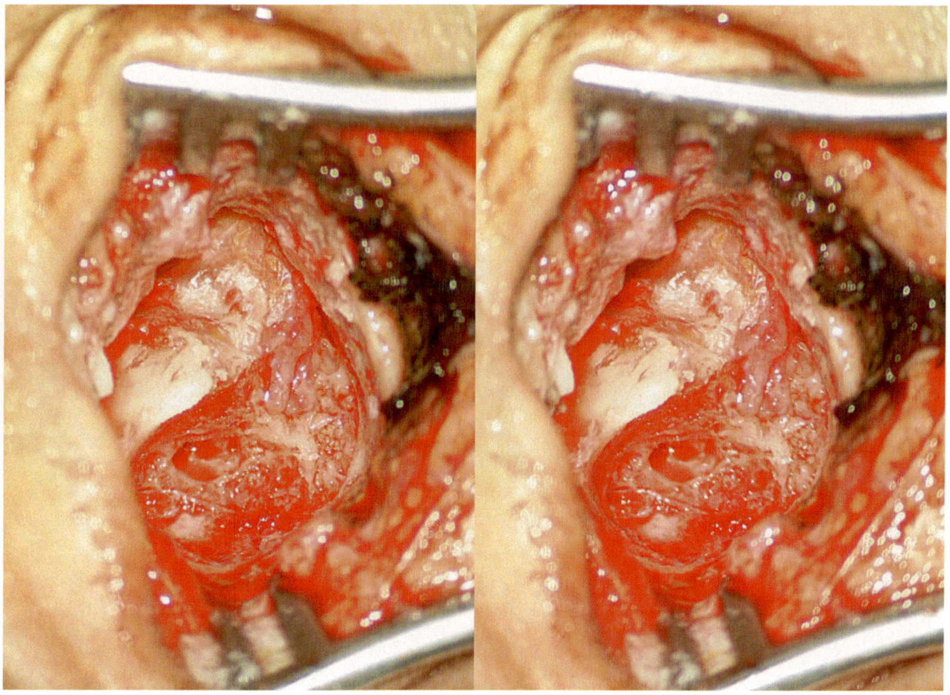

Fig. 2.156 Fashioning of mastoid cavity
The mastoid cavity is created with drilling of air cells and complete clearance of cholesteatoma

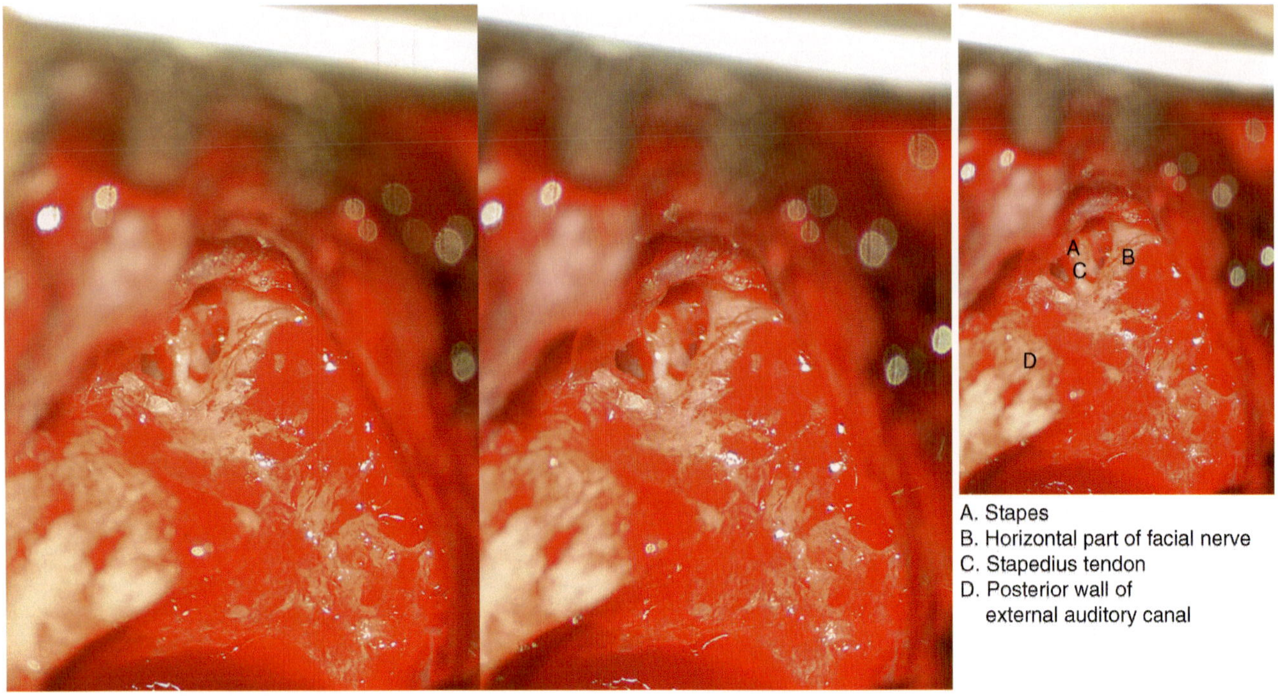

Fig. 2.157 Removal of incus and exposure of stapes
The incus is removed to expose the stapes. The stapes was intact and mobile. The middle ear cavity, attic and mastoid were seen to be free of cholesteatoma

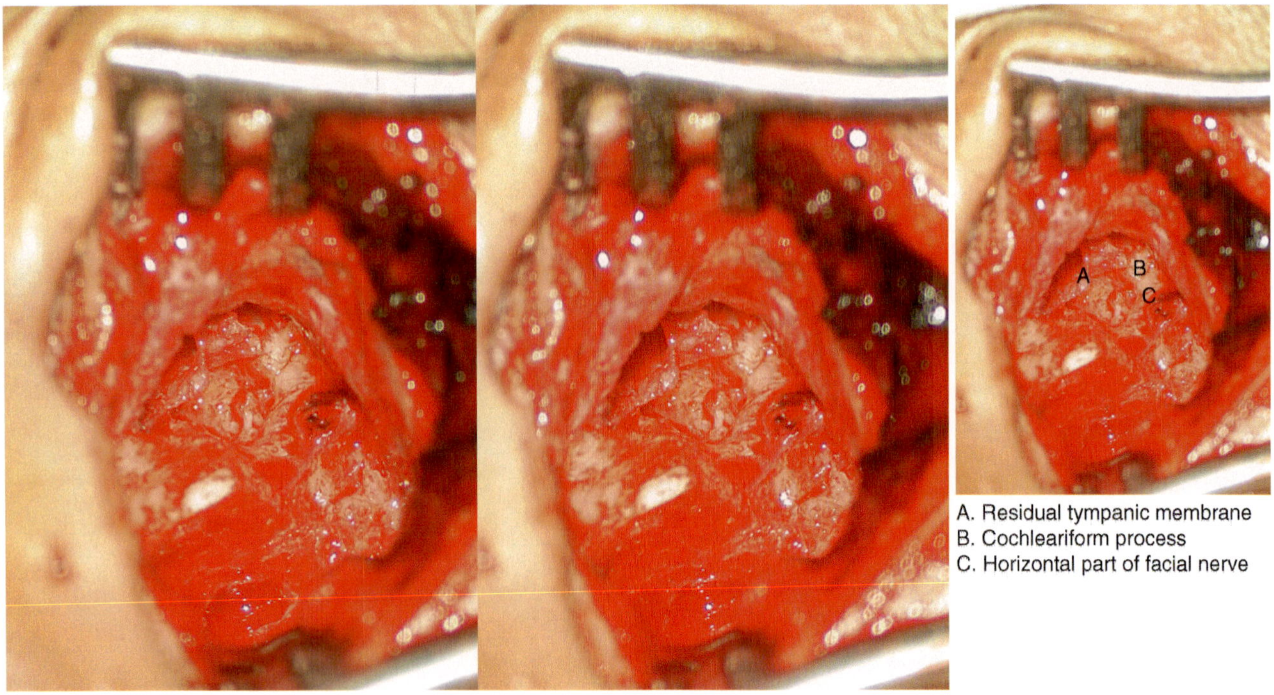

Fig. 2.158 Repair of tympanic membrane with temporalis fascia
The temporalis fascia is used to completely cover the tympanic membrane perforation on its medial side

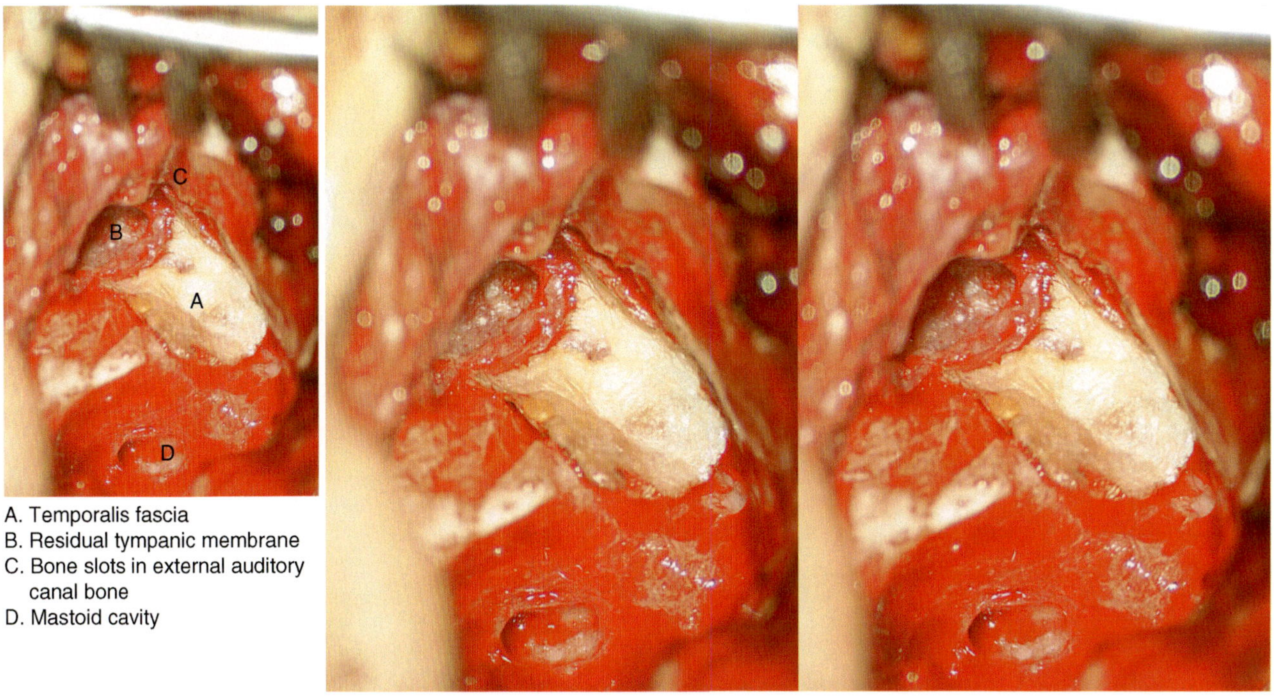

Fig. 2.159 Repair tympanic membrane with temporalis fascia
Perforation of tympanic membrane was repaired by temporalis fascia, and it's better to cover part of cartilage graft that was used for external ear canal reconstruction

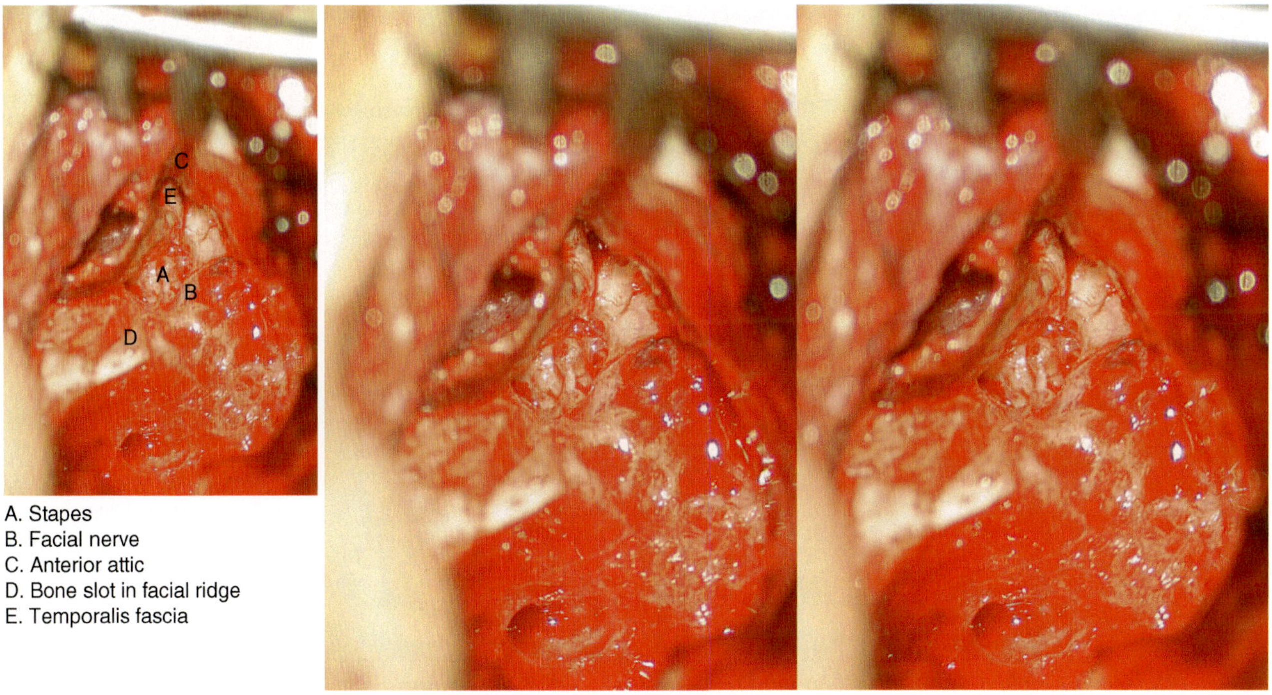

Fig. 2.160 Reconstruction of external auditory canal
Bone slots are drilled anteriorly between the attic and anterior wall of the ear canal and posteriorly on the upper part of the facial ridge to place the cartilage graft

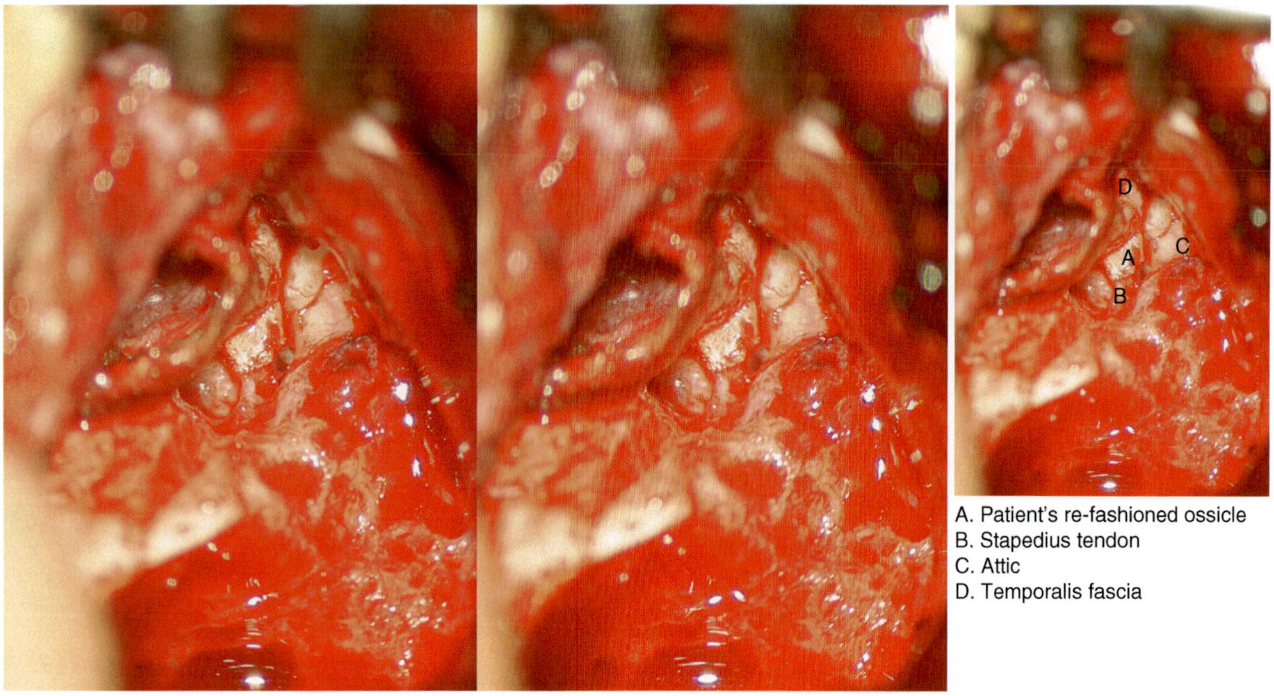

A. Patient's re-fashioned ossicle
B. Stapedius tendon
C. Attic
D. Temporalis fascia

Fig. 2.161 Rebuilding the ossicular chain
Drill the autologous ossicle to fit between the head of the stapes and the tympanic membrane. Position the ossicle and ensure it is stable

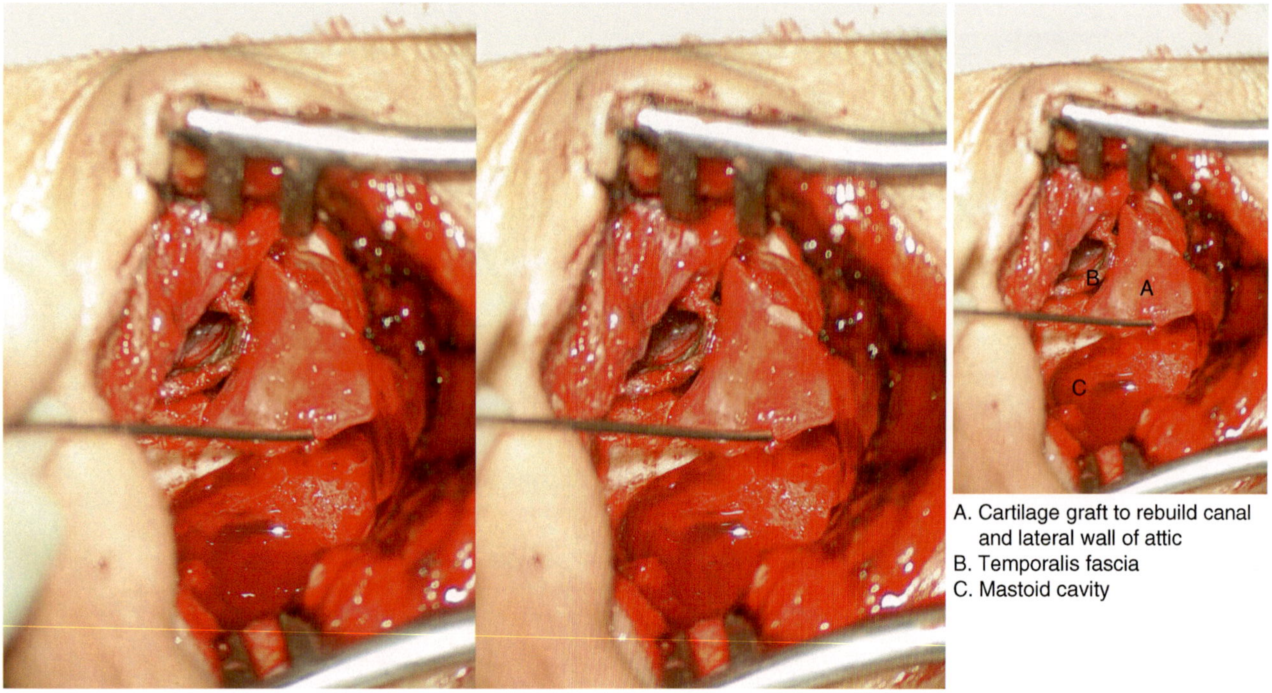

A. Cartilage graft to rebuild canal and lateral wall of attic
B. Temporalis fascia
C. Mastoid cavity

Fig. 2.162 Rebuild the lateral wall of the attic and the superior wall of the EAC
Place the free cartilage graft in the bone slots. Pack gelfoam into the attic and mastoid cavity. The cartilage graft is then covered with fascia and the tympanomeatal flap

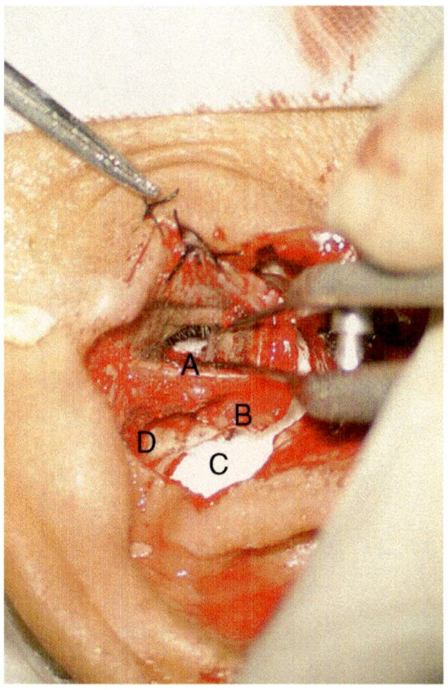

A. Meatal flaps
B. Extension of cartilage graft
C. Gelfoam in mastoid cavity and attic
D. Back wall of the bony external auditory canal

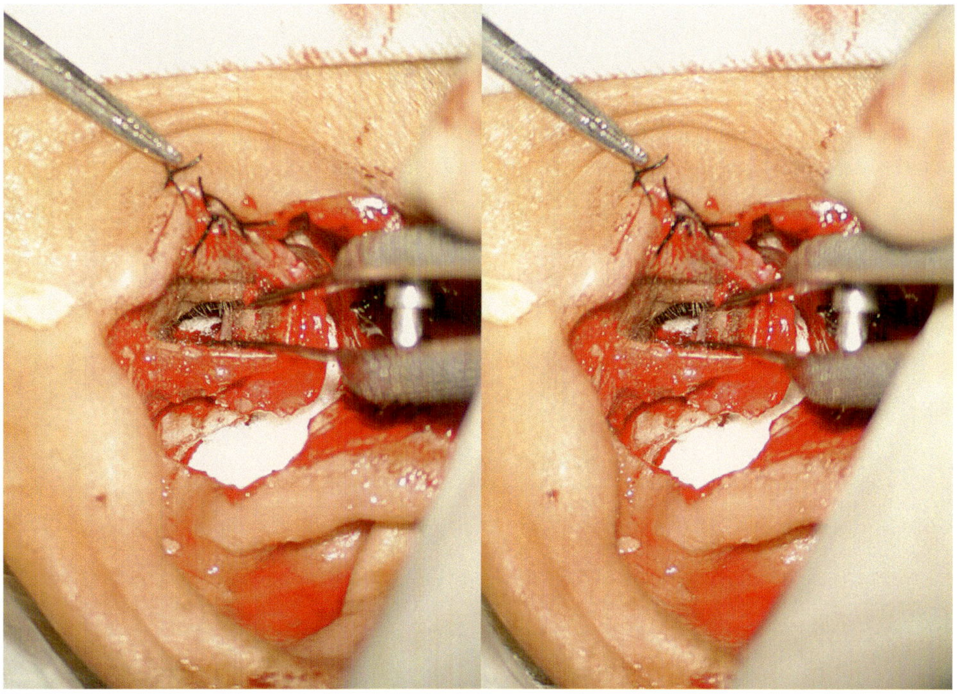

Fig. 2.163 Reposition meatal flaps
Cover with gelfoam then place iodoform gauze in the external auditory canal

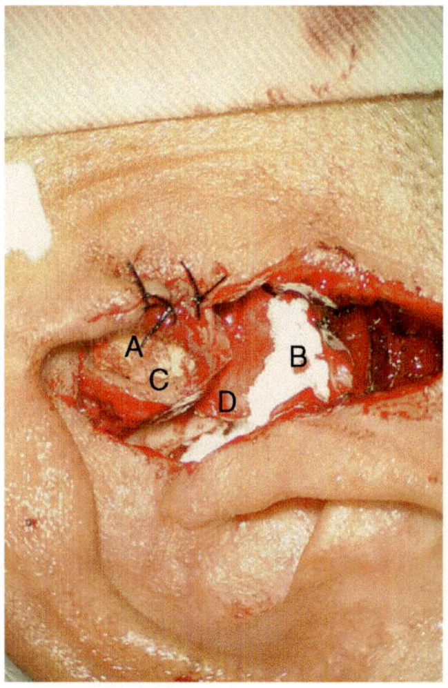

A. Iodoform gauze
B. Gelfoam
C. Meatal flaps
D. Cartilage graft

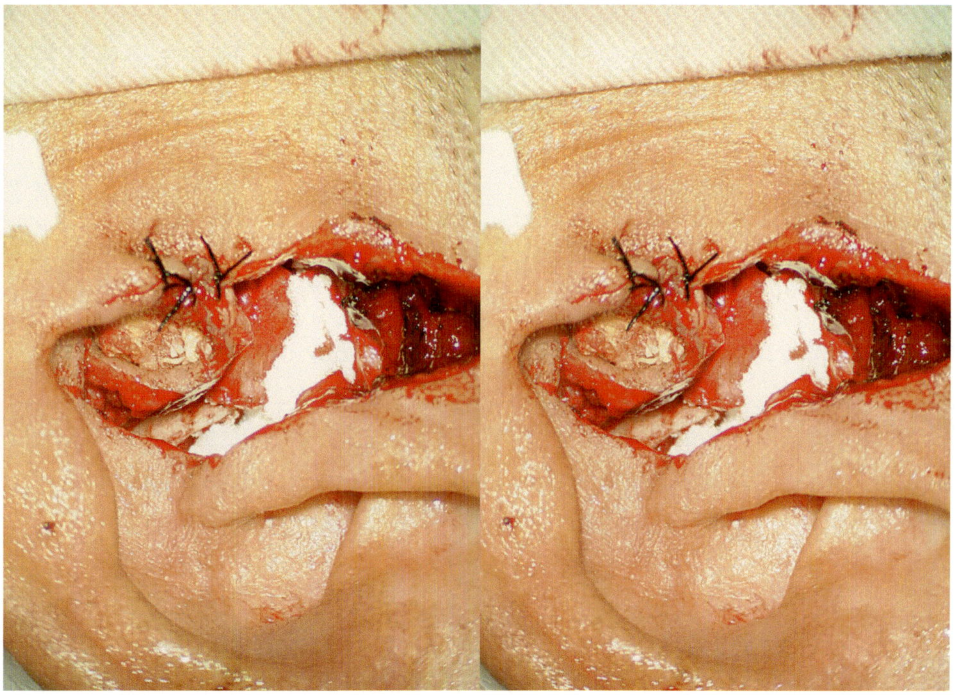

Fig. 2.164 Packing of external auditory canal
Pack iodoform gauze into external auditory canal and replace the flaps

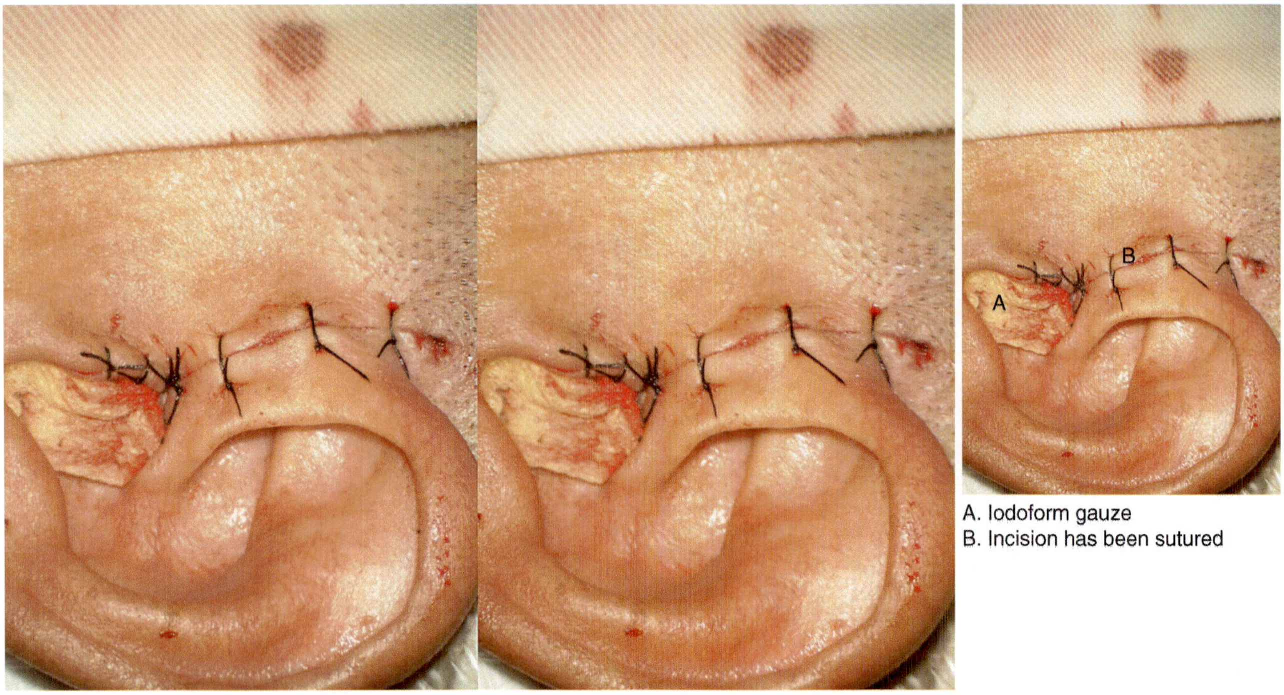

Fig. 2.165 Suturing the incision
After suturing the incision, the operation is complete

Surgery 3: Closed mastoidectomy with tympanoplasty and reconstruction of external auditory canal

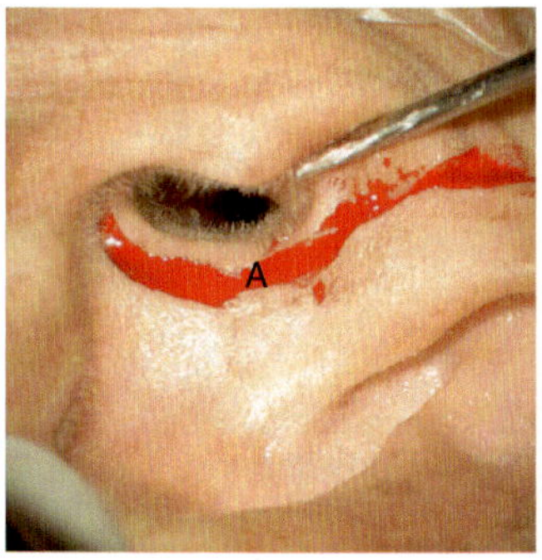

A. Incision
B. External auditory canal opening

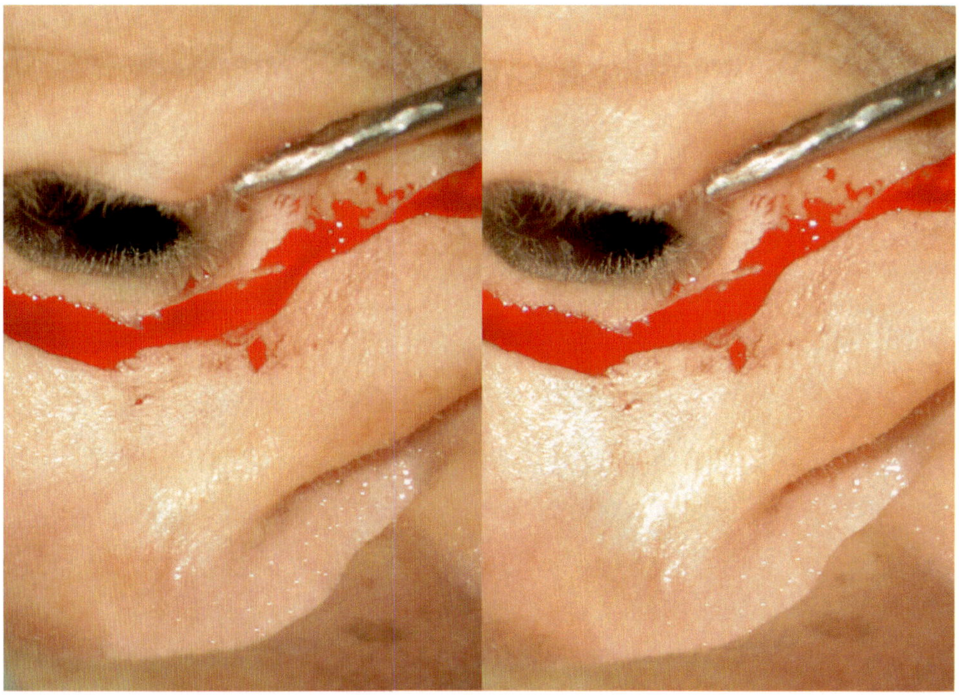

Fig. 2.166 Incision
The endaural incision is extended in to the external canal. The subcutaneous tissues are extensively removed

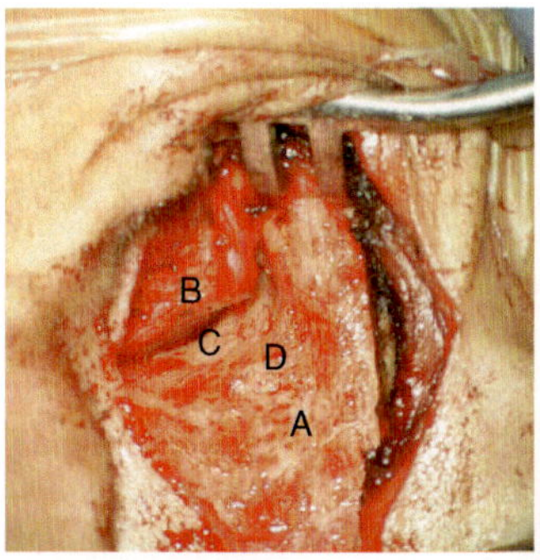

A. Cribriform area
B. Meatal flaps
C. Bony external auditory canal
D. Suprameatal spine of external auditory canal

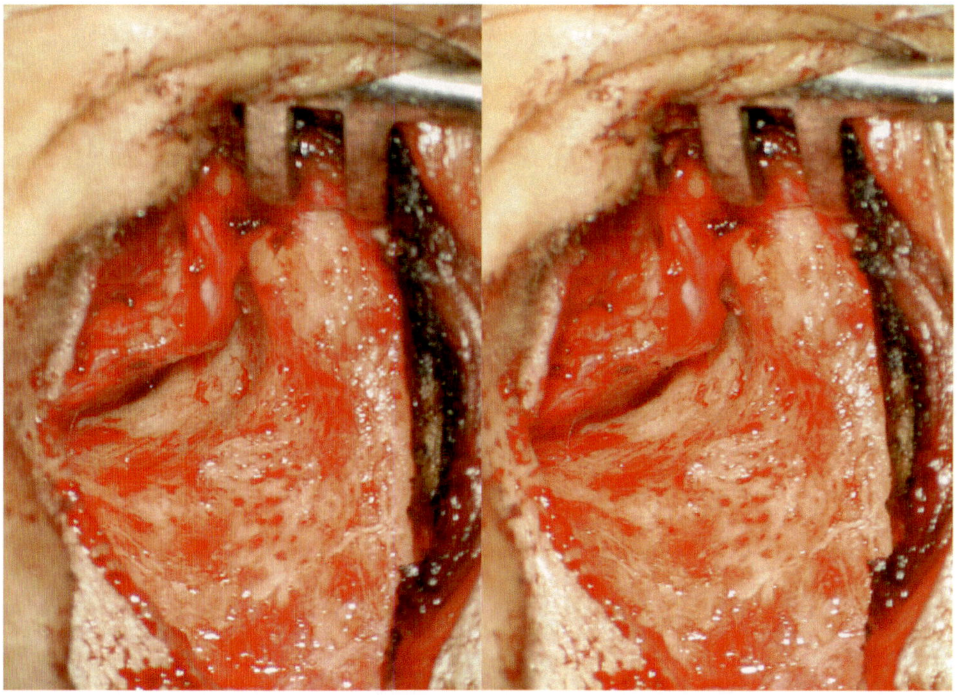

Fig. 2.167 Elevation of meatal flaps
Make the endaural incision, reflect the helix and subcutaneous tissues posteriorly to expose the posterior wall of the external auditory canal, the cribriform area and the mastoid cortex

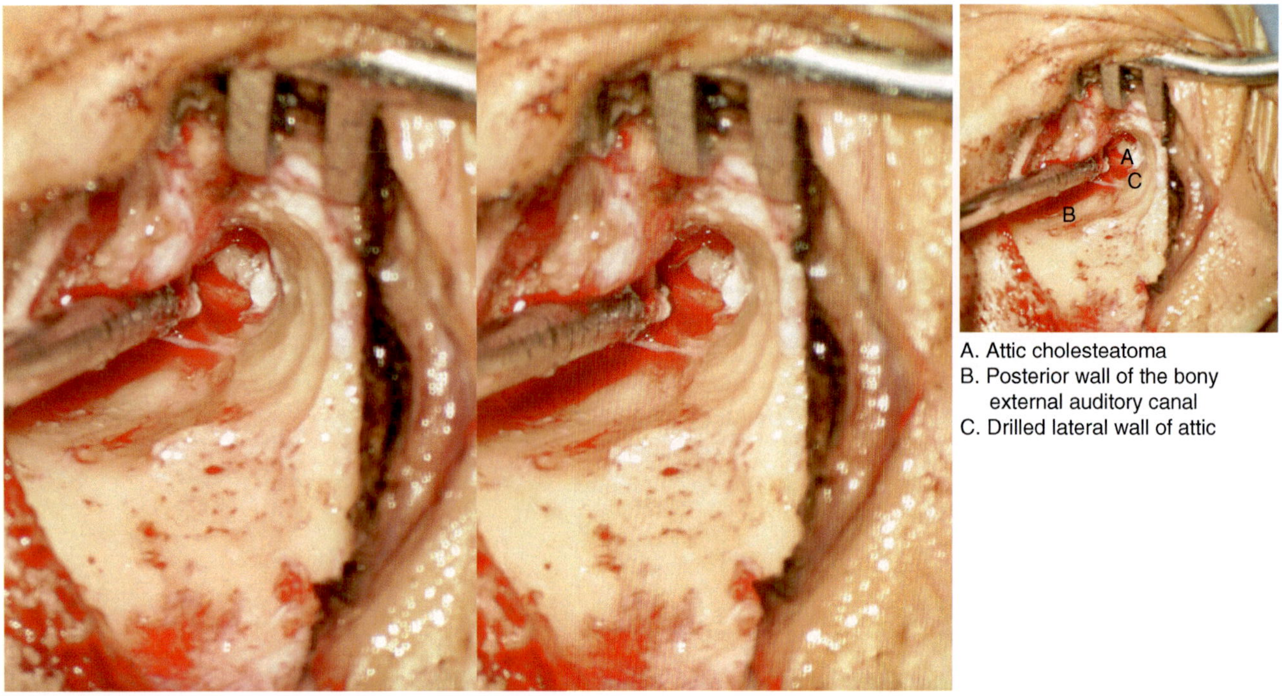

A. Attic cholesteatoma
B. Posterior wall of the bony external auditory canal
C. Drilled lateral wall of attic

Fig. 2.168 Opening the attic
Elevate the meatal flaps and tympanic membrane anteriorly. Drill down the lateral wall of the attic and expose it clearly. The attic here is filled with cholesteatoma

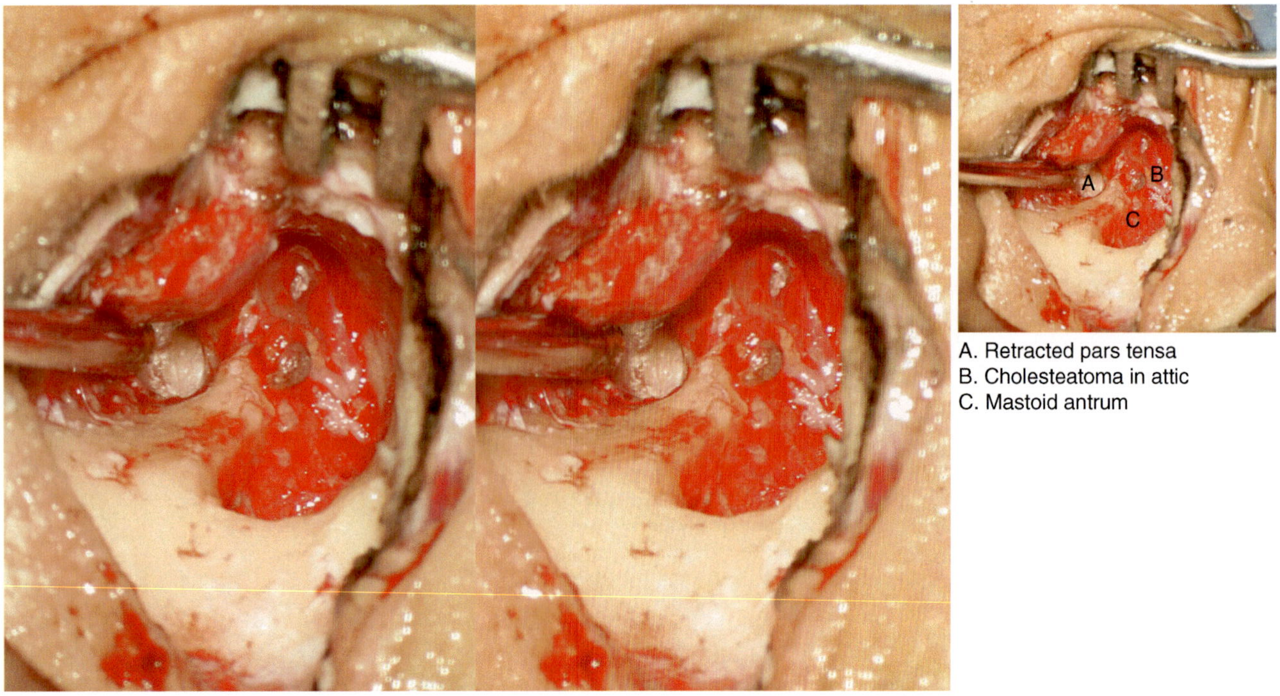

A. Retracted pars tensa
B. Cholesteatoma in attic
C. Mastoid antrum

Fig. 2.169 Exposure of mastoid antrum and tympanic cavity
Expose the attic, the antrum and tympanic cavity thoroughly. The tympanic membrane is intact but retracted

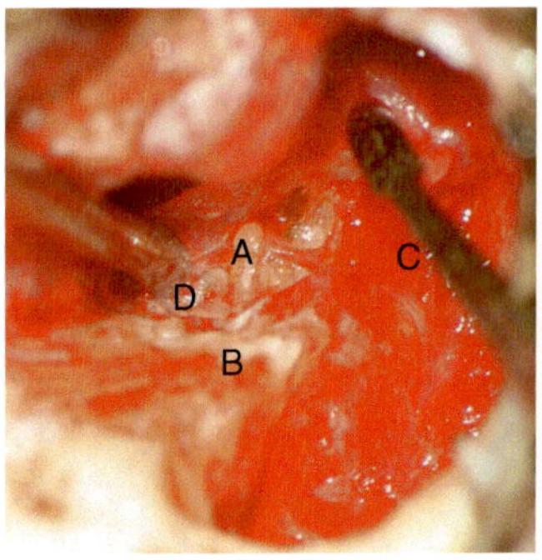

A. Stapes
B. Posterior wall of external auditory canal
C. Attic
D. Middle ear cavity

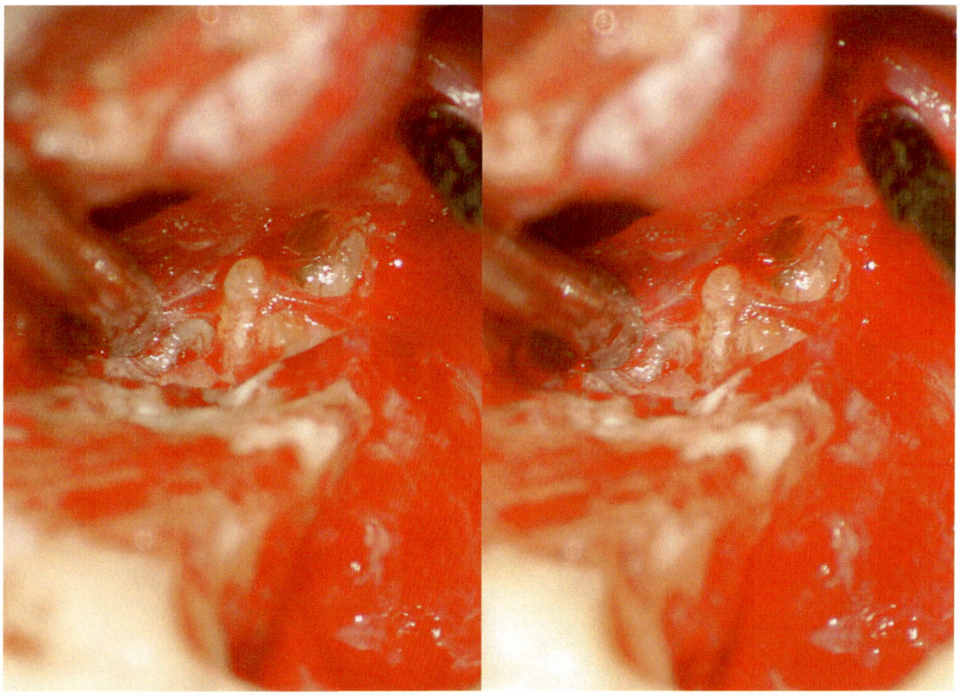

Fig. 2.170 Clear the cholesteatoma and elevate the tympanic membrane to expose the ossicular chain
Clear the cholesteatoma from the attic and mastoid antrum completely, elevate the tympanic membrane to expose the mesotympanum. The incus is absent and the stapes was normal. All cholesteatoma was removed

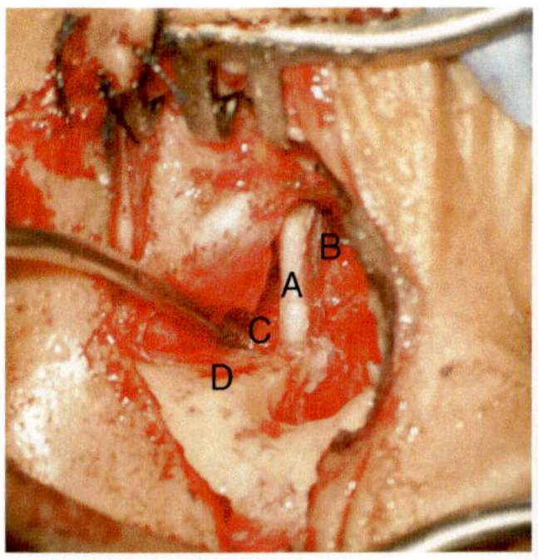

A. Free cartilage graft
B. Attic
C. Middle ear cavity
D. Posterior wall of the bony external auditory canal

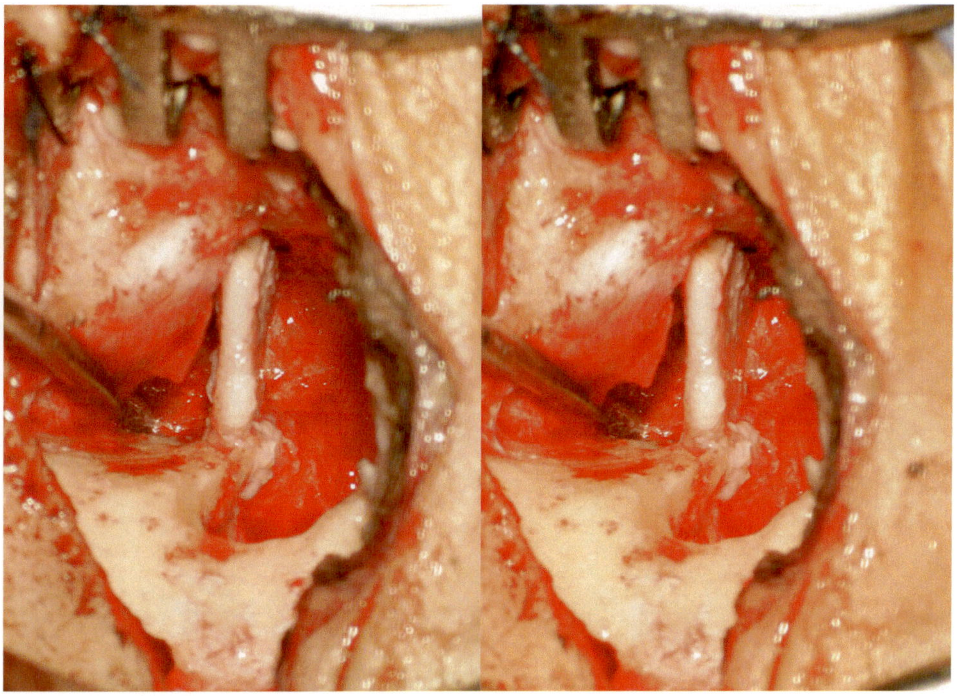

Fig. 2.171 Rebuild the superior wall of external auditory canal with cartilage graft
Place the free tragal cartilage graft in the bone slots to rebuild the external auditory canal wall

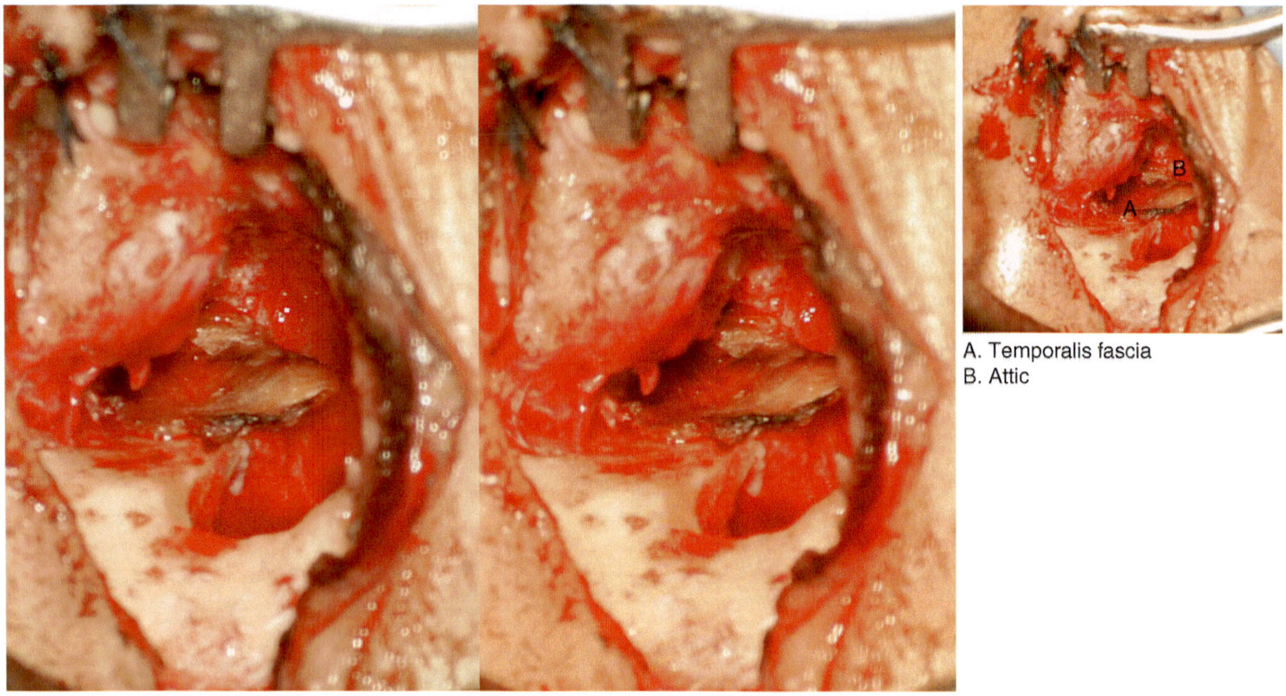

A. Temporalis fascia
B. Attic

Fig. 2.172 Repair the tympanic membrane
Reconstruct the tympanic membrane with temporalis fascia

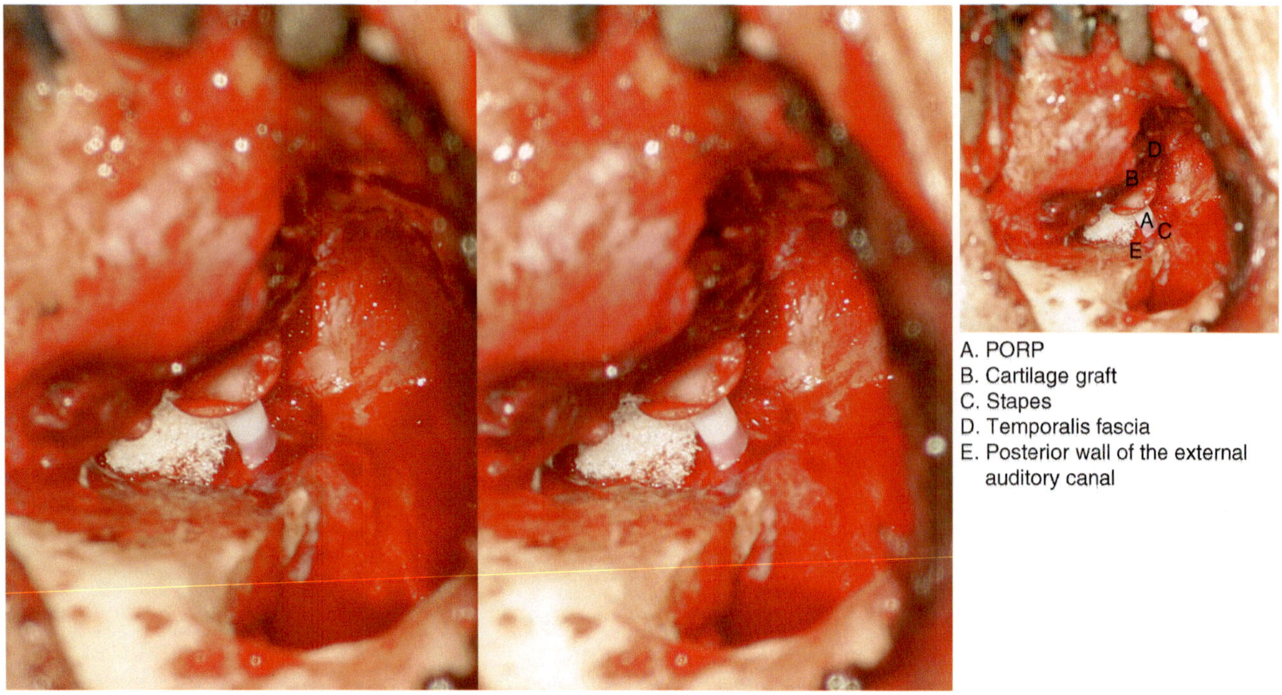

A. PORP
B. Cartilage graft
C. Stapes
D. Temporalis fascia
E. Posterior wall of the external auditory canal

Fig. 2.173 Rebuild the ossicular chain
Lift the fascial graft, trim the PORP to the correct length to fit between the head of stapes and the new tympanic membrane and rebuild the ossicular chain. Place the cartilage graft between the PORP and fascia

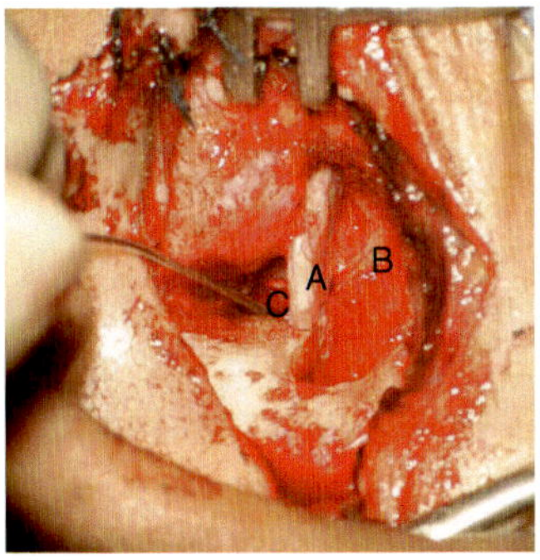

A. Free cartilage graft
B. Attic
C. Middle ear cavity

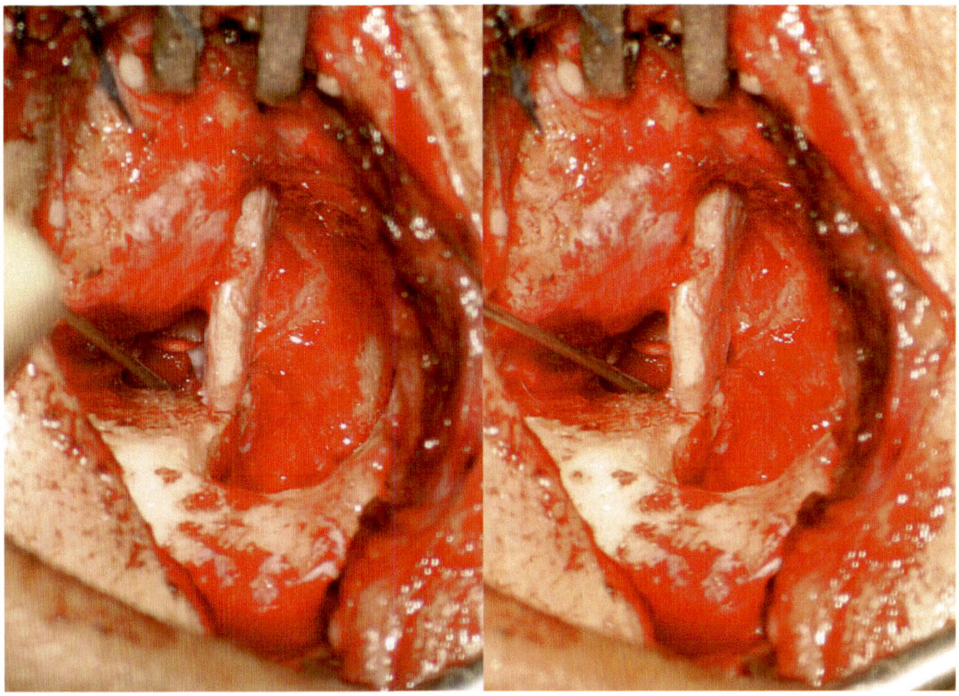

Fig. 2.174 Reconstruct the external auditory canal
Rebuild the external auditory canal wall with the free cartilage graft after the PORP has been positioned

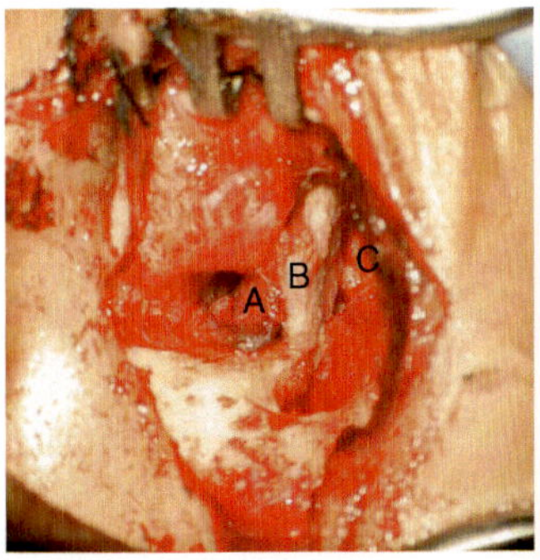

A. Transplanted temporalis fascia
B. Free cartilage flap
C. Attic

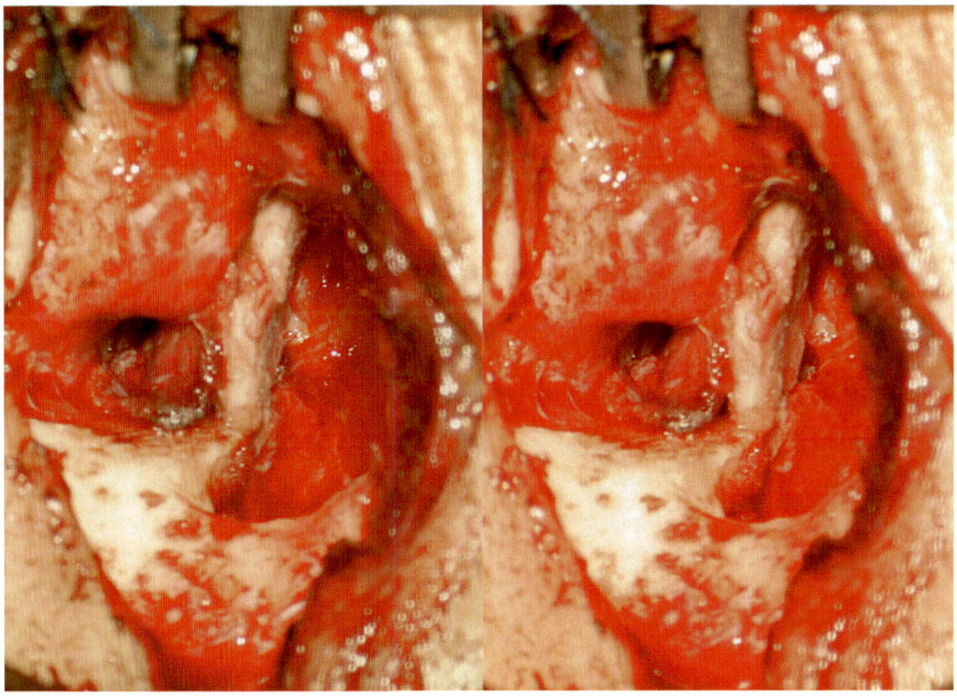

Fig. 2.175 Reposition the meatal flaps
Place the temporalis fascia on the canal side of the free cartilage graft and cover it with the meatal flap

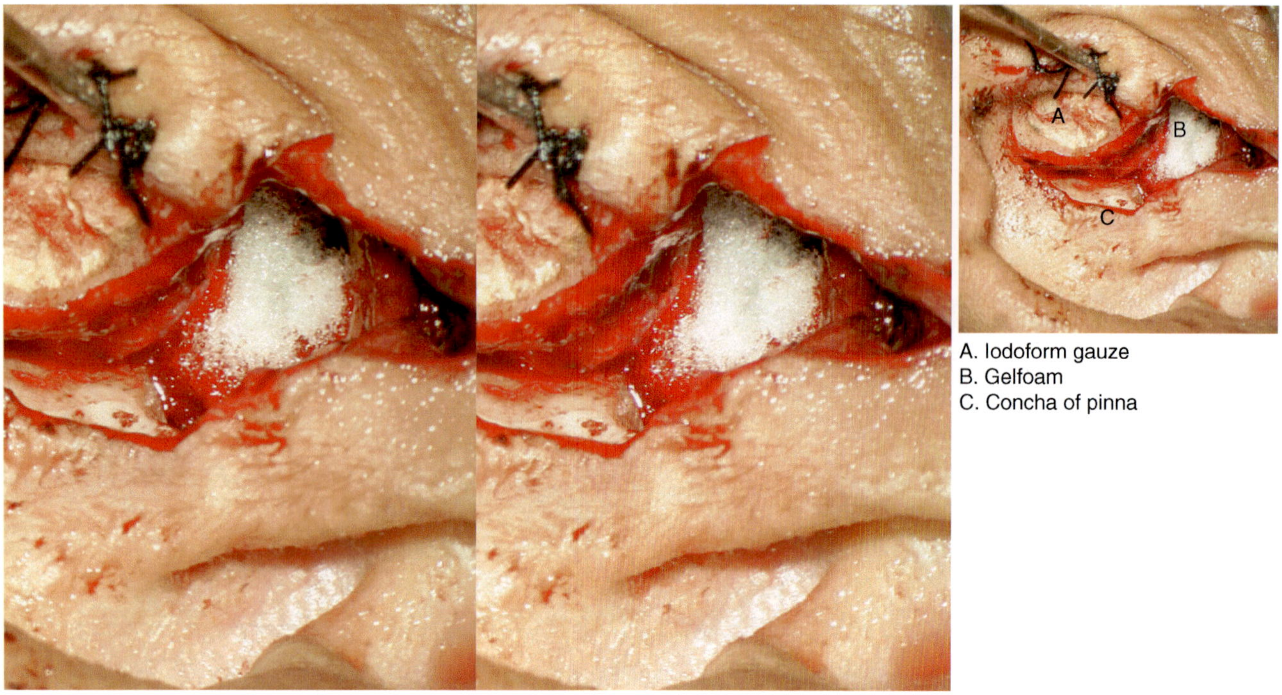

Fig. 2.176 Pack the external auditory canal and suture the incision
Place gelfoam into attic and mastoid cavity. Pack iodoform gauze into external auditory canal and suture the incision

Ossicular Chain Reconstruction for Congenital Deformity or Trauma

Bing Han, Pu Dai

Indications

1. Conductive hearing loss present at birth with normal tympanic membrane (usually symmetrical hearing loss)
2. Conductive hearing loss with intact tympanic membrane after minor trauma;
3. Conductive hearing loss with ossicular chain abnormality on CT scan.

Contraindications

1. Major round window malformation
2. Eustachian tube malformation or stenosis;
3. Patient unfit for operation.

Operative Procedures

1. Incise the skin in front of the helical crus. Carefully elevate a tympanomeatal flap to expose the middle ear. Bone may need to be curetted from the postero-superior wall to expose all of the oval window niche.
2. Assess the state of the ossicular chain and its mobility, with particular attention to the incus, the incudostapedial joint and stapes footplate.
3. Reconstruction of ossicular chain and choice of technique. If the stapes is present and mobile, the incus and head of malleus can be removed. Either the incus or a PORP can be positioned between the stapes head and tympanic membrane to reconstruct the chain. Where a PORP is used, a disc of cartilage should be placed between it and the drum to prevent extrusion. If the stapes footplate is fixed, stapedotomy or stapedectomy can be performed. If the incus long process is absent, the stapes prosthesis must be attached to the malleus handle. A small fat graft should be used to seal around the stapedotomy. If the oval window cannot be accessed, a fenestration of the lateral canal can be considered.
4. The tympanomeatal flap is repositioned. If the operation is done under local anesthesia, the improvement in hearing can be checked before packing the ear canal.

Special Comments

1. Take care not to damage the tympanomeatal flap. When a prosthesis is used, place a cartilage disc between it and the tympanic membrane to prevent secondary perforation and extrusion;
2. Ensure good mobility of the reconstructed chain;
3. Aspirate blood from the middle ear to reduce the formation of adhesions after operation;
4. Avoid injury of the mucous membrane around the Eustachian tube;
5. Check for a perilymph leak after stapedotomy or stapedectomy;
6. If the middle ear malformation is too severe, ossicular chain reconstruction may not be possible.

Complications

1. Facial paralysis: One should identify the position of the facial nerve clearly to avoid injury;
2. Sensorineural hearing loss: Care should be taken when drilling the stapes footplate and inserting the prosthesis of correct length to minimise trauma to the inner ear.
3. Cerebrospinal fluid otorrhea: This may occur if there is an abnormal communication between the inner ear and the subarachnoid space ("Gusher").
4. Perforation of tympanic membrane: Care should be taken to avoid perforation of the tympanic membrane. If it does occur it should be repaired immediately. Prostheses should not be placed in direct contact with the drum.

Surgery 1: ossiculoplasty of incus malformation (PORP)

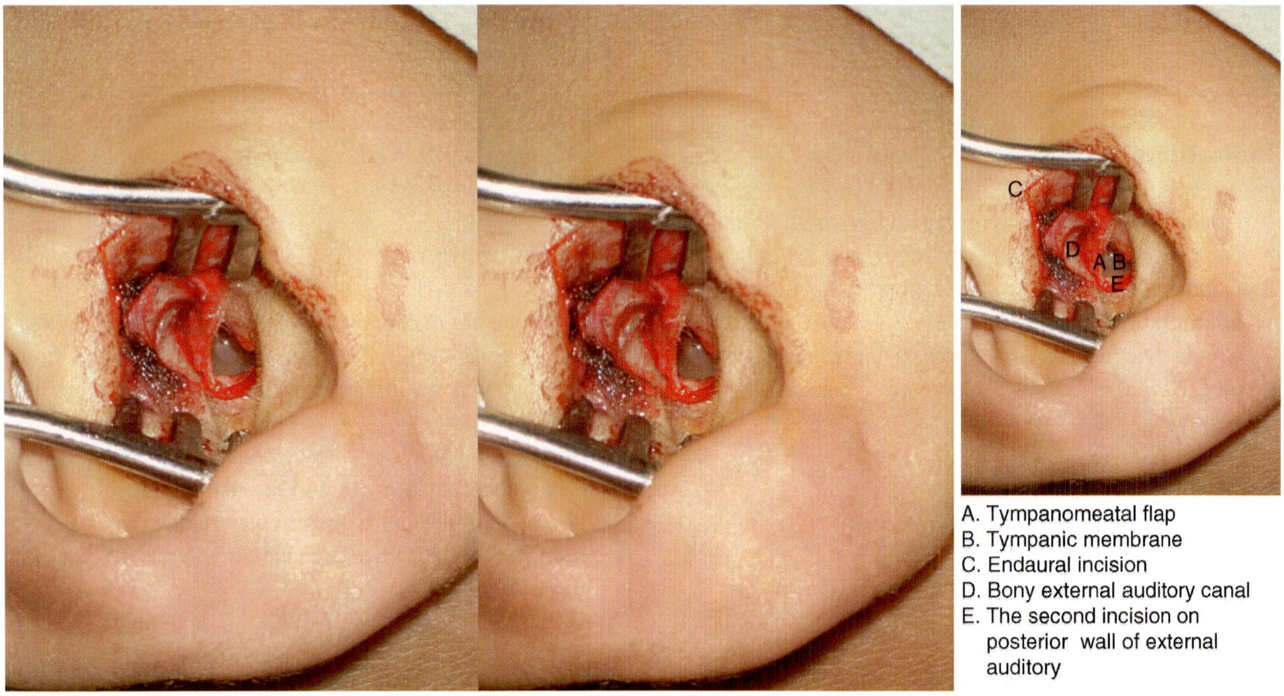

Fig. 2.177 Endaural incision
Incise the skin anterior to the helical crus and into the upper external auditory canal, elevate the tympanomeatal flap and tympanic membrane forward

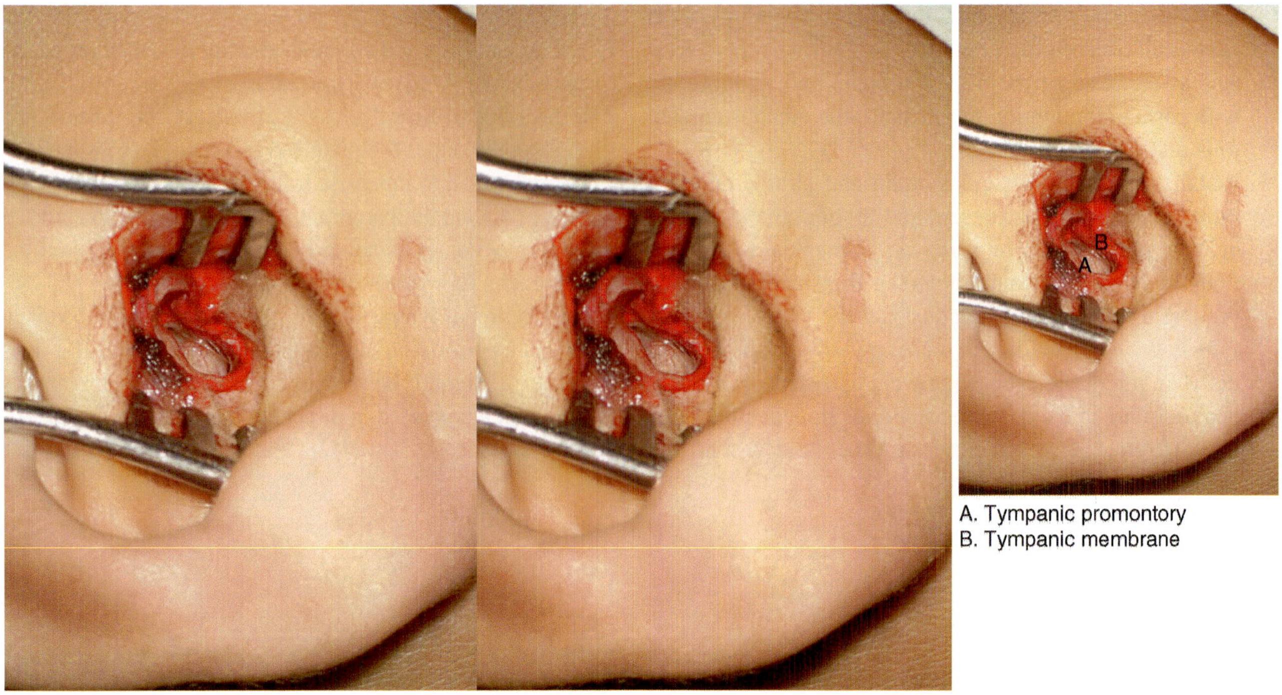

Fig. 2.178 Opening the tympanic cavity
Elevate the tympanomeatal flap and tympanic membrane to expose the tympanic cavity

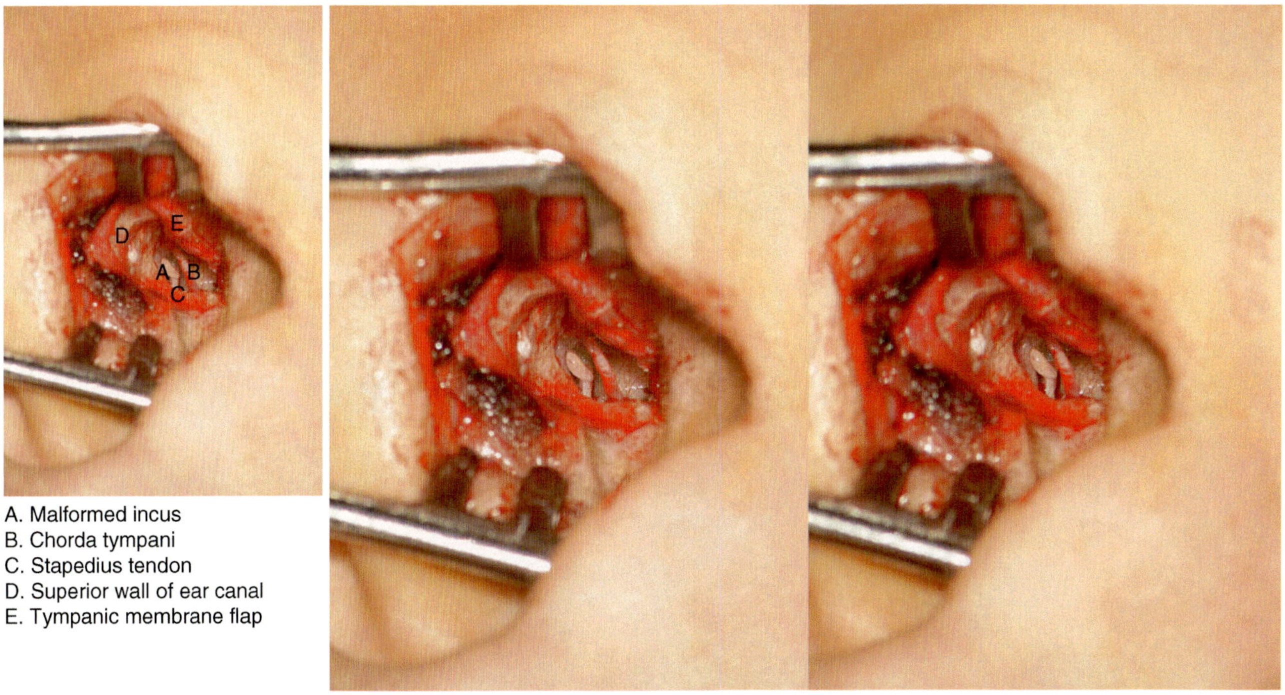

A. Malformed incus
B. Chorda tympani
C. Stapedius tendon
D. Superior wall of ear canal
E. Tympanic membrane flap

Fig. 2.179 Expose incudostapedial joint
Observe the chorda tympani nerve crossing the mesotympanum from back wall of external auditory canal. Adjust the angle of view of the microscope to display the incudostapedial joint. The long process of the incus is seen to be abnormal and separate from incus body

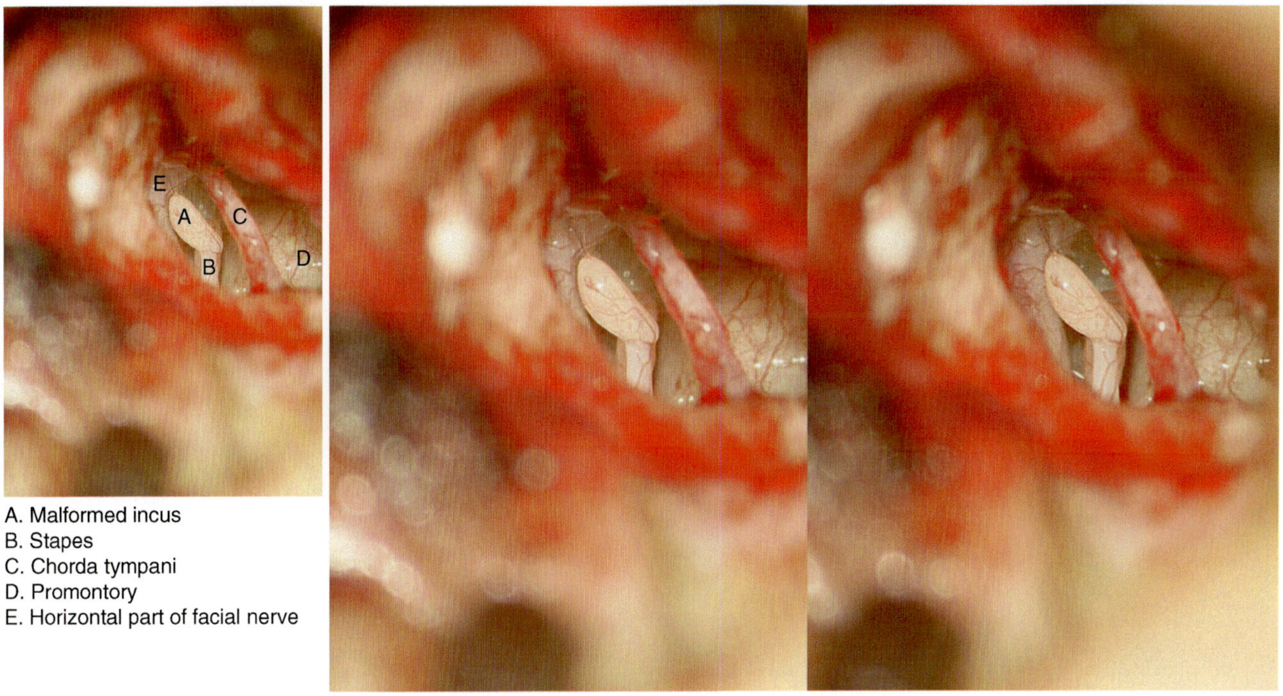

A. Malformed incus
B. Stapes
C. Chorda tympani
D. Promontory
E. Horizontal part of facial nerve

Fig. 2.180 Check for abnormalities
The ossicular chain malformation is shown under high power. The separate incus process, both stapes crura, the facial nerve canal and the footplate can be seen

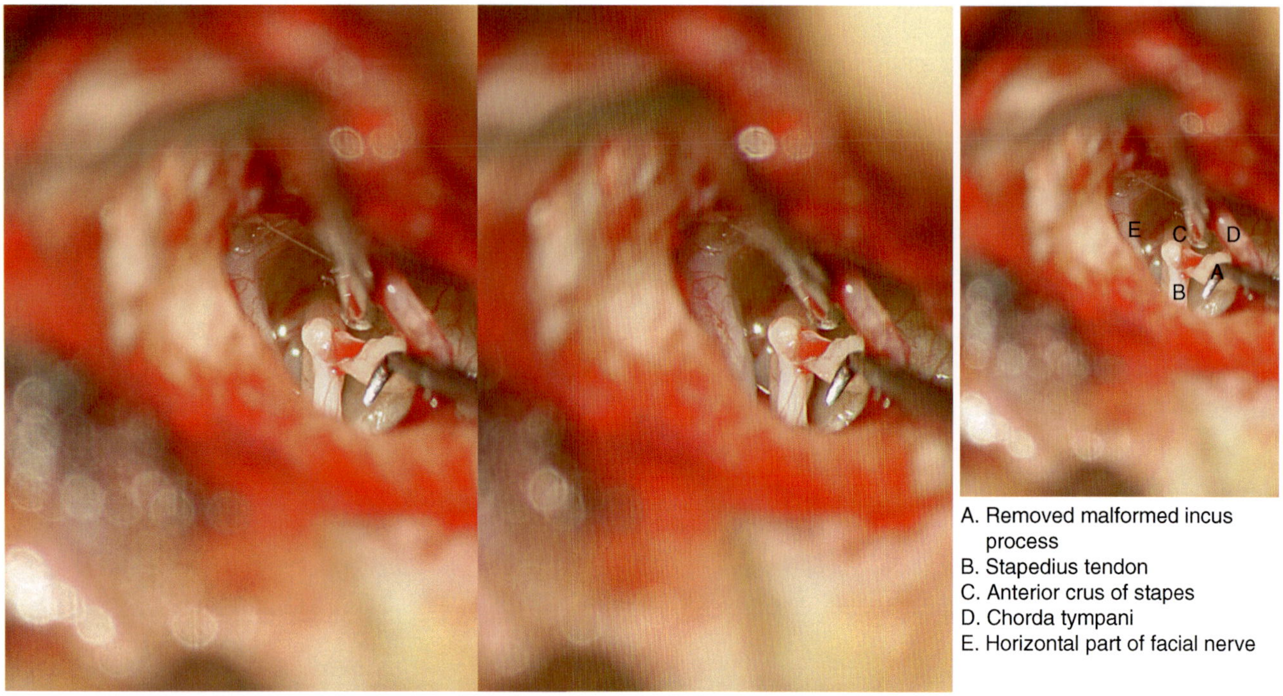

A. Removed malformed incus process
B. Stapedius tendon
C. Anterior crus of stapes
D. Chorda tympani
E. Horizontal part of facial nerve

Fig. 2.181 Remove abnormal incus
Use a hook to remove the abnormal incus process from head of stapes, check mobility of stapes

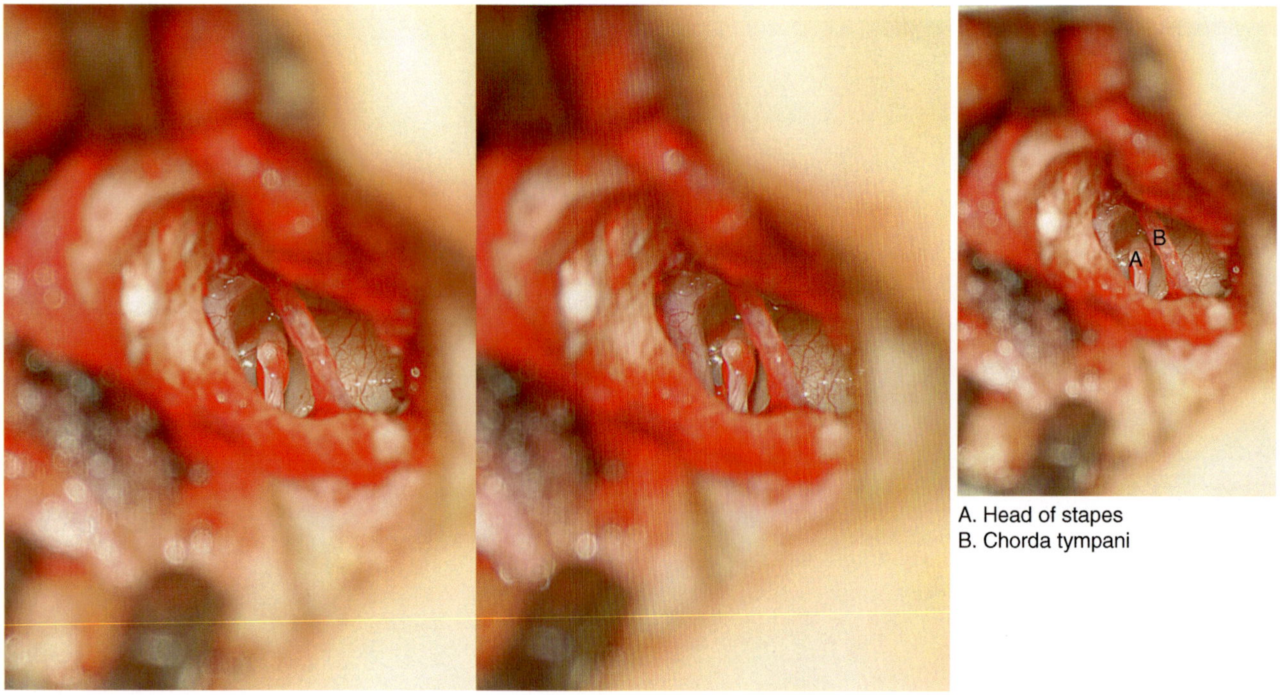

A. Head of stapes
B. Chorda tympani

Fig. 2.182 Check status of stapes
The stapes was intact and mobile. The chorda tympani should be preserved if possible. It can, sometimes be used to support the reconstructed ossicular chain

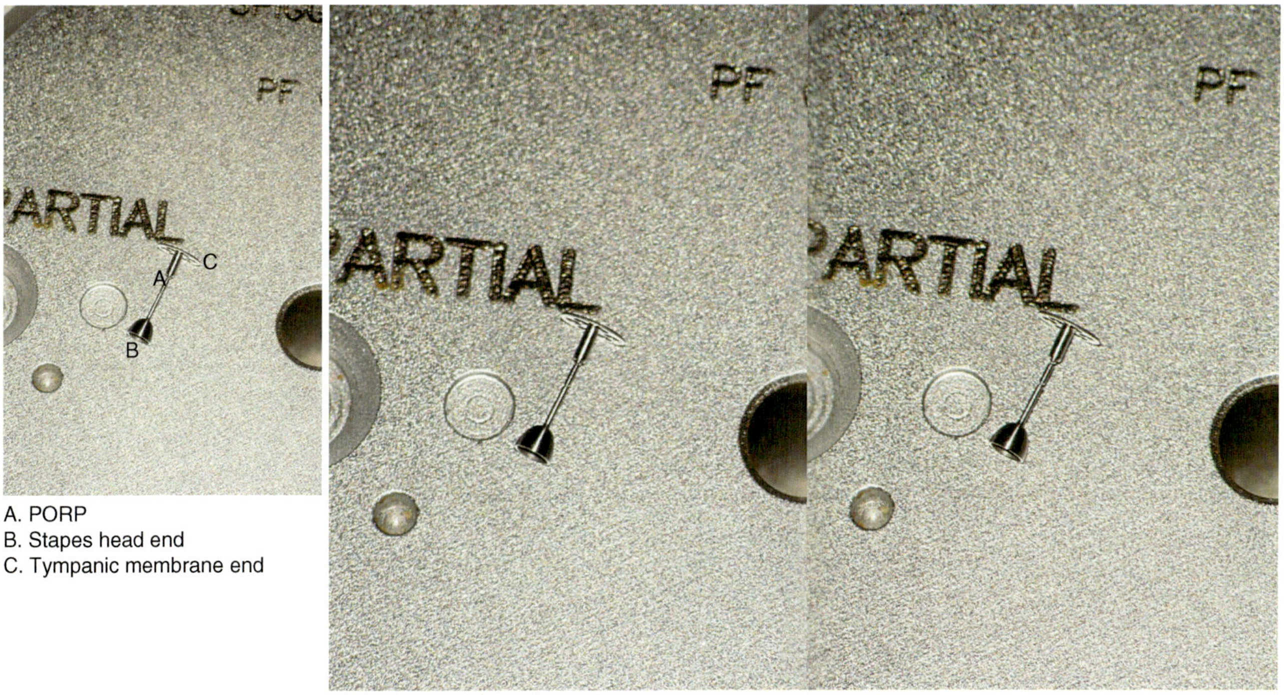

Fig. 2.183 PORP
The cupped end sits on the stapes head, and the disc end sits under the tympanic membrane. The connecting bar between the two ends can be trimmed to correct length

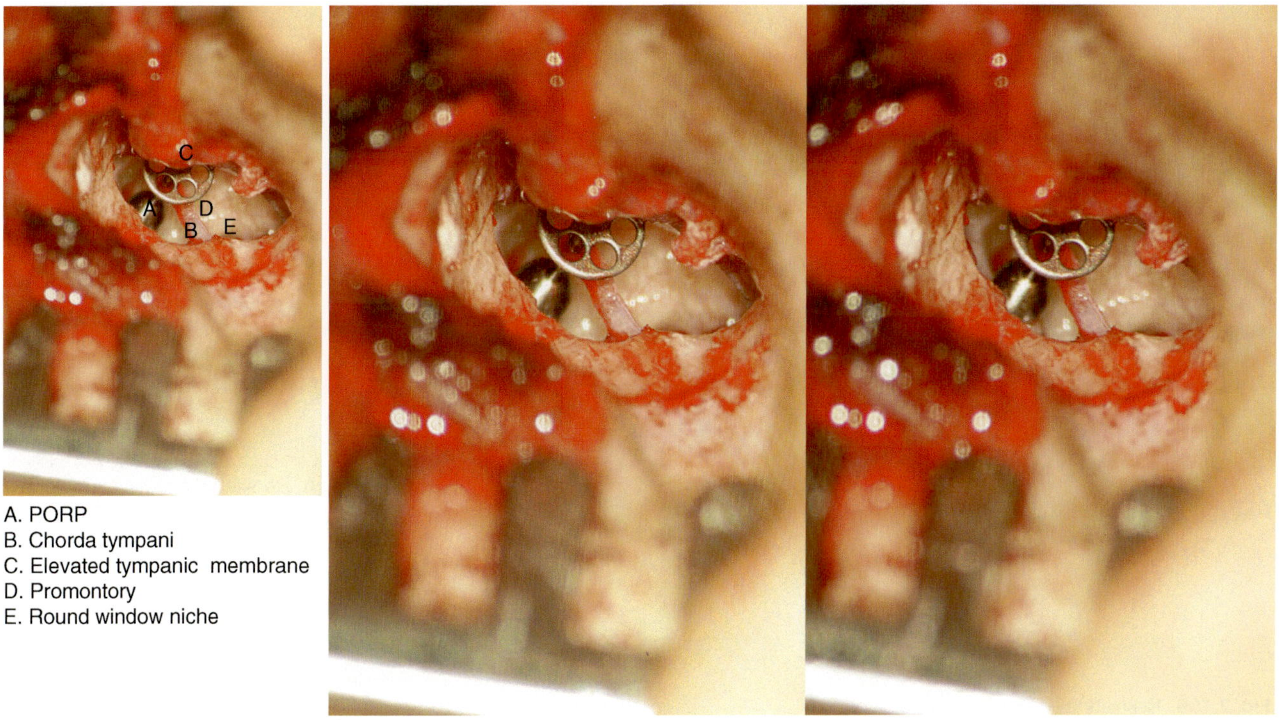

Fig. 2.184 Rebuilding ossicular chain
Once its shaft is trimmed to the correct length, the PORP can be placed between the stapes head and tympanic membrane. The shaft must be of optimal length for best hearing result

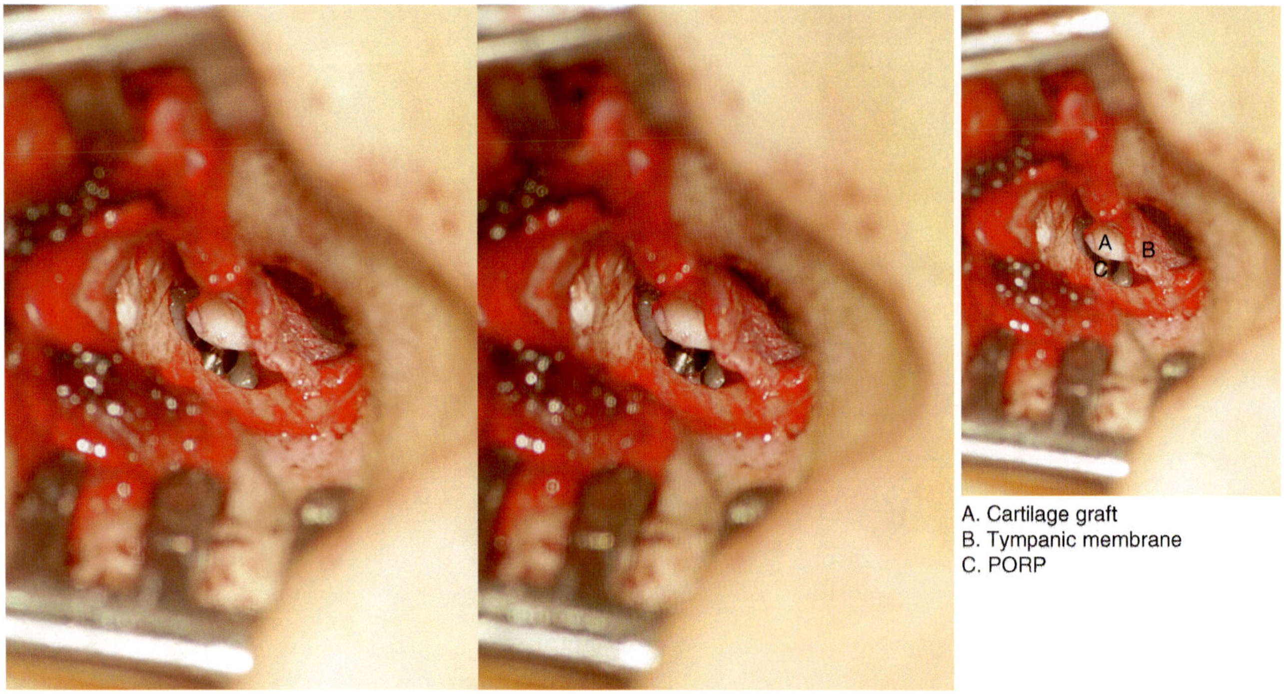

Fig. 2.185 Cover prosthesis with cartilage graft
Place the cartilage graft between PORP and tympanic membrane to prevent secondary perforation of tympanic membrane

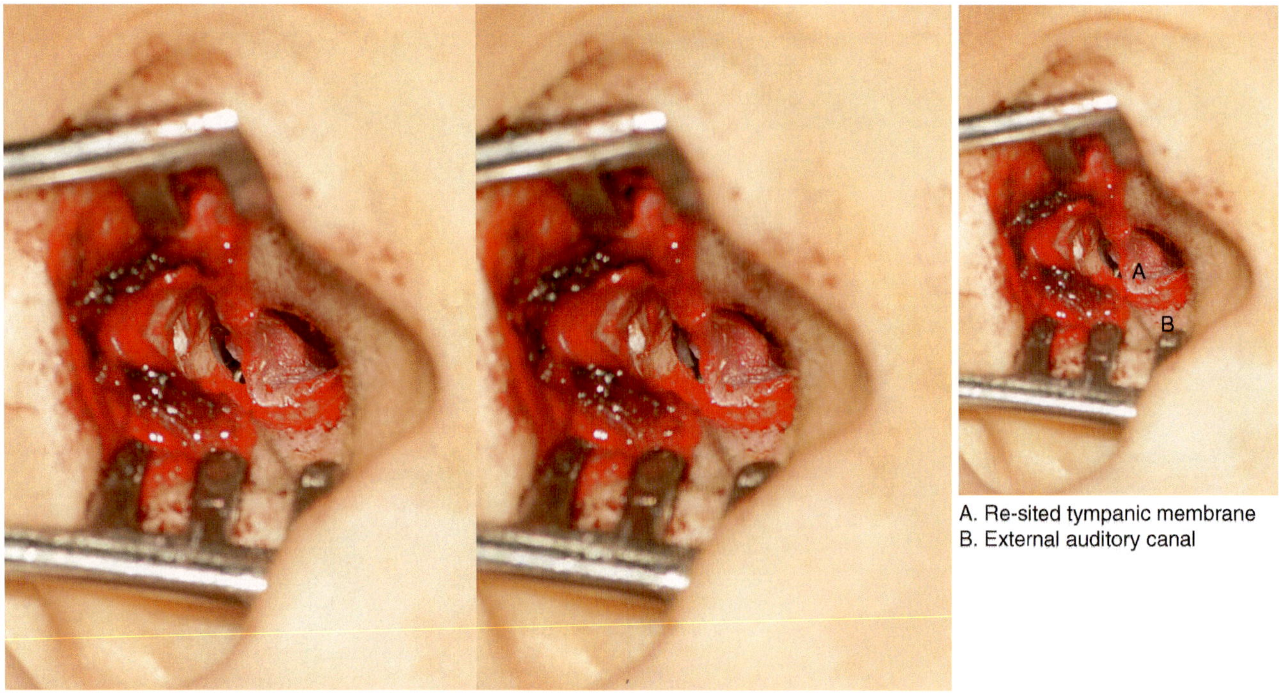

Fig. 2.186 Reposition tympanomeatal flap
Reposition the tympanic membrane and meatal flap in original position

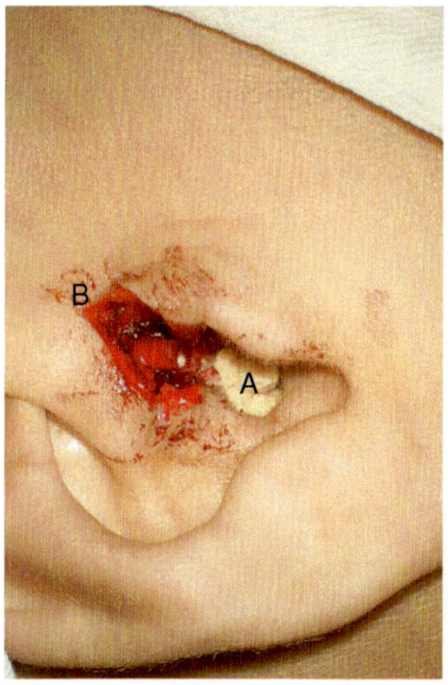

A. Iodoform gauze
B. Endaural incision

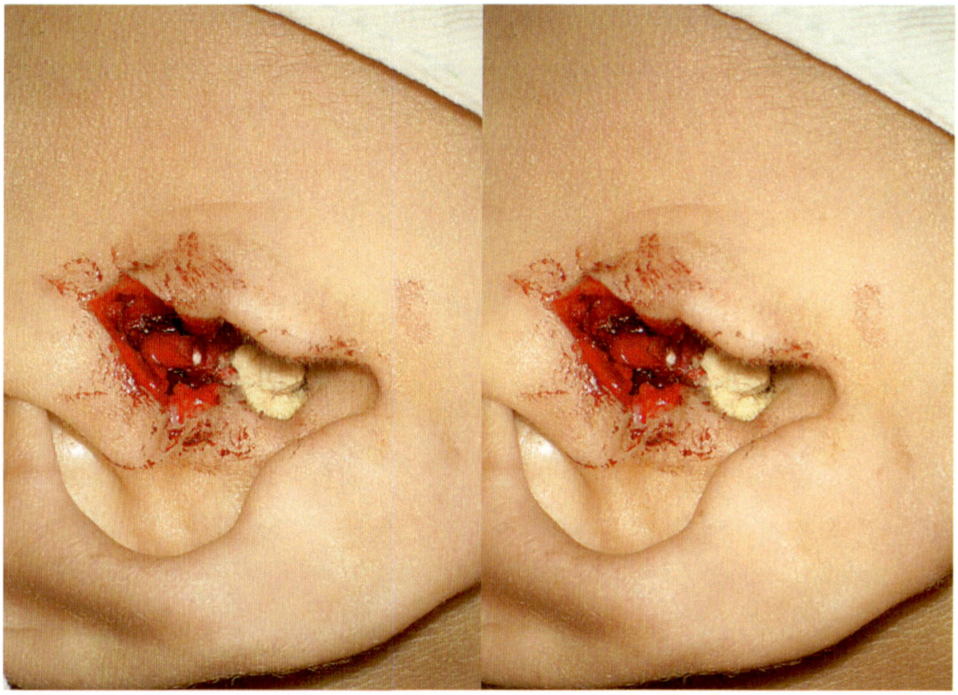

Fig. 2.187 Packing and closure
Pack iodoform gauze into external auditory canal and to sew up the incision. Cover the ear with an sterile dressing

Surgery 2: ossiculoplasty of incus malformation (autogenous ossicle)

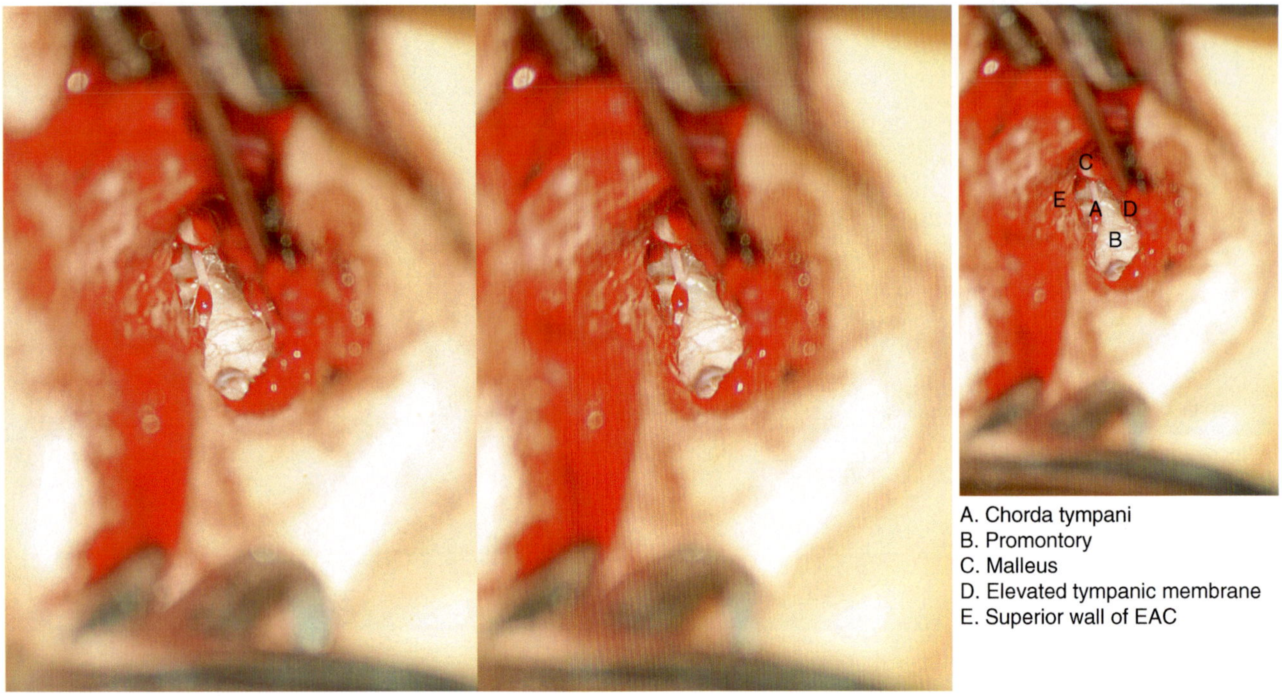

Fig. 2.188 Elevation of the tympanic membrane and exposure of the tympanic cavity
After the EAC incisions are made, the meatal flaps and tympanic membrane are elevated to expose the tympanic cavity. The promontory and round window niche are exposed

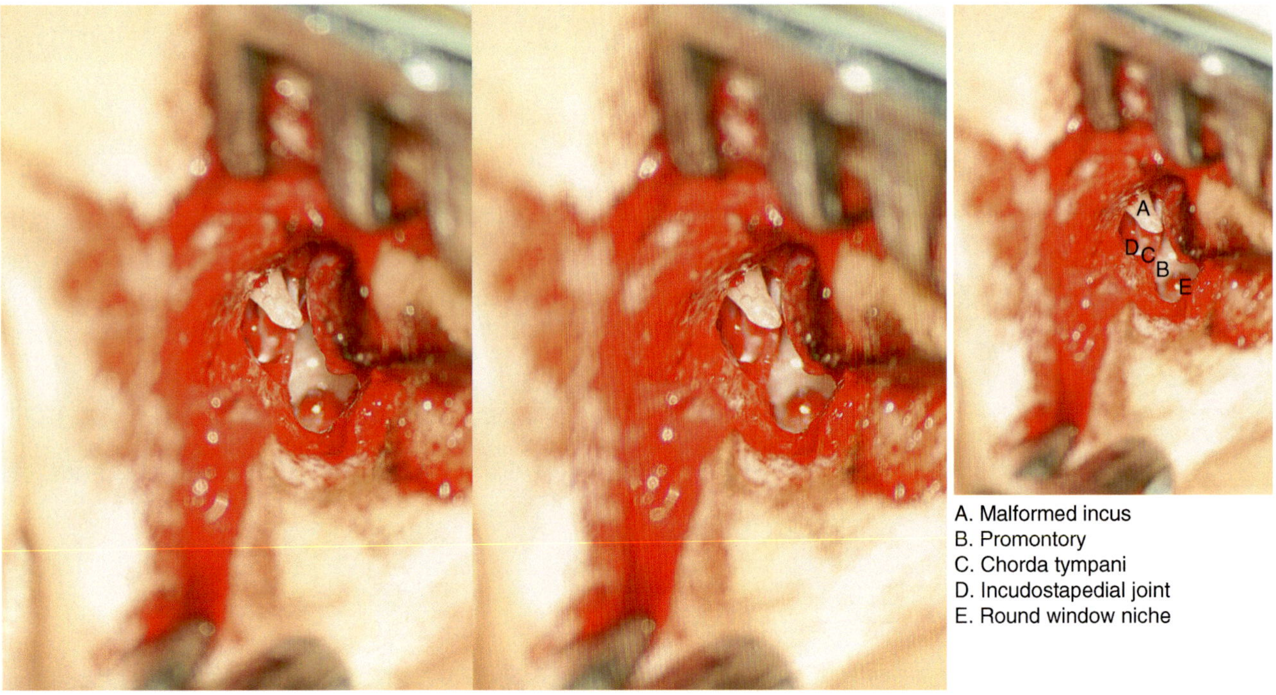

Fig. 2.189 Assessment of the ossicular chain
With adjustment of the microscope angle of view, the chorda tympani is seen to cross the tympanic cavity and the incus is noted to be markedly deformed

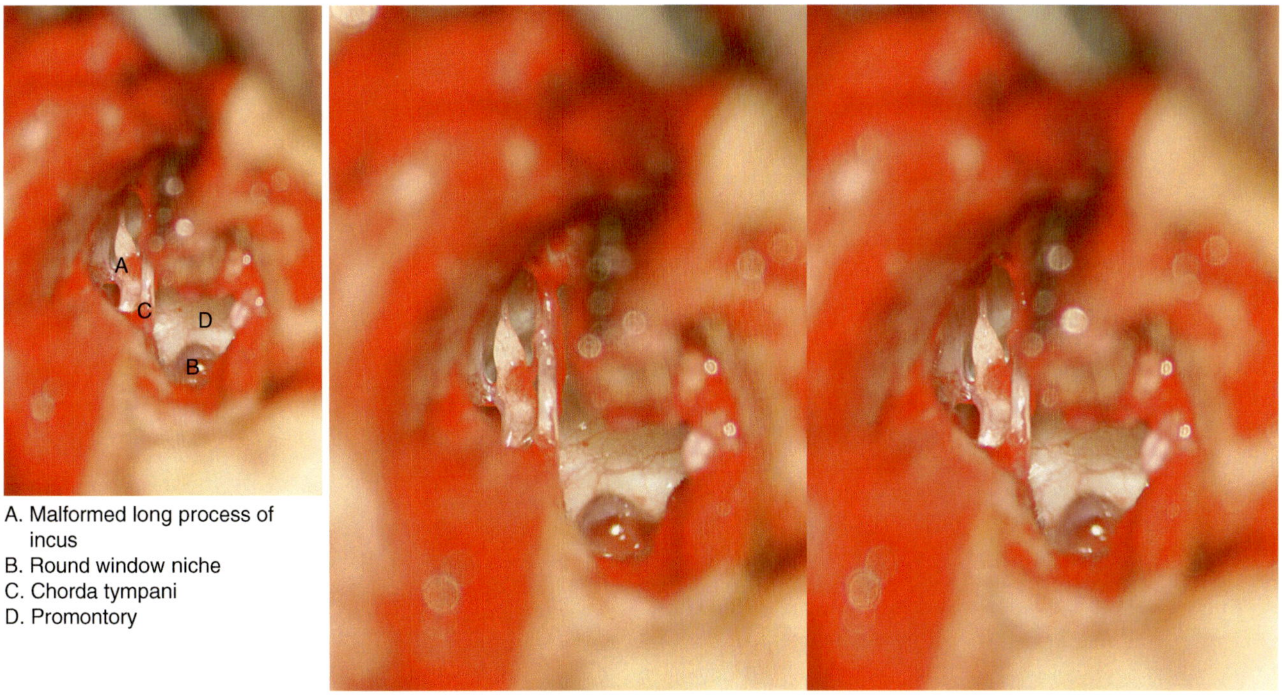

A. Malformed long process of incus
B. Round window niche
C. Chorda tympani
D. Promontory

Fig. 2.190 Examination of abnormal ossicular chain
The abnormal ossicular chain is assessed. There was only a segment of the abnormal long process of the incus on the head of stapes which did not connect with incus body. The stapes had a near normal shape but the crura were both thinner than normal

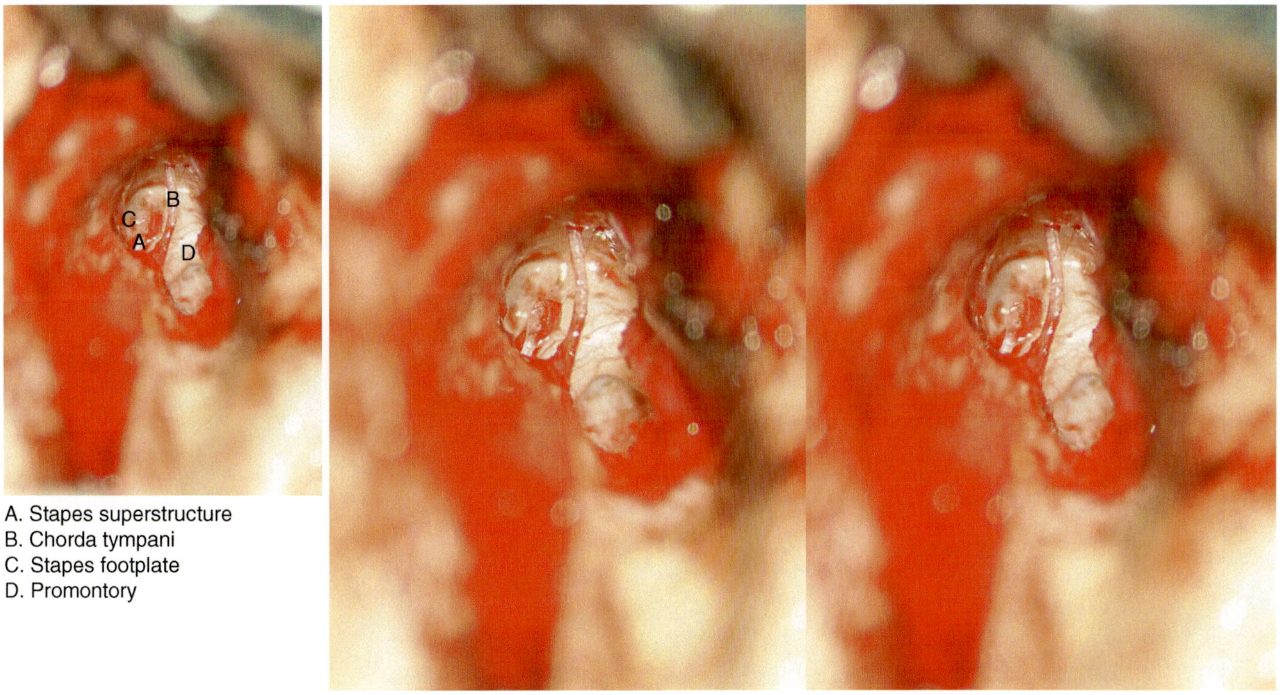

A. Stapes superstructure
B. Chorda tympani
C. Stapes footplate
D. Promontory

Fig. 2.191 Remove abnormal incus
Remove the abnormal segment of incus from the stapes head. The stapes mobility was seen to be normal

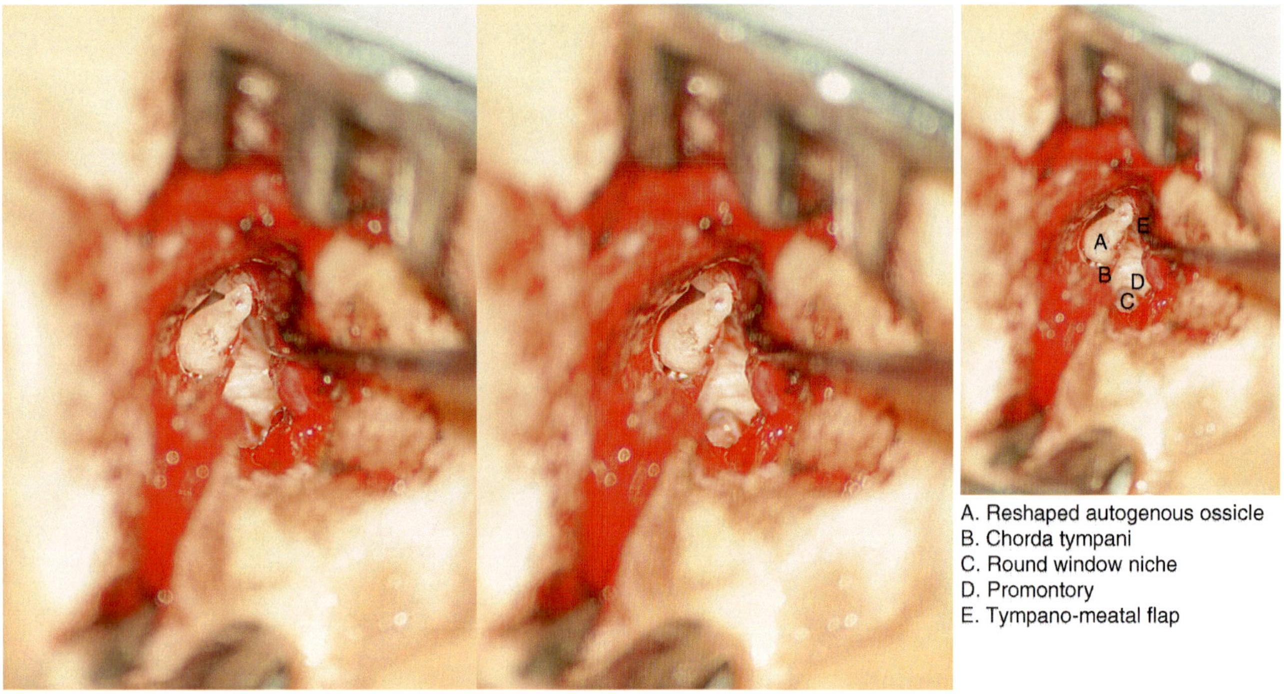

A. Reshaped autogenous ossicle
B. Chorda tympani
C. Round window niche
D. Promontory
E. Tympano-meatal flap

Fig. 2.192 Reconstruct the ossicular chain
Place the re-shaped autogenous ossicle between the stapes head and the tympanic membrane
Ensure that the grafted ossicle makes good contact with the stapes and is free of contact from all bony walls of the middle ear

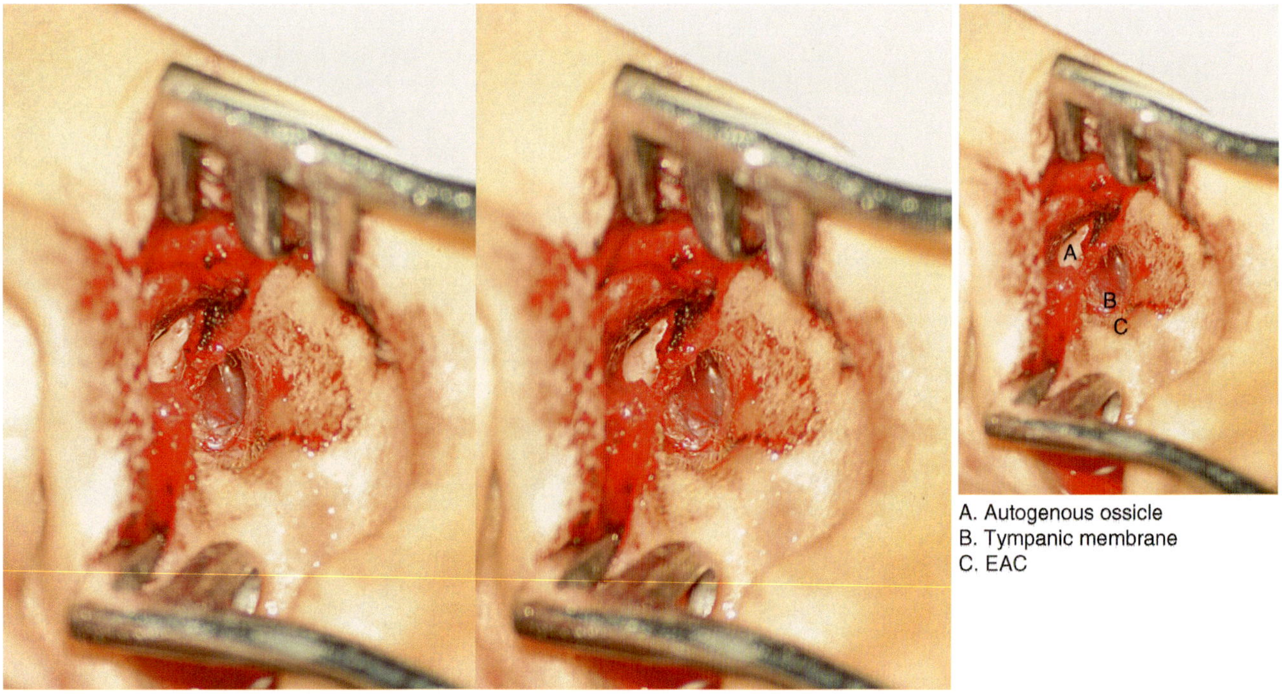

A. Autogenous ossicle
B. Tympanic membrane
C. EAC

Fig. 2.193 Replace tympanic membrane
Reposition the plastic meatal flaps and tympanic membrane in their correct position

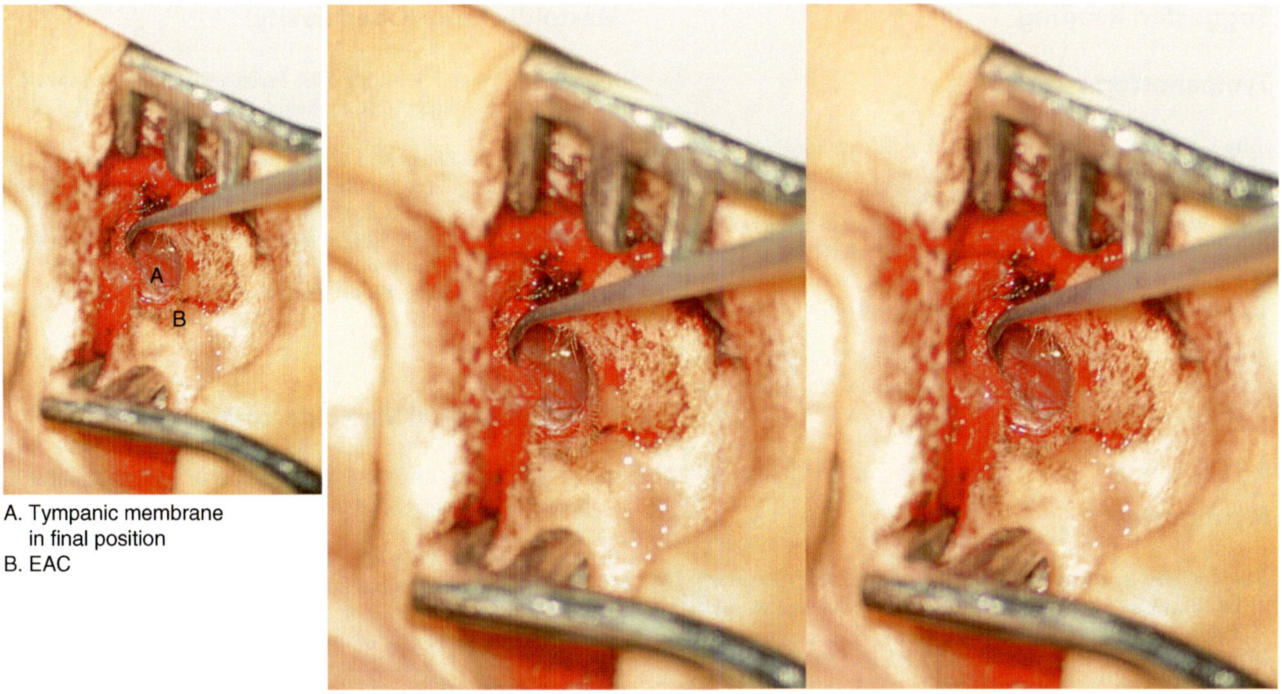

Fig. 2.194 Pack the external auditory canal and sew up the incision
Replace the plastic meatal flaps and tympanic membrane. Pack iodoform gauze into the external auditory canal and to sew up the incision. Cover the operation field with an aseptic dressing

Suggested Reading

Tympanostomy Tubes

Jiang S-C, Gu R, Zheng-Min W. Otorhinolaryngology – otology. 2nd ed. Shanghai: Shanghai Scientific and Technological Education Publishing House; 2002a. p. 754–75.

Kong WJ. Otorhinolaryngology head and neck surgery. Beijing: People's Medical Publishing House; 2005. p. 460–4.

Qian Y-Z, Fan Z, Li P-H. Otorhinolaryngology head and neck surgery manual. Beijing: People's Military Medical Press; 2000a. p. 26–31.

Zheng-Min W. Microsurgery of the ear. Shanghai: Shanghai Scientific and Technological Education Publishing House; 2004a. p. 125–41.

Myringoplasty

Jiang S-C, Gu R, Zheng-Min W. Otorhinolaryngology – otology. 2nd ed. Shanghai: Shanghai Scientific and Technological Education Publishing House; 2002b. p. 754–75.

Qian Y-Z, Fan Z, Li P-H. Otorhinolaryngology head and neck surgery manual. Beijing: People's Military Medical Press; 2000b. p. 26–31.

Zheng-Min W. Microsurgery of the ear. Shanghai: Shanghai Scientific and Technological Education Publishing House; 2004b. p. 125–41.

Tympanoplasty

Huang X-Z, Wang J-B, Kong W-J. Practice of otorhinolaryngology head and neck surgery. 2nd ed. Beijing: People's Medical Publishing House; 2008a. p. 888–965.

Jiang S-C, GU R, Zheng-Min W. Otorhinolaryngology – otology. 2nd ed. Shanghai: Shanghai Scientific and Technological Education Publishing House; 2002c. p. 754–75.

Zheng-Min W. Microsurgery of the ear. Shanghai: Shanghai Scientific and Technological Education Publishing House; 2004c. p. 125–41.

Reconstruction of Ossicular Chain/Ossiculoplasty

Huang X-Z, Wang J-B, Kong W-J. Practice of otorhinolaryngology head and neck surgery. 2nd ed. Beijing: People's Medical Publishing House; 2008b.

Javia LR, Ruckenstein MJ. Ossiculoplasty. Otolaryngol Clin North Am. 2006;39(6):1177–89.

McGee M, Hough JV. Ossiculoplasty. Otolaryngol Clin North Am. 1999;32(3):471–88.

Samy RN, Pensak ML. Revision ossiculoplasty. Otolaryngol Clin North Am. 2006;39(4):699–712.

Yang W-Y, Zhai S-Q. Head-neck dissection and temporal surgery. Beijing: People's Military Medical Press; 2002.

Yu Y-J, Dai P, Liu Z. Stereo anatomical and surgical atlas of temporal bone. Beijing: People's Military Medical Press; 2006a.

Mastoidectomy (Open Cavity)

Huang X-Z, Wang J-B, Kong W-J. Practice of otorhinolaryngology head and neck surgery. 2nd ed. Beijing: People's Medical Publishing House; 2008c.

Jiang S-C, Gu R, Zheng-Min W. Otorhinolaryngology – otology. 2nd ed. Shanghai: Shanghai Scientific and Technological Education Publishing House; 2002d.

Jiang S.-C, Yang W.-Y, Gu R. Operative surgery of otorhinolaryngology head and neck department. In: The complete works of operative surgery. 2nd ed. Beijing: People's Military Medical Press; 2005.

Modified Radical Mastoidectomy

Huang X-Z, Wang J-B, Kong W-J. Practice of otorhinolaryngology head and neck surgery. 2nd ed. Beijing: People's Medical Publishing House; 2008d.

Jiang S.-C, Yang W.-Y, Gu R. Operative surgery of otorhinolaryngology head and neck department. In: The complete works of operative surgery. 2nd ed. Beijing: People's Military Medical Press; 2005.

Sanna M, et al. The temporal bone a maunal for dissection and surgical apporaches. New York: Thieme; 2005.

Yu Y-J, Dai P, Liu Z. Stereo anatomical and surgical atlas of temporal bone. Beijing: People's Military Medical Press; 2006b.

Mastoidectomy (Closed Cavity)

Coker NJ, Jenkins HA. Atlas of otologic surgery. Philadelphia: Saunders; 2001.

Jiang S.-C, Yang W.-Y, Gu R. Operative surgery of otorhinolaryngology head and neck department. In: The complete works of operative surgery. 2nd ed. Beijing: People's Military Medical Press; 2005.

Yu Y-J, Dai P, Liu Z. Stereo anatomical and surgical atlas of temporal bone. Beijing: People's Military Medical Press; 2006c.

Mastoid Obliteration, Canal Wall Reconstruction and Tympanoplasty

Della Santina CC, Lee SC. Ceravital reconstruction of canal wall down mastoidectomy: long-term results. Arch Otolaryngol Head Neck Surg. 2006;132(6):617–23.

Ni Y, Hirsch BE, Da-zhang Y, et al. Outcome analysis of 40 ossiculoplasty cases. Chinese J Otol. 2005;3(2):100–3.

Ucar C. Canal wall reconstruction and mastoid obliteration with composite multifractured osteoperiosteal flap. Eur Arch Otorhinolaryngol. 2006;263(12):1082–6.

Ossicular Chain Reconstruction for Congenital Deformity or Trauma

Bahmad Jr F, Merchant SN. Histopathology of ossicular grafts and implants in chronic otitis media. Ann Otol Rhinol Laryngol. 2007;116(3):181–91.

Brackmann D, Shelton C, Arriaga MA. Otologic surgery. 2nd ed. Philadelphia: Saunders; 2001.

Caldart AU, Terruel I, Enge Jr DJ, Kurogi AS, Buschle M. Adriana Sayuri Kurogi, Maurício Buschle. Stapes surgery in residency – the ufpr clinical hospitalexperience. Braz J Otorhinolaryngol. 2007; 73(5):647–53.

Elsheikh MN, Elsherief H, Elsherief S. Physiologic reestablishment of ossicular continuity during excision of retraction pockets: use of hydroxyapatite bone cement for rebridging the incus. Arch Otolaryngol Head Neck Surg. 2006;132(2):196–9.

Fenli X, Keli C. Clinical study of congenital middle ear malformations. J Clin Otorhinol. 2004;18(10):586–9.

Hu U, Qiu-ju W, Dong-yi H. Clinical classification and relationship with conductive deafness of congenital middle ear malformations. Chinese J Otorhinol Head Neck Surg. 2005;40(12):893–5.

Lesinskas E, Vainutiene V. Closed tympanoplasty in middle ear cholesteatoma surgery. Medicina (Kaunas). 2004;40(9):856–9.

Facial Nerve Surgery

3

Pu Dai, Yong-yi Yuan, and Guo-jian Wang

Facial Nerve Decompression via Transmastoid Approach

Yong-yi Yuan and Pu Dai

Indications

This approach is used in patients with normal hearing, with the pathology confined to the vertical and horizontal segment, and not the geniculate ganglion or labyrinthine segment of the facial nerve (FN). It is only used in patients with peripheral facial paralysis, for example, Bell palsy, Ramsay-Hunt syndrome, temporal bone fracture, chronic otitis media and facial paralysis secondary to operation on the middle ear and mastoid.

Contraindications

1. It may be difficult in patients with poorly pneumatised mastoids and especially in those with a forward lying sigmoid sinus or low placed middle cranial fossa.
2. Facial paralysis appearing within 10 days of an attack of acute otitis media may be due to edema or inflammation of FN in its bony canal. Early treatment is indicated if the paralysis is not improving;
3. In patients with no muscle tonus, no reaction of the muscle to direct current, no random action or the fibrillation potential in electromyography, FN Decompression is contraindicated.
4. In patients with major temporal bone fractures, management of the potential life threatening head injury takes precedence. The facial paralysis can be addressed when the patient is stable again.
5. Patients with facial paralysis as well as Progressive Muscular Atrophy, hematological disease, or who are physically weak are unlikely to require FN decompression.

Operative Procedures

1. Incisions: The incision is placed 5–10 mm posterior to the postauricular sulcus. The skin and subcutaneous tissues are elevated from the periosteum overlying the mastoid cortex, and from the level of the top of the pinna to the mastoid tip.
2. Intact canal mastoidectomy: After drilling the mastoid cortex, the mastoid antrum is opened, then by thinning the posterior wall of EAC, access is enabled to the of tympanic cavity. The sigmoid sinus and middle cranial fossa plate, the ridge of the digastric muscle, the horizontal semicircular canal and short process of incus are all identified. The short process of incus should be protected to avoid dislocation and subsequent conductive hearing loss.
3. Exposure of the vertical segment of FN: The bony canal of FN is thinned from stylomastoid foramen to the bottom of short process of incus. The digastric ridge is a landmark for FN at stylomastoid foramen. When skeletonising the bony canal, one should use a diamond bur and drill along the longitudinal axis of FN. The blood vessels in the FN sheath give a pink colour through the bone, allowing early identification of the line and depth of the nerve. The vertical segment of FN can also be exposed via facial recess approach.
4. Exposure of the horizontal segment of FN: The posterior tympanic cavity is opened via a facial recess approach. The facial recess is a triangular area bounded by the chorda tympani nerve anterior-inferiorly, the superior part of the vertical segment of FN posterior-inferiorly and the fossa of the incus superiorly. An open facial recess provides access to the ossicles, stapedial tendon,

P. Dai, MD (✉) • Y.-y. Yuan, MD • G.-j. Wang, MD
Department of Otolarygngology Head and Neck Surgery,
Chinese PLA General Hospital, Beijing 100853, China
e-mail: daipu301@vip.sina.com

P. Dai et al. (eds.), *Stereo Operative Atlas of Micro Ear Surgery*, DOI 10.1007/978-981-10-2089-6_3

round window, oval window, bony canal of the horizontal segment of FN and the cochleariform process. The FN segment from cochleariform process to geniculate ganglion can be approached through the area surrounded by the body of incus, the horizontal semicircular canal and dural plate of middle cranial fossa. The ampulla of the horizontal and superior semicircular canal should be carefully protected. Decompression of the tympanic segment of FN canal can be performed by thinning the bony canal from the inferior surface of the curve of the second genu of the nerve to the cochleariform process. After removing bone along the canal inferiorly, the pyramid segment, the vertical segment and chorda tympani nerve can be decompressed.

5. When the ossicular chain is intact, only a small diamond bur should be used inferiorly to the incus in the facial recess. Separation of the incudostapedial joint is usually not necessary. Sometimes the incus could be removed temporarily and stored in physiological saline. The head of malleus can then be displaced laterally or drilled down. The lateral wall of the bony canal of the horizontal segment is removed as far as the geniculate ganglion. Once the decompression of the nerve is complete, the incus is repositioned.
6. Spiral thinning of the bony canal of FN : The bone of the canal is thinned from the posterior part of FN canal in the vertical segment, the lateral part in the pyramid segment and inferior part in the horizontal segment in a spiral fashion to protect neighboring structures. The chorda tympani nerve may be injured if the decompression is performed laterally in the vertical segment. The horizontal semicircular canal may be injured if the decompression is performed posteriorly in the pyramid segment. The superior semicircular may could be injured if the decompression is performed posterior superiorly in the horizontal segment. A diamond bur is used to delineate the course of the nerve, but leaving an eggshell layer of bone. When the light pink FN is identified through the eggshell thick bone, the nerve can be exposed with gentle removal of the bone using a micro elevator. The nerve is exposed across its full width and for at least 5 mm beyond the pathology at each end of the decompression. The bone chips, granulation tissue and cholesteatoma are all removed from the FN.
7. Dissecting the FN sheath: The FN sheath is opened with a sharp knife or hook to decompress the FN. Fibrous adhesions around the nerve fibre must be divided.
8. Closing the operative cavity: After the FN decompression, the operative cavity is irrigated with physiological saline, clearing bone and blood debris. Gelatin sponge soaked with dexamethasone is placed on the vertical segment of FN. In an open mastoid cavity, the skin flap of the external acoustic meatus is used to cover the FN. Finally, the cavity is gently packed with iodoform gauze and the incision is sutured step by step.

Special Comments

1. If the patient has nearly normal hearing, the ossicular chain should be protected as far as possible during FN decompression to avoid sensorineural and conductive hearing loss.
2. Avoid contact with the incus when working close to the horizontal semicircular canal. The bone of the facial nerve canal is also thin in this region and one needs to be careful to avoid damaging the nerve and the chorda tympani.
3. A diamond bur should be used in a spiral fashion to drill the bone of the FN canal with suction and liberal irrigation to avoid heat and to clear bone dust, thus improving identification of the nerve through the bone. When opening the FN sheath attention should be paid not to injure the stylomastoid artery.
4. When dissecting the thinned bone over the sheath, care should be taken not to lever on the nerve or injure it with the dissector.
5. If a bone spicule is found in the FN, it should be removed and the integrity of the nerve should be assessed. If the nerve is substantially intact, the sheath should be opened to decompress the nerve. If there is separation of the nerve, it should be repaired with re-routing and primary repair or grafting with a nerve cable graft. Re-routing is the first option as there will be only one anastomosis. This must be done without tension, and if this is not possible, a cable graft is used.

Complications

1. Sensorineural hearing impairment due to direct injury to inner ear or drill contact with the incus causing transmitting intense vibration to the inner ear.
2. Vertigo due to injury of the semicircular canals.
3. Conductive hearing impairment. There are two mechanisms:
   a. The removal of incus or head of malleus to facilitate the decompression of horizontal segment of FN will affect sound conduction. Reconstruction of the ossicular chain after decompression will then be necessary.
   b. Fibrous scarring and fixation as a result of hemorrhage at operation or effusion after operation, will have an effect on sound conduction.

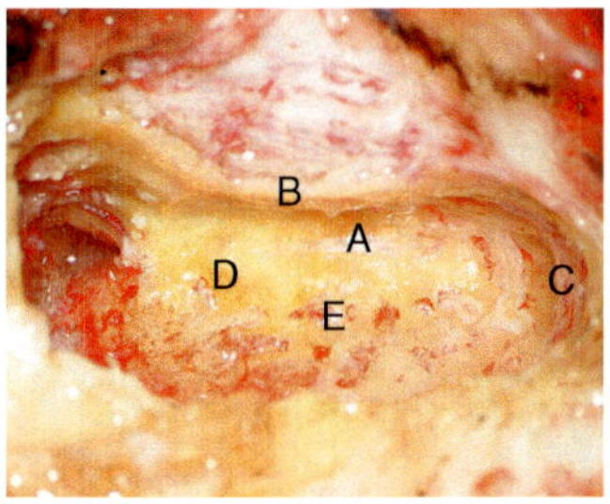

A. Chorda tympani
B. Posterior wall of EAC
C. Mastoid tip
D. Facial recess
E. Facial nerve

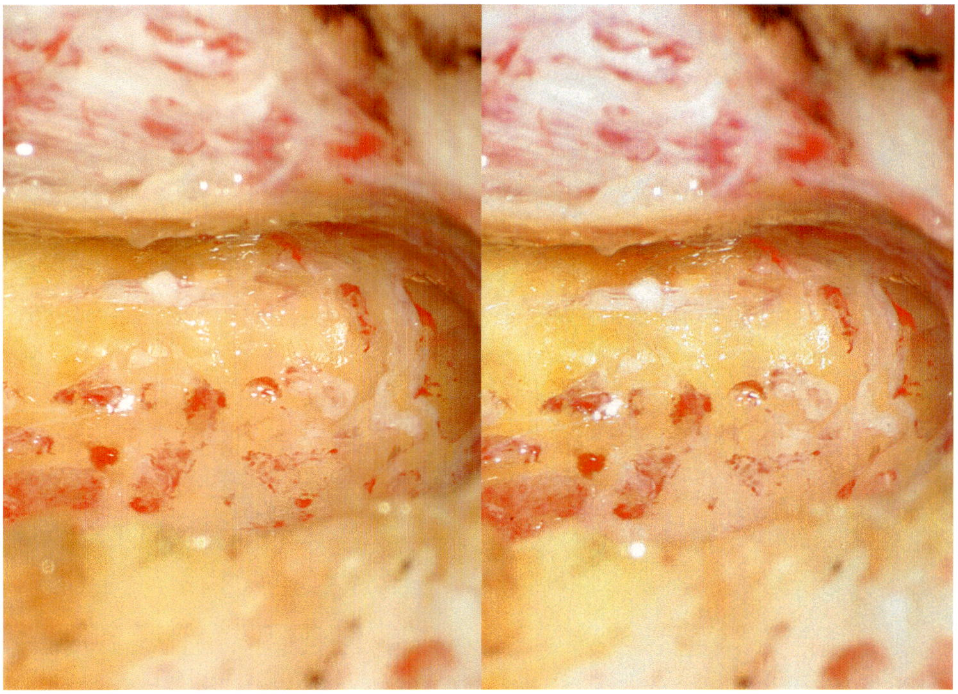

Fig. 3.1 Skeletonization of mastoid with intact posterior wall of EAC
The posterior wall of EAC is skeletonized and thinned down but kept intact. The digastric ridge is exposed and used as a landmark for finding the stylomastoid foramen. The vertical segment of FN is found by drilling superiorly from this area. The chorda tympani nerve is identified. The fossa between chorda tympani and the FN is the facial recess

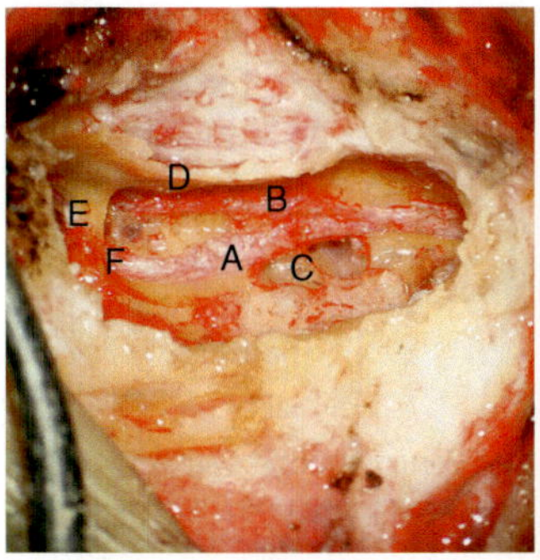

A. Swollen vertical segment of FN (the bone has been removed but the sheath is still intact)
B. Chorda tympani nerve
C. Retrofacial air cells
D. Posterior wall of EAC
E. Incus buttress
F. Pyramid segment of FN

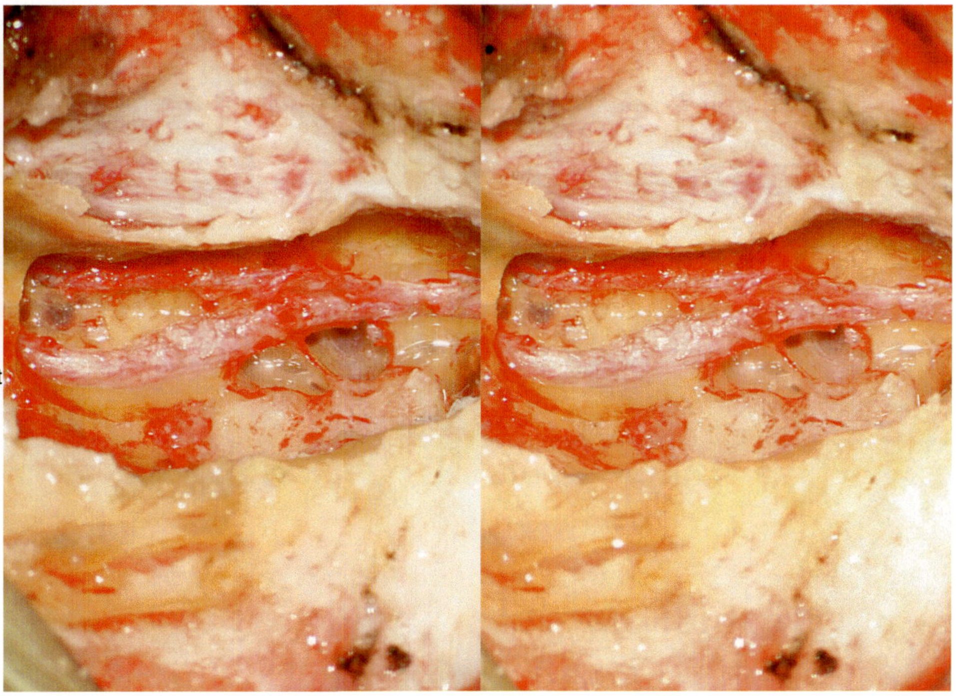

Fig 3.2 Exposure of the vertical segment of FN
The bone of the canal of the vertical segment of FN is thinned like an egg shell. On removal of the bone, the FN sheath is exposed and both the chorda tympani and FN are found to be swollen

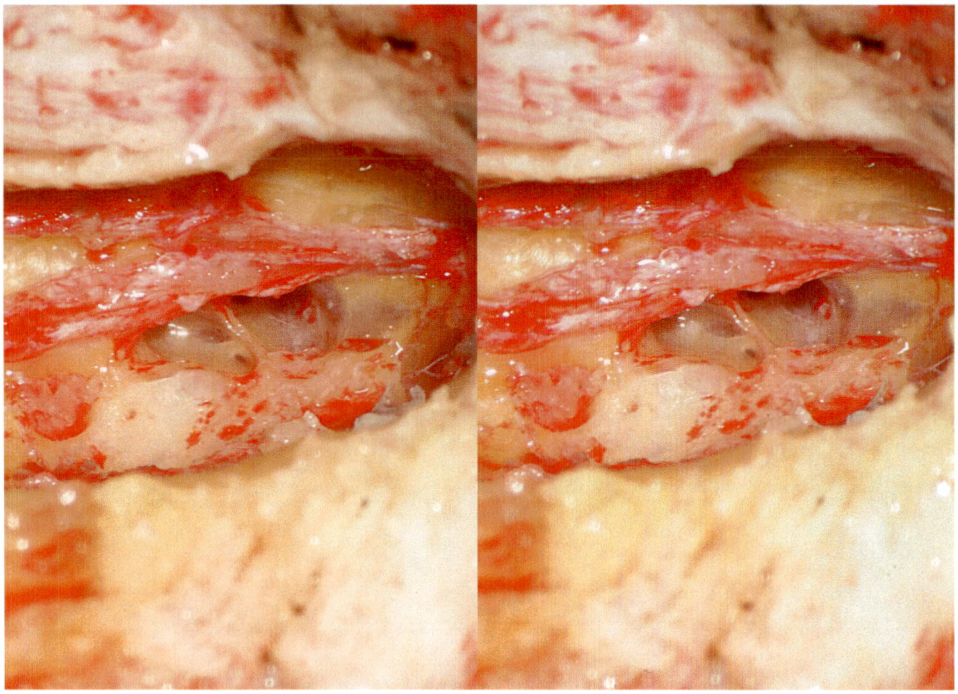

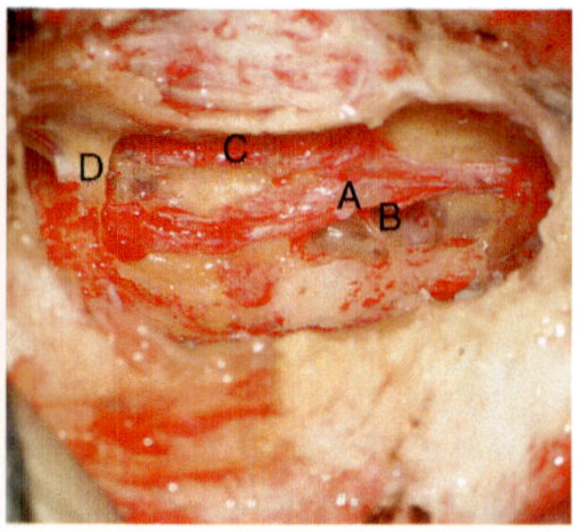

A. Swollen vertical segment of FN (the canal bone has been removed and the nerve sheath is still intact)
B. Retrofacial air cells
C. Chorda tympani
D. Posterior arch buttress

Fig. 3.3 Decompression of the vertical segment of FN
The FN sheath is opened longitudinally with a fractured razor in order to relieve the compression of the nerve within

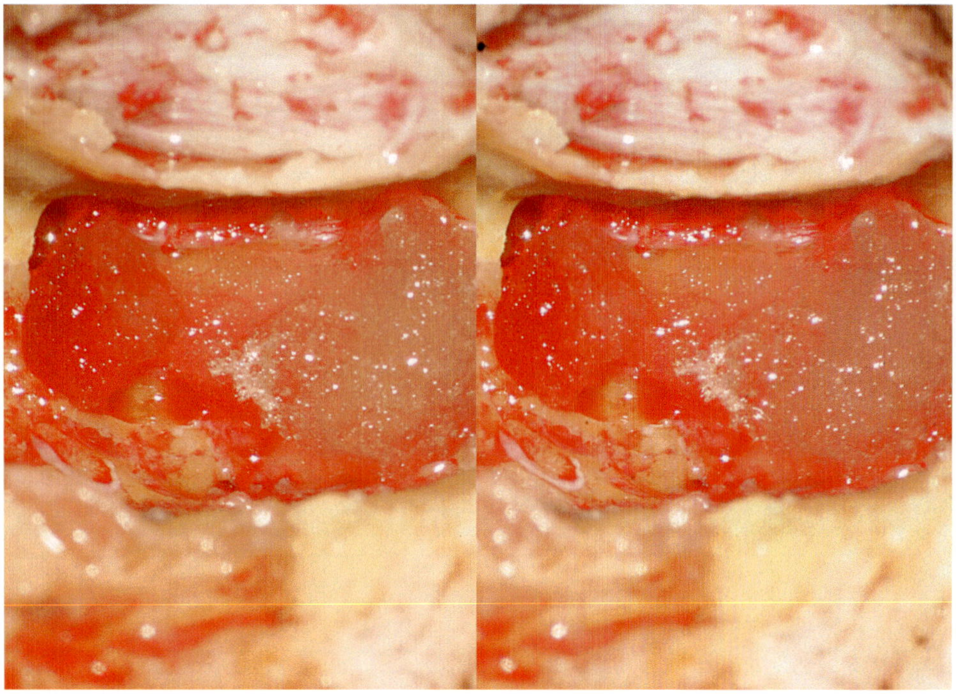

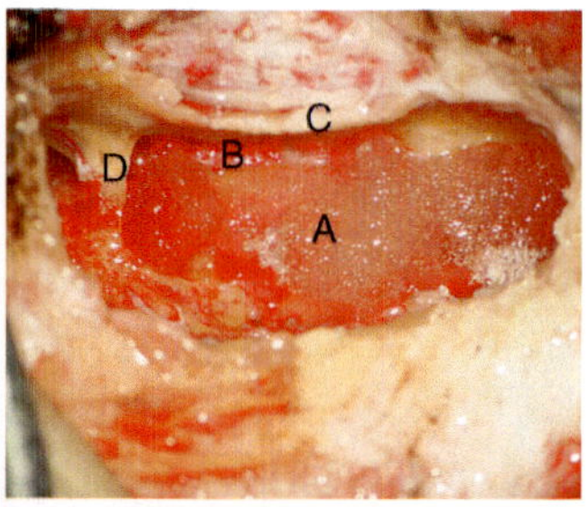

A. Gelatin sponge soaked with dexamethasone
B. Chorda tympani
C. Posterior wall of EAC
D. Incus buttress

Fig 3.4 Opening of the FN sheath and application of dexamethasone
The cavity is liberally irrigated to clear bone dust and blood. Gelatin sponge soaked with dexamethasone is placed on the vertical segment of FN

Facial Nerve Decompression via Translabyrinthine Approach

Yong-yi Yuan and Pu Dai

Indications

This technique is used in patients with facial paralysis but no useful inner ear function.

Contraindications

1. It may be difficult in patients with poorly pneumatised mastoids and especially in those with a forward lying sigmoid sinus or low placed middle cranial fossa.
2. Facial paralysis appearing within 10 days of an attack of acute otitis media may be due to edema or inflammation of FN in its boney canal. Early treatment is indicated if the paralysis is not improving;
3. In patients with no muscle tonus, no reaction of the muscle to direct current, no random action or the fibrillation potential in electromyography, FN Decompression is contraindicated.
4. In patients with major temporal bone fractures management of the potential life threatening head injury takes precedence. The facial paralysis can be addressed when the patient is stable again.
5. Patients with facial paralysis as well as Progressive Muscular Atrophy, hematological disease, or who are physically weak are unlikely to require FN decompression.

Operative Procedures

1. Incision: The post auricular incision is the same as that for the transmastoid approach for decompression of the facial nerve.
2. Mastoidectomy and decompression of the vertical segment of the facial nerve: The posterior and superior walls of the external auditory canal are preserved and the upper tympanic cavity is exposed. The procedure is facilitated with removal of the incus and head of the malleus. The area to be exposed is bounded by the vertical segment of the facial nerve anteriorly, the middle cranial fossa dural plate superiorly, the skeletonized sigmoid sinus posteriorly, and the digastric ridge inferiorly. The decompression of the vertical segment of the facial nerve is then completed.
3. Labyrinthectomy: The three semicircular canals are identified then drilled out. The vestibule is opened. The lateral wall of the vestibule is removed and its medial wall is exposed. The posterior wall of the internal acoustic canal is skeletonized before opening.
4. Opening the internal acoustic canal: After drilling the whole posterior wall on the internal acoustic canal, the dura is opened along the line of the inferior vestibular nerve. The transverse crest separates the upper and lower parts of the canal. A vertical crest (Bill's bar) divides the lateral part of the canal into an anterior section containing the facial nerve and a posterior segment containing the superior vestibular nerve. The cochlear nerve is located in the anterior part below the transverse crest. The inferior vestibular nerve is located in the posterior part below the crest. The labyrinthine segment, geniculate ganglion and horizontal segment of the facial nerve can be exposed by drilling along the facial nerve anterior and lateral to the fundus of the internal auditory canal (IAC). This is the most important part of a translabyrinthine decompression of the facial nerve.
5. If there were no injury to the facial nerve localized at the bottom of the internal acoustic canal, the internal acoustic canal can be kept intact. Drill the bone gradually along the interior wall of the anterior semicircular canal ampulla to expose the labyrinthine segment of the facial nerve. The labyrinthine segment of the facial nerve is thin and in a narrow bony canal and care needs to be taken not to injure it with the drill or other instruments.
6. The procedure of decompression of the facial nerve is the same as that of the transmastoid decompression of the facial nerve. If the facial nerve is severed or a segment is missing, rerouting or grafting should be performed.
7. Closing the operative cavity: After opening the internal auditory canal, the temporal fascia or autogenous fat is used to pack it to prevent a cerebrospinal fluid leak and this is covered with compressed gelfoam. The mastoid cavity is filled with fat and a drainage is placed. The incision is then closed step by step.

Special Comments

1. To improve exposure of the internal auditory canal, the bone over the sigmoid sinus should be removed. The sinus can then be depressed to give better access to the inferior part of the canal.
2. To avoid cerebrospinal fluid otorrhea, pay attention not to drill the bony bottom of internal acoustic canal too much.
3. Facial nerve monitoring should be used if possible to localize the nerve and assess its function, especially in cases of congenital deformity, and in revision mastoid procedures.

4. A diamond bur should be used in a spiral fashion to drill the bone of the FN canal with suction and liberal irrigation to avoid heat and to clear bone dust, thus improving identification of the nerve through the bone. When opening the FN sheath, attention should be paid not to injure the stylomastoid artery.
5. When dissecting the thinned bone of the sheath, care should be taken not to lever on the nerve or injure it with the dissector.
6. If a bone spicule is found in the FN, it should be removed and the integrity of the nerve should be assessed. If the nerve is substantially intact, the sheath should be opened to decompress the nerve. If there is separation of the nerve it should be repaired with re-routing and primary repair or grafting with a nerve cable graft. Re-routing is the first option as there will be only one anastomosis. This must be done without tension, and if this is not possible, a cable graft is used.

Complications

Cerebrospinal fluid otorrhea or rhinorrhea, cerebrospinal fluid leakage by incision due to breaching the bottom of internal acoustic canal and laceration of the cerebral dura mater.

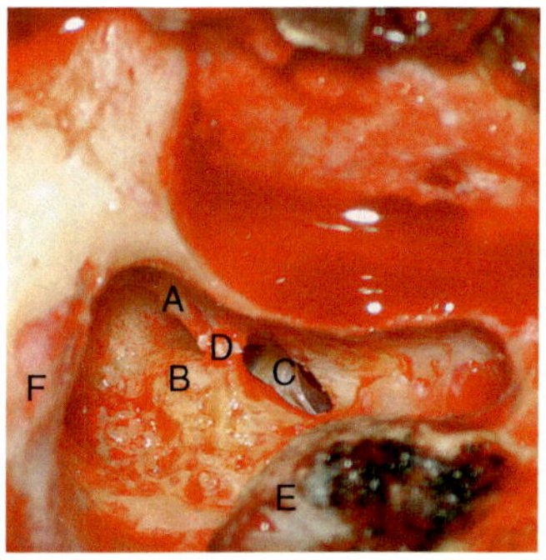

A. Short process of incus
B. Eminence of the horizontal semicircular canal
C. Facial recess
D. Incus buttress
E. Anterior wall of sigmoid sinus
F. Dural plate of middle cranial fossa

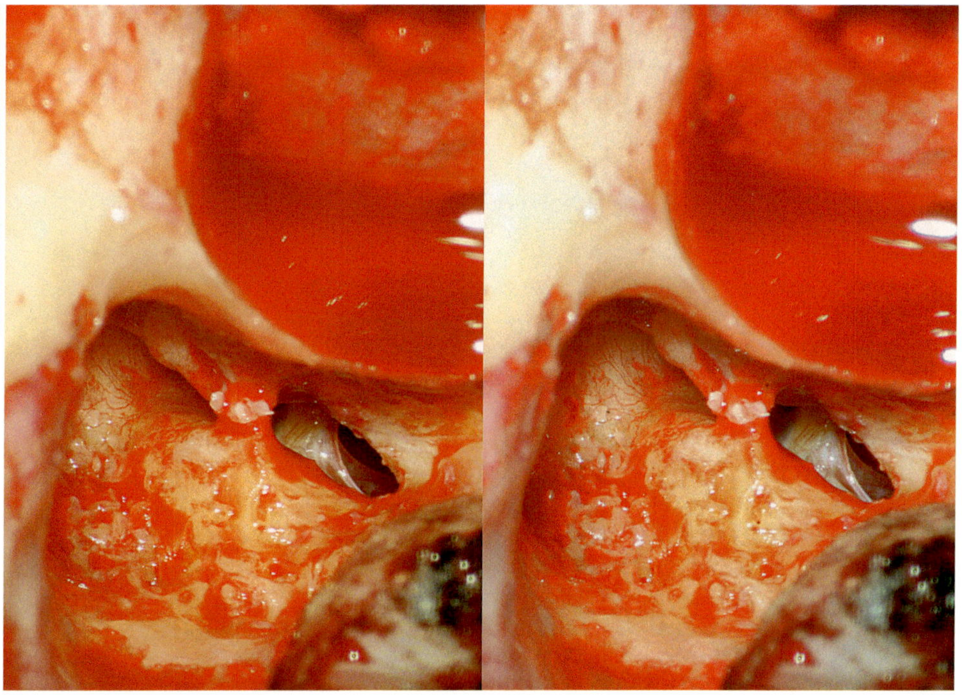

Fig. 3.5 Opening of the facial recess
Having localized the vertical segment of the facial nerve and chorda tympani, the facial recess is opened. Due to the anterior position of the sigmoid sinus, its bony covering is removed to improve exposure

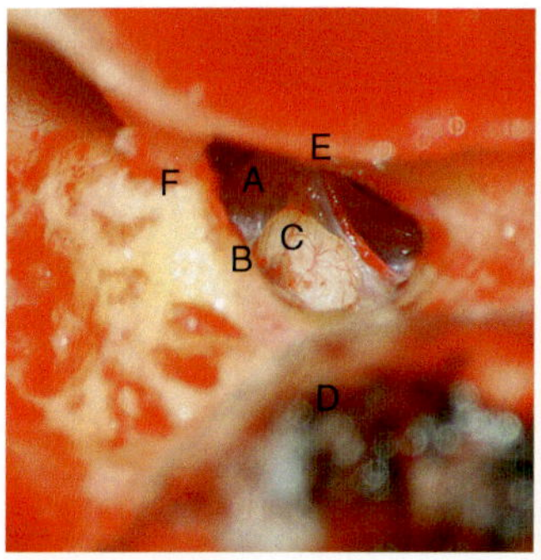

A. Facial recess
B. Bony facial canal
C. Bone fragment of fracture of the promontory
D. Anterior wall of sigmoid sinus
E. Posterior wall of external auditory canal
F. Incus buttress

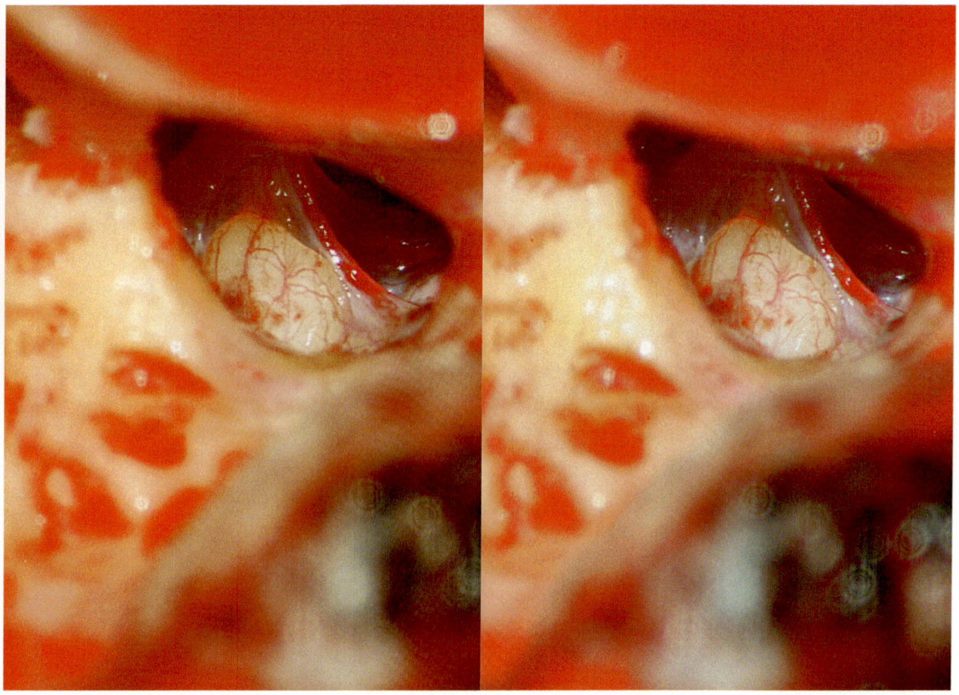

Fig. 3.6 Exposure of the promontory
The promontory is exposed after opening out the facial recess approach. A large mobile bone fragment is identified, indicating a major injury of the inner ear

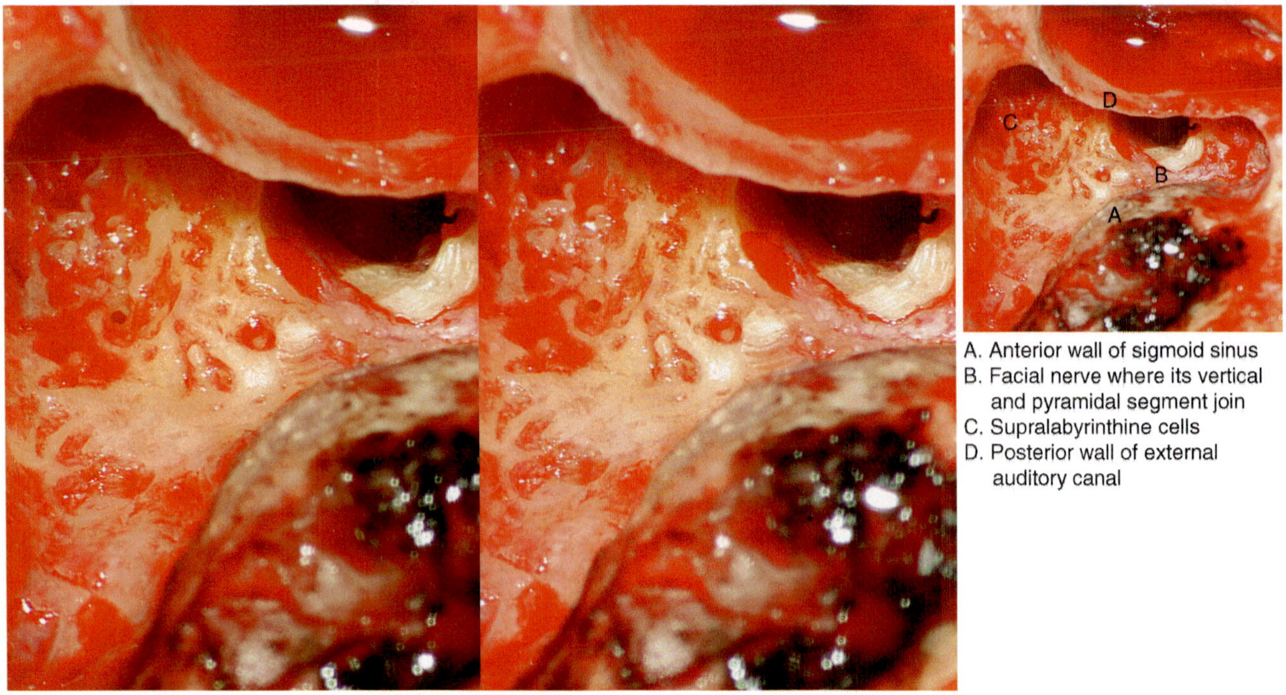

A. Anterior wall of sigmoid sinus
B. Facial nerve where its vertical and pyramidal segment join
C. Supralabyrinthine cells
D. Posterior wall of external auditory canal

Fig. 3.7 Exposure of the superior vertical and pyramid segments of the facial nerve
The bone of anterior and posterior margins of the facial recess thinned down. The vertical segment is exposed and found to be normal in this case. When working more superiorly, the pyramid segment of the facial nerve is identified

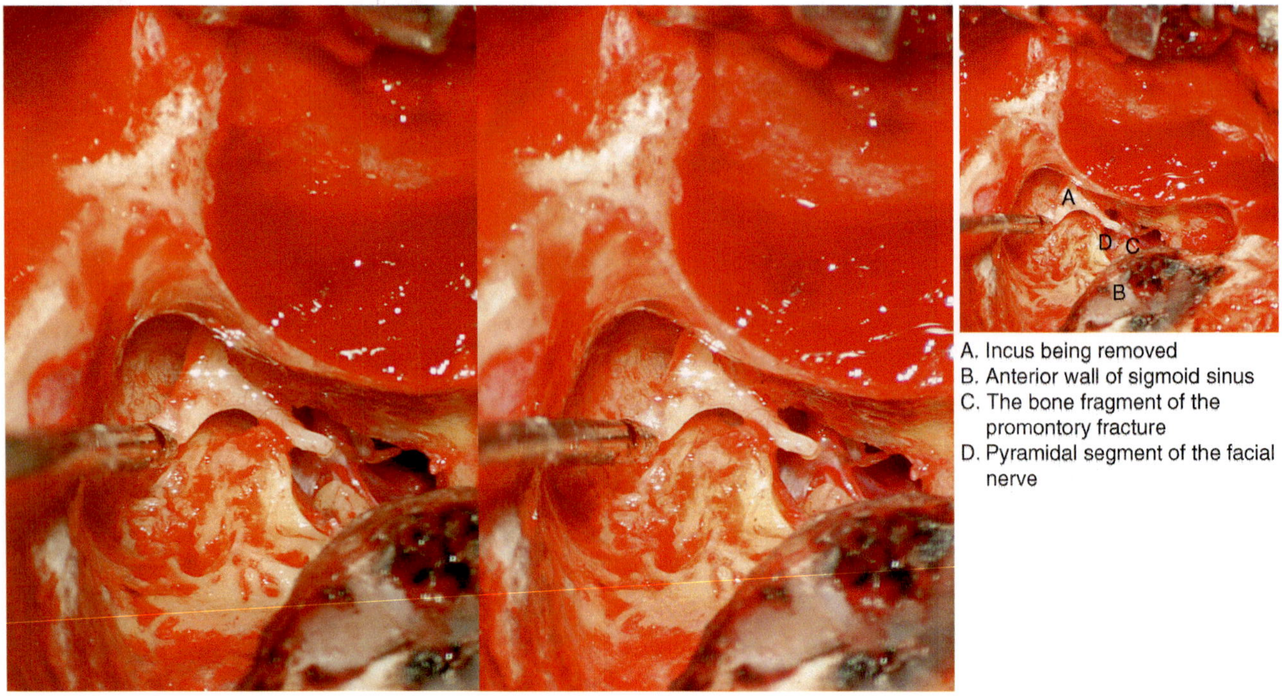

A. Incus being removed
B. Anterior wall of sigmoid sinus
C. The bone fragment of the promontory fracture
D. Pyramidal segment of the facial nerve

Fig. 3.8 Removal of the incus buttress and incus
As the inner ear is fractured, the incus buttress and incus are removed in order to expose the horizontal semicircular canal, horizontal segment of the facial nerve and geniculate ganglion

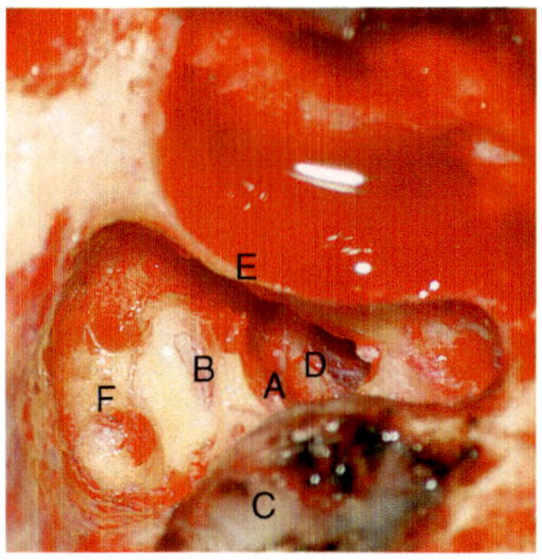

A. Pyramidal segment of the facial nerve
B. Fibrotic horizontal semicircular canal
C. Anterior wall of sigmoid sinus
D. Promontory covered with mucosa and fibrous tissue
E. Posterior wall of external auditory canal
F. Superior semicircular canal

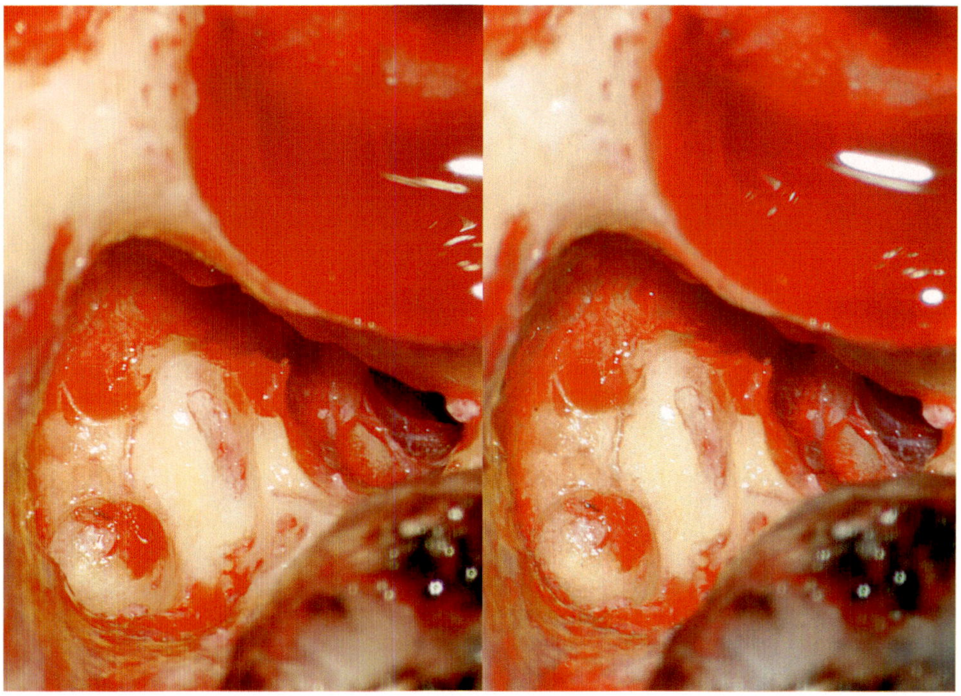

Fig. 3.9 Dissection of the semicircular canal
The compact bone of the horizontal semicircular canal is drilled down. Under normal circumstances the blue line of the semicircular canal would be seen. The inner ear and canal in this case are totally fibrosed. The ampulla of the canal is exposed in this operating procedure

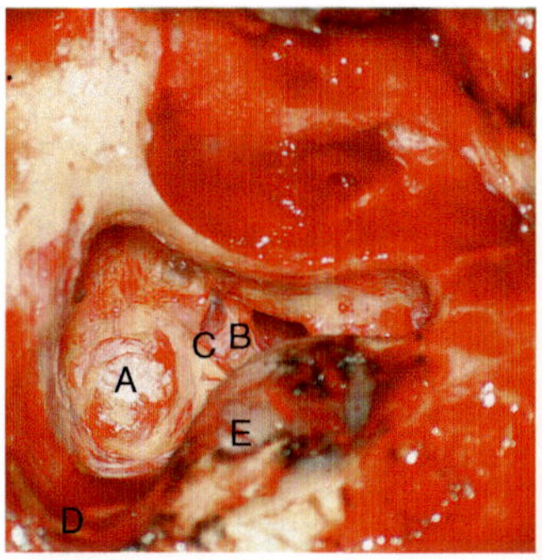

A. Fibrotic vestibule
B. Fibrosis over the promontory
C. Pyramidal segment of the facial nerve
D. Sinodural angle
E. Anterior wall of sigmoid sinus

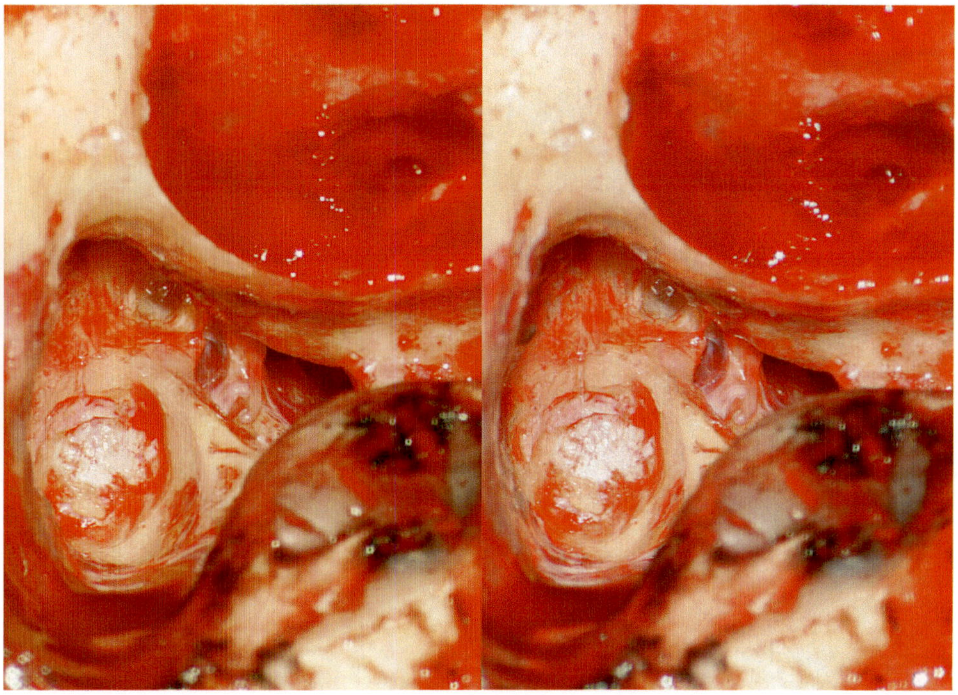

Fig. 3.10 Opening of the vestibule
The horizontal semicircular canal and part of the ampulla of the superior semicircular canal are removed. With further drilling the vestibule is opened. This is also found to be filled with fibrous tissue. The geniculate ganglion and the labyrinthine segment of the facial nerve can be exposed through this approach

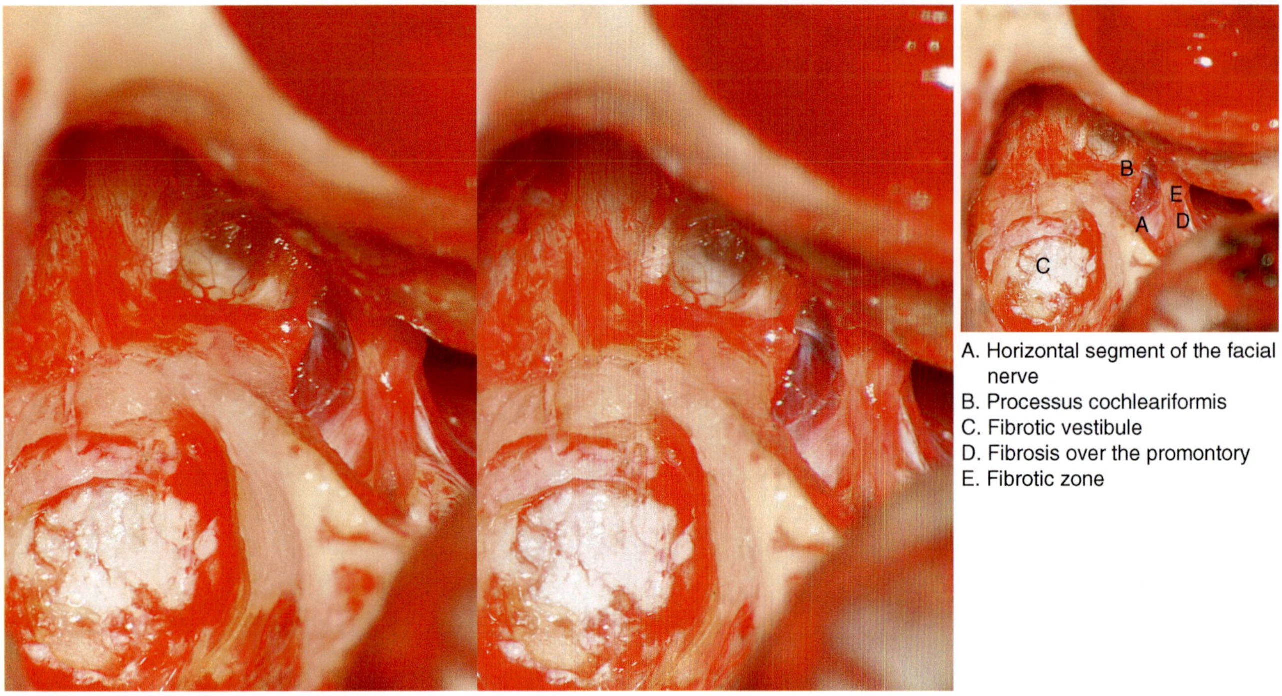

A. Horizontal segment of the facial nerve
B. Processus cochleariformis
C. Fibrotic vestibule
D. Fibrosis over the promontory
E. Fibrotic zone

Fig. 3.11 Exposure of the horizontal segment of the facial nerve
The horizontal segment of the facial nerve is seen when drilling up from the pyramidal. Bone chips is found ahead of the horizontal segment of the facial nerve

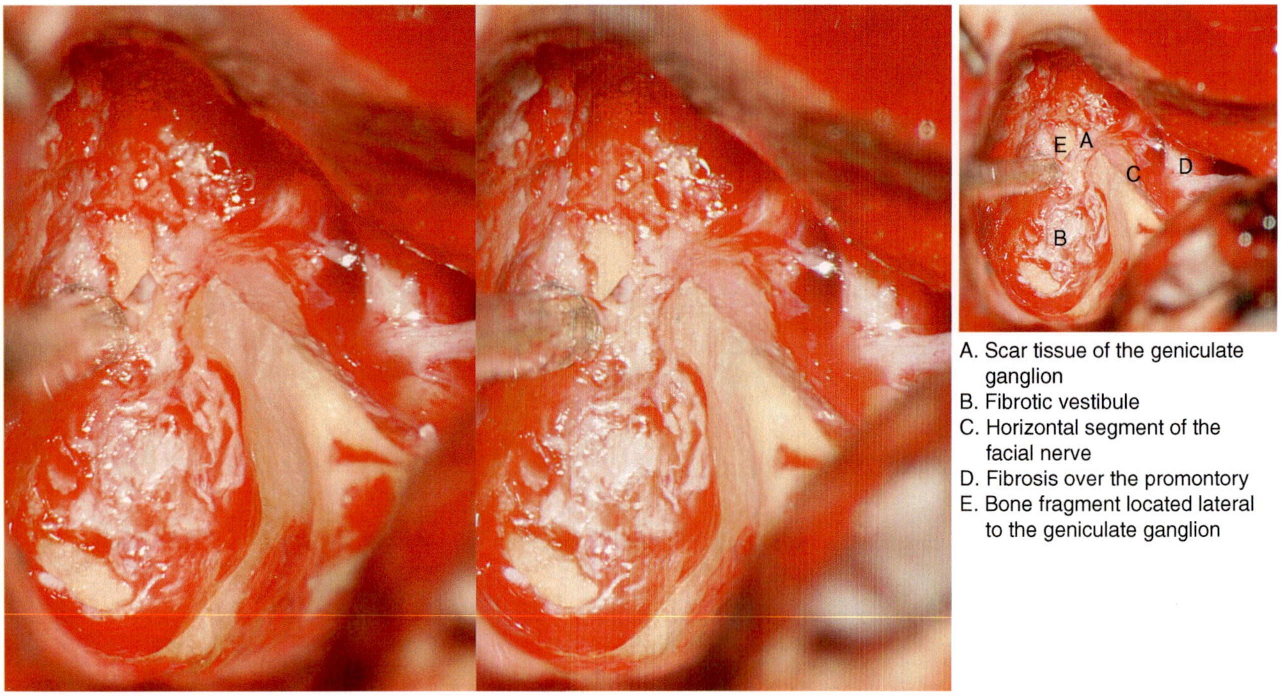

A. Scar tissue of the geniculate ganglion
B. Fibrotic vestibule
C. Horizontal segment of the facial nerve
D. Fibrosis over the promontory
E. Bone fragment located lateral to the geniculate ganglion

Fig. 3.12 Exposure of the geniculate ganglion
The bone around the geniculate ganglion is fractured. The geniculate ganglion is found compressed by bone fragments laterally. The geniculate ganglion is wholly replaced by fibrous tissue. The scar tissue of the geniculate ganglion is dissected layer by layer and no nerve fibres are found

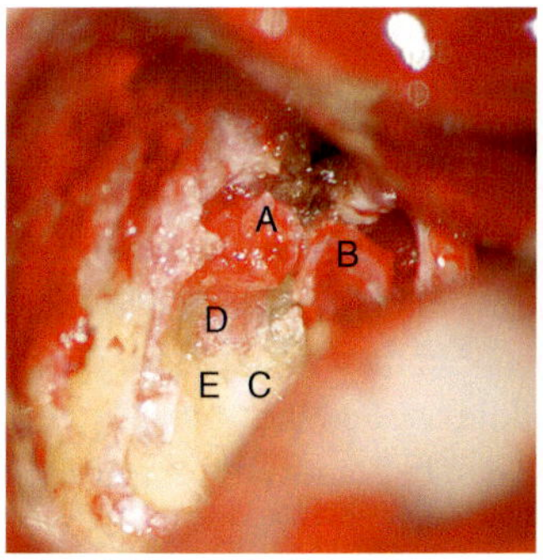

A. The amputated stump between the geniculate ganglion and labyrinthine segment of the facial nerve
B. The amputated stump between the geniculate ganglion and horizontal segment of the facial nerve
C. Medial wall of vestibule
D. The terminal of labyrinthine segment of the facial nerve close to cranial cavity
E. Scar close to the bottom of internal acoustic canal

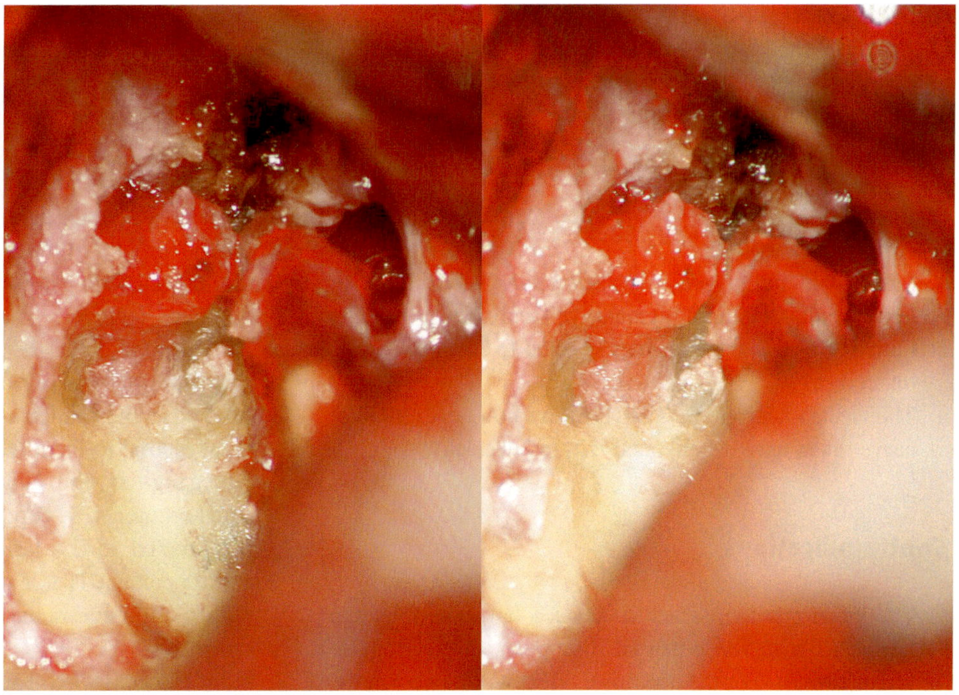

Fig. 3.13 Exposure of the labyrinthine segment of the facial nerve
The fibrous tissue in the vestibule is removed and the labyrinthine segment of the facial nerve is exposed gradually until its portion near the inner acoustic canal is seen. Having removed the scar tissue of the geniculate ganglion, the facial nerve is found to be fully divided. There is a loss of 2 mm of the nerve between the labyrinthine and horizontal segments of the facial nerve

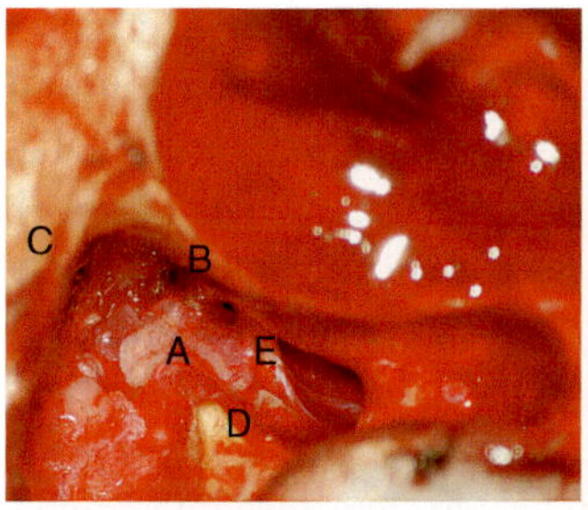

A. The greater auricular nerve is transplanted, fixed by biogel and covered with a vein flap.
B. Posterior wall of external auditory canal
C. Dural plate of middle cranial fossa
D. Pyramid segment of the facial nerve
E. Fibrosis over the promontory

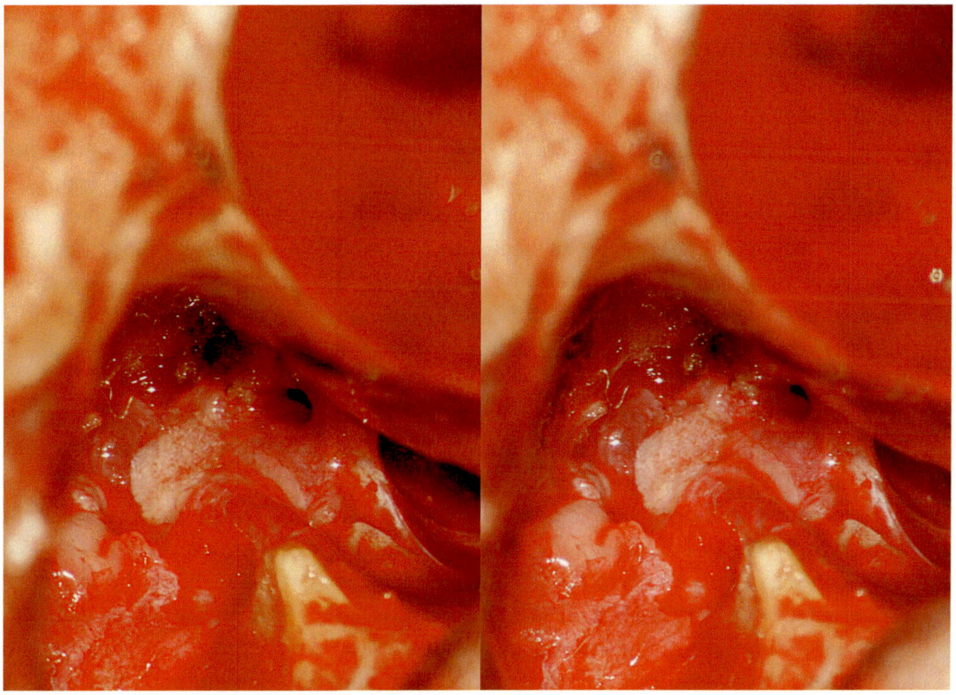

Fig. 3.14 Grafting of the facial nerve
A segment of the greater auricular nerve to repair the defect between the labyrinthine and horizontal segments of the facial nerve. The graft is fixed by biogel and covered with a vein flap. The function of the facial nerve begins to recover 6 months after operation

Middle Cranial Fossa Approach Decompression of Facial Nerve

Guo-jianWang and Pu Dai

Indications

1. Lesions involving geniculate ganglion, labyrinthine or internal auditory canal segments of facial nerve;
2. Function of facial nerve not expected to recover despite intact trunk;
3. The electro-neurogram (ENOG) shows that over 90 % of nerve fibers have degenerated within 2 weeks.

Contraindications

1. The facial muscle has lost its tension but to atrophy and fibrosis, fibrillation potential disappears in electromyogram (EMG); (For the operating effect will be poor if the patient's facial nerve is in this status.)
2. Other life threatening injuries must be managed first;
3. Patient's general health not sufficient for operation to be performed safely.

Operative Procedures

Supine position, affected ear side up, the surgeon seated at the top of patient's head.

1. Incision: A vertical incision is commonly used, which is 6–8 cm long and 2 cm in front of tragus, and approximately at right angles to the root of the zygoma. An inverse L-shaped incision may also be used, which is like the vertical incision inferiorly but turns forwards in the upper part.
2. The skin, temporal muscle and periosteum are incised vertically and elevated using blunt dissection to expose the squamous part of temporal bone;
3. Above the zygomatic arch and temporal line, 4 holes are drilled in the bone of the squamous part of the temporal bone forming a 3 cm × 4 cm rectangle, of which the front 2/3 is anterior to a vertical line crossing the front wall of external auditory canal. The lower edge of the 'window' is near the zygomatic arch or temporal line. The bone between the holes is cut to form a rectangle with a fret-saw or trephine, and bone flap is removed leaving a 'window' craniotomy.
4. An elevator or brain spatula is used to detach the dura of middle cranial fossa from the superior surface of petrosal bone; three important anatomic marks on base of middle cranial fossa are carefully identified: the middle meningeal artery, the greater superficial petrosal nerve and the arcuate eminence.
5. The bone covering the greater superficial petrosal nerve is removed from front to back to expose the geniculate ganglion; and medial to this, the labyrinthine and internal auditory canal segments can then be exposed. If necessary, the roof of the middle ear and the bone posterior to the geniculate ganglion can be removed to expose the tympanic segment.
6. If the landmarks of the base of middle cranial fossa are not clear, the roof of tympanum can be firstly removed to expose the malleus and incus. The horizontal segment medial to them is identified, and then the geniculate ganglion, the labyrinthine and internal auditory canal segments are exposed in turn. If there is no pathology medial to the labyrinthine segment, the internal auditory canal is not necessarily opened, in order to reduce the occurrence of postoperative cerebrospinal otorrhea.
7. After the geniculate ganglion, labyrinthine and internal auditory canal segments are exposed, the sheath of facial nerve (and dura of internal acoustic meatus if necessary) is dissected with a sharp blade to reduce pressure on the nerve;
8. The decompressed facial nerve is covered with gelatin sponge soaked in dexamethasone to prevent and reduce edema. If the roof of tympanic cavity has been removed, the attic should be sealed with a temporalis musculofascial flap; and if the dura of internal acoustic meatus is opened, temporalis muscle is used to gently pack it to prevent a CSF leak.
9. The bone flap previously removed is replaced and fixed with skull locking rivets;
10. The cavity is liberally irrigated, any bleeding is controlled, a drain tube is inserted, the wound is closed and a dressing is applied.

Special Comments

1. The proper location of the 'bone window' is important for best exposure of the operative field. 2/3 of the bone window should be in front of the vertical line crossing the front wall of the external of the auditory canal. The lower edge is near the zygomatic arch or temporal line mark the base of middle cranial fossa.
2. Occasionally, the bone covering of the geniculate ganglion is absent; so elevation of the dura from the superior surface of the temporal bone should be done with care to prevent injury to the nerve.
3. Before elevating the dura, mannitol can be administered to reduce intracranial pressure. The dura should be

separated carefully, particularly medially to prevent injury to the superior petrosal sinus.

4. The roof of the tympanic cavity is located at the posterior end of the root of the zygoma, 18 mm medial to the lateral bone plate of the squamous part of the temporal bone.
5. The labyrinthine segment is located between the cochlea and superior semicircular canal, 4 mm in front of the semicircular canal and 1 mm behind the cochlea. When removing the bone covering the labyrinthine and internal auditory canal segments, care should be taken to avoid injury of these parts.
6. When decompressing the facial nerve, bone should be removed from at least half of the circumference of the canal, and the nerve should be exposed back to normal tissue at each end of the decompression.

Complications

1. Conductive deafness: if the attic is exposed, the middle fossa contents may herniate through the defect in the roof of the middle ear and impede normal movement the ossicular chain.
2. Sensorineural hearing impairment: due to direct injury of inner ear or vibration damage to the inner ear as a result of drilling contact with the ossicles.
3. Leakage of cerebrospinal fluid due to the tearing of dura, which is handled with repairing dura, sealing the attic and plugging the operative cavity with a temporal musculofascial flap, fat or fascia lata.
4. Vertigo due to injury of the semicircular canals or vestibule.
5. Direct nerve injury due to burn from drilling or contusion by forceps.

Surgery 1: Middle cranial fossa approach decompression of facial nerve

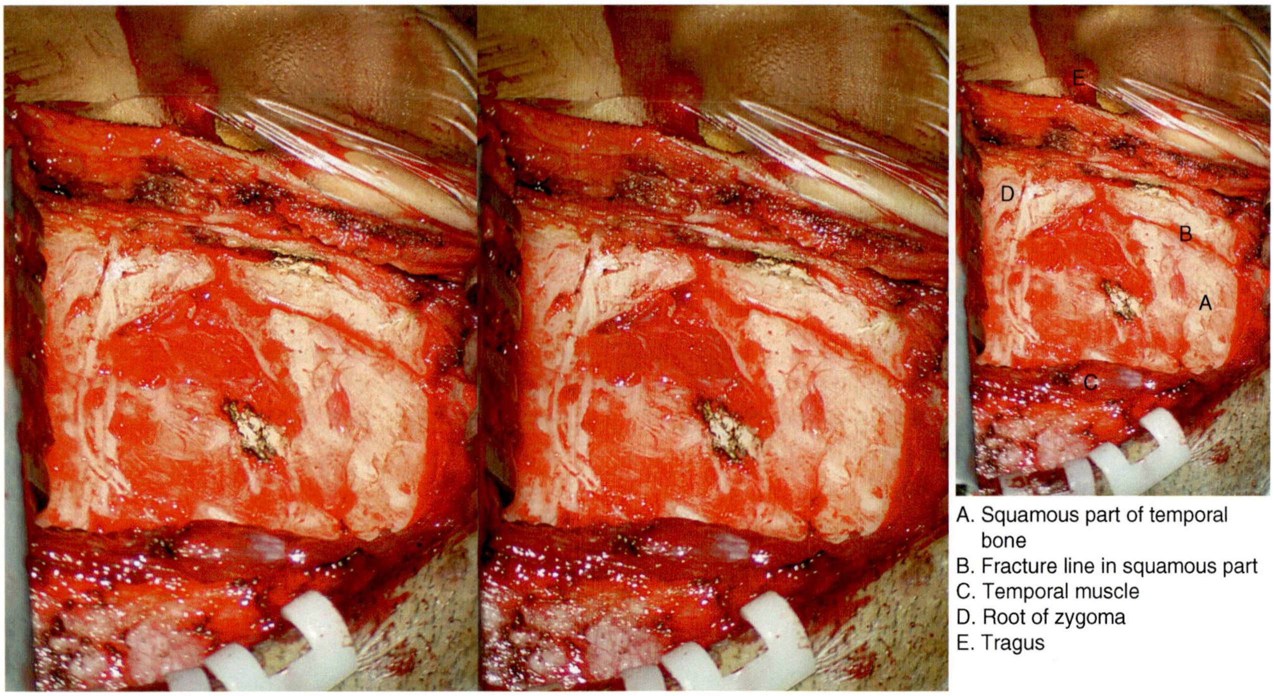

Fig. 3.15 Incision of skin and subcutaneous tissue, exposing squamous part of temporal bone
Inverse L-shaped incision is used, which is 6–8 cm long and is made 2 cm in front of tragus approximately at right angles to the root of zygoma in its lower part, and turns upwards and forwards in the upper part. The skin, temporal muscle and periosteum are incised and elevated with blunt dissection. A retractor is placed to expose the squamous part of temporal bone. A temporal musculofascial flap attached to the zygoma can be dissected in parallel to help exposure. Bleeding of edge can be stopped with scalp clamps

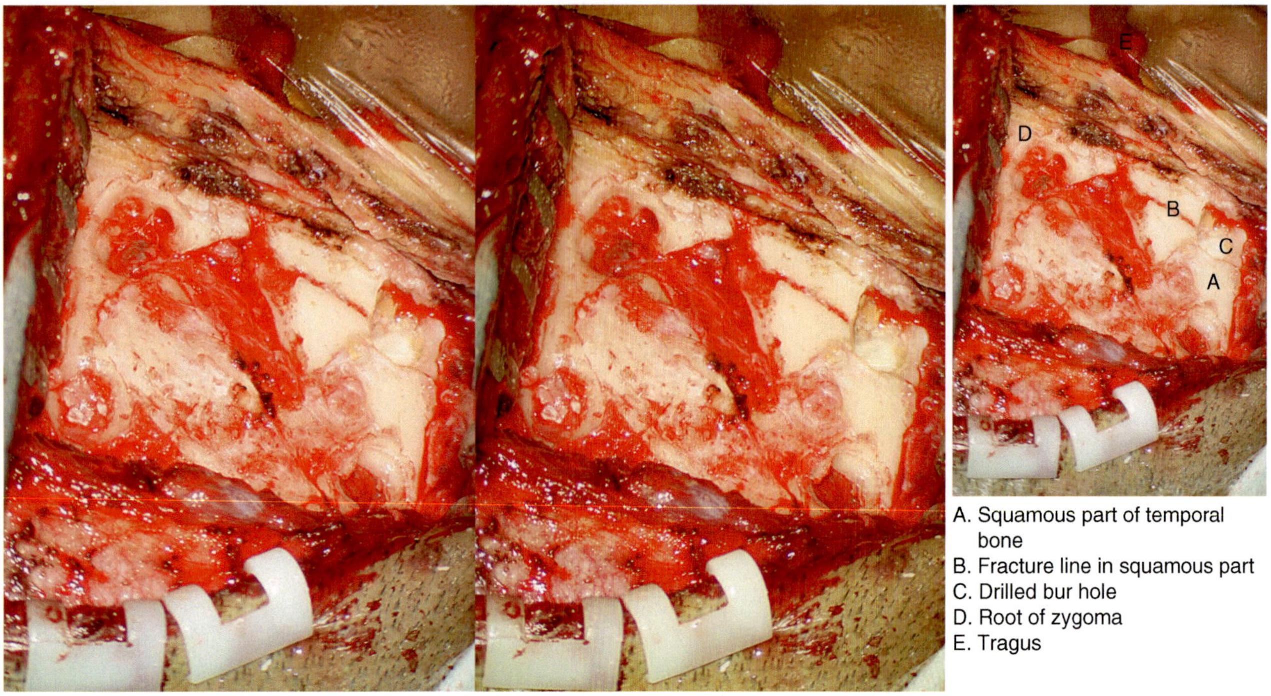

Fig. 3.16 Removing bone to form a 'window' in the temporal bone, and exposing the base of middle cranial fossa
Above the zygomatic arch, 4 holes are drilled in the bone forming a 3 cm × 4 cm rectangle, which should be as low as possible. The bone along the margins of the rectangle is sawed with a fretsaw or a trephine, and the bone flap is removed leaving a 'bone window' in the squamous part of the temporal bone. The anterior 2/3 of the window should be in front of the vertical Line crossing the anterior wall of the external auditory canal. The low edge includes the zygomatic arch or temporal line. An elevator or brain retractor blade is used to detach the dura of middle cranial fossa from the superior surface of petrosal bone

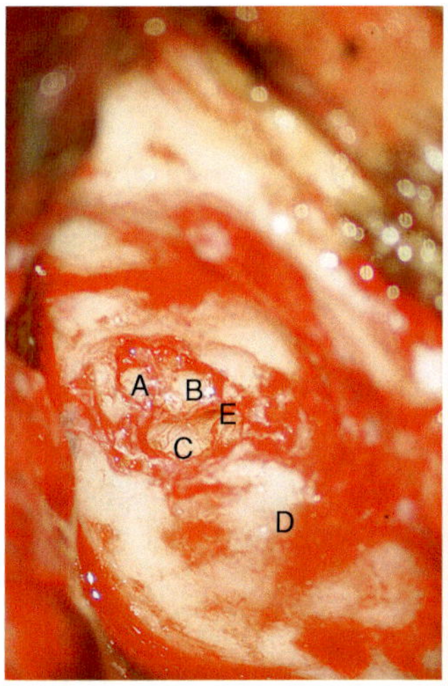

A. Malleus
B. Incus
C. Lateral semicircular canal
D. Surface of base of middle cranial fossa
E. Aditus ad antrum

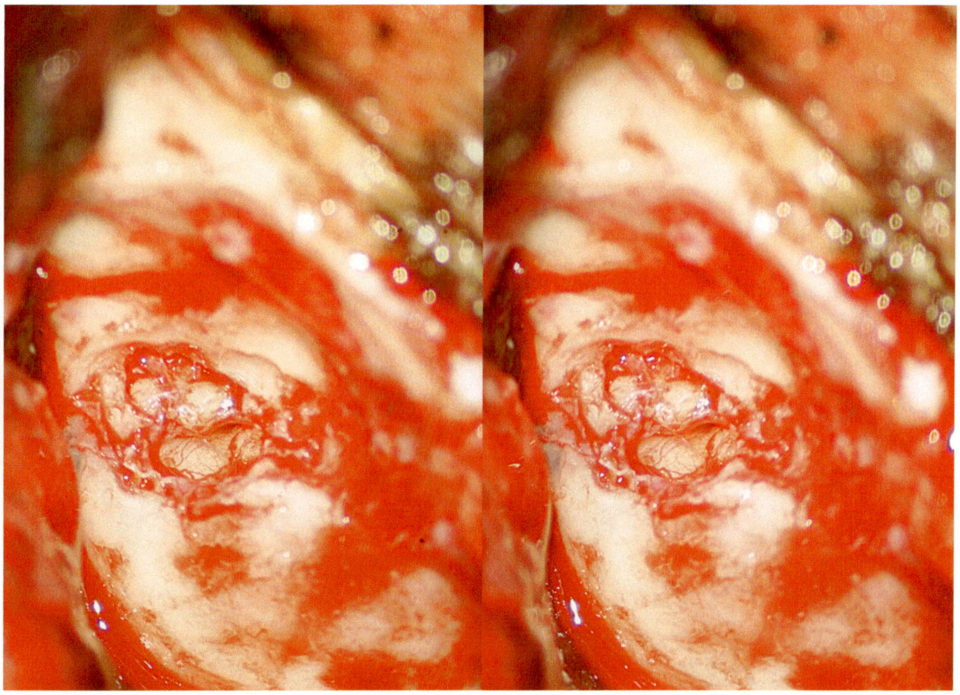

Fig. 3.17 Removing the tegmen of attic; exposing the tympanic segment of facial nerve
If the landmarks of the floor of the middle cranial fossa are not clear, the tegmen of the attic can firstly be removed to expose the contents of the attic such as the malleus and incus, medial to which the horizontal segment of the facial nerve is identified. The tegmen of the attic is located at the posterior end of the root of zygoma, 18 mm medial to the lateral surface of the squamous part of temporal bone

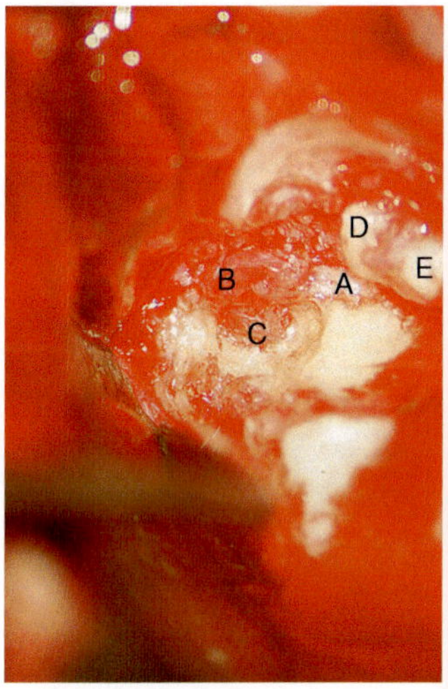

A. Horizontal segment of facial nerve
B. Geniculate ganglion
C. Labyrinthine segment
D. Malleus
E. Incus

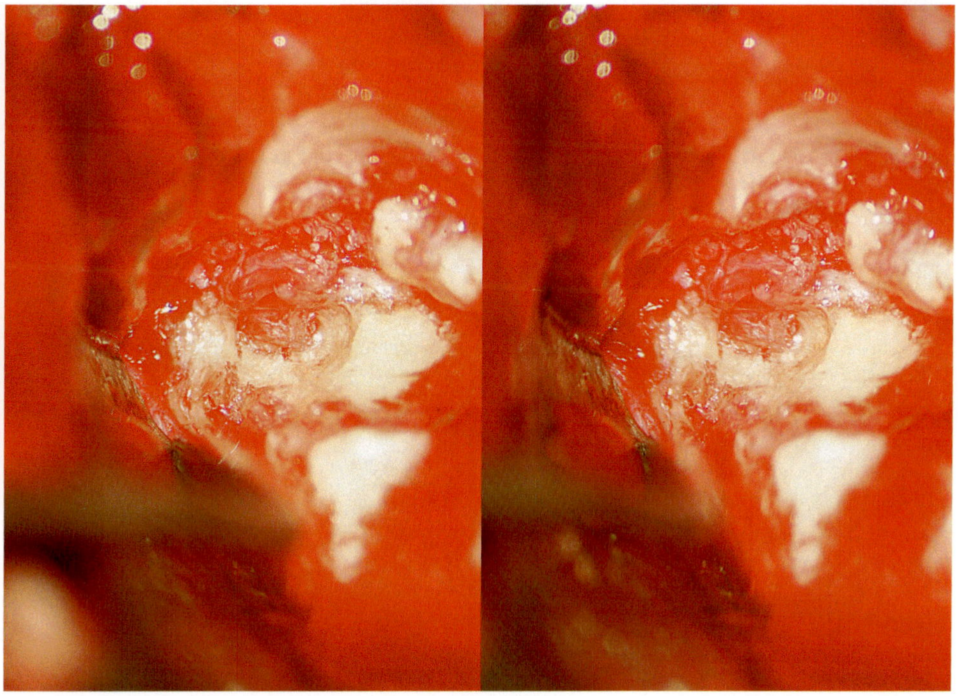

Fig. 3.18 Exposing horizontal segment, geniculate ganglion and labyrinthine segment of facial nerve
The canal of facial nerve medial to ossicles is opened to expose the horizontal segment of the facial nerve. Drilling forwards allows identification of the geniculate ganglion. The labyrinthine segment is medial and forms an angle of 60° with the horizontal segment. It is exposed by drilling medial to the ganglion

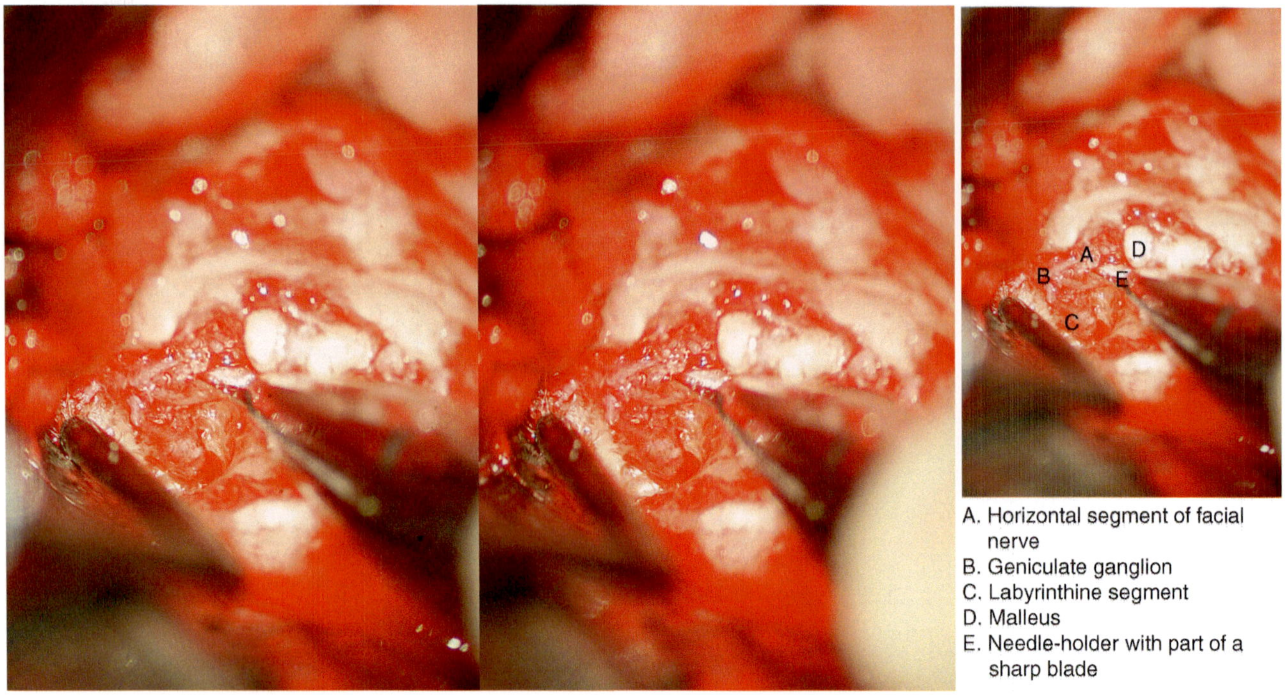

Fig. 3.19 Opening the sheath of facial nerve
The sheath of the facial nerve is divided along the long axis of the nerve with a sharp blade to relieve pressure, allowing the nerve to bulge. Great care should be taken to avoid secondary injury to the facial nerve

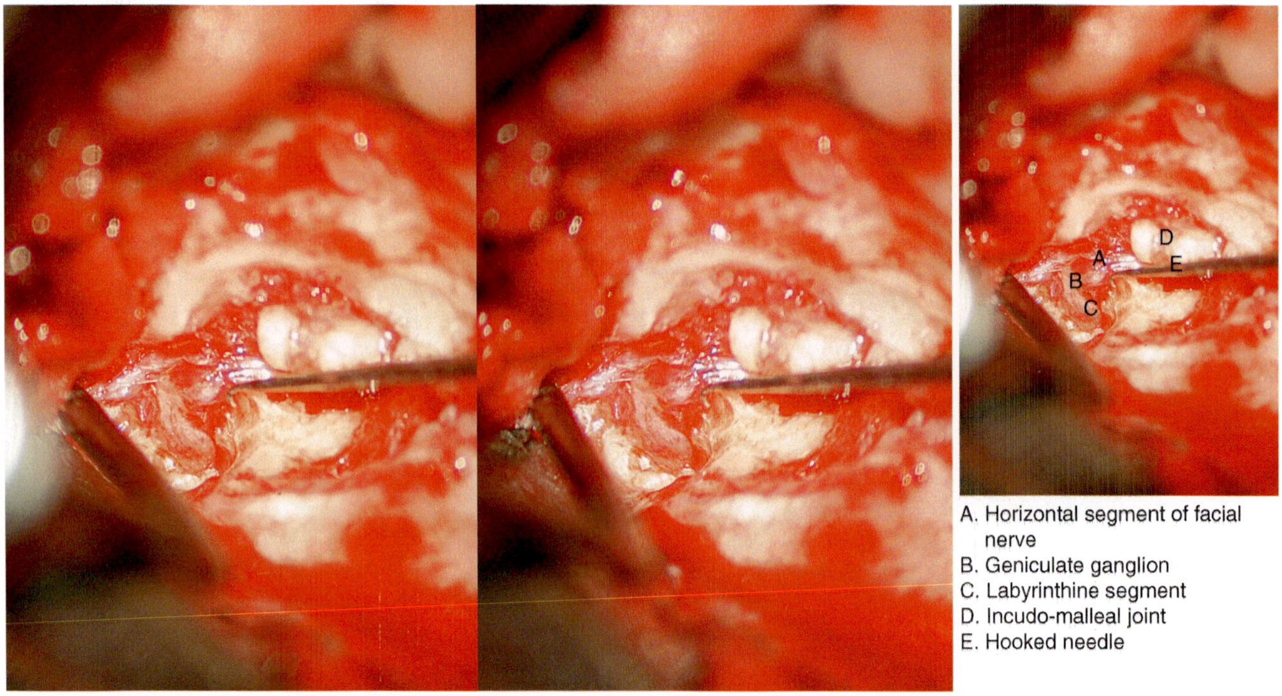

Fig. 3.20 Opening the sheath of the horizontal and labyrinthine segments and geniculate ganglion
The sheath of the horizontal and labyrinthine segments and the geniculate ganglion has been opened to fully relieve the pressure inside. The geniculate ganglion and the front-end of horizontal segment are clearly observed to swell

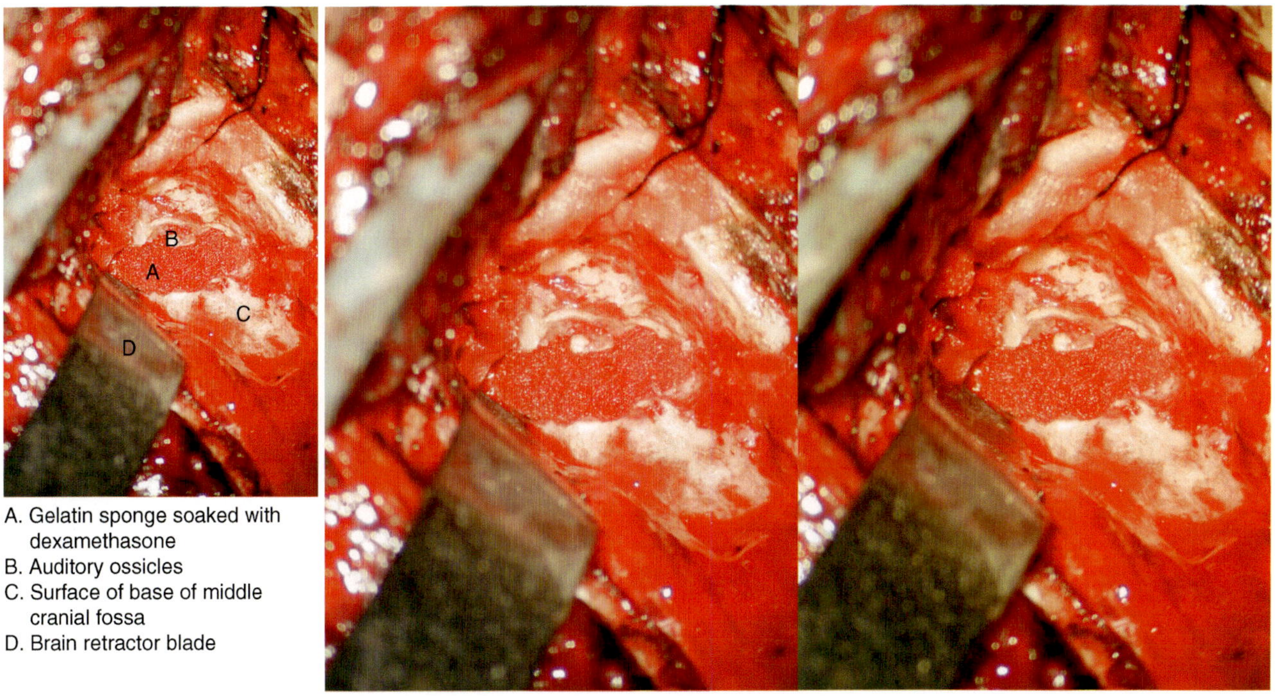

Fig. 3.21 The decompressed facial nerve is covered by gelatin sponge soaked with dexamethasone
The decompressed facial nerve is covered by gelatin sponge soaked with dexamethasone to reduce the edema of the nerve

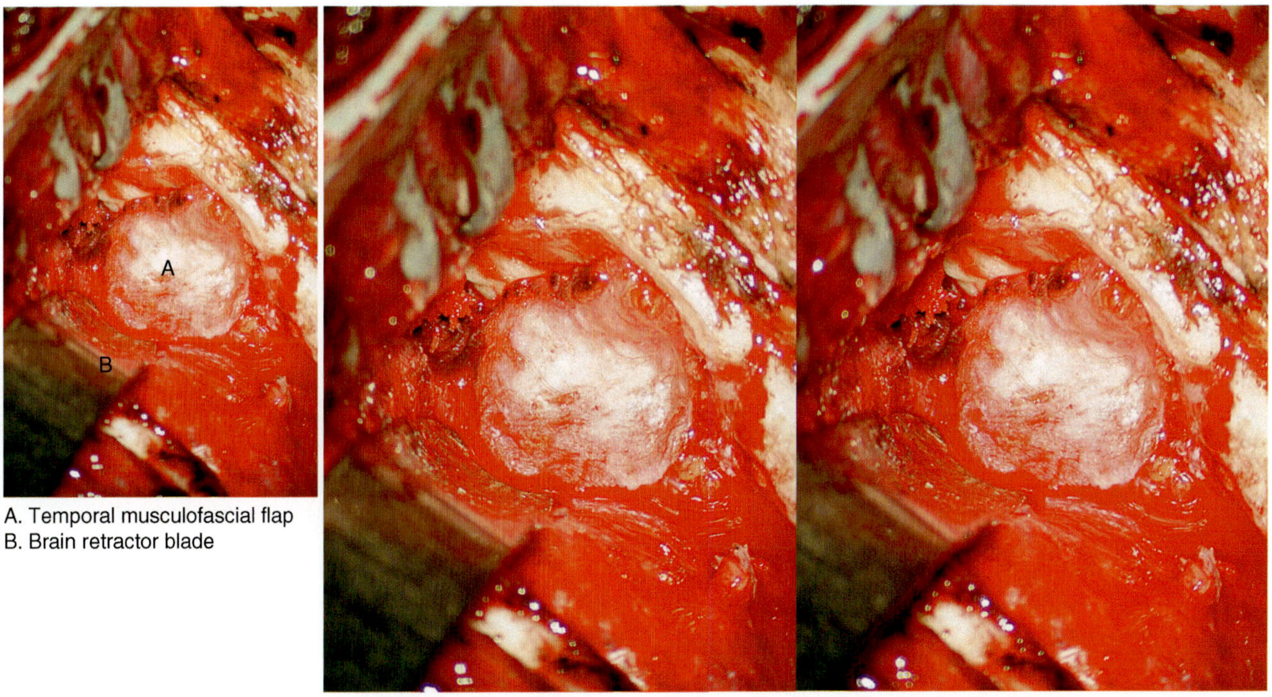

Fig. 3.22 The attic is sealed with a piece of temporal musculofascial flap
All bleeding is controlled, particularly checking for bleeding of the middle meningeal artery after the brain retractor blade is removed. Temporal musculofascial flaps are used to cover the surface of the decompressed facial nerve and seal the attic

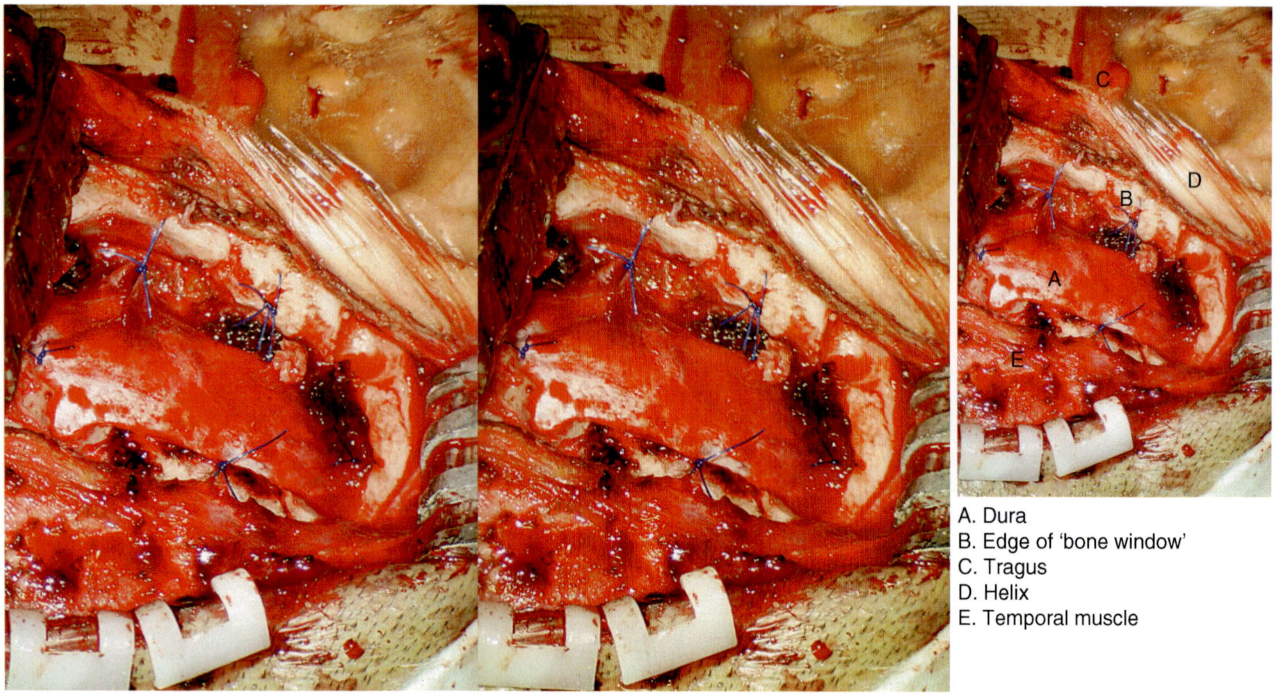

A. Dura
B. Edge of 'bone window'
C. Tragus
D. Helix
E. Temporal muscle

Fig. 3.23 Fixing the dura
Remove the brain retractor blade, place gelatin sponge between dura and skull, and fix the dura to the periosteum of the bone margin with nylon thread in order to prevent the occurrence of epidural hematoma

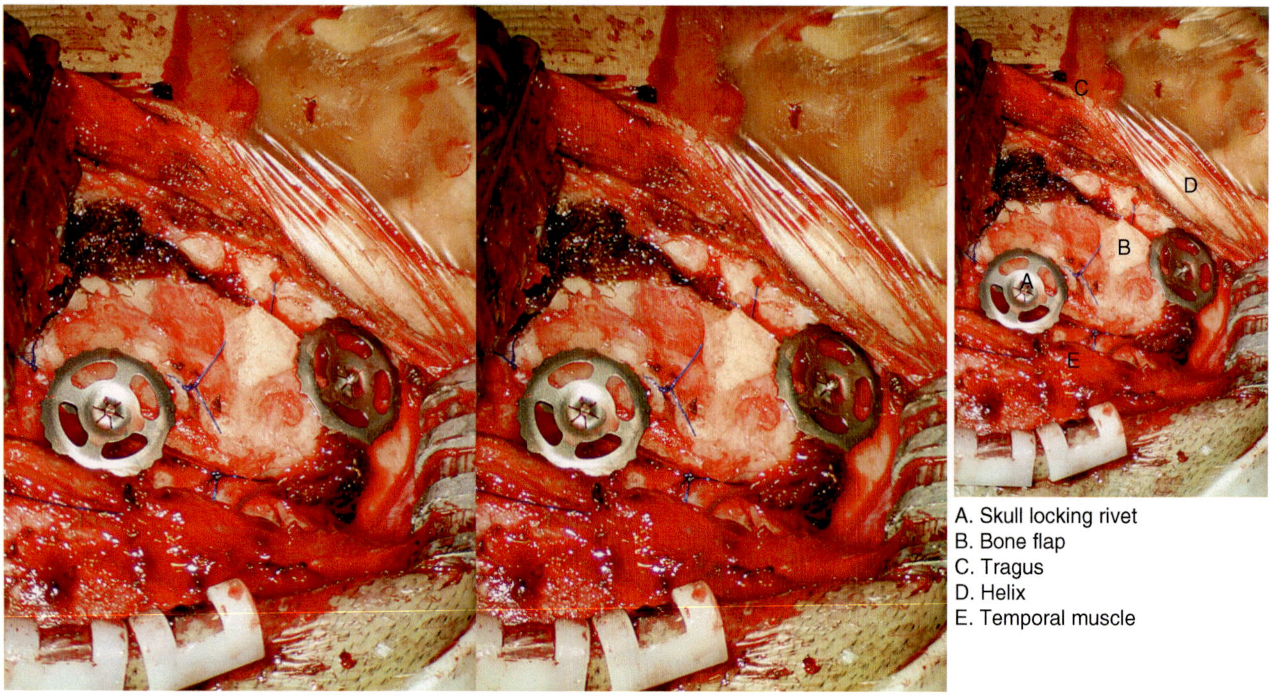

A. Skull locking rivet
B. Bone flap
C. Tragus
D. Helix
E. Temporal muscle

Fig. 3.24 Replacement and fixation of bone flap
The free bone flap is replaced and fixed with skull locking rivets

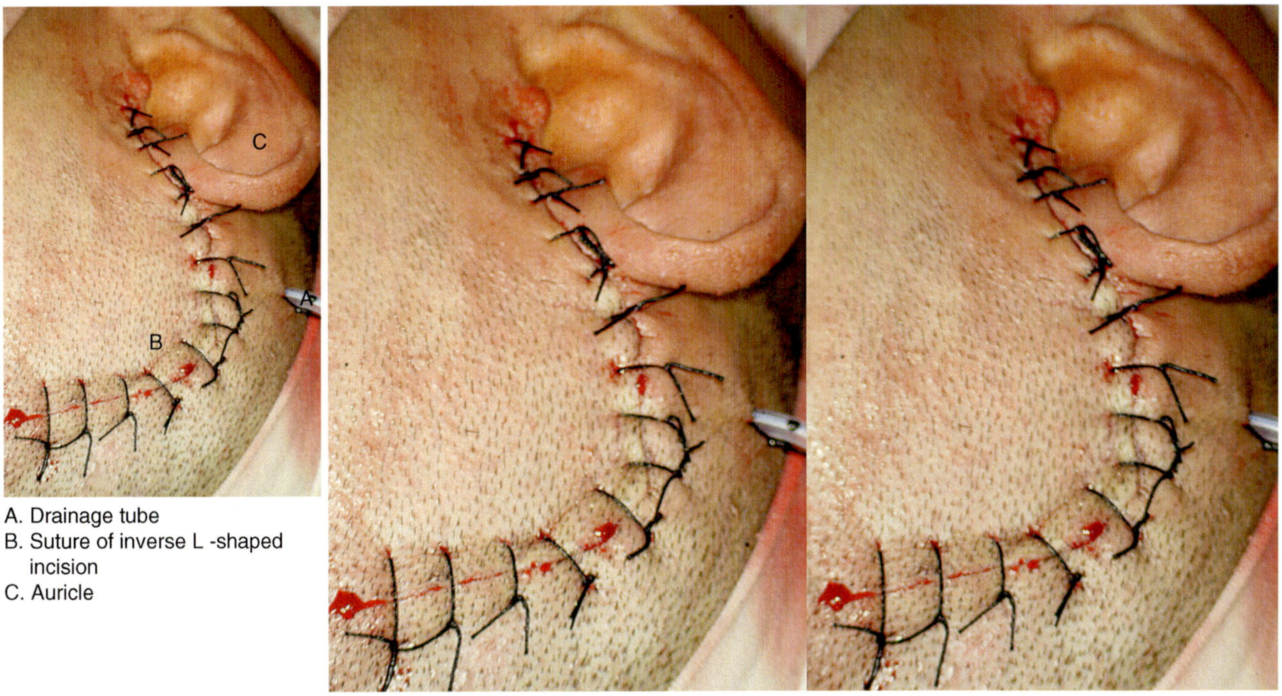

A. Drainage tube
B. Suture of inverse L -shaped incision
C. Auricle

Fig. 3.25 Suture of the subcutaneous tissue and skin
Liberally irrigate the cavity, control any bleeding, insert a drainage tube into the cavity via the skin and 2 cm behind the incision, close the skin and apply a dressing

Surgery 2: Middle cranial fossa approach decompression of facial nerve

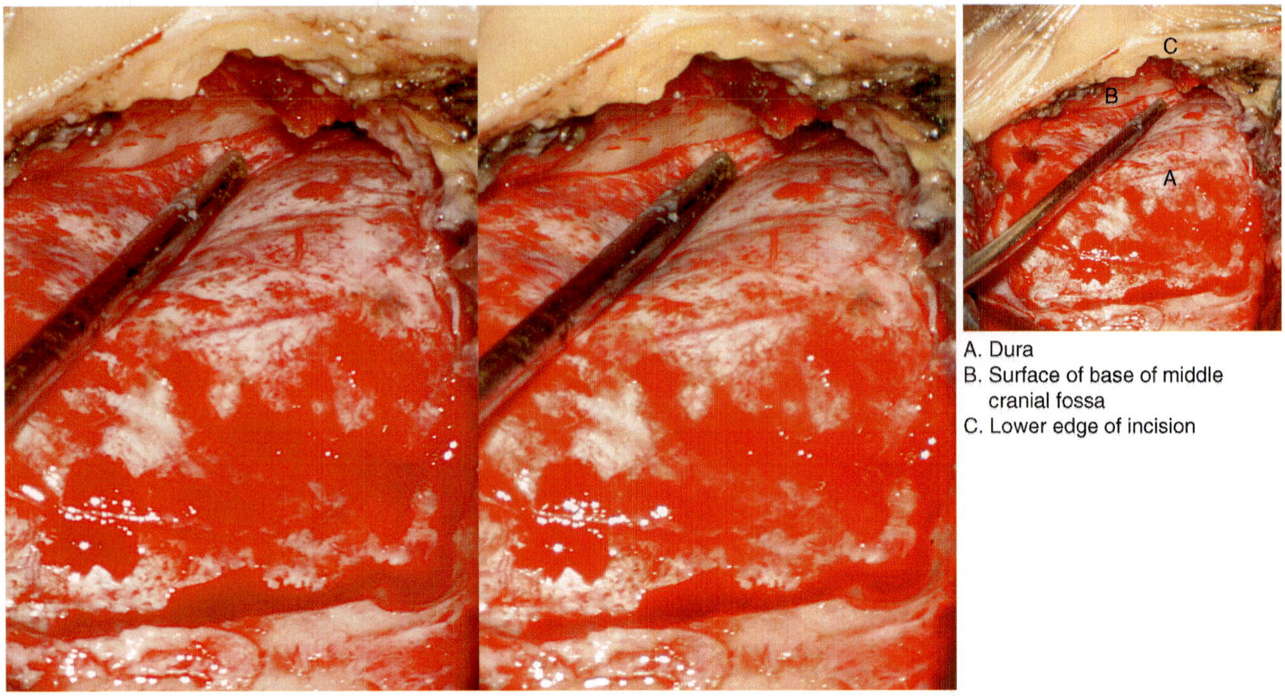

A. Dura
B. Surface of base of middle cranial fossa
C. Lower edge of incision

Fig. 3.26 Exposure the surface of base of middle cranial fossa
The bone is removed from the squamous part of temporal bone forming a 'bone window'; the dura of middle cranial fossa is detached from the superior surface of petrosal bone carefully, and the important landmarks of the middle cranial fossa floor are identified. If intracranial pressure is raised making it difficult to elevate the dura, mannitol should be administered to reduce intracranial pressure; the dura should be separated carefully and not dissected too far medially avoiding injury of the superior petrosal sinus

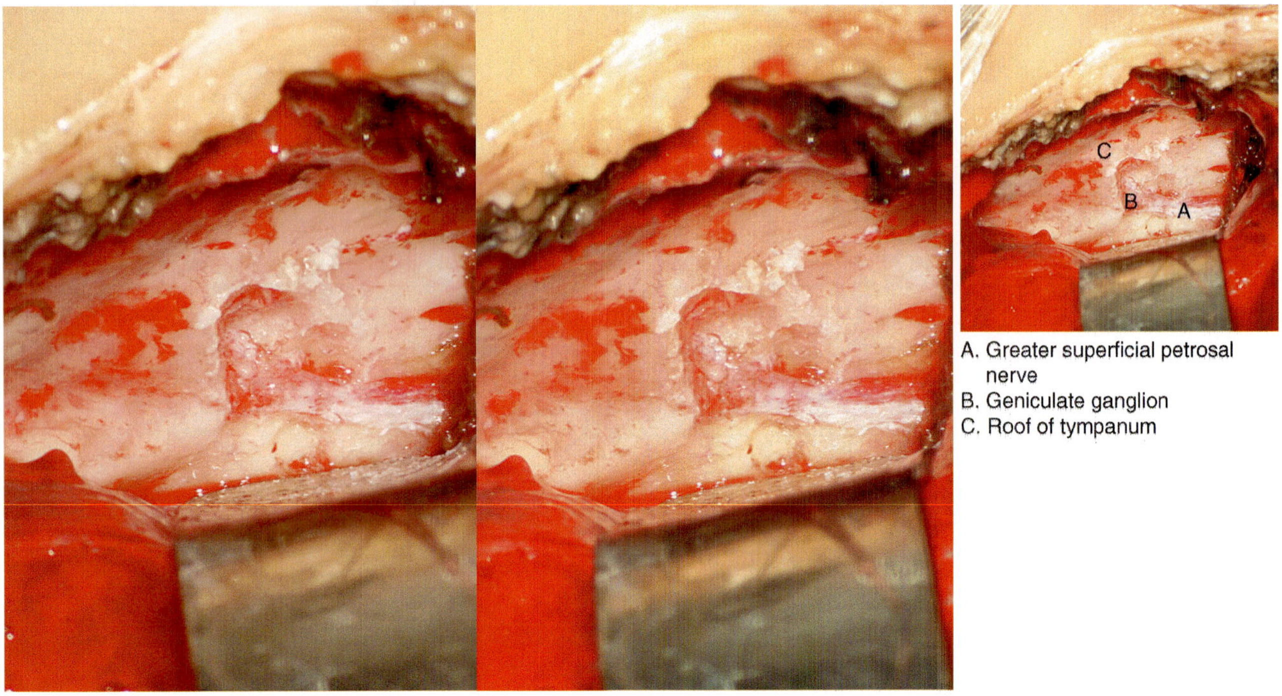

A. Greater superficial petrosal nerve
B. Geniculate ganglion
C. Roof of tympanum

Fig. 3.27 Exposure of geniculate ganglion along greater superficial petrosal nerve
Firstly, the greater superficial petrosal nerve should be identified, and the bone covering is removed from front to back to expose the geniculate ganglion. In few cases, the bone over geniculate ganglion is absent; the geniculate ganglion should be carefully protected when exposed

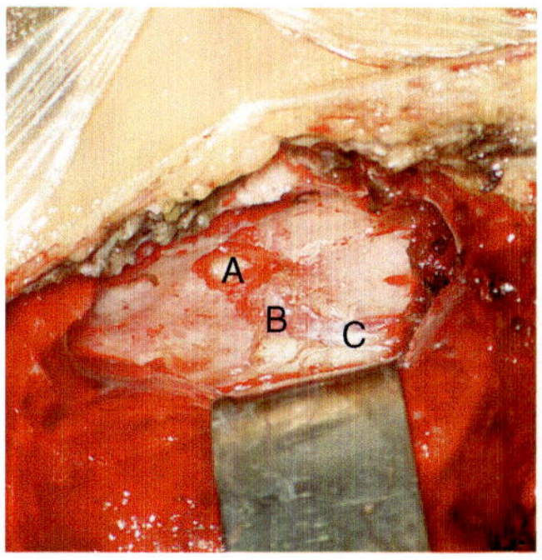

A. Incudo-malleal joint
B. Geniculate ganglion
C. Greater superficial petrosal nerve

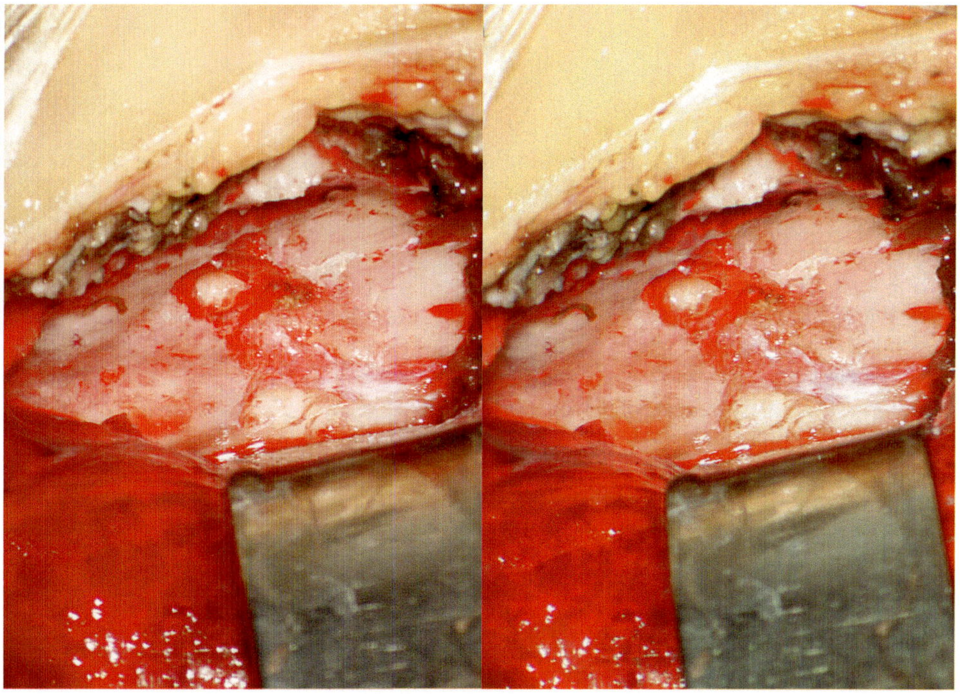

Fig. 3.28 Removing the roof of tympanum, exposure of the ossicles and the horizontal segment of facial nerve
Before the horizontal segment of facial nerve is exposed by drilling backwards from the geniculate ganglion, the upper parts of the malleus and incus should be exposed

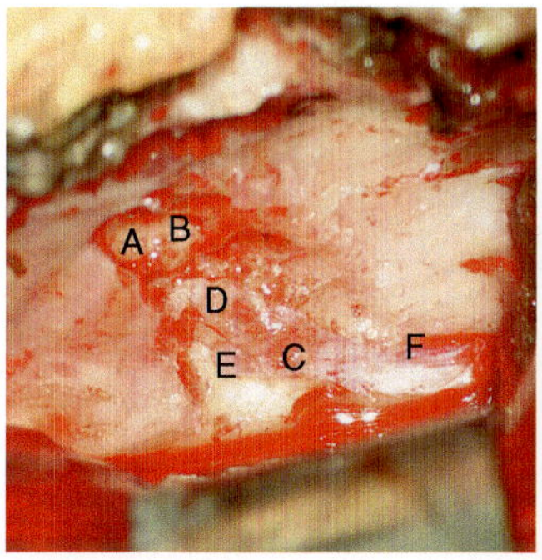

A. Incus
B. Malleus
C. Geniculate ganglion
D. Horizontal segment of facial nerve
E. Labyrinthine segment
F. Greater superficial petrosal nerve

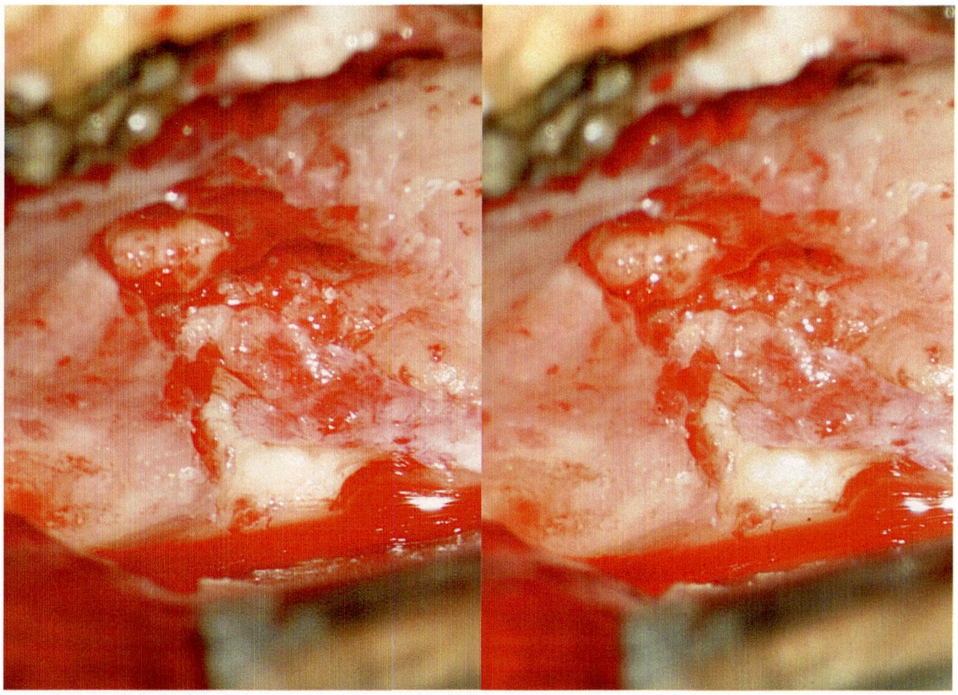

Fig. 3.29 Exposure of labyrinthine segment and internal acoustic meatus
The front half of horizontal segment has been exposed, the sheath of the junction of the geniculate and horizontal segment is found out to be injured, which is considered to be the cause of the facial paralysis due to the swollen fibers of the facial nerve seen through it. The bone medial to the geniculate ganglion is removed to expose the labyrinthine segment. If drilling is continued, the internal auditory foramina will be exposed

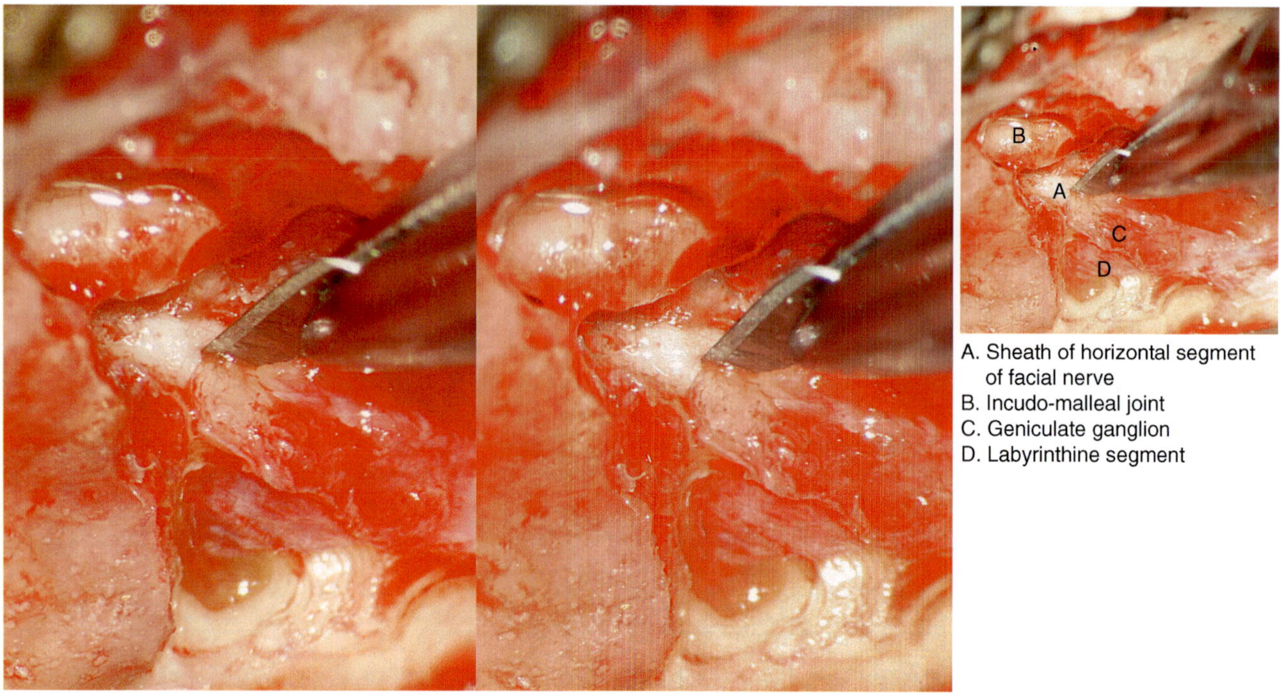

A. Sheath of horizontal segment of facial nerve
B. Incudo-malleal joint
C. Geniculate ganglion
D. Labyrinthine segment

Fig. 3.30 Incision of the sheath of facial nerve
A longitudinal incision of the sheath of geniculate ganglion, labyrinthine and horizontal segments of the facial nerve is made with a sharp blade

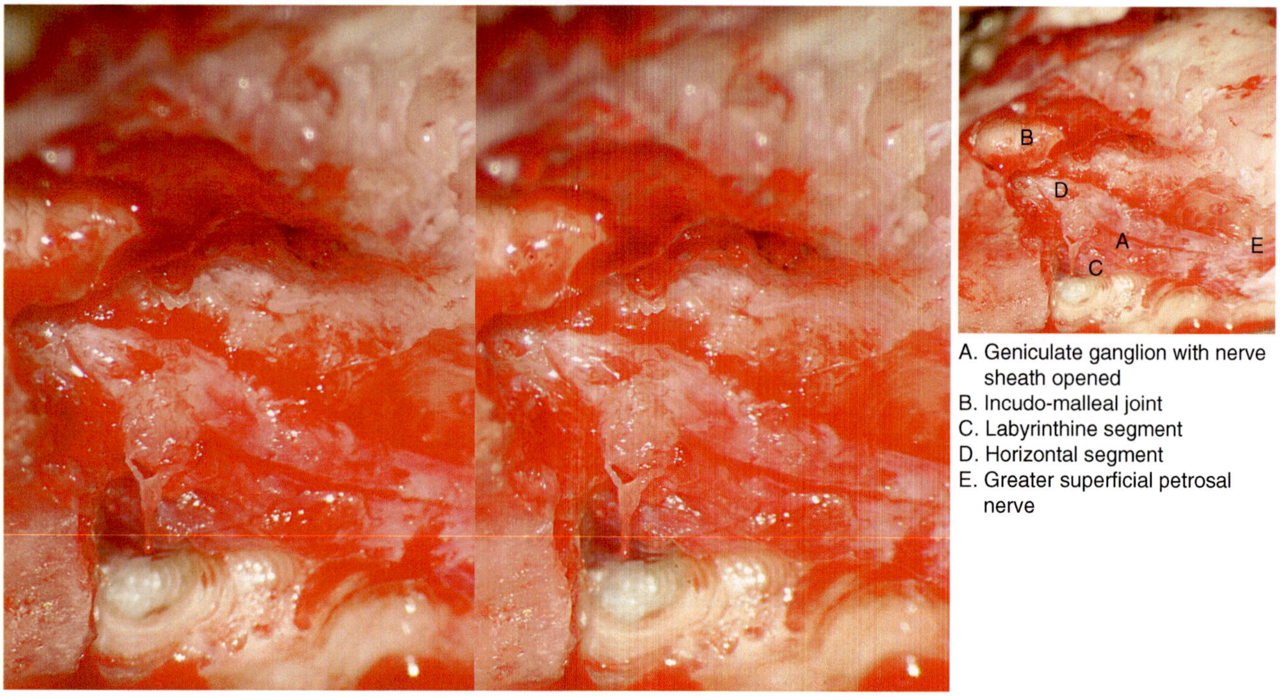

A. Geniculate ganglion with nerve sheath opened
B. Incudo-malleal joint
C. Labyrinthine segment
D. Horizontal segment
E. Greater superficial petrosal nerve

Fig. 3.31 The facial nerve with opened nerve sheath
The facial nerve with opened sheath clearly shows the site of nerve fibers with edema and distortion. Since the continuity of the facial nerve is preserved well with only a small proportion of injured fibers, the prognosis after decompression is favorable

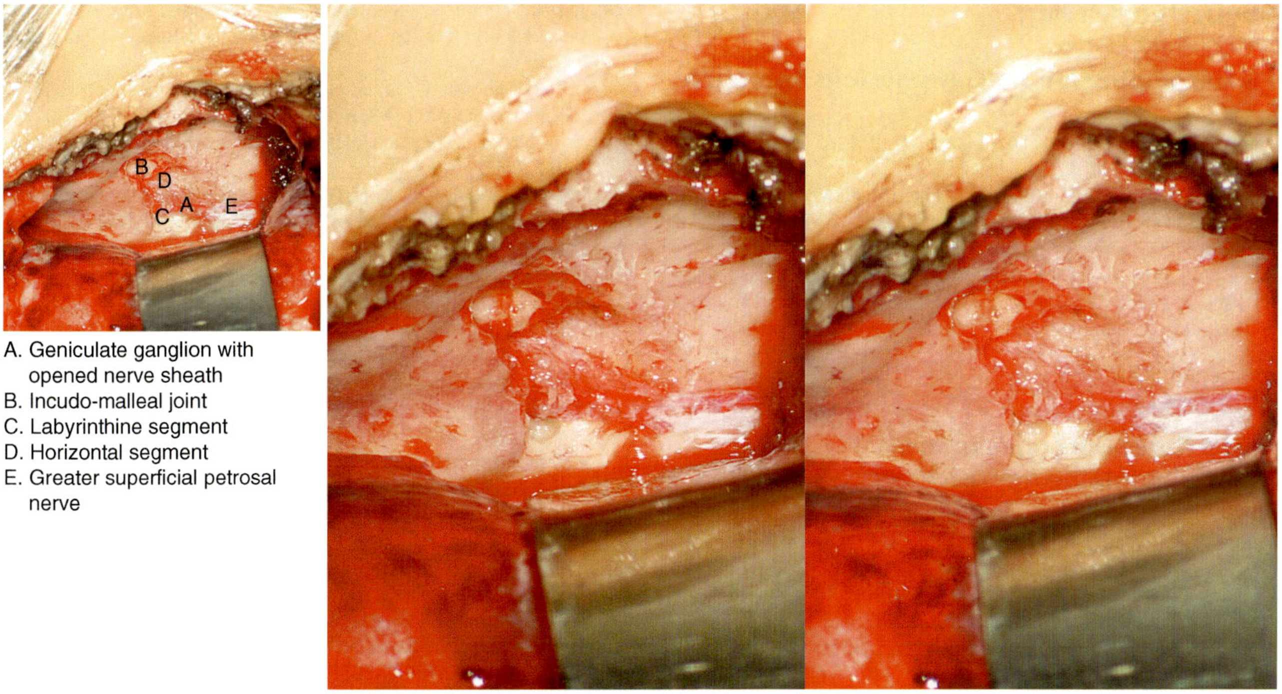

A. Geniculate ganglion with opened nerve sheath
B. Incudo-malleal joint
C. Labyrinthine segment
D. Horizontal segment
E. Greater superficial petrosal nerve

Fig. 3.32 The facial nerve with nerve sheath opened
The procedure is complete after the responsible site is identified and decompressed. In the operative field, the superior parts of malleus and incus can be observed through the defect of tegmen tympani. The middle part of the horizontal segment is located medial to the ossicles, whilst the front part of horizontal segment and geniculate ganglion are anterior and medial to the ossicles

Suggested Reading

FN Decompression via Transmastoid Approach

Han D-Y. Nerve otology and Lateral skull base surgery. Beijing: Science Press; 2008a.

Huang X-Z, Wang J-B, Kong W-J. Practice of otorhinolaryngology head and neck surgery. 2nd ed. Beijing: People's Medical Publishing House; 2008a.

Jiang S-C, Yang W-Y,Gu R Operative surgery of otorhinolaryngology head and neck Department. 2nd ed. The complete works of operative surgery. Beijing: People's Military Medical Press; 2005.

Facial Nerve Decompression via Translabyrinthine Approach

Huang X-Z, Wang J-B, Kong W-J. Practice of otorhinolaryngology head and neck surgery. 2nd ed. Beijing: People's Medical Publishing House; 2008b.

Yang W-Y, Zhai S-Q. Head-neck dissection and temporal surgery. Beijing: People's Military Medical Press; 2002a.

Middle Cranial Fossa Approach Decompression of Facial Nerve

Catalano PJ, Eden AR. An external reference to identify the internal auditory canal in middle fossa surgery. Otolaryngol Head Neck Surg. 1993;108(2):111–6.

Dongyi H, Shiming Y, Wenming W, et al. Resection of acoustic neurinoma and preservation of function of the facial nerve. Chin J Otol. 2004;2(1):1–3.

Green Jr JD, Shelton C, Brackmann DE. Iatrogenic facial nerve injury during otologic surgery. Laryngoscope. 1994;104:922–6.

Han D-Y. Nerve otology and lateral skull base surgery. Beijing: Science Press; 2008b.

Huang X-Z, Wang J-B, Kong W-J. Practice of otorhinolaryngology head and neck surgery. 2nd ed. Beijing: People's Medical Publishing House; 2008c.

Jiang S-C. Ear anatomia and temporal bone histopathology. Beijing: People's Military Medical Press; 1999.

Jiang S-C, Gu R, Zheng-Min W. Otorhinolaryngology – otology. 2nd ed. Shanghai: Shanghai Scientific and Technological Education Publishing House; 2002.

Jiang S-C, Yang W-Y, GU R. Operative surgery of otorhinolaryngology head and neck Department. 2nd ed. The complete works of operative surgery. Beijing: People's Military Medical Press; 2005.

Pulec JL. Total facial nerve decompression: technique to avoid complications. Ear Nose Throat J. 1996;75(7):410–5.

Yang W-Y, Zhai S-Q. Head-neck dissection and temporal surgery. Beijing: People's Military Medical Press; 2002b.

Yong Z, Xiaofeng M, Hong W, et al. Reasons and prevention of facial paralysis in tympanomastoid surgery. Chin Arch Otolaryngol-Head Neck Surg. 2000;7:199–201.

Yu Y-J, Dai P, Liu Z. Stereo anatomical and surgical atlas of Temporal bone. Beijing: People's Military Medical Press; 2006.

Inner Ear Surgery

4

Pu Dai, Jian-zhong Li, Fei Yu, Song Gao, Yi Jiang, Wei-dong Shen, Jian-dong Zhao, Sha-sha Huang, and Yi-hui Zou

Stapedectomy

Jian-zhong Li and Pu Dai

Indications

1. Stapedial Otosclerosis, air conduction hearing levels (Pure Tone threshold on average) >30 dB with conductive hearing loss >15 dB.
2. Late stage otosclerosis.
3. Fixation of the footplate by tympanosclerosis with an intact or repaired tympanic membrane.
4. Congenital anomalies with fixation of the footplate.

Contraindications

1. Infection in the external auditory canal or middle ear.
2. Perforated tympanic membrane.
3. High-resolution computer tomography scan showing absence of the bony partition between the fundus of the internal auditory canal and the vestibule or the cochlea.
4. Dysfunction of the Eustachian tube.
5. Gusher in the contralateral ear.
6. Advanced cochlear otosclerosis.

Operative Procedures

1. Make the first incision: Cut the skin, subcutaneous tissue, and periosteum of the external auditory canal (EAC) at the anterior notch of the ear laterally, and extend the incision medially, to the junction of cartilage and bone.
2. Make the second incision: Begin from the 6 o'clock position, 5–6 mm lateral to the fibrous annulus, along the posterior meatal wall in an ascending spiral fashion, to meet the first incision at its medial end.
3. Elevate the tympanomeatal flap: The meatal flap is elevated to the tympanic sulcus with a blunt elevator and the fibrous annulus is then elevated from the sulcus with the same instrument. The tympanomeatal flap is pushed forward over the edge of bony sulcus. Special care should be taken to avoid tearing the flap.
4. To gain adequate exposure to the oval window and stapes, 2–4 mm of postero-superior bony canal rim must be removed with an angled middle ear curette or chisel, taking care not to injure the surrounding structures. Bone should be removed until the facial nerve, footplate of stapes, stapedius tendon, and pyramidal eminence can be seen.
5. Evaluate the mobility of each of the three ossicles.
6. Measure the distance between the undersurface of the long process of the incus and the footplate.
7. Cut the stapedius tendon.
8. Separate the incudostapedial joint.
9. Removal of the stapes: The stapes superstructure is down-fractured toward the promontory and taken out, the footplate is fenestrated in its midportion. A fine hook is used to remove the entire footplate (total stapedec-

P. Dai, MD (✉) • F. Yu, MD • W.-d. Shen, MD • J.-d. Zhao, MD
S.-s. Huang, MD • Y.-h. Zou, MD
Department of Otolaryngngology Head and Neck Surgery, Chinese PLA General Hospital, Beijing 100853, China
e-mail: daipu301@vip.sina.com

J.-z. Li, MD
Department of Otolaryngology Head and Neck Surgery, Fuzhou General Hospital of Nanjing Command, Chinese PLA, Fuzhou 350025, China

S. Gao, MD
Department of Otolaryngology, The 175th Hospital of Chinese PLA, Zhangzhou 363000, China

Y. Jiang, MD
Department of Otolaryngology, Fujian Provincial Hospital, Fuzhou 350001, China

P. Dai et al. (eds.), *Stereo Operative Atlas of Micro Ear Surgery*, DOI 10.1007/978-981-10-2089-6_4

tomy) or the anterior half of the footplate (partial stapedectomy).

10. Placement of prosthesis: The crook of the prosthesis is adequately crimped onto the long process of the incus with a crimper. The prosthesis should pass into the vestibule for about 0.25 mm, not more than 0.5 mm.
11. A small piece of fat is applied to seal the opening of the oval window around the prosthesis.
12. Return the tympanomeatal flap to its original position. Rinne's test is performed to assess the hearing gain in patients where local anesthesia has been used. If Rinne's test is negative, the position of the prosthesis should be re-checked and adjusted if necessary.
13. The EAC is packed with gelatin sponge and iodoform gauze, suture the first incision.

Special Comments

1. Expose the oval window, long process of the incus, and facial canal adequately.
2. The mobility of all three ossicles should be assessed.
3. Pay attention to the integrity of the facial canal and its relationship with the oval window.
4. Avoid applying epinephrine cotton ball for hemostasis in tympanic cavity after opening of the oval window.
5. Avoid using suction directly over the opening of the oval window.
6. The mucosa of the oval window niche should be removed before sealing the oval window with fat.
7. The length of the prosthesis should be long enough for its medial end to enter the perilymph fluid without contacting the membranous labyrinth.
8. The crook of the prosthesis should be crimped on the long process of the incus adequately to avoid incus erosion.
9. Bed rest for 3 days after operation, avoiding straining and nose blowing.
10. Avoid air travel for at least 1 month to reduce the risk of significant changes in middle ear pressure and displacement of the tympanic membrane and prosthesis.

Complications

1. Sensorineural hearing loss: It is usually irreversible. Trauma to the inner ear should be avoided during operation.
2. Vertigo or dizziness: This symptom is not common after surgery, but may be due to loss of perilymph fluid, surgical trauma, protrusion of prosthesis to the utricle, or serous labyrinthitis.
3. Loss or distortion of taste affecting the tongue on the side of the operation: This symptom is caused by severance of or trauma to the chorda tympani nerve. Care should be taken not to injure the chorda tympani when removing the posterosuperior bony canal rim,
4. Facial paralysis: resulting from injury to the facial nerve. A dehiscent, prolapsed facial nerve protruding over the footplate is prone to injury. It is very important to obtain full exposure of facial canal and identify any abnormal course of facial nerve and its canal.
5. Perilymph fistula: resulting from failure to seal the oval window. The mucosa of the oval window niche should be removed before sealing the window with fat or fascia.
6. Tympanic membrane perforation: due to failure to effectively repair a torn tympanic membrane. Special care should be take not to tear the tympanic membrane when elevating the annulus. If a tear does occur, it can be repaired with a piece of fascia or fat.
7. Prosthesis displacement: This is usually caused by a short prosthesis slipping out of the oval window.
8. Distortion of sense of voice may be experienced by vocal musicians after the operation.
9. Labyrinthitis: This may be caused by a failure to maintain proper asepsis during the operation and failure to seal the oval window effectively.

Surgery 1: Total Stapedectomy and Piston Prosthesis (artificial stapes) Implantation

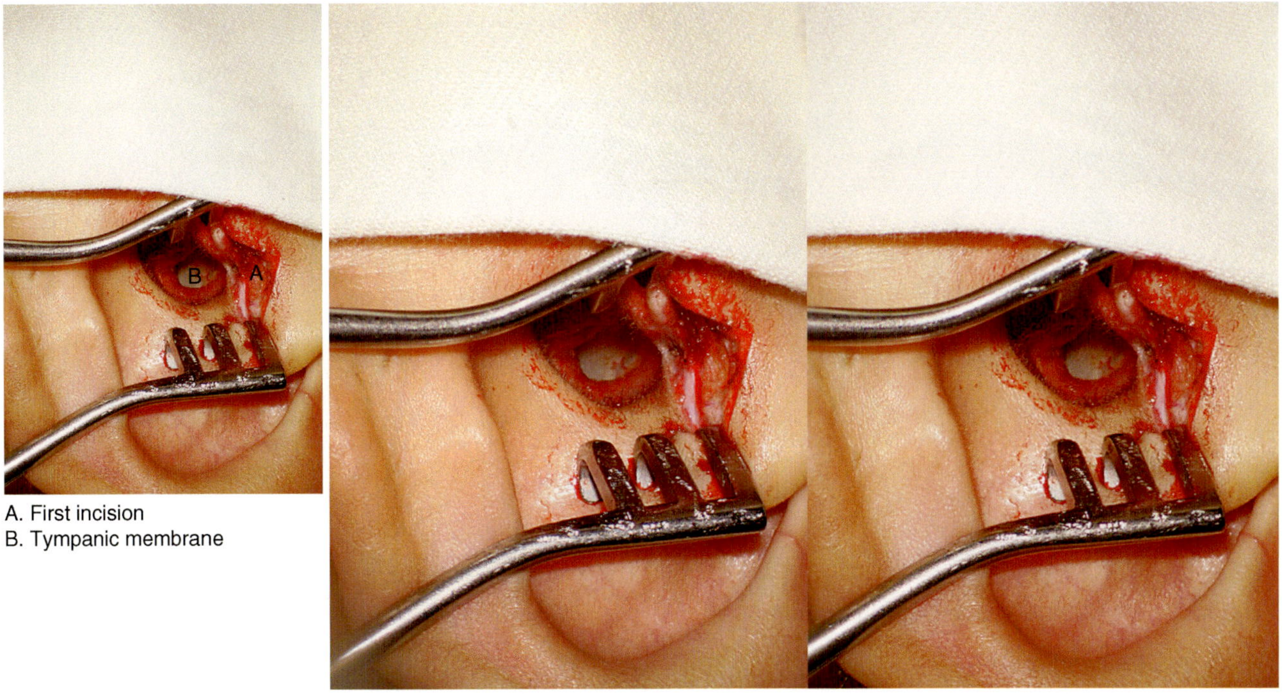

Fig. 4.1 Make the first incision
The first skin incision starts from the 12 o'clock position of EAC and is carried down to the bone. It is extended laterally between the tragus and the root of helix for about 0.5–1.0 cm and medially to a point 6–8 mm lateral to the pars flaccida membrane

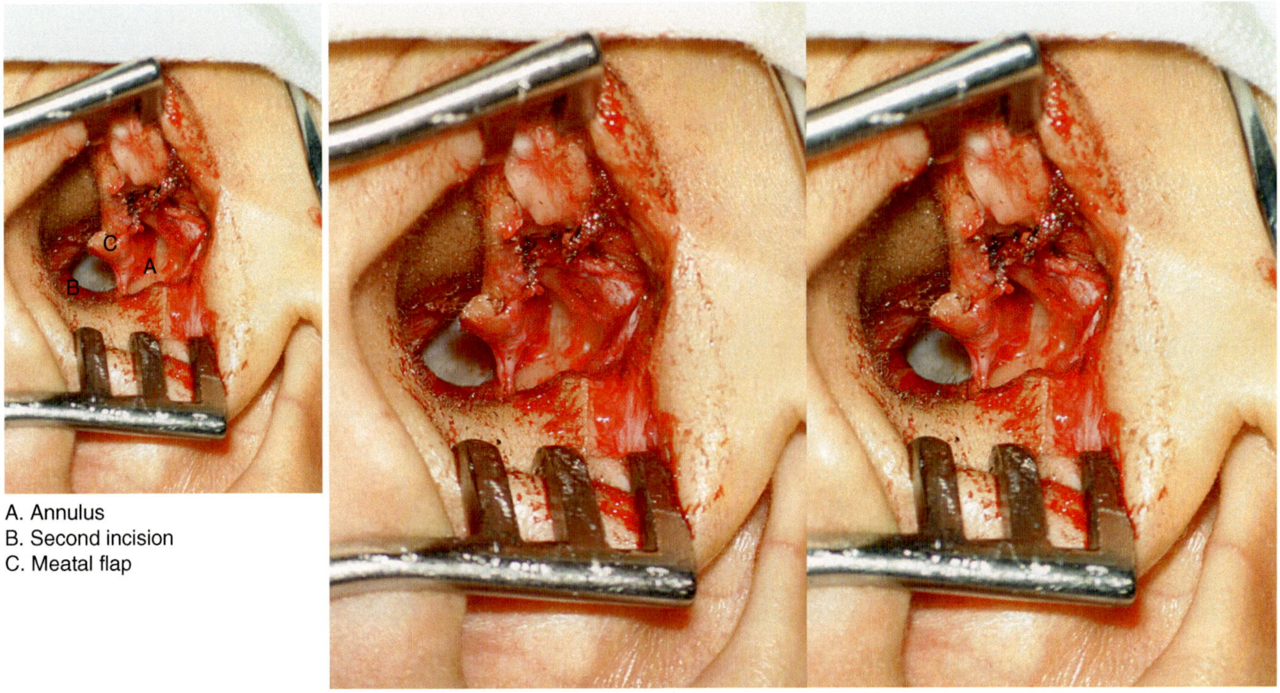

Fig. 4.2 Make the second incision and elevate the meatal flap
Make the second incision to connect the 6 o'clock point, running 5–6 mm lateral to the annulus, and the medial end of the first incision. The meatal flap is elevated with a micro-elevator to the posterior sulcus and notch of Rivinus. The skin of the bony external auditory canal can be very thin in patients with otosclerosis. A small suction tube is used, avoiding tearing of the flap by not sucking directly on it. Remove the overhanging suprameatal spine to get better exposure using a diamond burr or chisel if necessary

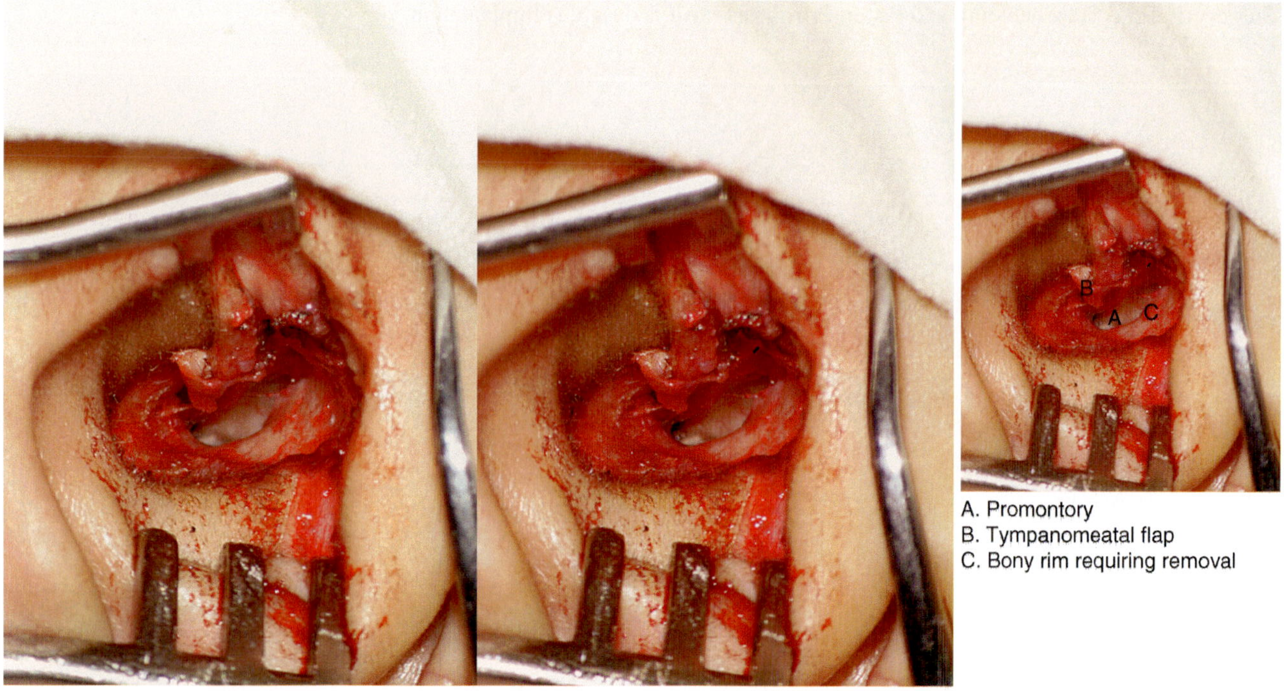

Fig. 4.3 Enter the tympanic cavity
The fibrous annulus is elevated from the tympanic sulcus from the 12 to 6 o'clock position with a blunt elevator. The tympanomeatal flap is pushed forward to expose the tympanic cavity. Care should be taken not to tear the flap

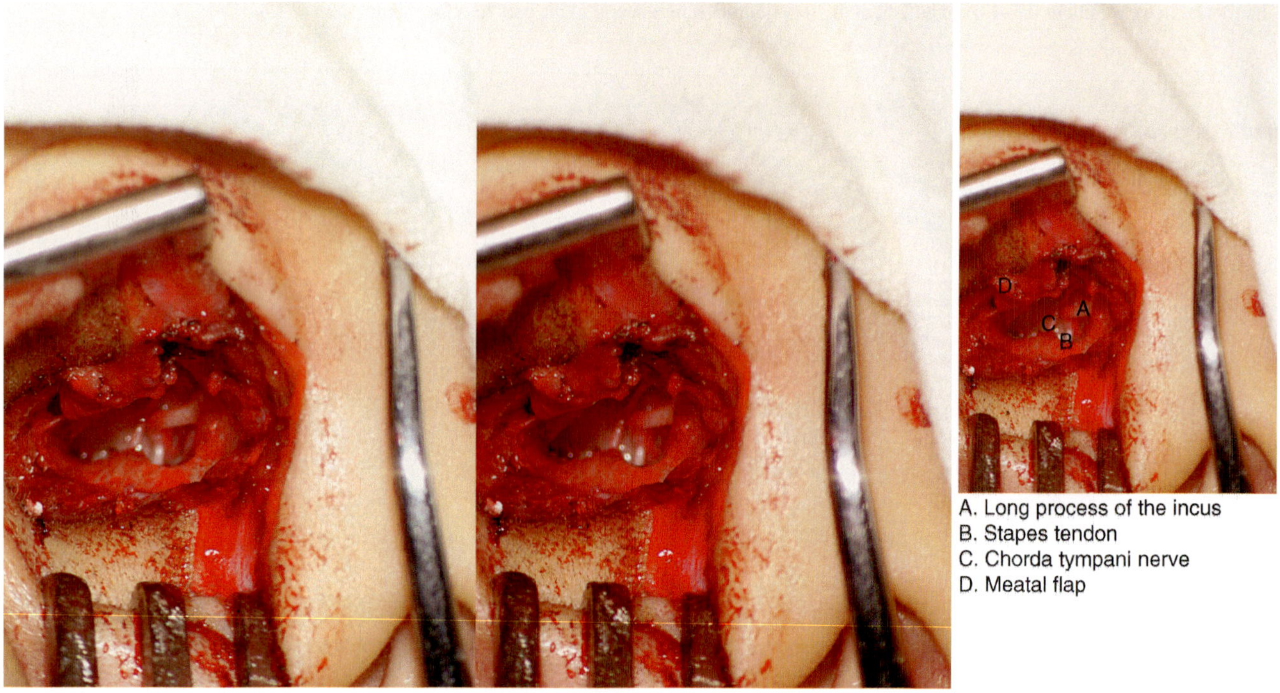

Fig. 4.4 Exposure of the oval window
2–4 mm of postero-superior bony canal rim is removed with an angled middle ear curette or chisel to fully expose of the incudostapedial joint, the long process of the incus, the stapedius tendon, the anterior and posterior crura, the oval window, and the horizontal segment of the facial nerve. The mobility of the three ossicles is evaluated. Care is taken to assess whether the facial nerve has an aberrant course or if the nerve is dehiscent and overhanging too much to allow the procedure to continue

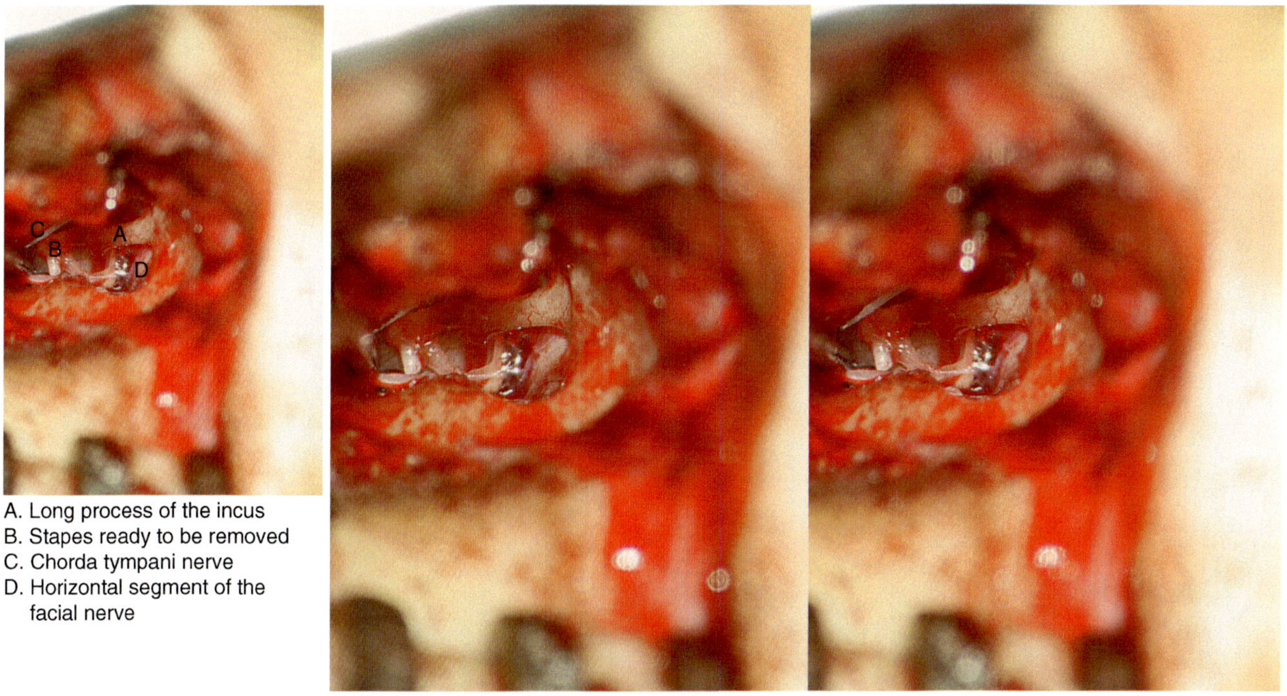

Fig. 4.5 Total stapedectomy
After confirming the mobility of the incus and malleus, the stapes is removed. The chorda tympani nerve is pushed forward and downward, the distance between the undersurface of the long process of the incus and the footplate is measured with a measuring rod, the stapes tendon is cut with delicate scissors, the incudostapedial joint is disconnected with a micro hook, and the stapes is mobilized and taken out totally

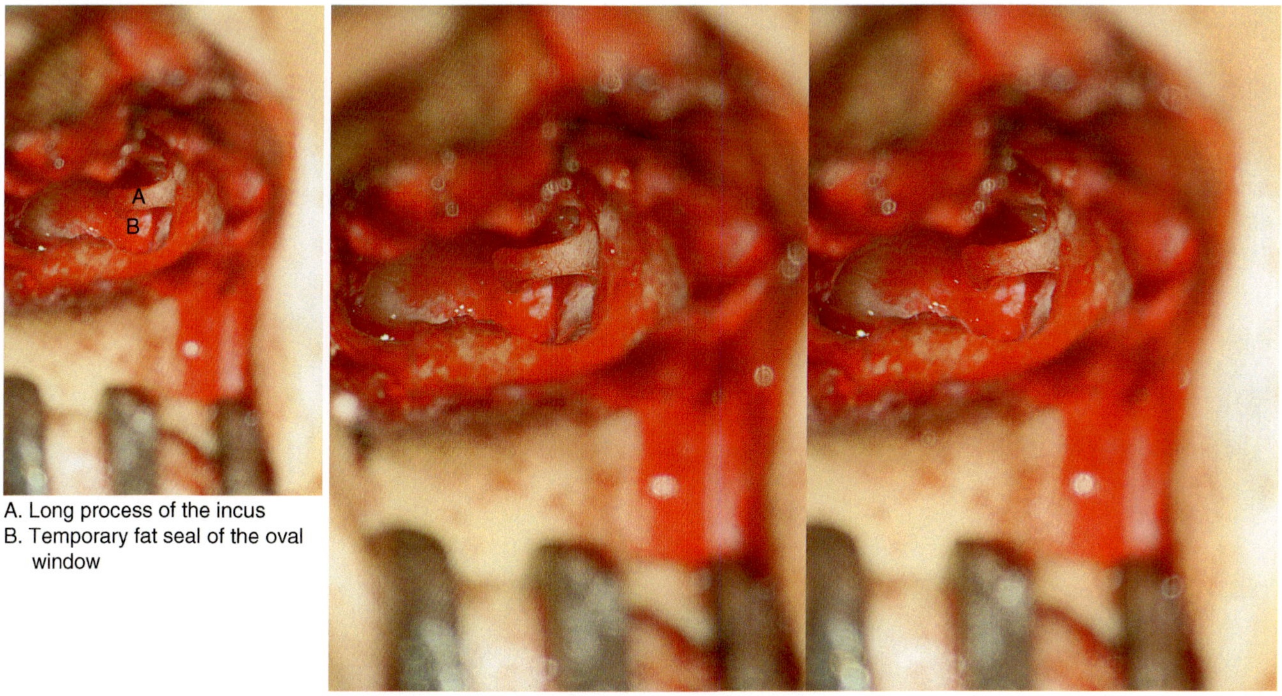

Fig. 4.6 Seal the oval window temporarily with a piece of fat
After removal of the stapes, the opening of the oval window is immediately sealed with an adequately sized piece of fat to prevent blood from entering the labyrinth and loss of perilymphatic fluid. After opening the oval window, a saline (rather than adrenaline) soaked cotton ball is applied to stop bleeding. Meanwhile, the prosthesis is cut to suitable length based on the measurement of the distance between the undersurface of the long process of the incus and the footplate

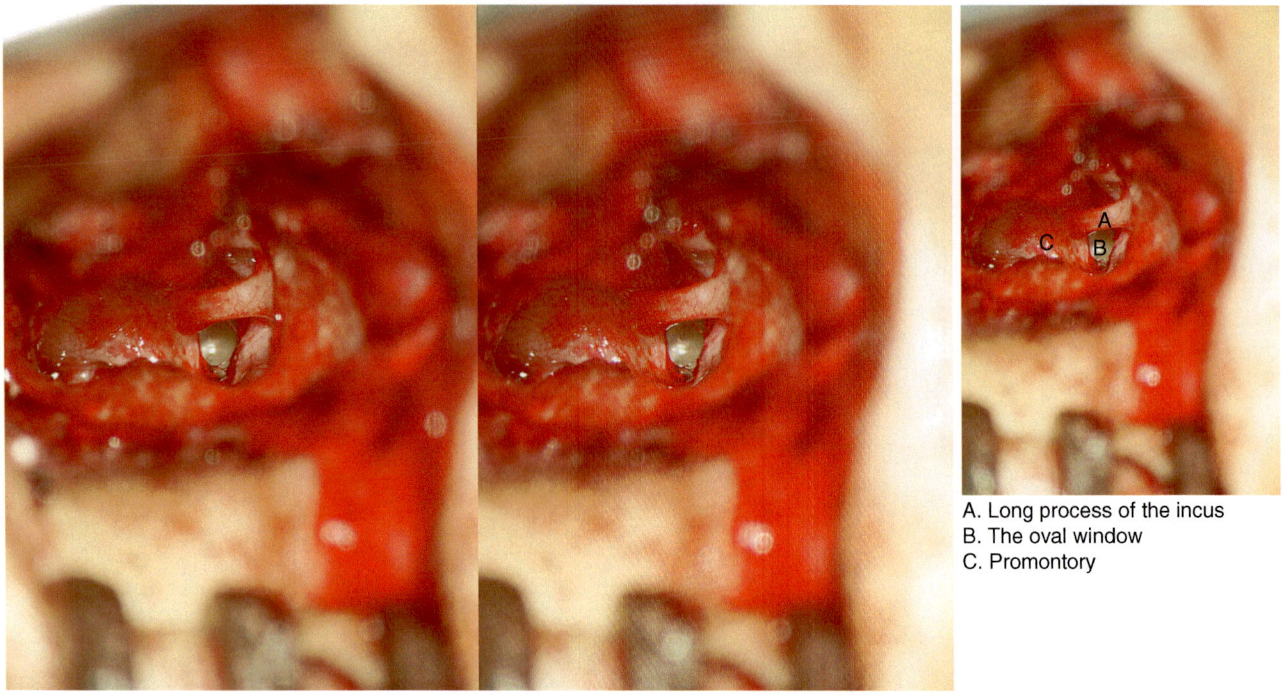

Fig. 4.7 Get ready to place the prosthesis
Take the fat out gently in order not to interfere with the perilymphatic space. The opening of the oval window looks light blue and clear. Direct suction in the opening of the oval window must be prohibited to avoid loss of the perilymph and damage to the inner ear

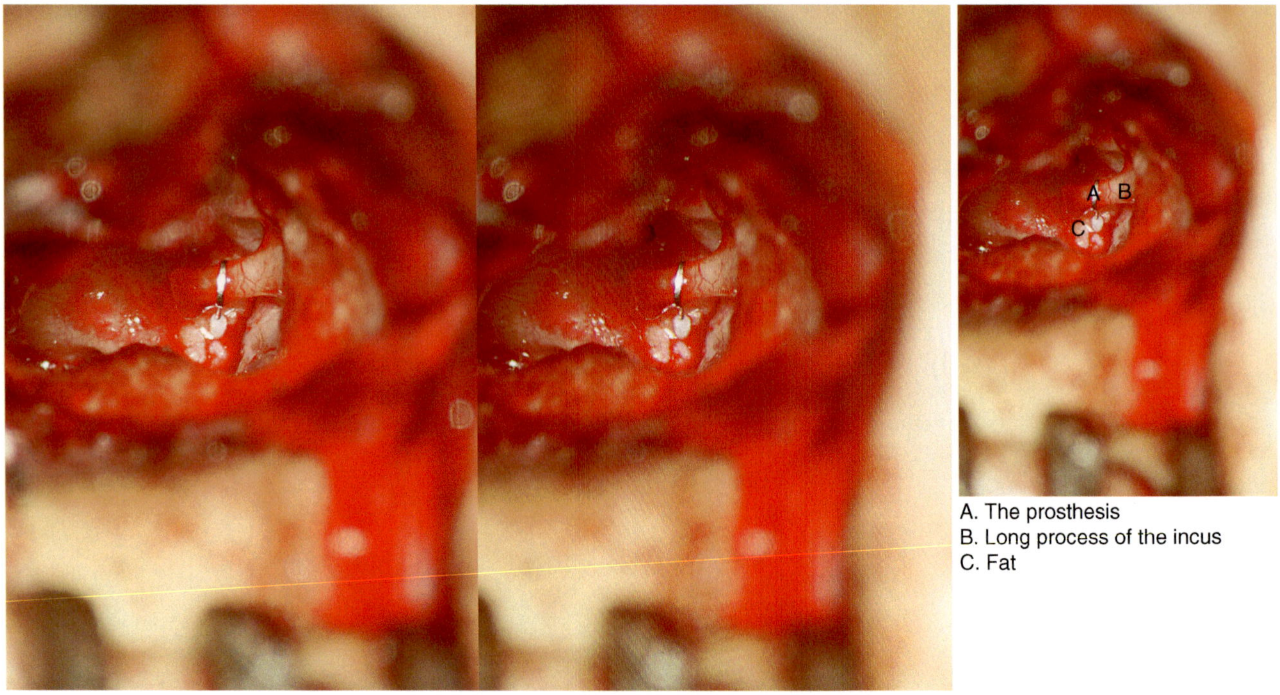

Fig. 4.8 Placement of the prosthesis
The wire of the prosthesis is hooked over to the long process of the incus at the junction of its middle and lower thirds. The medial end of the prosthesis is placed at the center of the oval window. The wire is fixed properly with a crimper. One or two adequate sized pieces of fat are applied to seal the oval window

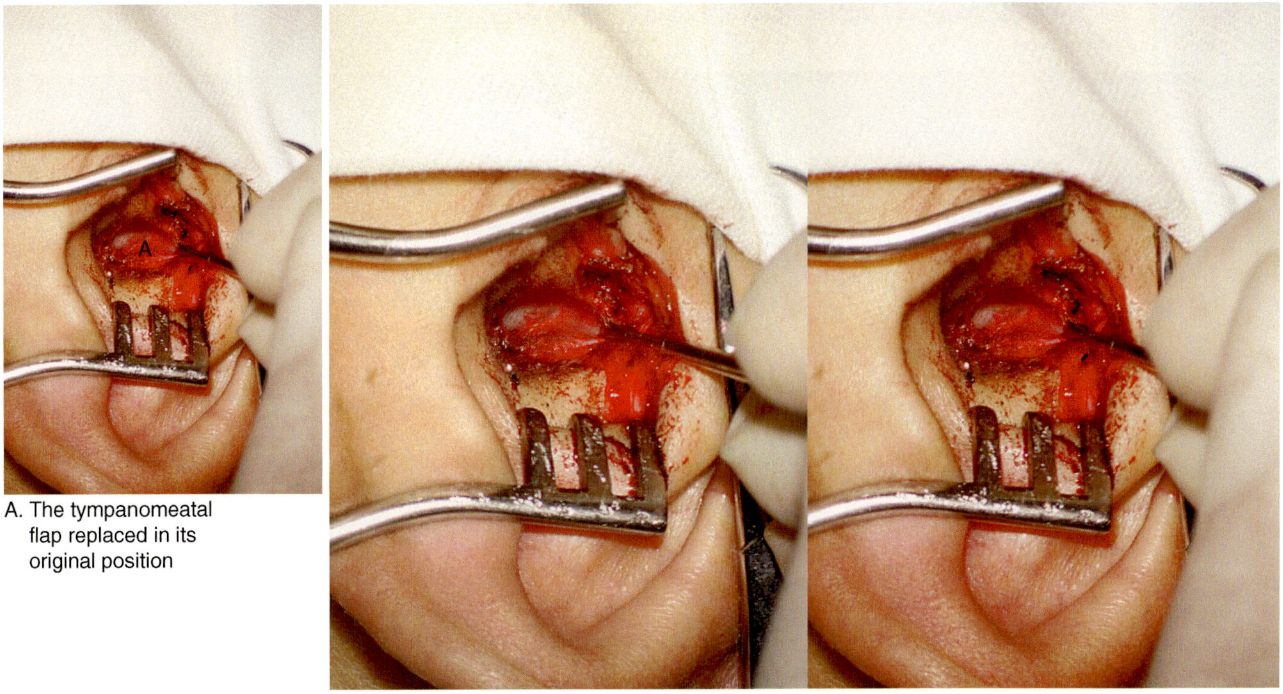

Fig. 4.9 Replace the tympanomeatal flap in its original position
Replace the tympanomeatal flap in its original position. Rinne's test is performed in patients under local anesthesia to assess the hearing gain. If Rinne's test is negative, the mobility of malleus and incus and position of the prosthesis should be checked again

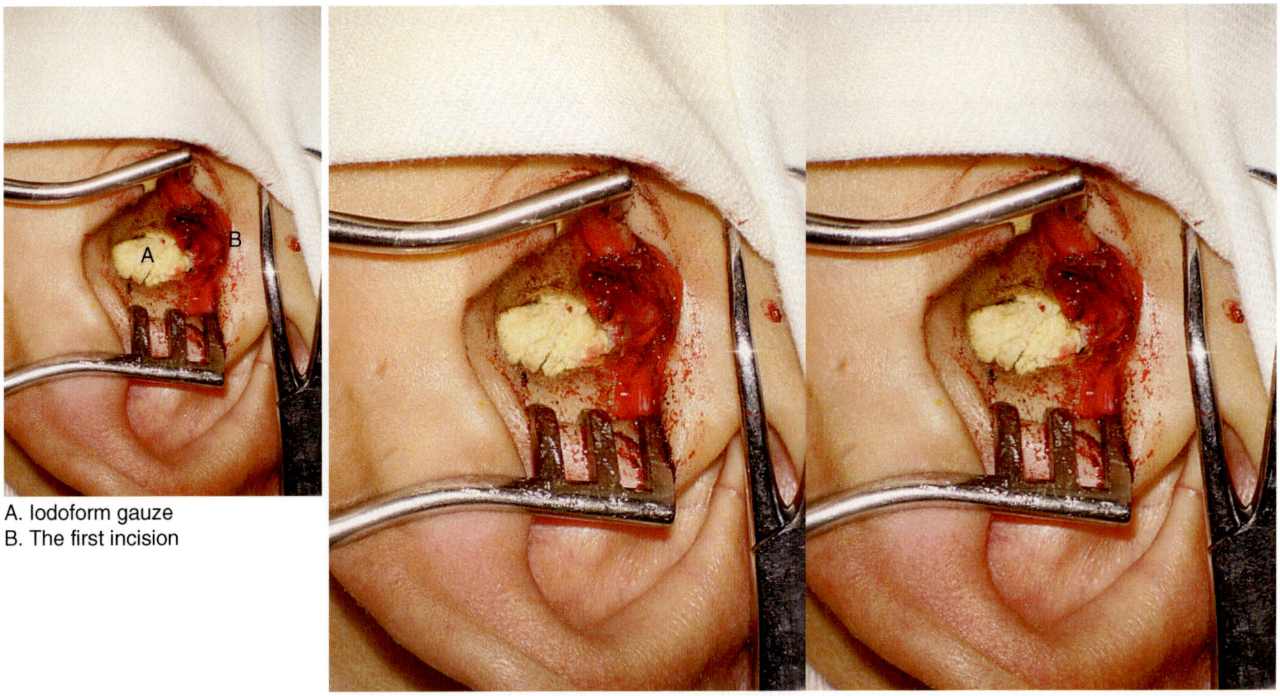

Fig. 4.10 Packing of the external auditory canal and suturing the incision
After re-positioning of the flap, the external auditory canal is packed with gelatin sponge and iodoform gauze. After loosening the self-retaining retractor, there may be some bleeding, which can be stopped by bipolar coagulation. The first incision is sutured

Surgery 2: Total Stapedectomy and Implantation of Piston Prosthesis

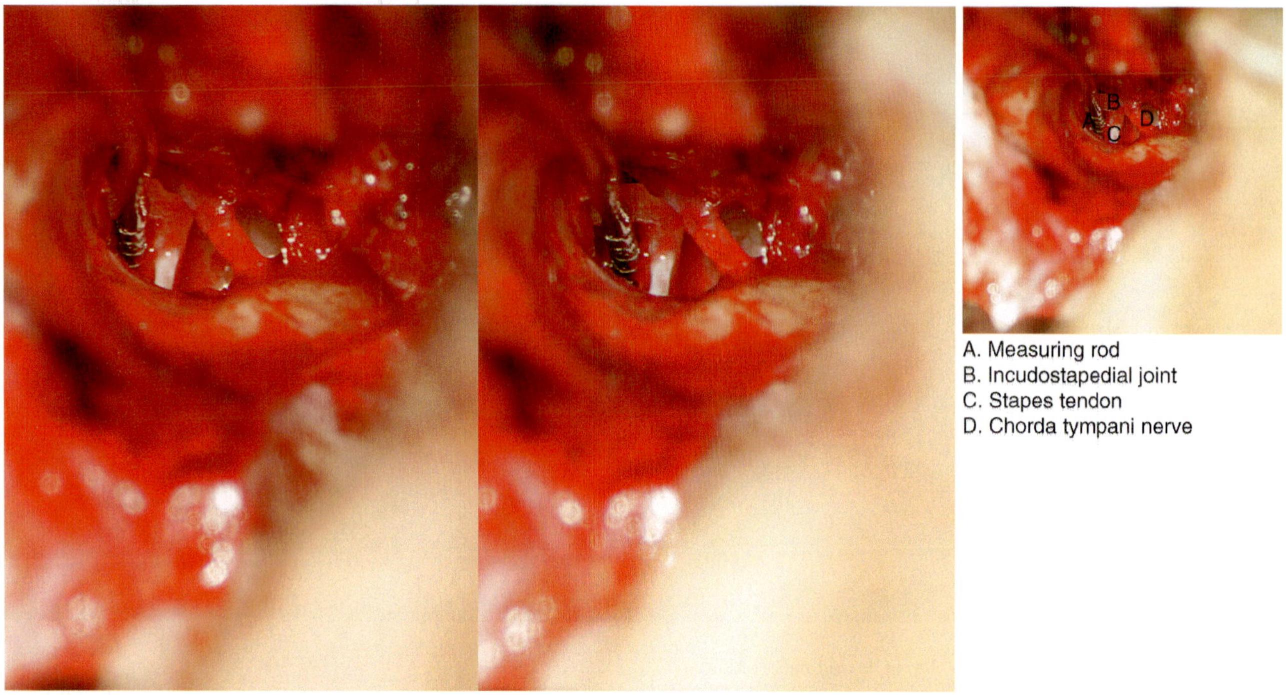

Fig. 4.11 Measuring the distance between the footplate and the undersurface of the long process of the incus
Measure the distance between the footplate and the undersurface of the long process of the incus with the measuring rod. The distance is about 4 mm in this case. This step should be performed before removal of the stapes in case of alteration of the position of the incus

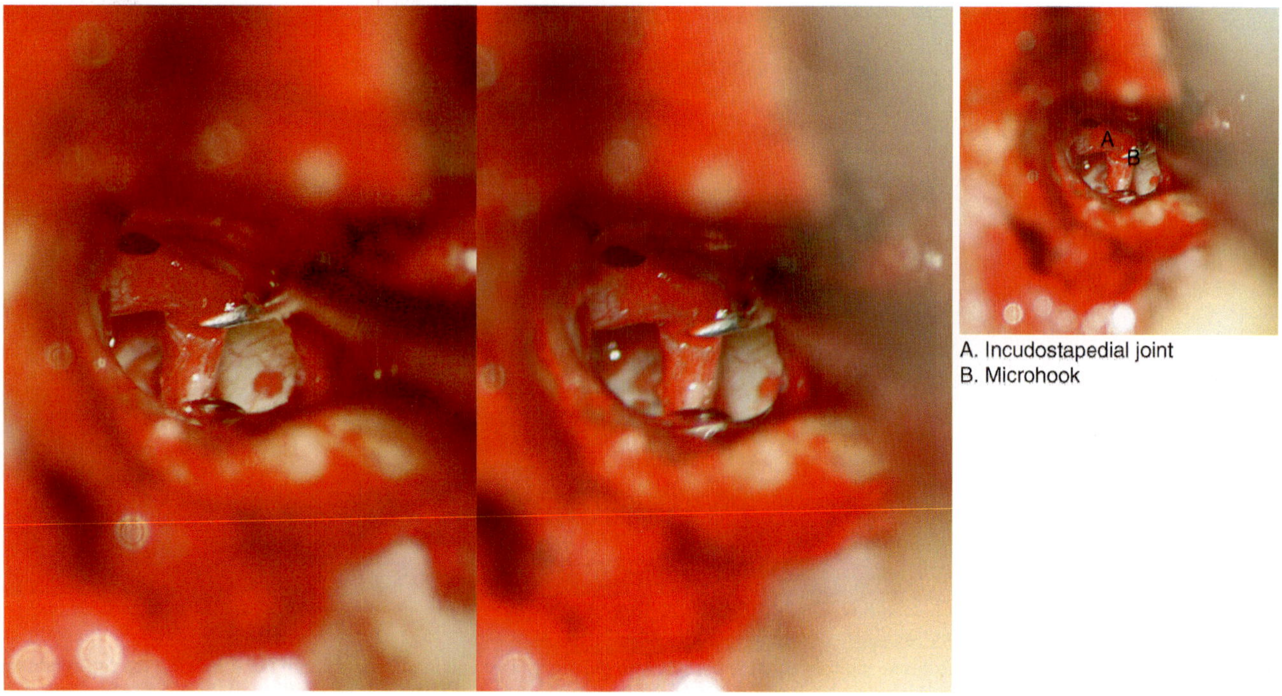

Fig. 4.12 Disconnection of the incudostapedial joint
After the stapes tendon is cut with delicate scissors, a micro hook is inserted into the incudostapedial joint space to disconnect the joint by gently moving the micro hook in a direction parallel with the articular surface. Care should be taken not to displace the incus

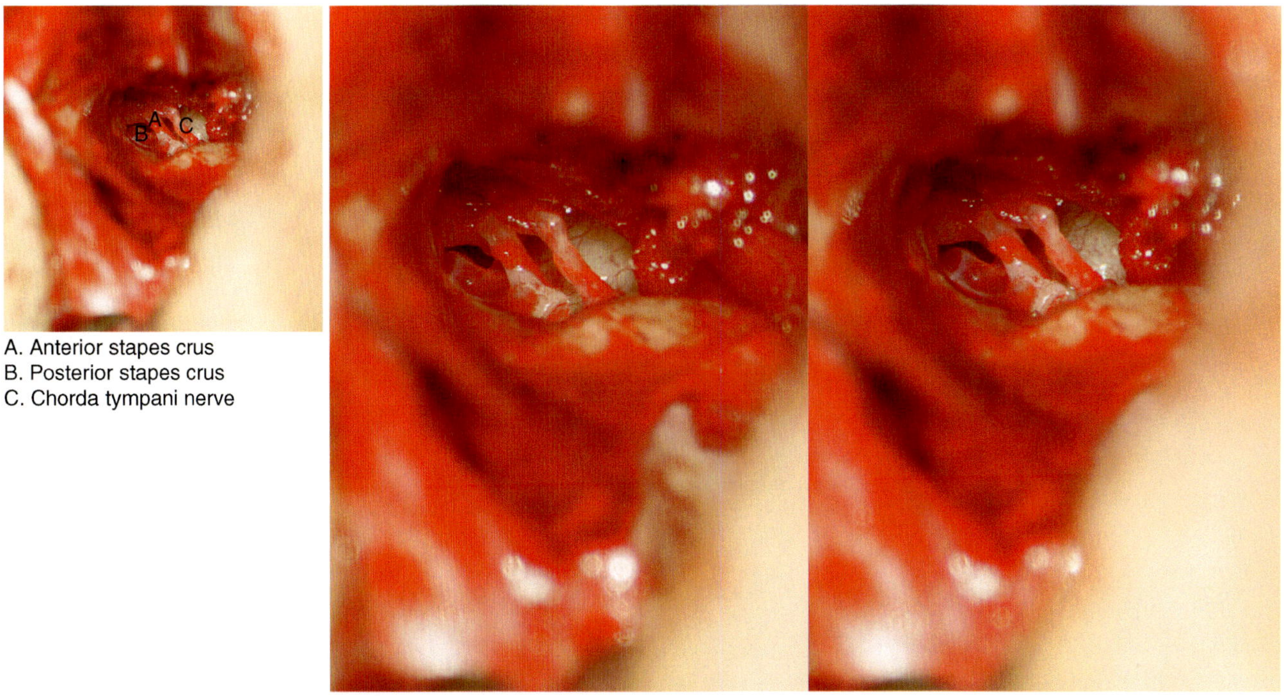

Fig. 4.13 Removal of the superstructure of the stapes
Push the anterior and posterior stapes crura down toward the promontory with a right angled microhook to fracture them or cut them with a set of stapes scissors. Do not push the superstructure of stapes upward in case of injury of the facial nerve. Then remove the superstructure and make a fenestration in the center of the footplate. Use micro hook to take the footplate out

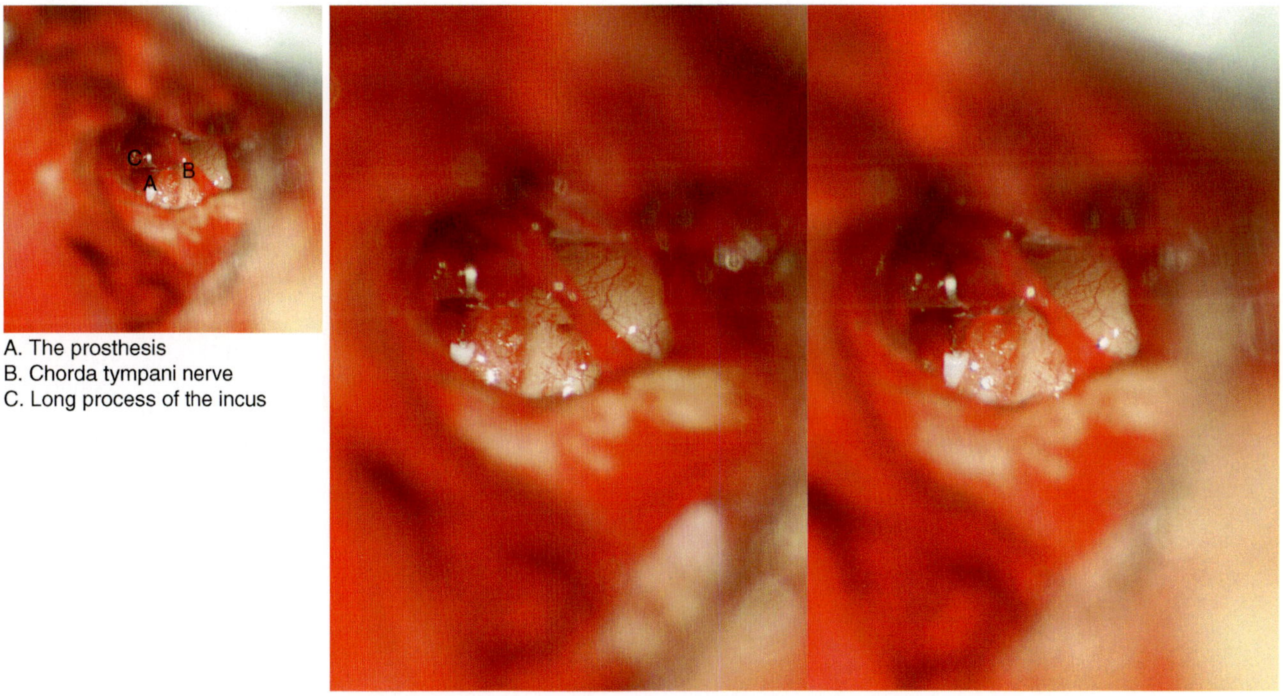

Fig. 4.14 Placement of the prosthesis
The wire of the prosthesis is hooked over to the long process of the incus at the junction of its middle and lower thirds. The medial end of the prosthesis is placed at the center of the oval window. The wire is fixed properly to the incus with a crimper. One or two adequate sized pieces of fat are applied to seal the oval window tightly

Surgery 3: Partial Stapedectomy and Implantation of Piston Prosthesis

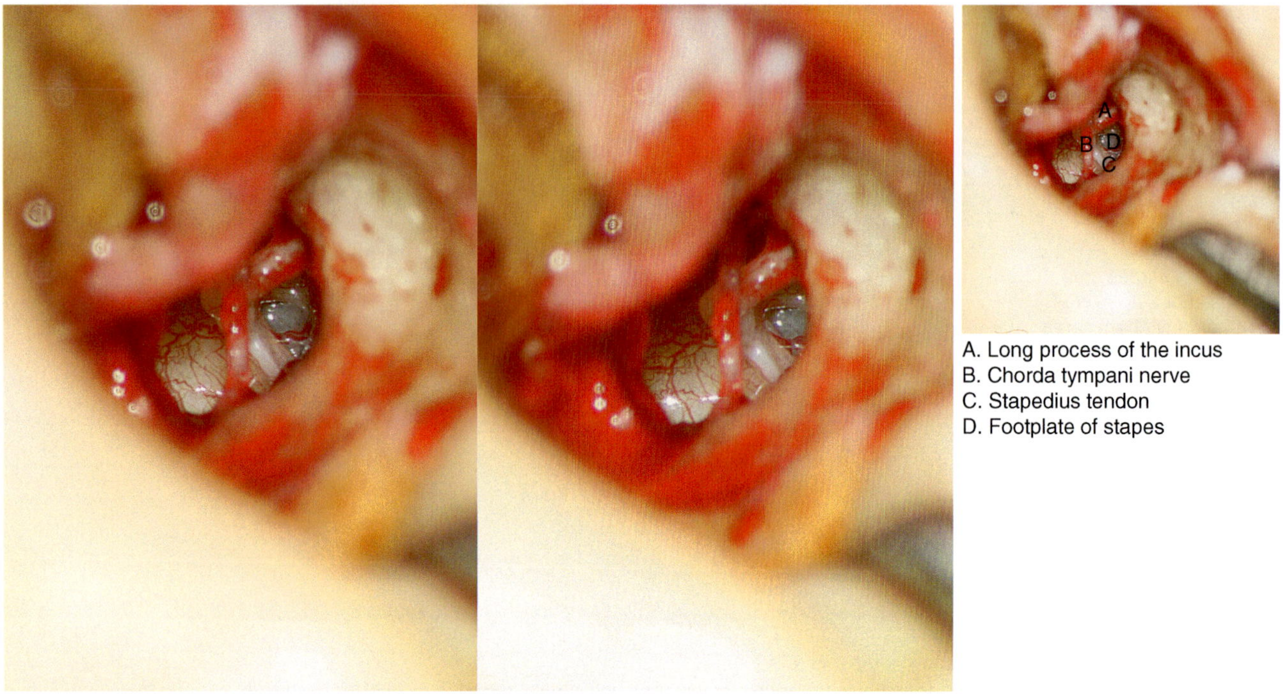

Fig. 4.15 Exposure of the oval window and the long process of the incus
2–4 mm of posterior superior bony canal rim is removed with an angled middle ear curette or chisel to fully expose of the long process of the incus, stapes tendon, the oval window, and the horizontal segment of the facial nerve. The mobility of the three ossicles is evaluated. Slippage of the chisel may damage important structures such as facial nerve, incus, stapes and inner ear

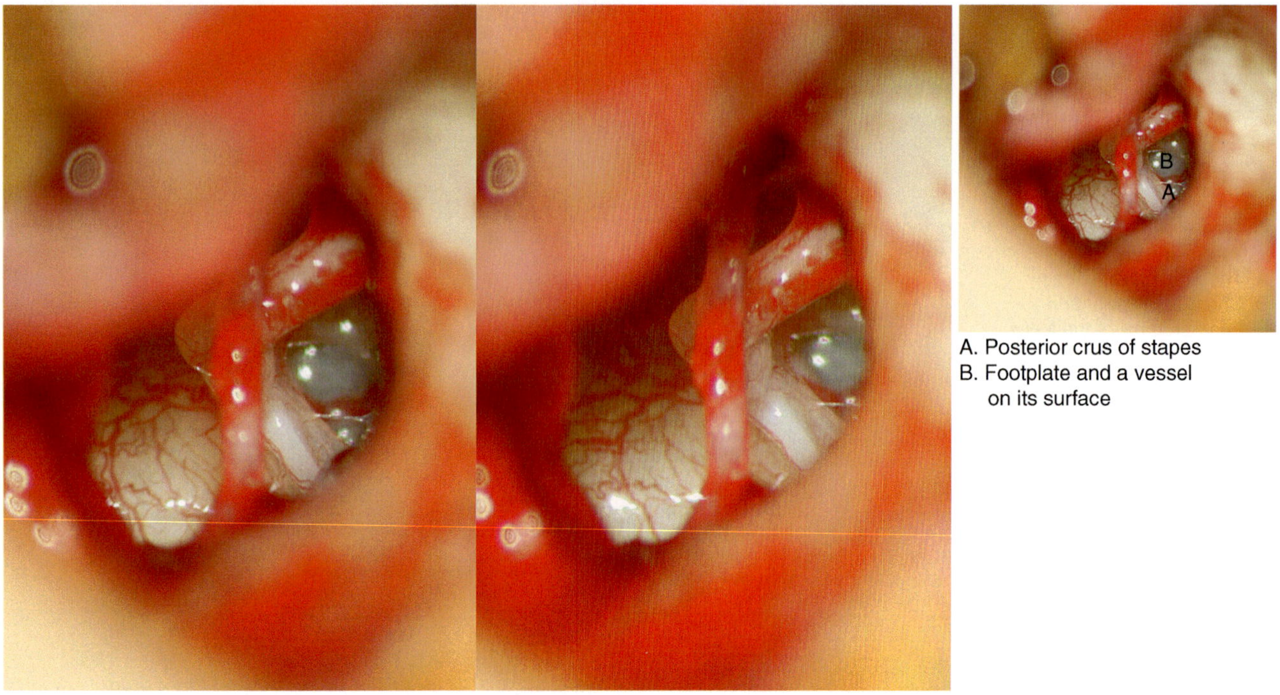

Fig. 4.16 The oval window and stapes (with high magnification)
Fully expose the incudostapedial joint, the long process of the incus, stapes tendon, anterior and posterior crura, the oval window, and the horizontal segment of the facial nerve. The footplate looks lustrous. There is a relatively large vessel on the footplate. The vessel should be treated before fenestration of the footplate using micro-bipolar coagulation or by applying an adrenaline cotton ball after removal of the mucosa of the oval window

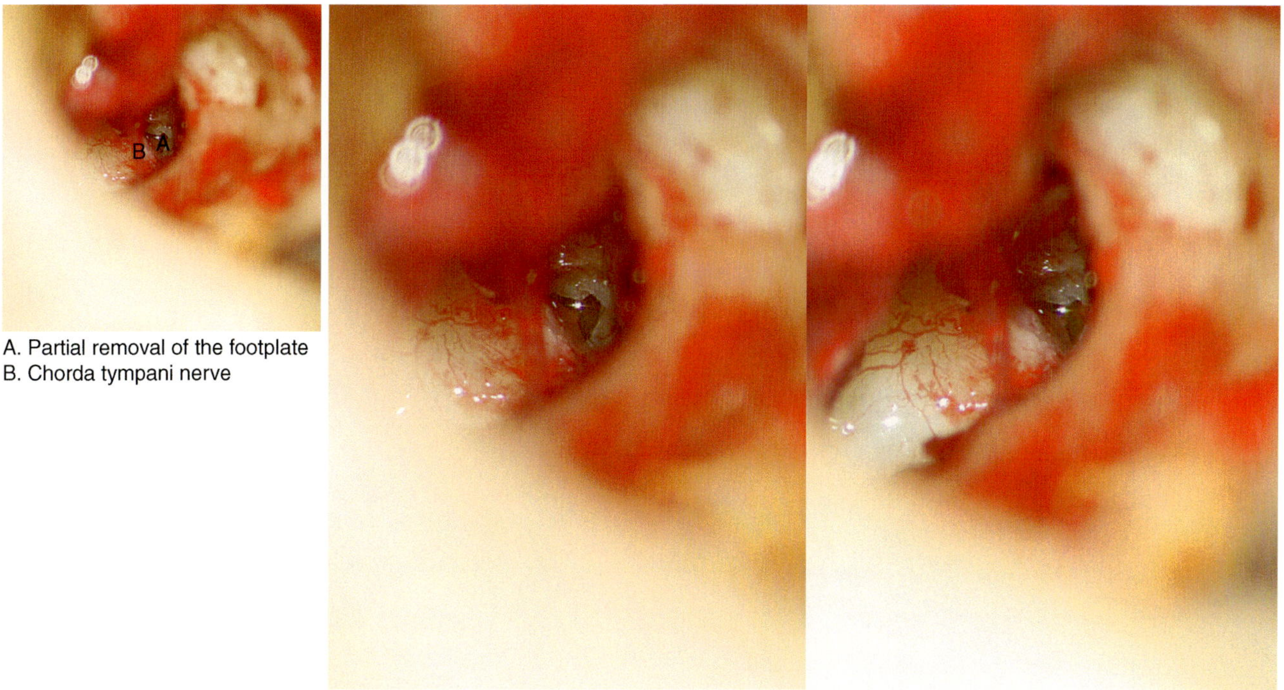

A. Partial removal of the footplate
B. Chorda tympani nerve

Fig. 4.17 Remove part of the footplate
After taking out the superstructure of the stapes, a hole is made in the center of the footplate with a three-sided perforator or with a micro bur. Then enlarge the hole with a special micro hook to remove the central part of the footplate

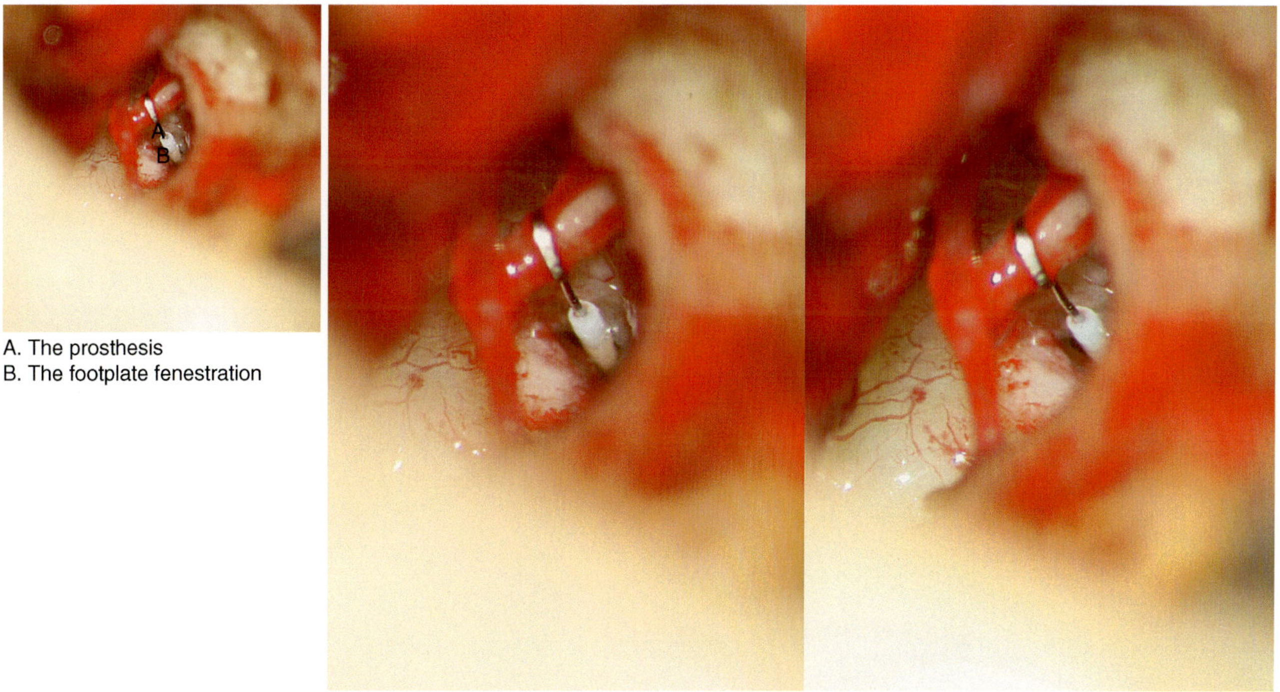

A. The prosthesis
B. The footplate fenestration

Fig. 4.18 Placement of the prosthesis
The medial end of the prosthesis makes contact with the perilymph through the opening of the footplate. The prosthesis should extend into the vestibule for about 0.25 mm, and not more than 0.5 mm. The wire of the prosthesis is hooked over the long process of the incus and fixed to it properly with a crimper. An adequate sized piece of fat is applied to seal the opening of the footplate

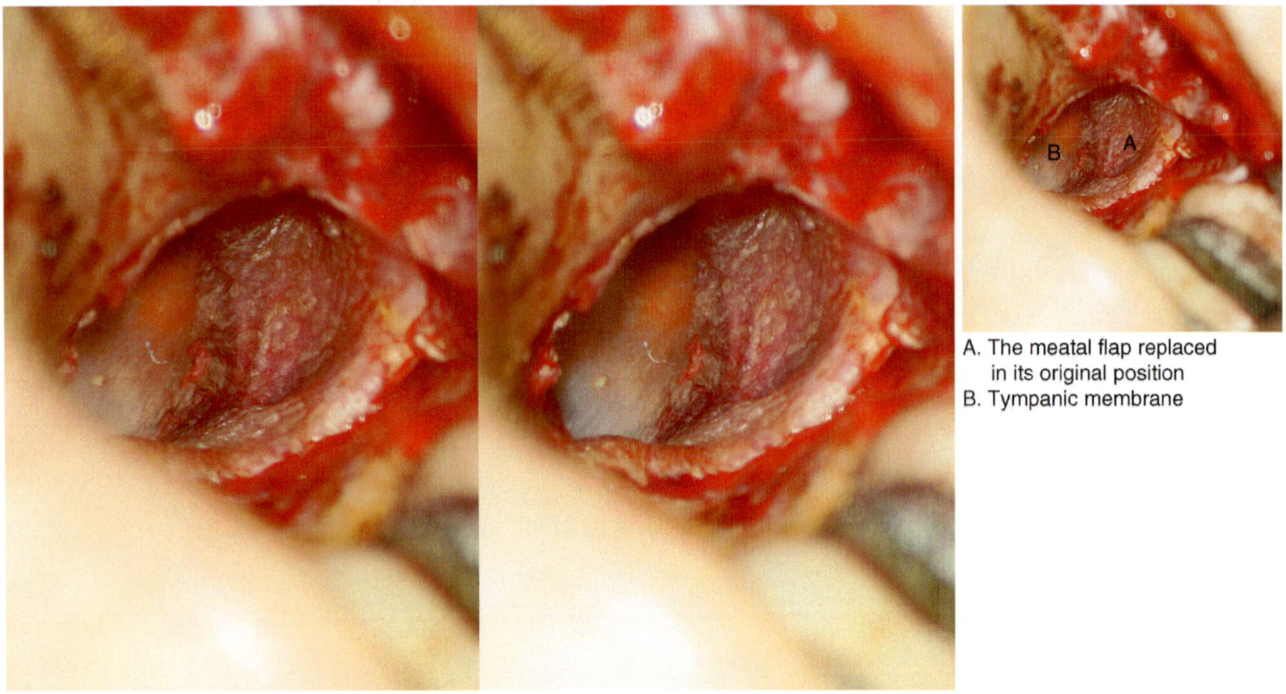

Fig. 4.19 Replace the meatal flap
Replace the meatal flap in its original position. Check the integrity of the tympanic membrane. The external auditory canal is packed with gelatin sponge and iodoform gauze and the first incision is sutured

Fenestration of Stapes and Implantation of Stapes Prosthesis

Fei Yu and Pu Dai

Indications

1. Stapedial otosclerosis, air conduction hearing levels (Pure Tone threshold on average) >30 dB with conductive hearing loss >15 dB.
2. Tympanosclerosis or adhesive otitis media with fixation of stapes but good Eustachian tube function.
3. Congenital stapes malformation.
4. Age range of 5–80 years.

Contraindications

1. Poor general health.
2. Sensorineural hearing loss of a moderate or worse degree.
3. Conductive hearing loss less than 15 dB.
4. Dysfunction of Eustachian tube.
5. Acute upper respiratory infection.
6. Small children or elderly patients.
7. Active menstruation in women
8. Certain professions such as pilots or those who work at heights.

Operative Procedures

1. Endaural incision. First, a longitudinal incision should be made anterior to the root of the helix toward the junction of bone and cartilage in the upper part of the external auditory canal (EAC). A second circumferential incision is made under the microscope from the 6 o'clock position inferiorly, 4 mm posterior to the tympanic ring and extending superiorly to meet the first incision.
2. Elevation of tympano-meatal flap. Dissection should be across a wide front from lateral to medial, elevating the flap from the bony canal wall and taking care to keep it intact. Hemostasis can be achieved with adrenalin soaked cotton or bipolar coagulation. The superior meatal spine can be curetted away if necessary.
3. Entering the middle ear. Elevation of the flap continues to the tympanic ring, where the annulus is elevated with vertical dissection to enter the middle ear.
4. Explosion of middle ear cavity. Part of the postero-superior wall of the EAC may need to be curetted to provide good visualization of the incus long process, the stapes, the stapedius tendon, the pyramidal eminence, and the horizontal part of facial nerve. The ossicles are then assessed for shape (in case of congenital malformation) and mobility. In otosclerosis, the malleus and incus are normally mobile but the stapes footplate fixed.
5. Removal of stapes superstructure. The incudostapedial joint are separated and the stapedius tendon is severed close to the pyramidal eminence. The anterior and posterior crura of the stapes are down fractured and the superstructure is removed.
6. Perforation of stapes footplate. A pinhole of about 1 mm diameter is made in the center of the stapes footplate using a mini drill, a triangle shaped perforator or a laser, and the perilymph is visible.
7. Setting prosthesis. A Teflon and wire prosthesis can be used. The Teflon end can be trimmed for the appropriate overall length (usually between 3.75 and 4.5 mm). The Teflon end is placed in the stapedotomy, the wire hook is placed over the incus long process and crimped firmly. The mobility of the prosthesis is confirmed.
8. Sealing footplate opening. The footplate opening around the piston is sealed with small pieces of fat taken from the skin wound to minimize perilymph leak.
9. Most otosclerosis patients' eardrum are intact, so it is unnecessary for them to require repair of the eardrum. Conversely, intact eardrum is seldom seen in tympanosclerosis, we prefer to restore the eardrum at a first stage operation and do stapes surgery at later time.
10. Reposition the tympano-meatal flap and pack the canal with erythromycin soaked gelatin sponge or other absorbable material then pack the external auditory canal with iodoform gauze.
11. Suture the incision using interrupted sutures and apply a sterile dressing

Special Comments

1. Ensure good expose of the stapes.
2. Protect facial nerve to avoid injury and facial paralysis.
3. Sever the stapedius tendon close to the pyramidal eminence to ensure good exposure of the posterior crus.
4. Dissection near the stapes footplate and its fenestration needs to be done with great care to avoid its mobilization or dislocation and consequent inner ear injury.
5. Measure the distance from the incus to the stapes footplate exactly to assess the appropriate length of the piston.
6. The footplate fenestration around the piston is sealed with fat to prevent perilymph leak. The fat should be placed carefully to prevent it entering the vestibule.
7. If a gusher is encountered, the oval window should be sealed and the procedure terminated.

Complications

1. Hemorrhage and infection. The operation is carried out under sterile conditions, with thorough hemostasis and using post-operative antibiotics.
2. Deafness or severe hearing loss. Avoid injury to the membranous labyrinth.
3. Facial paralysis. Facial nerve decompression is performed immediately if the facial nerve is injured during the operation or peripheral facial paralysis is present immediately after the procedure.
4. Vertigo. Mild vertigo will occur in some patients after operation. This may be present for days but rarely more than 1 week. If it persists, re-operation should be considered, especially if it is accompanied by hearing loss and/or tinnitus.
5. Perilymphorrhea. The fenestration around the piston should be re-sealed with fat.
6. Taste disturbance is common and due to dissection of the chorda tympani nerve during surgery. This usually recovers within 1 month.
7. Persistent middle ear blood clot or fluid. This usually resolves with time and gentle Eustachian tube inflation.
8. If a tympanic membrane perforation occurs, it should be repaired immediately.

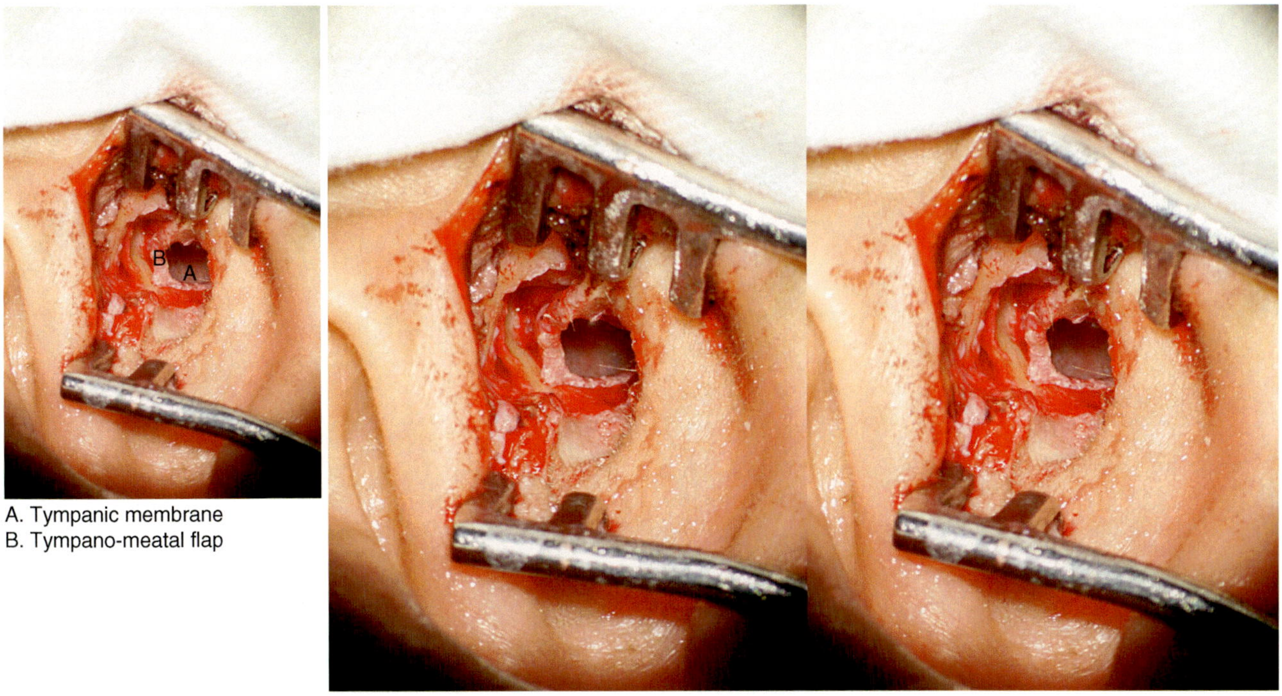

A. Tympanic membrane
B. Tympano-meatal flap

Fig. 4.20 Incision, dissection of tympano-meatal flap
A vertical incision is made anterior to the root of the helix and extended to the bony-cartilage junction of the external auditory canal. A circumferential incision is made under the microscope. It starts at the 6 o'clock point inferior, passes 4–5 mm from the annulus and extends superiorly to meet the first incision. The tympano-meatal flap is then elevated

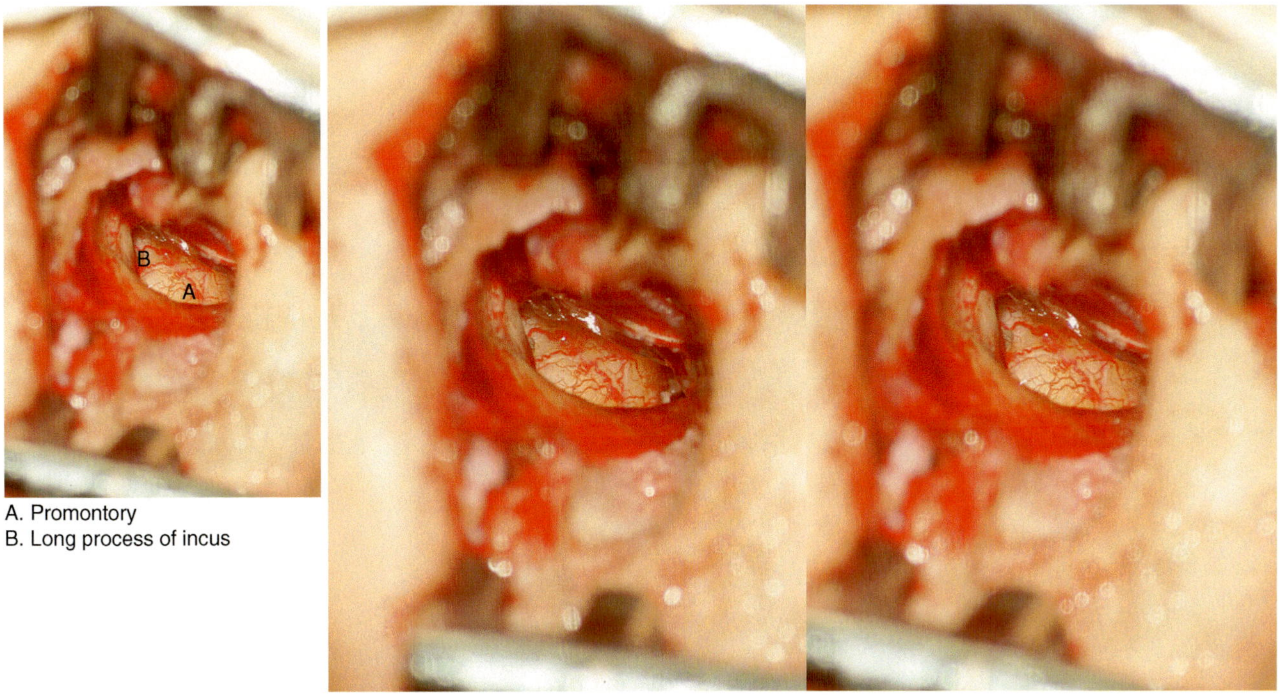

A. Promontory
B. Long process of incus

Fig. 4.21 Exposure of tympanic cavity
Elevate the annulus from the tympanic sulcus superiorly and inferiorly. Reflect the tympano-meatal flap forward to expose the middle ear cavity. Curette the superior meatal spine if necessary. The lenticular process of the incus is identified and the blood vessels over the promontory are clearly seen

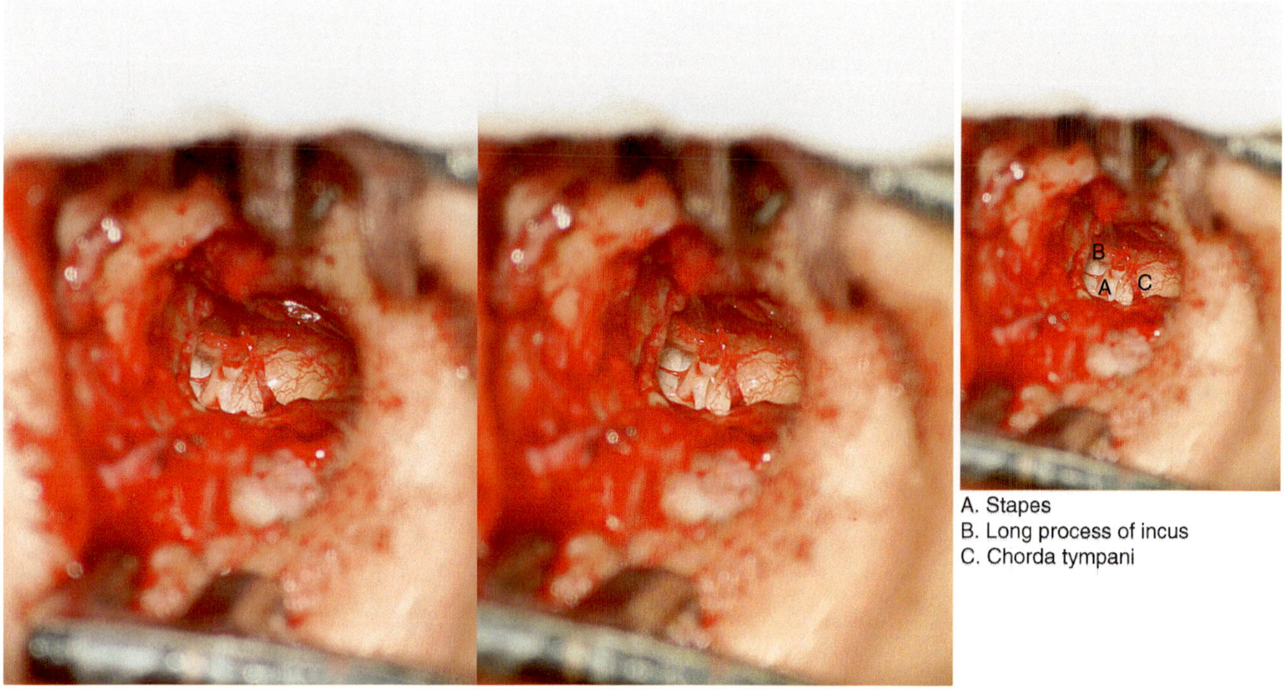

Fig. 4.22 Exposure of the stapes
Curette part of the postero-superior EAC wall to expose the long process of the incus. The chorda tympani and the horizontal part of facial nerve is seen

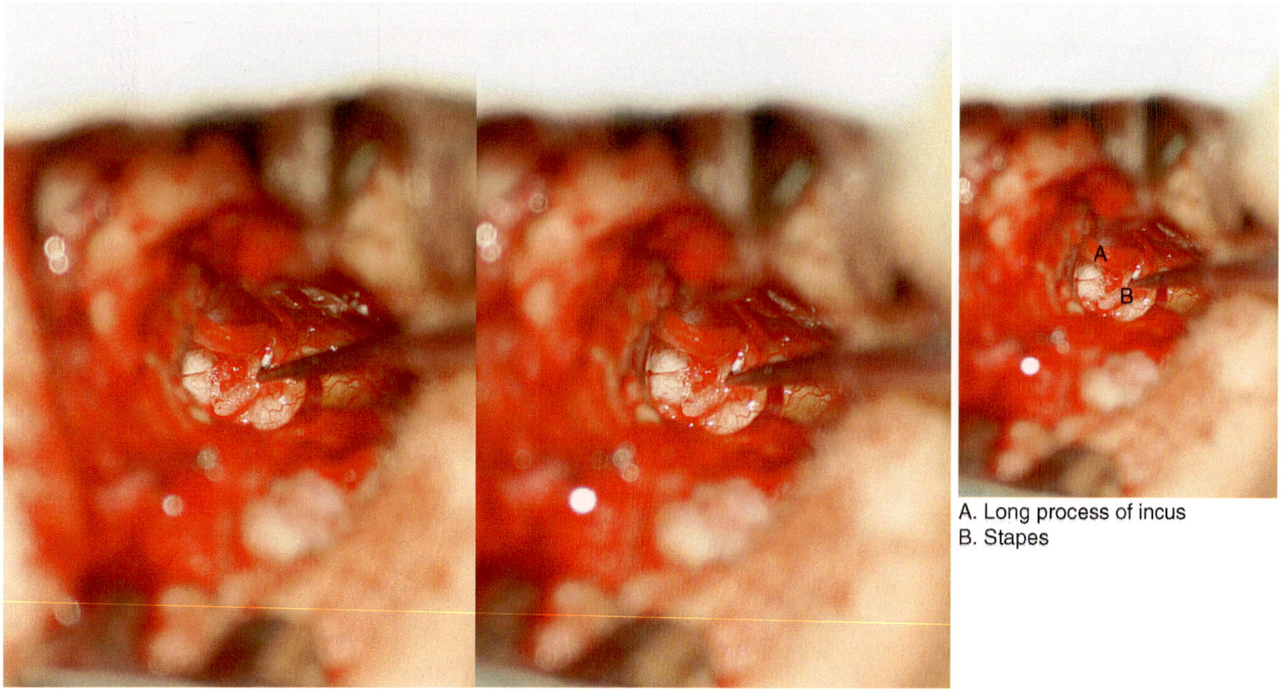

Fig. 4.23 Stapes superstructure removal
Protect the chorda tympani. Confirm the stapes fixation. Disconnect the incudostapedial joint. Sever the stapedius tendon close to the pyramidal eminence. Down fracture the anterior and posterior crura of the stapes. Remove the superstructure of the stapes

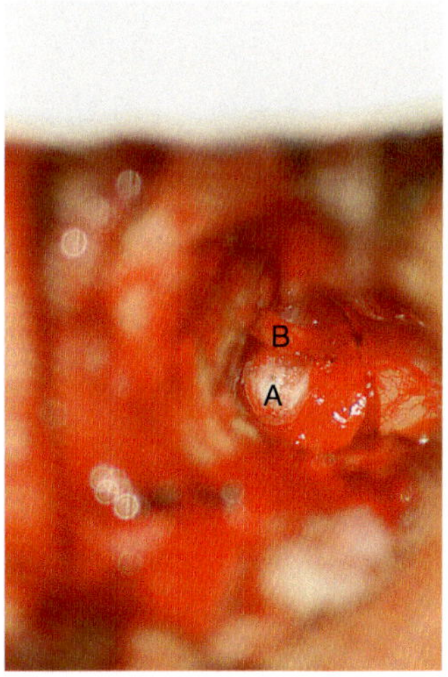

A. Stapes footplate
B. Long process of incus

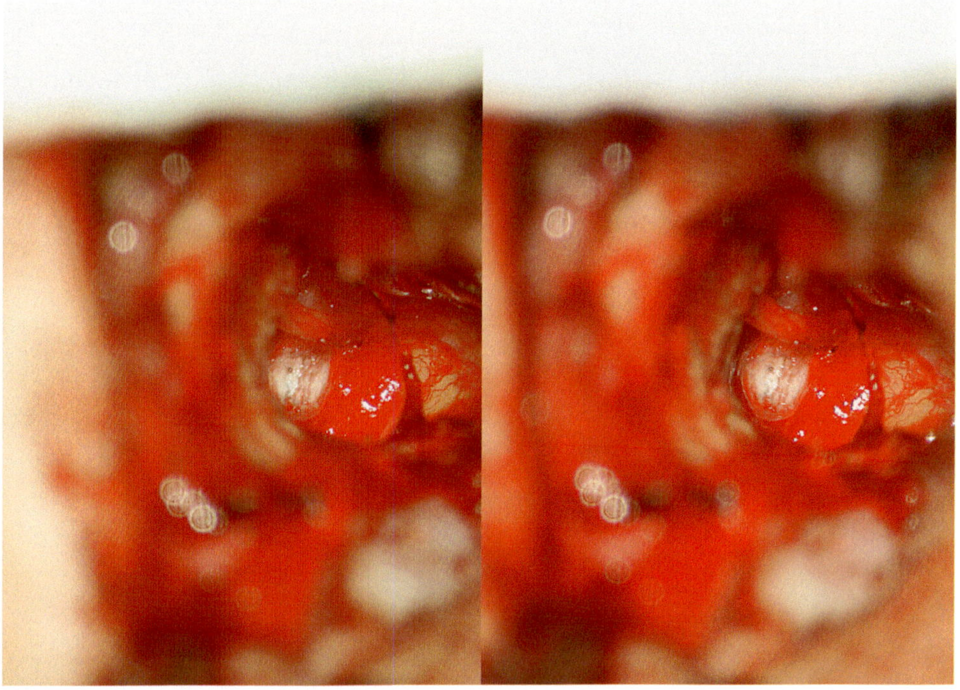

Fig. 4.24 Exposure of stapes footplate
The stapes footplate fixation is confirmed

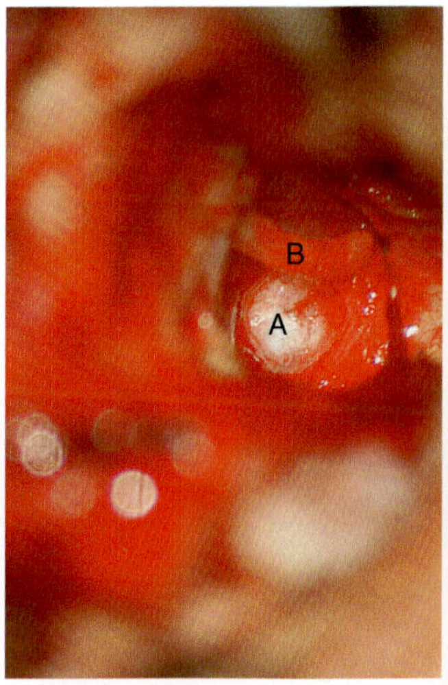

A. Drilling a pinhole in the stapes footplate
B. Long process of incus

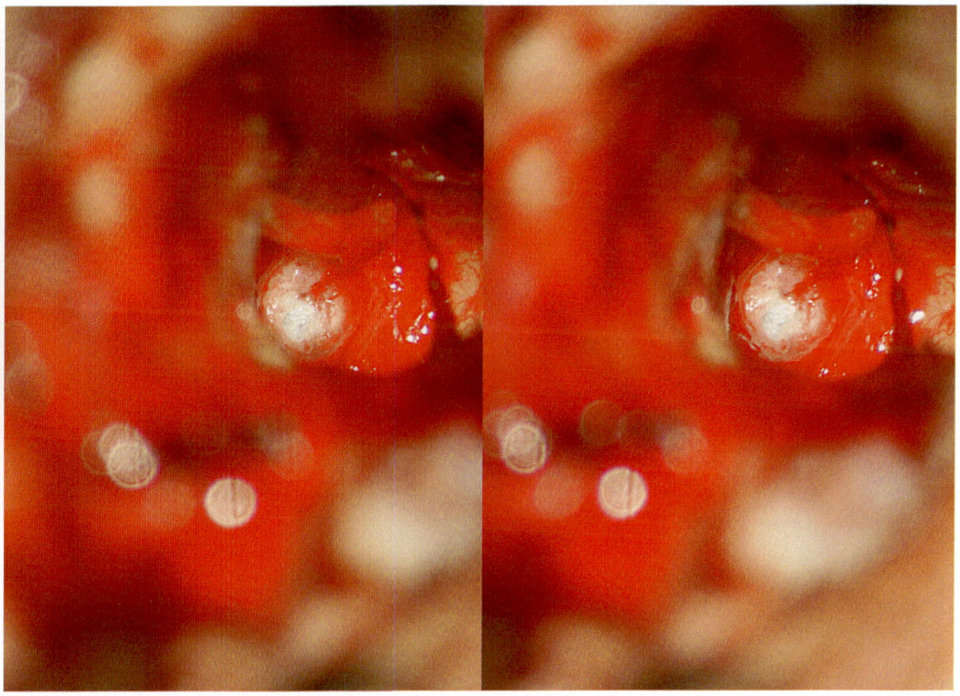

Fig. 4.25 Fenestration of stapes footplate
The blue appearance of the oval window is apparent through the fenestration

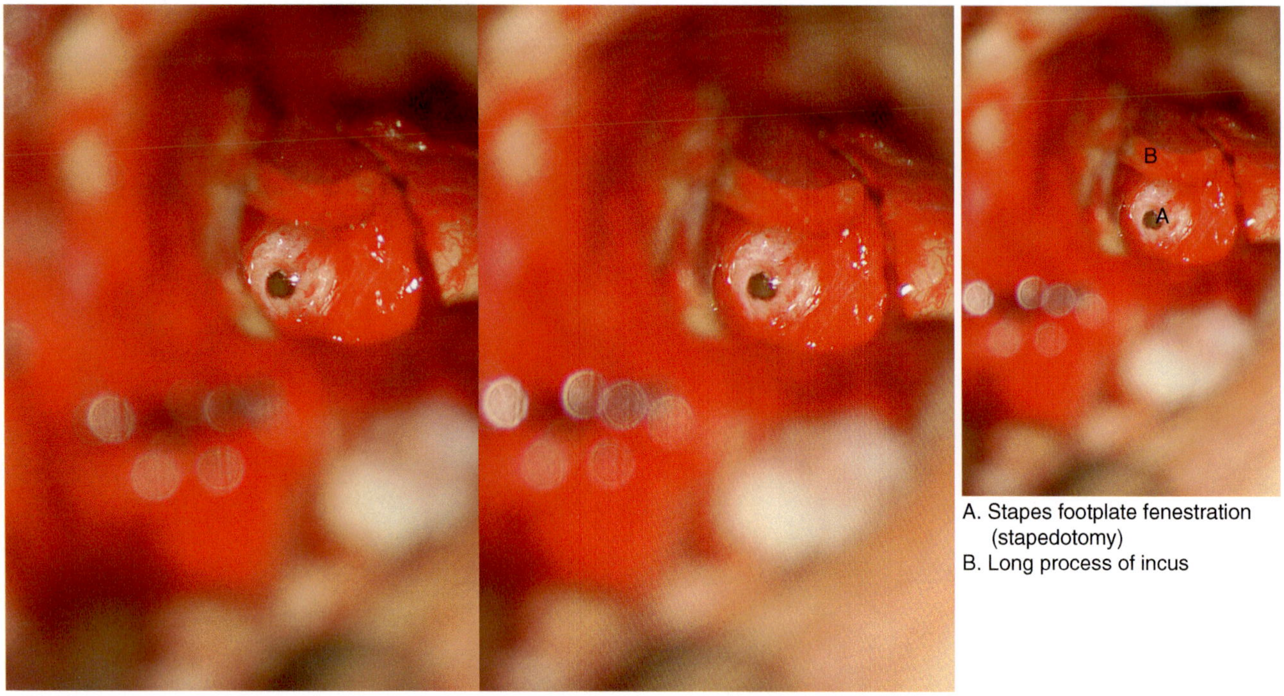

A. Stapes footplate fenestration (stapedotomy)
B. Long process of incus

Fig. 4.26 Fenestration of stapes footplate
Clear perilymph is seen through the footplate opening

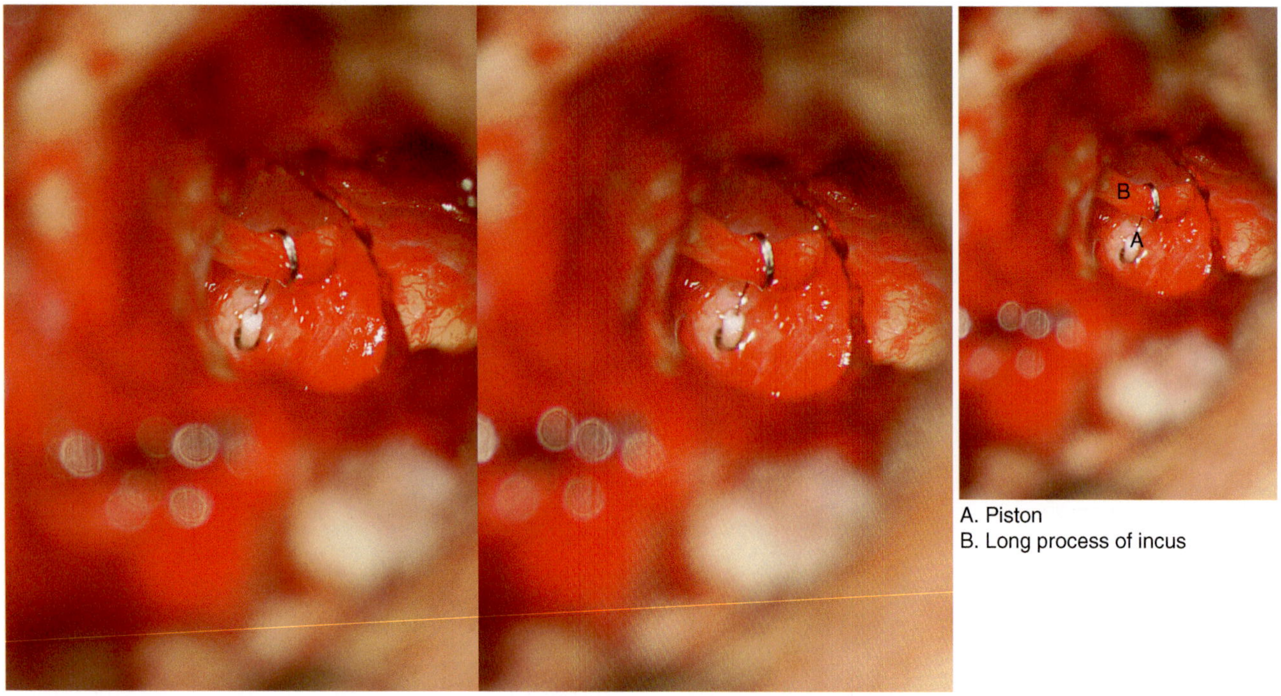

A. Piston
B. Long process of incus

Fig. 4.27 Implantation of stapes prosthesis
The Teflon end of the piston is trimmed to appropriate overall length (3.75–4.5 mm). The Teflon end is placed in the stapedotomy, the wire hook is placed over the incus long process and crimped firmly. The mobility of the prosthesis is confirmed

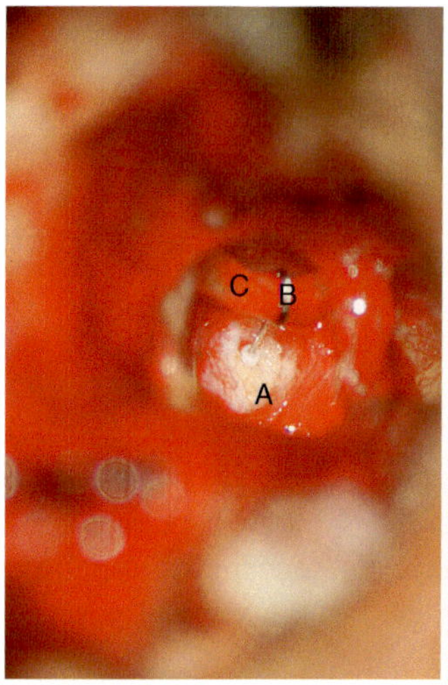

A. Fat
B. Piston
C. Long process of incus

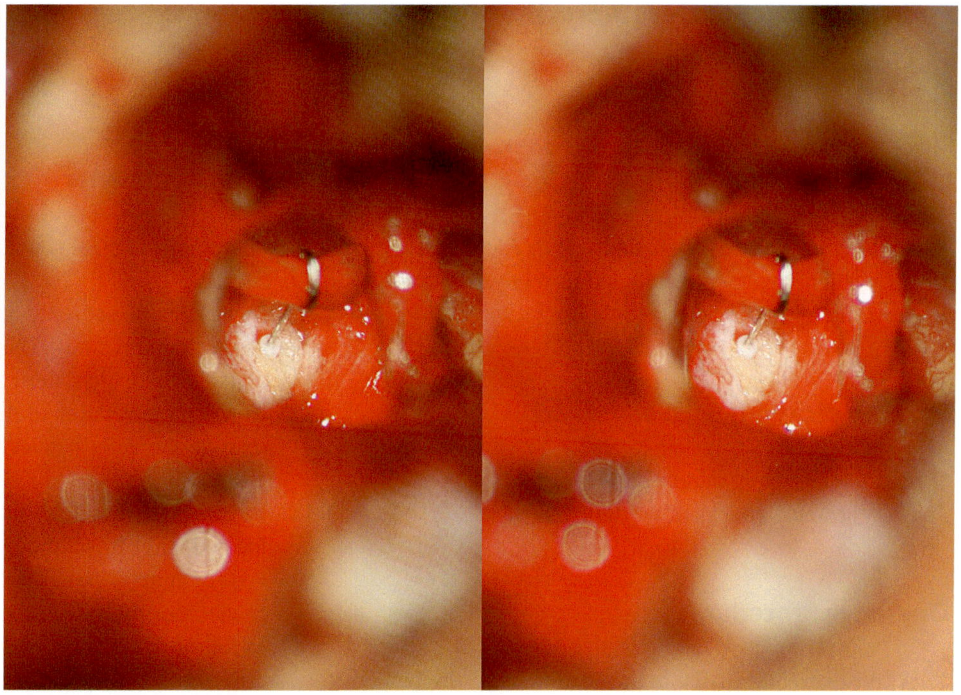

Fig. 4.28 Seal the oval window
The footplate opening around the piston is sealed with small pieces of fat from the skin wound to minimize perilymph leak

Endolymphatic Sac Decompression

Song Gao and Pu Dai

Indications

This procedure is used in patients with Meniere's disease where medical treatment has failed to relieve the frequency and severity of the vertigo.

Contraindications

1. Acute infection in middle ear.
2. Current Acute attacks of vertigo.

Operative Procedures

1. A postauricular incision is made from the superior extremity of the auricle to the mastoid tip, about 10 mm posterior to the postauricular crease. Incise the skin, subcutaneous tissue, and periosteum of the mastoid to expose the entire mastoid cortex.
2. Using a cutting bur, the mastoid cortex is removed from the cribriform area to expose the mastoid antrum which lies 10–15 mm deep to Macewen's triangle.
3. A complete mastoidectomy is performed and the lateral semicircular canal, posterior semicircular canal, sigmoid sinus, sinodural angle and facial nerve canal are exposed. The posterior fossa dural plate lies deep to the Trautmann triangle which lies between the mastoid tegmen, sigmoid sinus, posterior semicircular canal.
4. After completion of the mastoidectomy, the endolymphatic sac is located in a thickened portion of posterior fossa dura medial to the sigmoid sinus and inferior to the posterior semicircular canal, that is inferior to the Donaldson line. This line is an imaginary line extending through the long axis of the lateral semicircular canal and bisects the posterior semicircular canal. Using a diamond bur, remove the bone covering the posterior fossa dura over an area of approximately 1 cm × 2 cm.
5. Exposing the Sac. In the area of bone removal, separate the dura using a micro elevator, and expose the white sac and light blue dura.
6. Incising the Sac. After identifying the Sac, cut its lateral surface with small sickle-shaped knife. A little fluid may be seen. In order to ensure smooth drainage, the incision should be large enough or a segment of the lateral wall of the sac can be elevated and rolled over or excised.
7. The wound is thoroughly irrigated with saline and the mastoid cavity is filled with gelfoam. The wound is sutured in layers.

Special Comments

1. A complete mastoidectomy is the first step of this surgery.
2. Remove bone but leave an "eggshell" bone on the surface of the sigmoid sinus. The sinus is retracted posteriorly to assist with identification of the endolymphatic sac.
3. Confirm the position of the lateral semicircular canal, and remove the cells between the facial nerve and posterior fossa dura.
4. It may be difficult to find the endolymphatic sac if it is located inferior to the posterior canal. The wall of the endolymphatic sac is thicker and whiter than dura. Sometimes the sac is positioned close to the jugular bulb. In this situation the operator should be careful when cutting the sac.
5. If the dura is lacerated by mistake, it is necessary to close it with sutures and muscle or fascia, in order to prevent a cerebrospinal fluid leak.

Complications

1. Sensorineural hearing impairment. This is due to an inner ear injury which is more likely to happen in a sclerotic mastoid where it is difficult to distinguish the semicircular canal from surrounding bone. If such an injury occurs, suctioning over the open semicircular canal is avoided. Plug the fenestration with either muscle, fascia or bone paste or bone wax as soon as possible. Sensorineural hearing impairment is also likely to occur if the surgery fails to control the disease.
2. Cerebrospinal fluid leak. This may occur when removing the bone over the posterior fossa and damaging the dura or incising the dura when trying to confirm the position of the sac. If this occurs, the injured dura should be closed directly or repaired with muscle or fascia.
3. Facial paralysis. In some patients, the space between the sigmoid sinus and the descending portion of the facial nerve is small, and injury to facial nerve is more likely to happen when removing the air cells in this region. Facial function usually returns within several weeks in mild injuries; but, facial nerve transplantation or facial nerve-hypoglossal nerve anastomosis will be necessary in severe injuries.

Surgery1: Endolymphatic Sac Decompression

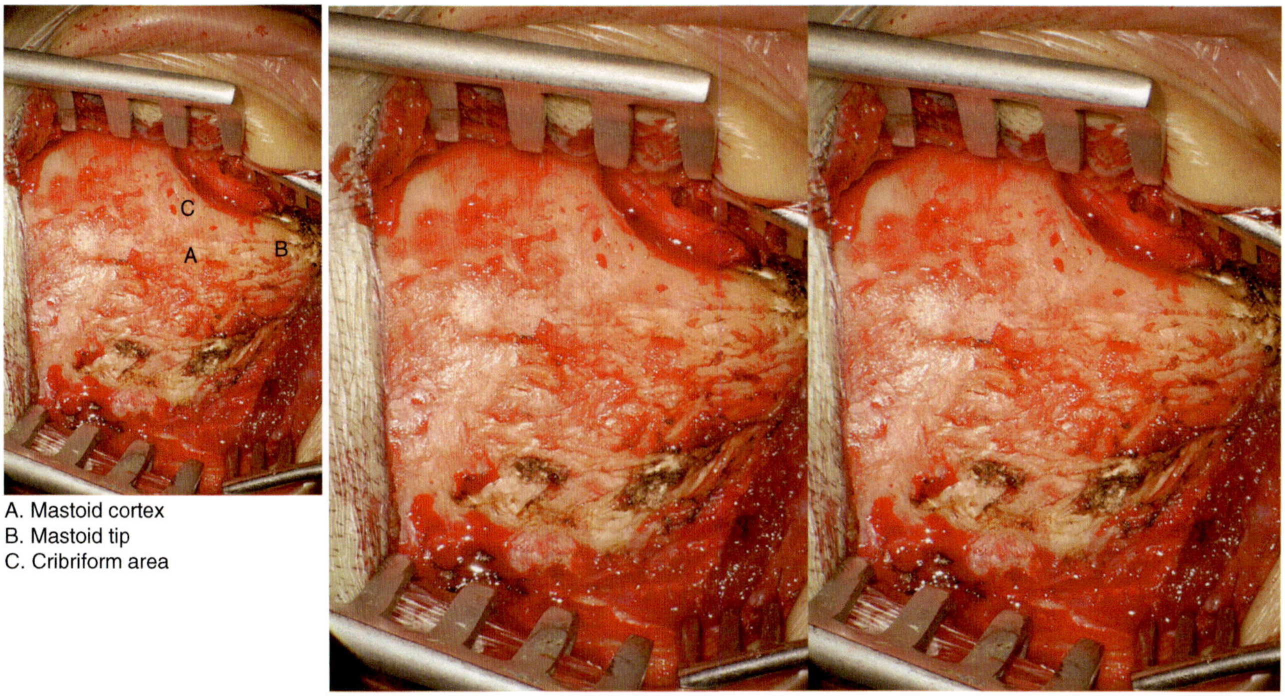

Fig. 4.29 Exposure of mastoid cortex
A postauricular incision is made from the superior extremity of the auricle to the mastoid tip, about 10 mm posterior to the postauricular crease. Incise the skin, subcutaneous tissue, and periosteum of the mastoid to expose the entire mastoid cortex

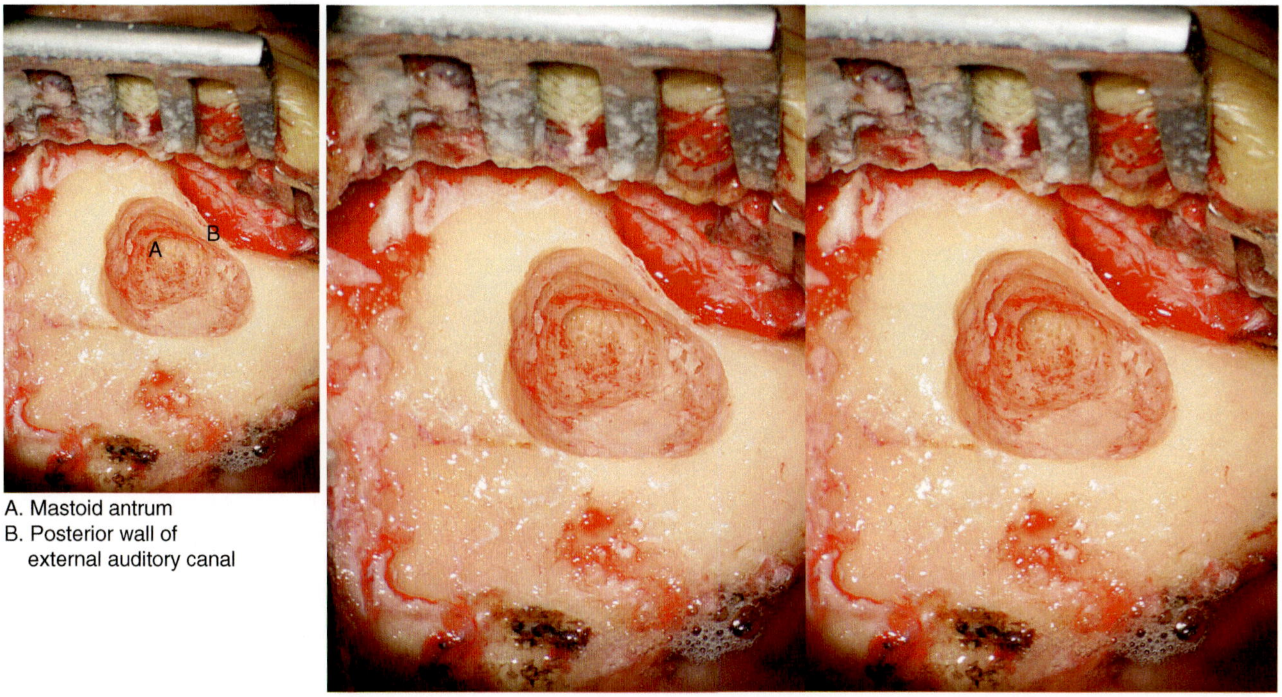

Fig. 4.30 Opening the mastoid antrum
The mastoid cortex is removed in a systematic fashion. The first cut is made along the temporalis line toward the sinodural angle. This line is the landmark of middle cranial fossa dura. A second cut perpendicular to the first is immediately posterior to the posterior external auditory canal wall toward the mastoid tip. The third cut connects the first two along the surface projection of the sigmoid sinus. Dissection parallel to a given landmark and removal of bone in layers is safe. Deep drilling at one single point must be avoided. Wide saucerization is necessary for adequate visualization of deeper structures

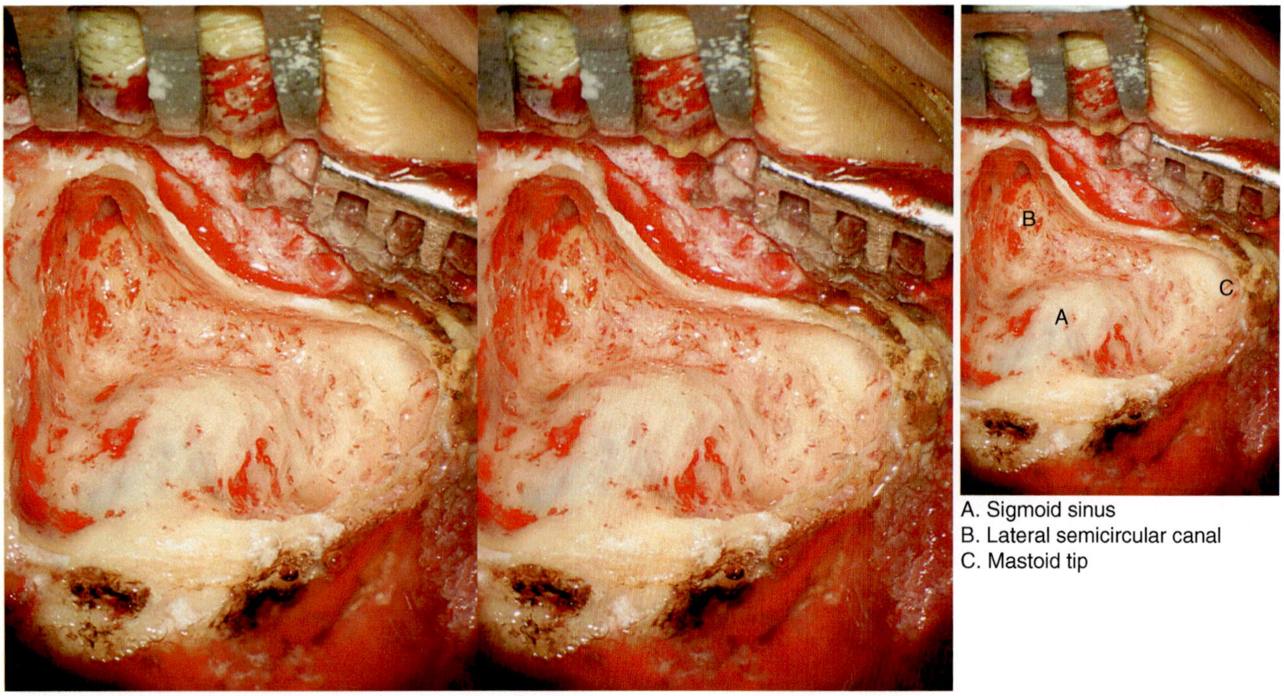

Fig. 4.31 Cavity saucerization
Cavity saucerization is completed. The posterior external canal wall should be thinned, and the mastoid tegmen exposed as is the mastoid tip. The area of bone removal posteriorly is larger than that of a normally saucerized mastoid cavity. The bone over the sigmoid sinus is thinned

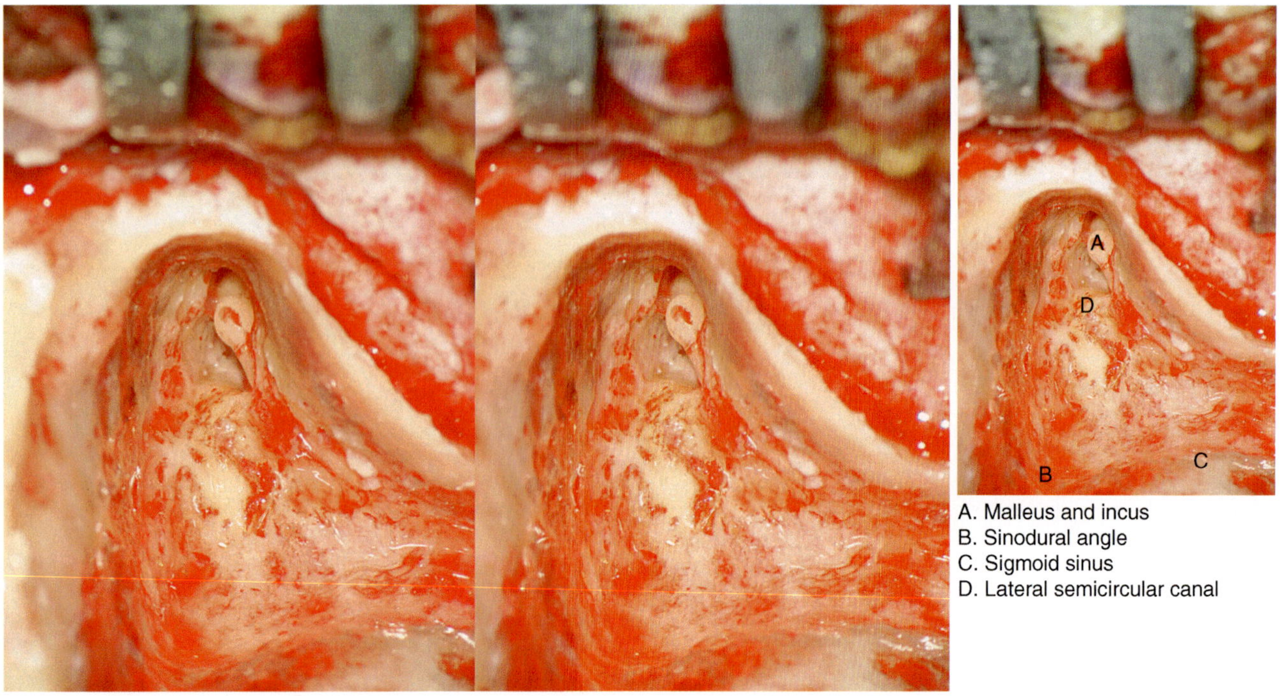

Fig. 4.32 Exposure of lateral semicircular canal
Enlarge the aditus ad antrum to promote drainage and ventilation between the middle ear and mastoid cavity, and avoid blockage of the aditus with granulation tissue post-operatively. To avoid injury to the labyrinth, the area of exposure should not be deeper than the prominence of lateral semicircular canal

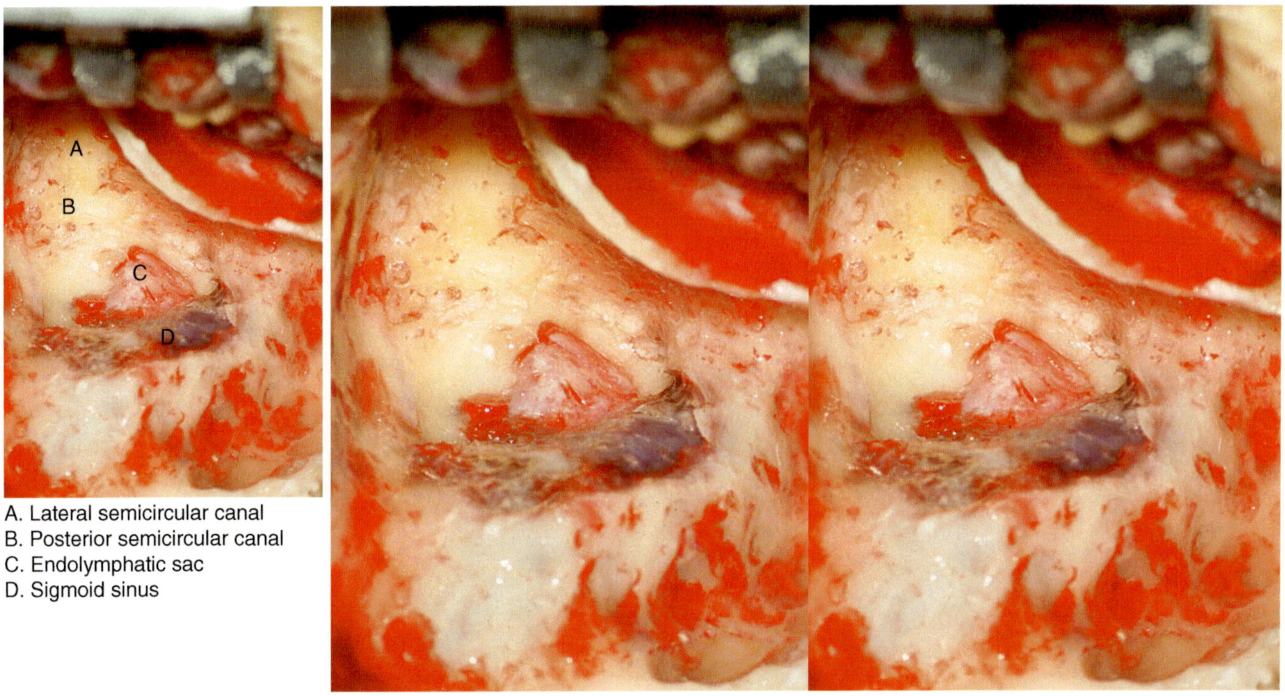

Fig. 4.33 Exposure of endolymphatic sac
The bone over the sigmoid sinus and posterior fossa dura is thinned and removed. The sigmoid sinus is retracted posteriorly. The bone between the sigmoid sinus and posterior semicircular canal removed. The posterior fossa dura is exposed and retracted posteriorly to identify the endolymphatic sac

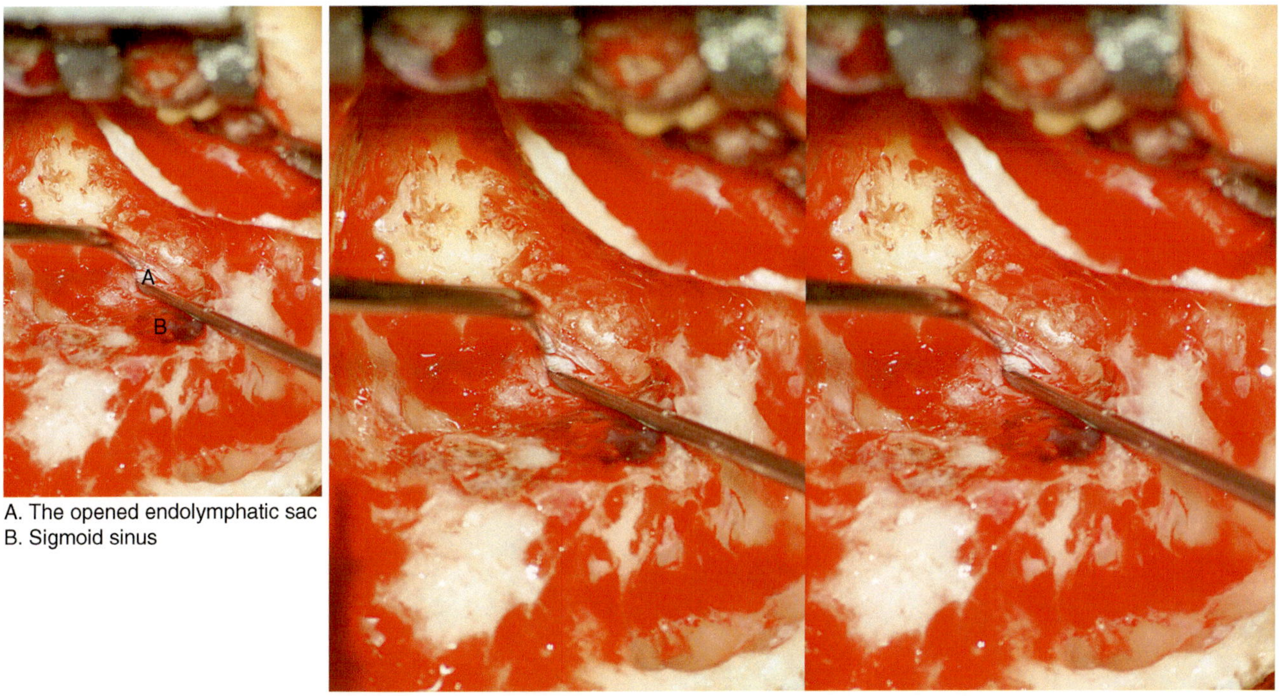

Fig. 4.34 Incising endolymphatic sac
The location of the endolymphatic sac is variable and there are several methods to confirm its position. A micro elevator can be delicately inserted between the posterior fossa dura and the posterior surface of the temporal bone. Passage of the elevator will be prevented by the endolymphatic duct. The white color of endolymphatic sac can help to confirm its position as the surrounding dura is light blue

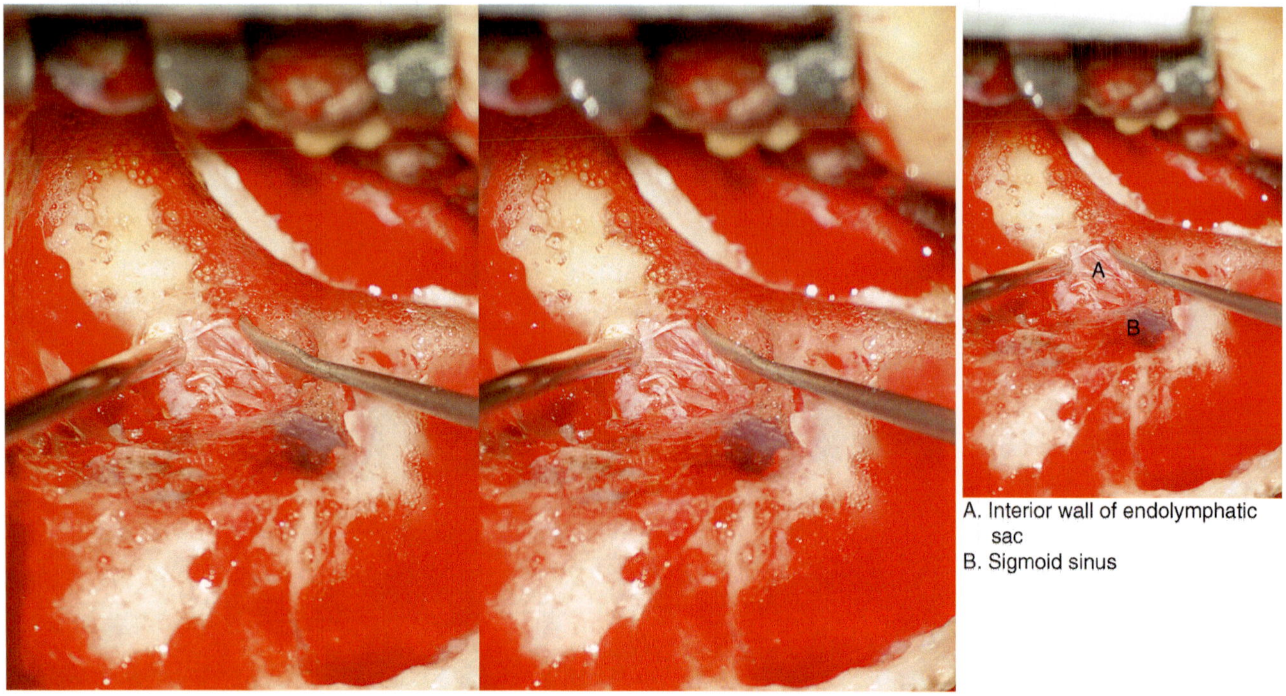

Fig. 4.35 Expose the cavity of the endolymphatic sac
The lateral wall of endolymphatic sac is incised and separated to confirm the lumen of the sac. Enlarge the incision or remove a part of the lateral wall to get adequate drainage

Surgery 2: Endolymphatic Sac Decompression

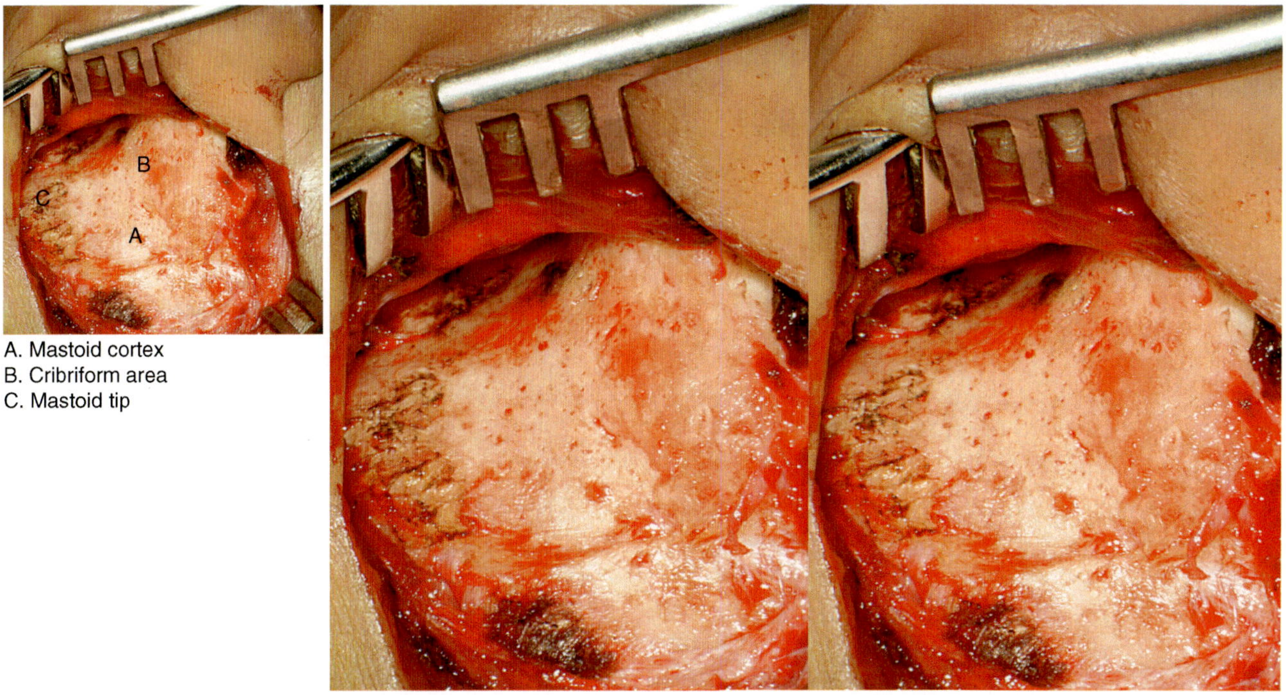

Fig. 4.36 Exposure of mastoid cortex
A postauricular incision is made as mentioned above, or in the postauricular crease. Incise the skin, subcutaneous tissue, and periosteum of the mastoid to expose the entire mastoid cortex

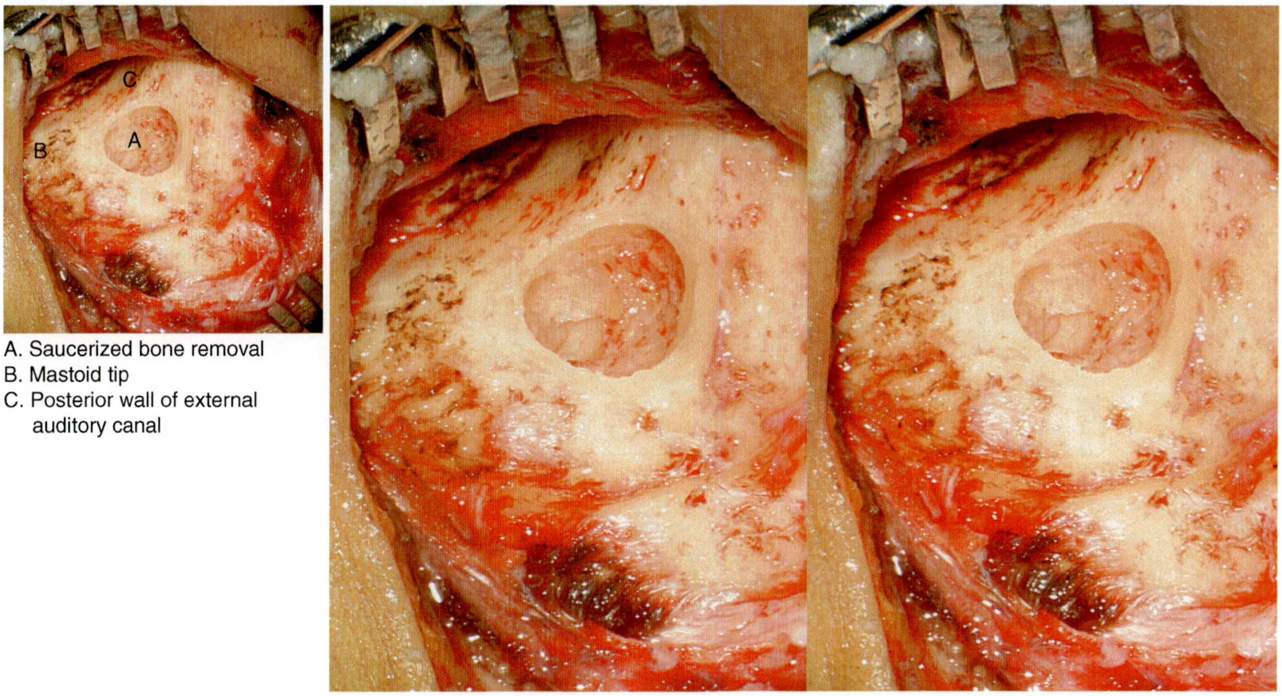

Fig. 4.37 Exposure of the mastoid antrum
The mastoid cortex is removed in a systematic fashion, saucerizing the cavity with a 5 or 7 mm cutting bur. Remove the bone over the mastoid tegmen and the anterior wall of sigmoid sinus. This is a safe approach when it is difficult to identify the sac

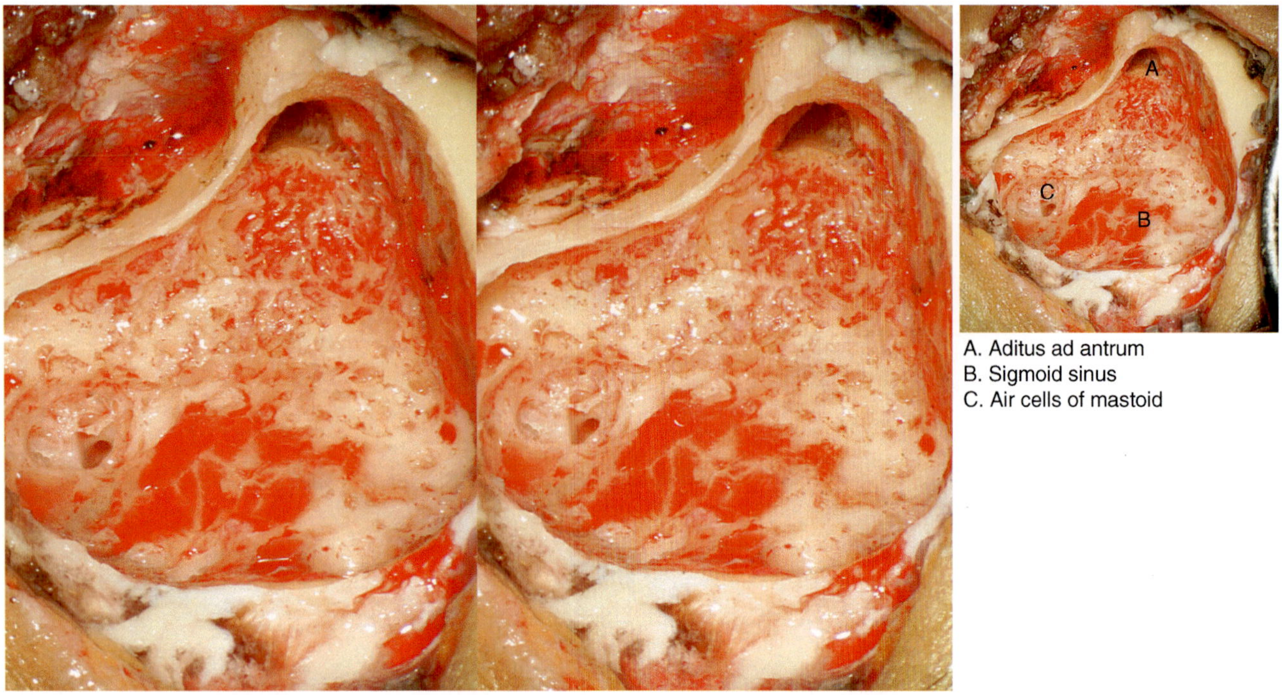

Fig. 4.38 Cavity saucerization
A wide saucerization is completed. Expose the aditus ad antrum and identify the short process of incus. The mastoid tegmen and the anterior wall of the sigmoid sinus are thinned, and the mastoid tip and digastric ridge are exposed

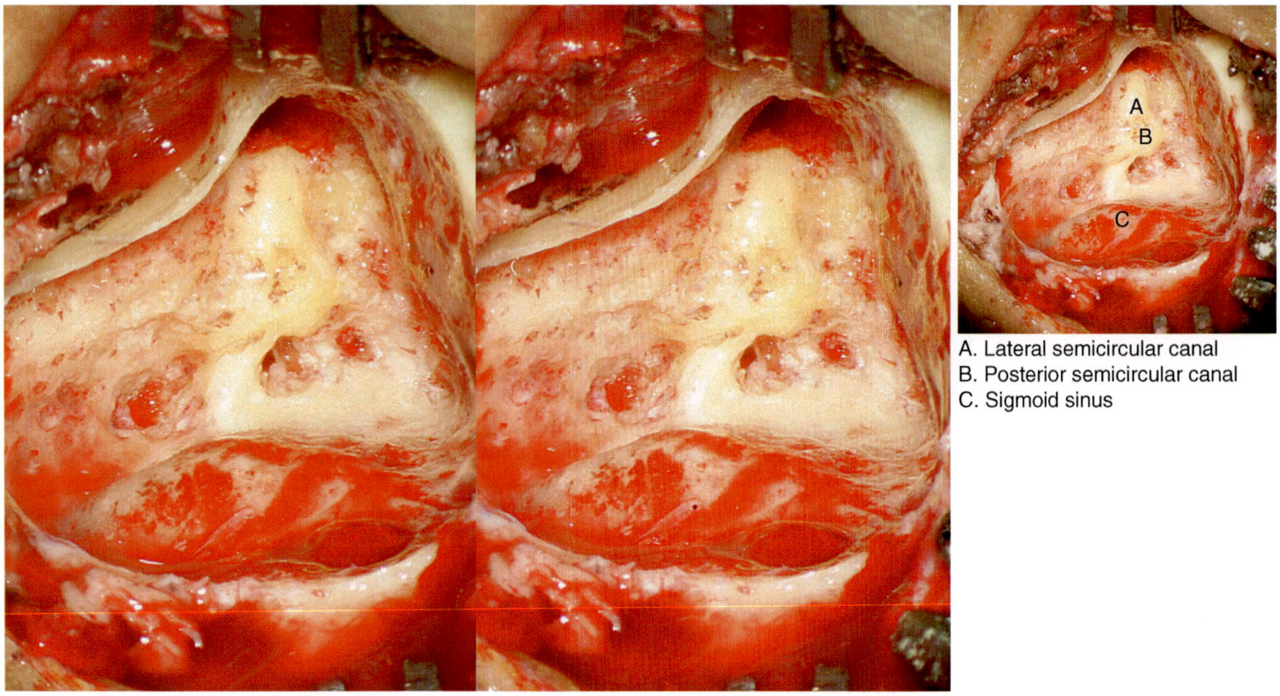

Fig. 4.39 Exposure of lateral and posterior semicircular canal
There are some large air cells between descending portion of facial nerve and posterior fossa dura in well pneumatized mastoids. Remove the air cells and expose the posterior fossa dura

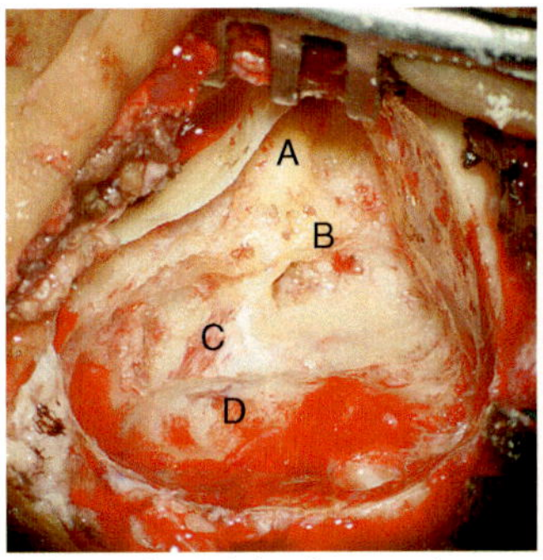

A. Lateral semicircular canal
B. Posterior semicircular canal
C. Endolymphatic sac
D. Sigmoid sinus

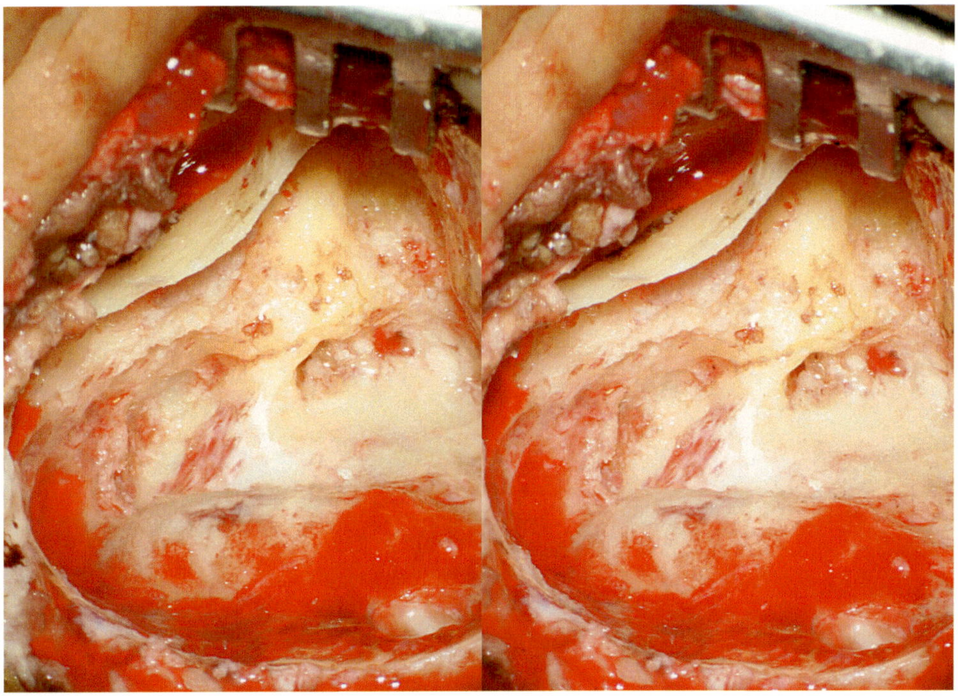

Fig. 4.40 Exposure of endolymphatic sac
Expose posterior fossa dura and look for endolymphatic sac. The wall of the sac is thicker and whiter than dura. There are few air cells inferior to the labyrinth in sclerotic mastoids. One must protect the facial nerve when exposing the posterior fossa dura. Temporal bone CT scanning is necessary to identify which type the mastoid process is before operation

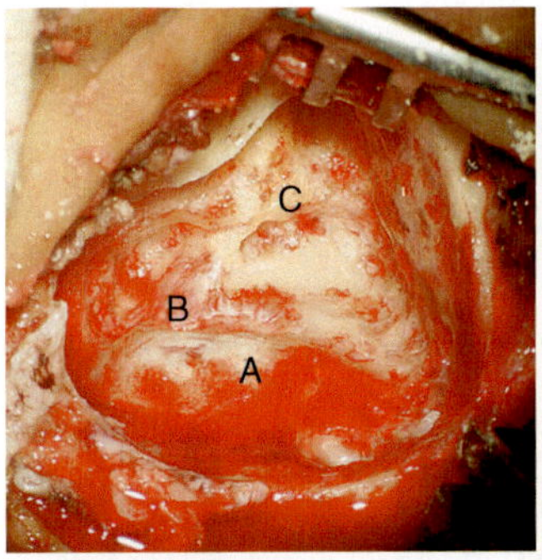

A. Sigmoid sinus
B. Endolymphatic sac
C. Posterior semicircular canal

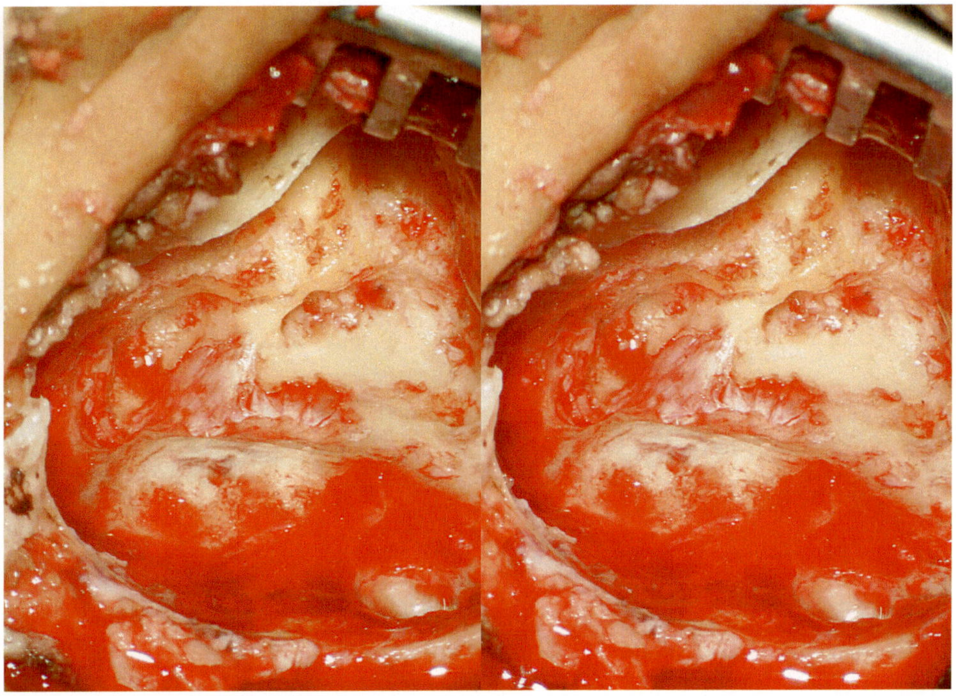

Fig. 4.41 Exposure of endolymphatic sac
In this, patient it is easy to expose the sac because the sigmoid sinus is posterior. Temporal bone CT scanning is necessary to identify where the sigmoid sinus is located before operation

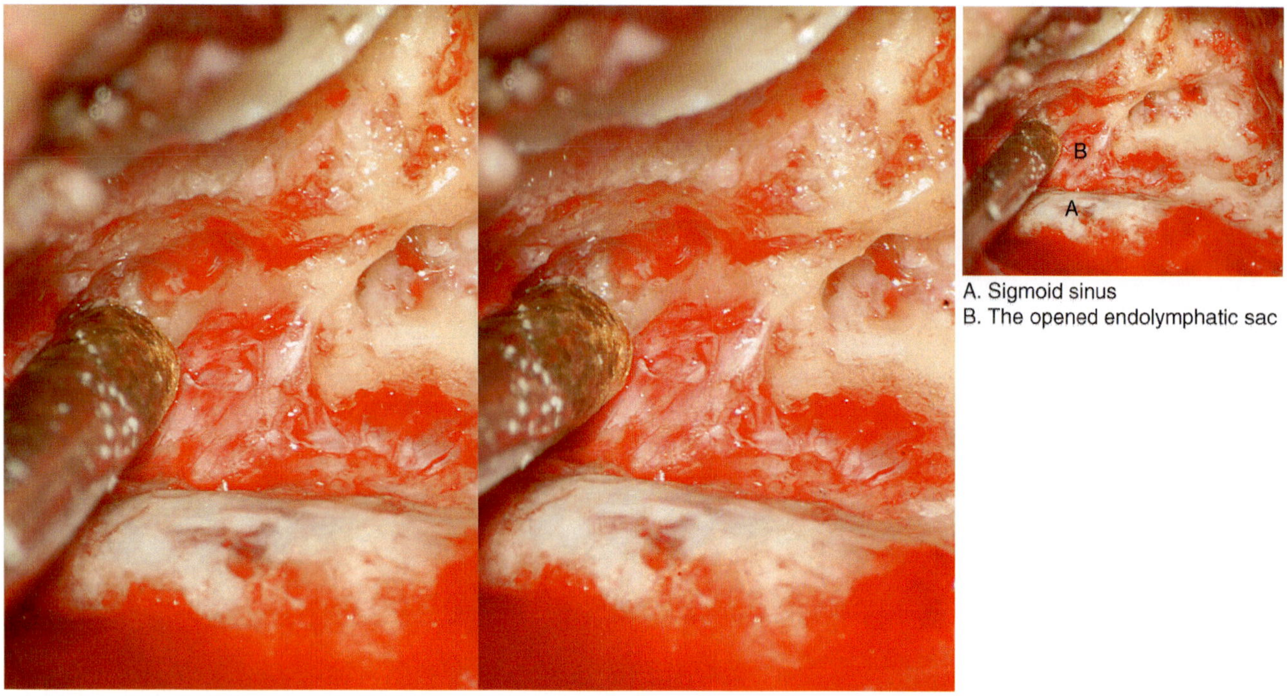

A. Sigmoid sinus
B. The opened endolymphatic sac

Fig. 4.42 Incising the endolymphatic sac
The cavity is thoroughly irrigated before incising the endolymphatic sac. Bone dust can enter the middle ear via the aditus ad antrum and accumulate in the oval window leading to fixation of the stapes or new bone formation

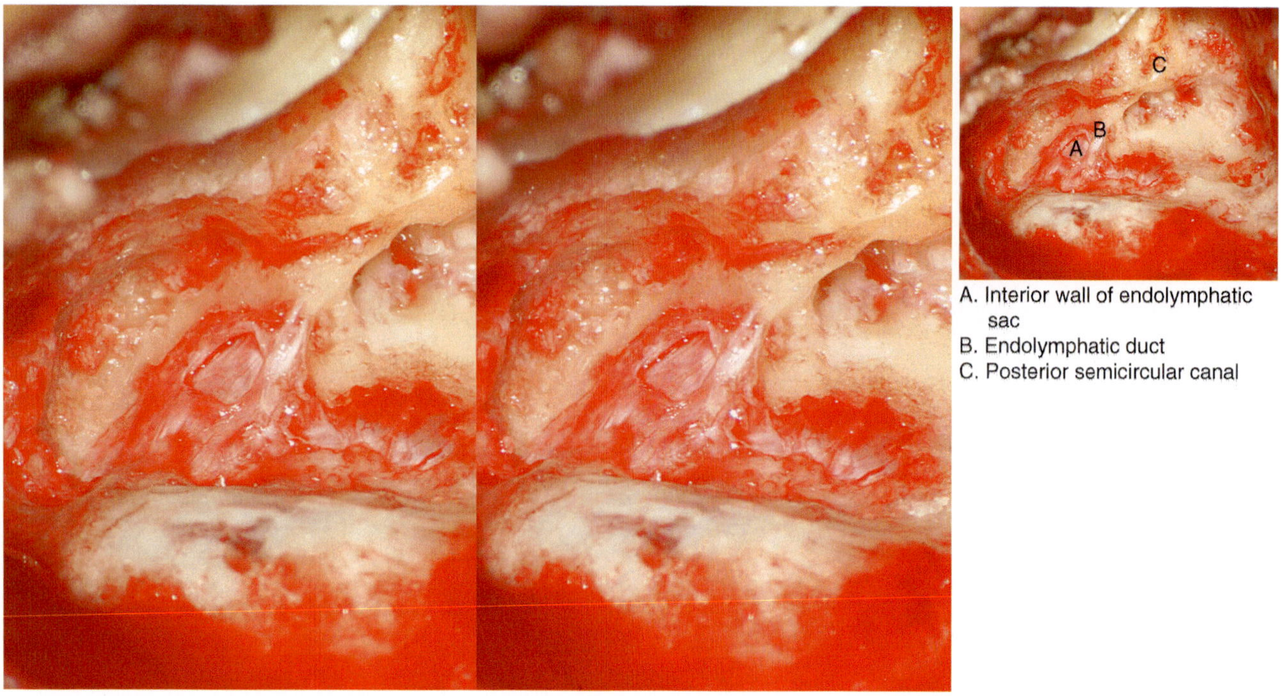

A. Interior wall of endolymphatic sac
B. Endolymphatic duct
C. Posterior semicircular canal

Fig. 4.43 Exposure of the lumen of the endolymphatic sac
Incise the endolymphatic sac, remove part of lateral wall of the sac and expose its lumen. Alternatively, one can turn the lateral surface of the sac over to get adequate drainage

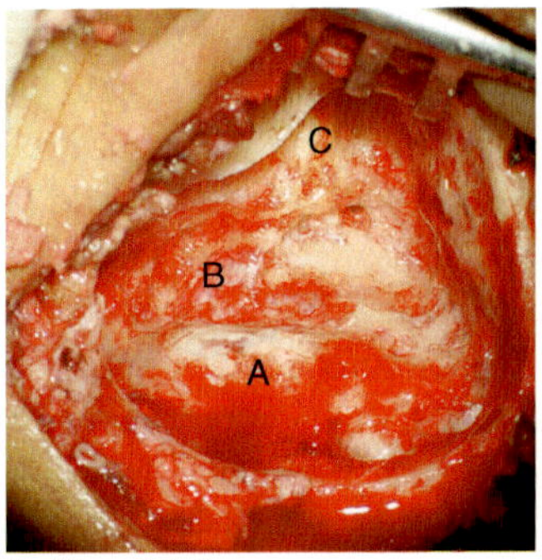

A. Sigmoid sinus
B. Endolymphatic sac removed part of laterior wall
C. Lateral semicircular canal

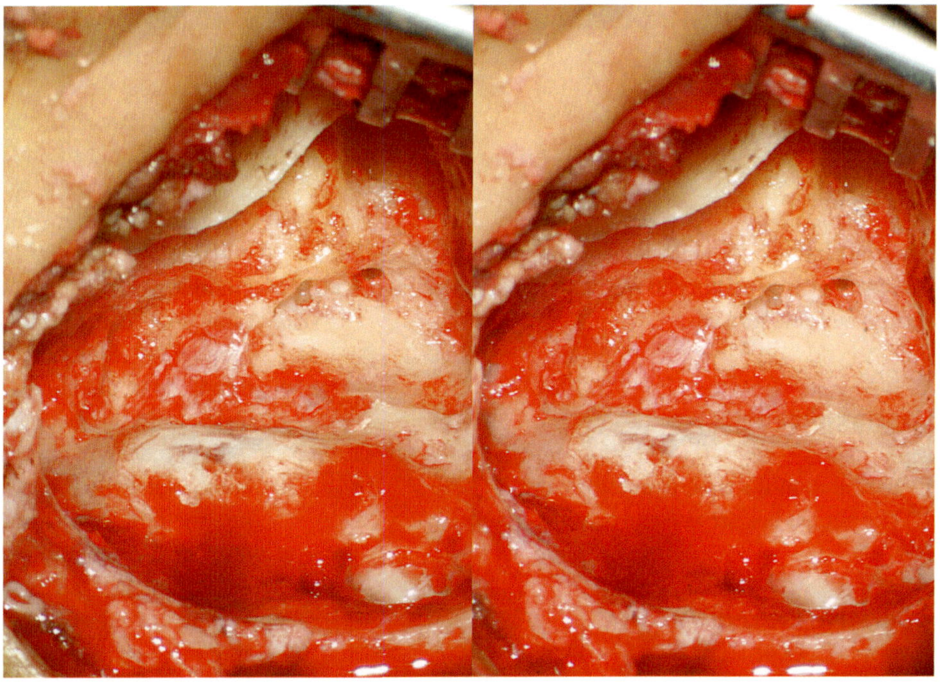

Fig. 4.44 Overview of cavity
The cavity is thoroughly irrigated, any bleeding is controlled to minimize bloody accumulating in the cavity. The wound is closed in layers

Transmastoid Labyrinthectomy

Wei-dong Shen and Pu Dai

Indication

Labyrinthectomy is indicated for unilateral Ménière's Disease that is refractory to medical management, and with non-serviceable hearing.

Contraindications

1. Patient unfit for general anesthesia.
2. The patient has serviceable hearing

Operative Procedures

1. Anesthesia and position: The patient is positioned supine and the operation is performed under general endotracheal anesthesia.
2. Skin Incision: A post-auricular skin incision is made approximately 1 cm behind the sulcus.
3. Mastoidectomy: A cortical mastoidectomy is performed with identification of the short process of the incus, the lateral semicircular canal and vertical portion of facial nerve.
4. Identify the lateral semicircular canal and the course of facial nerve. Dissect the air cells surrounding the labyrinth and the retro-facial cells. The bone of the three semicircular canals is drilled until the membranous labyrinth is identified, initially as a "blue line".
5. Dissection of the semicircular canals and vestibule neuroepithelium: Identify the lateral semicircular canal (LSC), and then the posterior semicircular canal (PSC) which lies posterior and inferior to it. Follow the posterior canal superiorly to the common crus and then the superior semicircular canal (SSC). Generally, the lateral canal lumen is opened first, followed by the posterior and then the superior semicircular canals.

   Follow the posterior canal anteriorly and inferiorly to find its ampulla which is located medial to mastoid portion of facial nerve. Carefully drill away the semicircular canals, but preserve the medial wall of superior and lateral canals, and the inferior wall of posterior canal. The labyrinthine portion of the facial nerve is located under the ampulla of superior semicircular canal. The jugular bulb may be just inferior to the ampulla of posterior semicircular canal. The posterior canal ampulla and the common crus lead to the vestibule. Removal of the bone joining the three ampullae exposes the vestibule. Once this is done the cupulae of each semicircular canal, the utricle, and the saccule can all be seen. The neuroepithelium of these five structures is removed with a right-angle hook and suction tip. Care should be taken to not perforate the thin bone of the lateral end of the internal auditory canal while removing the neuroepithelium. Note that the medial wall of vestibule is also the lateral wall of IAC.
6. Wound closure: Close the wound in layers after making sure there is no CSF leakage.

Special Comments

1. Intraoperative monitoring of facial nerve function is used to improve the safety of the operation and reduce complications.
2. All three semicircular canals must be exposed to allow a complete labyrinthectomy.
3. All neuroepithelium is removed under high magnification of the microscope.
4. The aditus ad antrum is sealed and the mastoid is obliterated with abdominal fat to prevent CSF leak if necessary.
5. In general, labyrinthectomy destroys more than 95 % of residual vestibular function

Complications

1. Facial nerve injury
2. Cerebrospinal fluid otorrhea
3. Meningitis
4. Incomplete labyrinthectomy

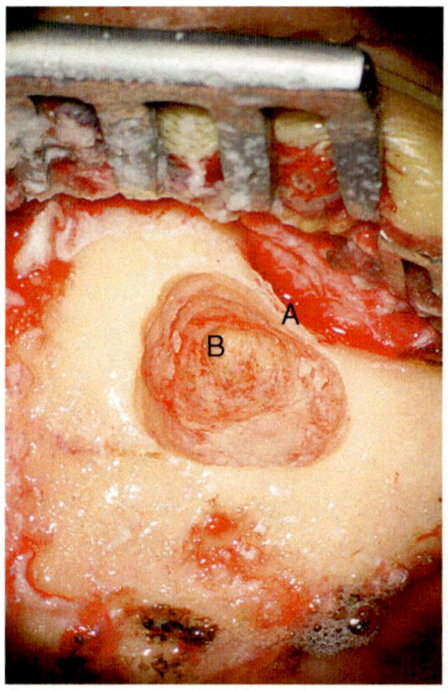

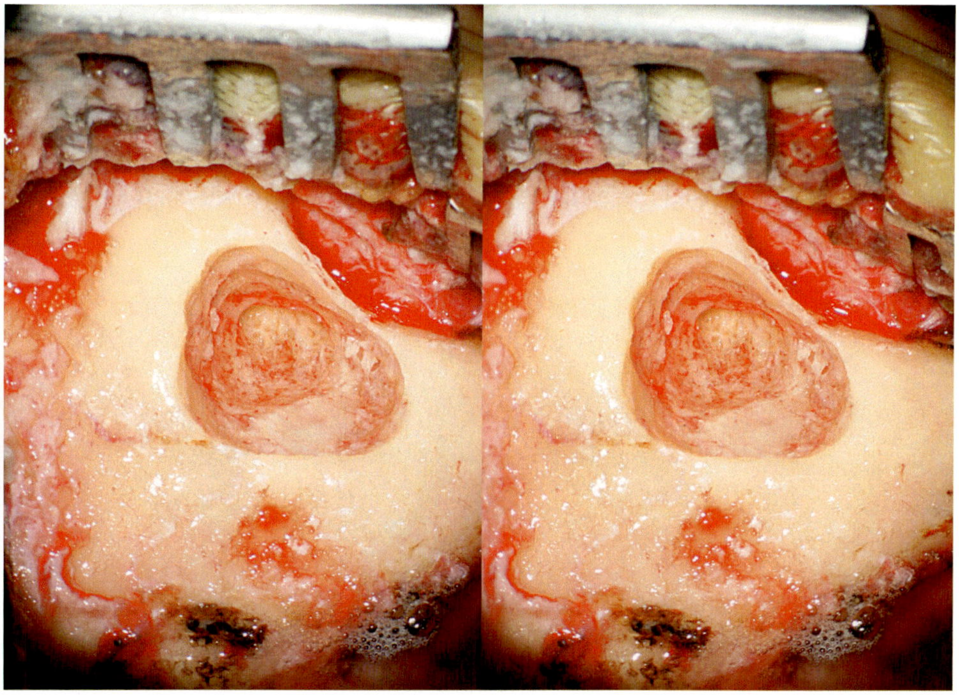

A. Posterior wall of external auditory canal
B. Aditus ad antrum

Fig. 4.45 Enter mastoid via the cribriform area
After the incision is made and the mastoid cortex is exposed, raise the meatal flap for only a short distance, identify the anatomical landmarks on the surface of mastoid. Drill the bone of cribriform area and enter the antrum

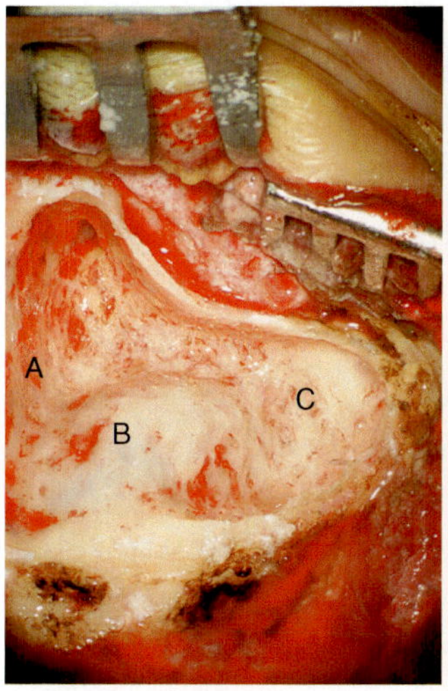

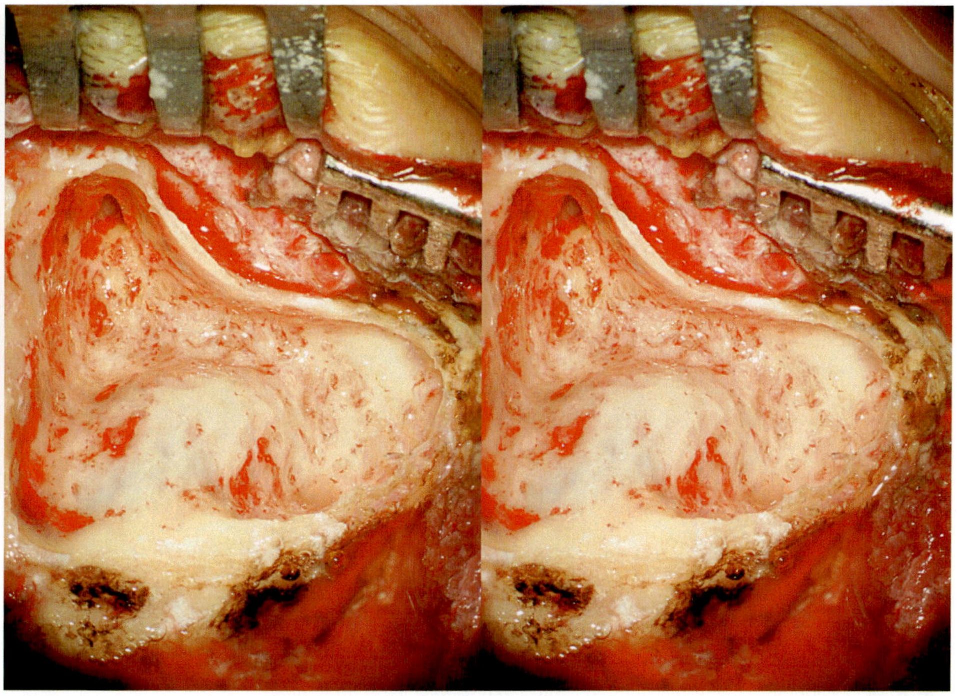

A. Tegmen of mastoid
B. Skeletonized sigmoid sinus
C. Digastric ridge

Fig. 4.46 Mastoidectomy
Perform a standard mastoidectomy removing air cells and delineate the tegmen, sigmoid sinus and digastric ridge, thinning out the posterior wall of the external auditory canal (EAC). Expose the attic, the short process of the incus, the fossa incudis and lateral semicircular canal as markers to locate the facial nerve

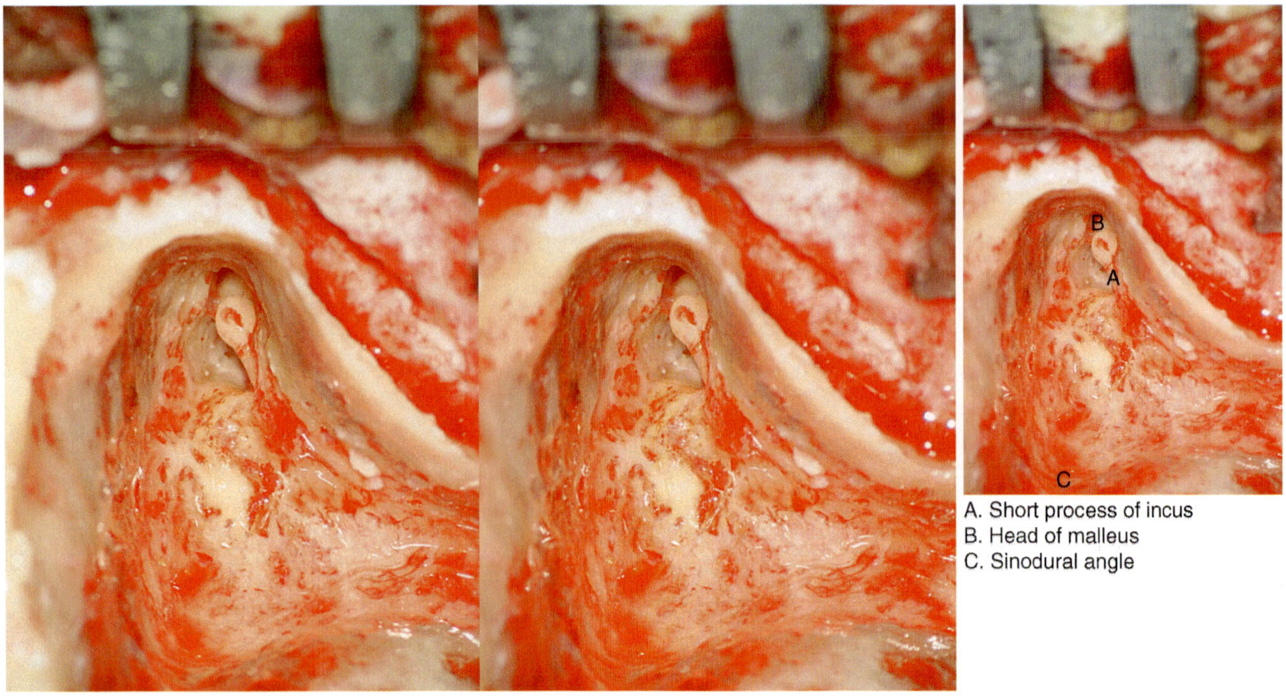

Fig. 4.47 Epitympanectomy
After removal of the lateral wall of attic, identify the short process and body of the incus, and the head of malleus in epitympanum. Expose the tegmen of the mastoid, the sinodural angle and the lateral semicircular canal

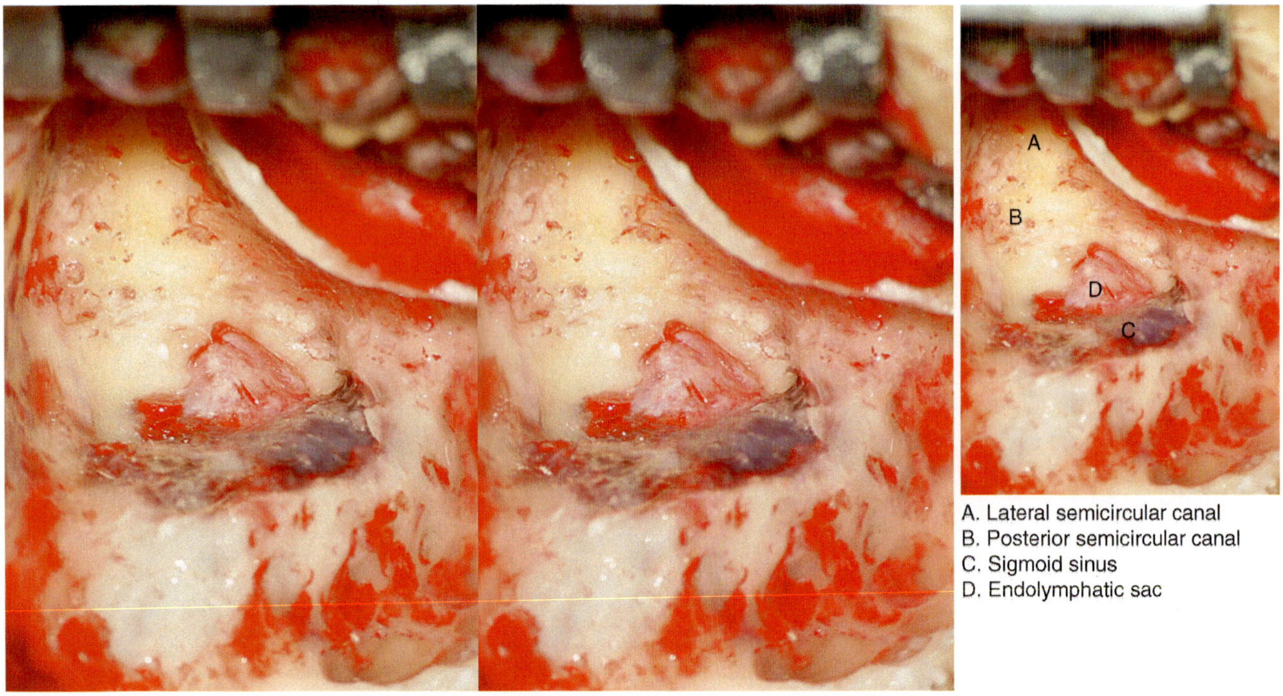

Fig. 4.48 Decompression of the sigmoid sinus and posterior fossa dural plate
After a wide mastoidectomy and atticotomy are performed, the lateral semicircular canal is used as a landmark. The peri-labyrinthine air cells are removed to expose the lateral and posterior semicircular canals with solid angle and the thin plate of bone over the dura of the posterior cranial fossa. The endolymphatic sac may be uncovered to aid with identification of the posterior semicircular canal

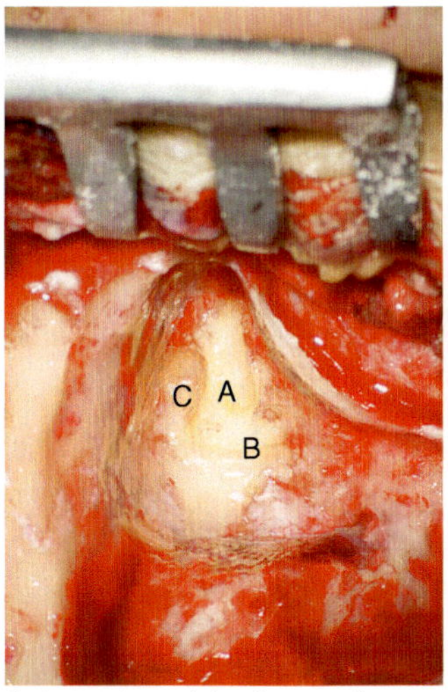

A. Lateral semicircular canal
B. Posterior semicircular canal
C. Superior semicircular canal

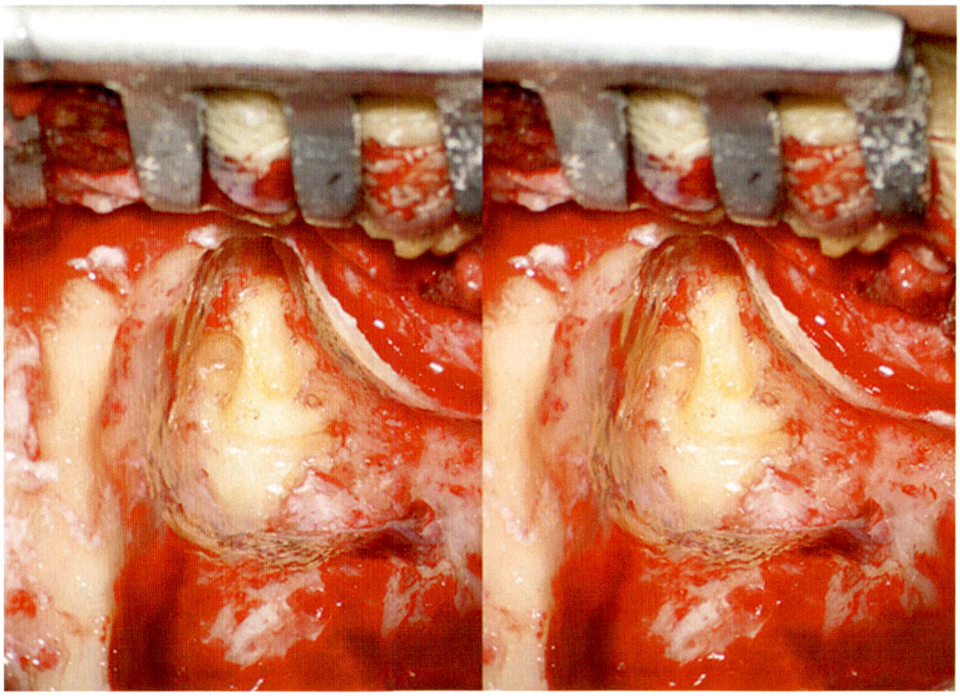

Fig. 4.49 Skeletonized semicircular canals
The three canals are identified after removal of the perilabyrinthine air cells, skeletonizing the lateral semicircular canal until the membranous labyrinth is identified through the bone as a thin "blue line"

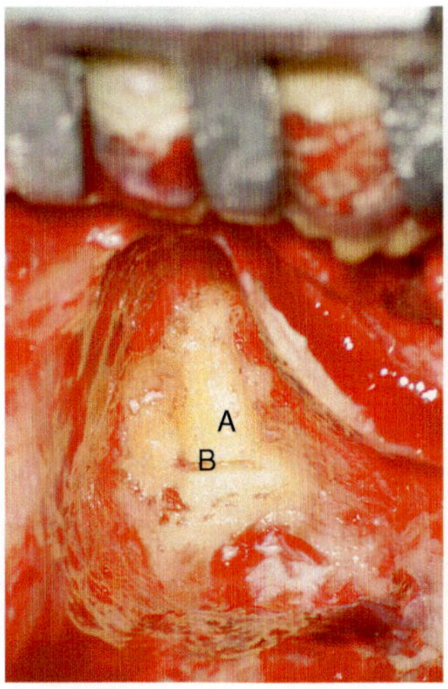

A. Lateral semicircular canal opened
B. Posterior semicircular canal opened

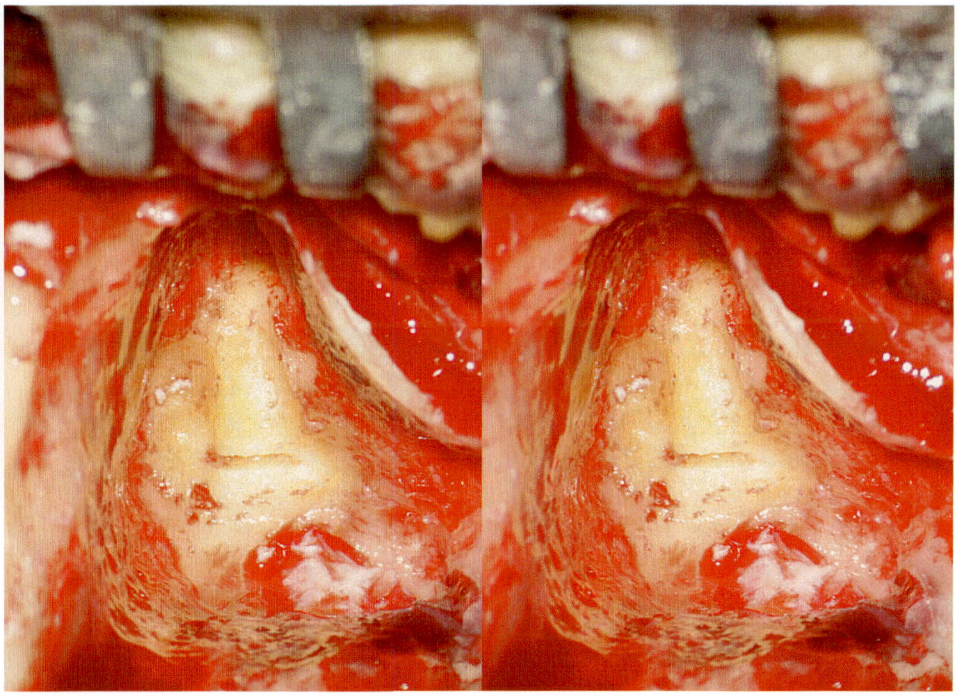

Fig. 4.50 Opening the semicircular canals
The lateral semicircular is delineated and opened first, followed by the posterior semicircular canal. After opening the osseous semicircular canal, the membranous labyrinth is identified within. The facial nerve is located just anterior and inferior to the LSC and PSC at this point. The bone covering the external genu of the facial nerve should be thinned but preserved when the anterior and inferior portion of the posterior canal is opened to the ampulla to avoid the possible damage to the nerve

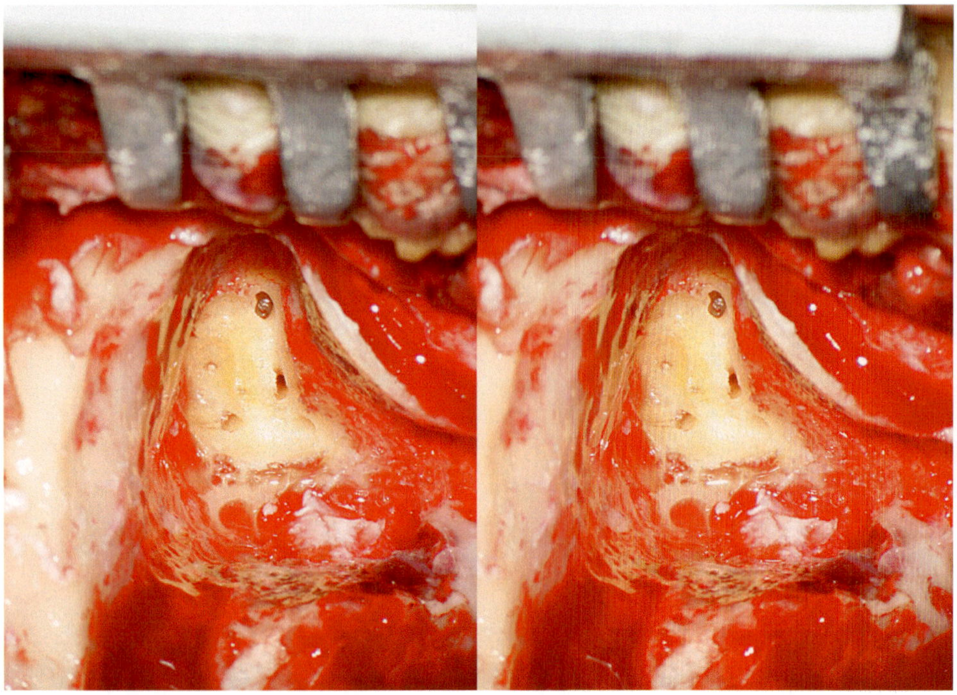

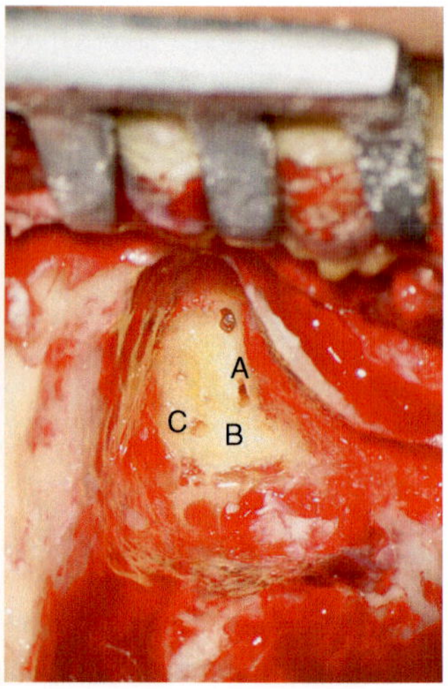

A. Lateral semicircular canal opened
B. Posterior semicircular canal opened
C. Superior semicircular canal opened

Fig. 4.51 Opening the semicircular canals
Follow the opened lateral canal, drill away the bone of labyrinth towards the ampulla and the non-ampullary end of the canal which connect to the vestibule. The non-ampullary ends of the superior and posterior semicircular ducts unite to form the common crus

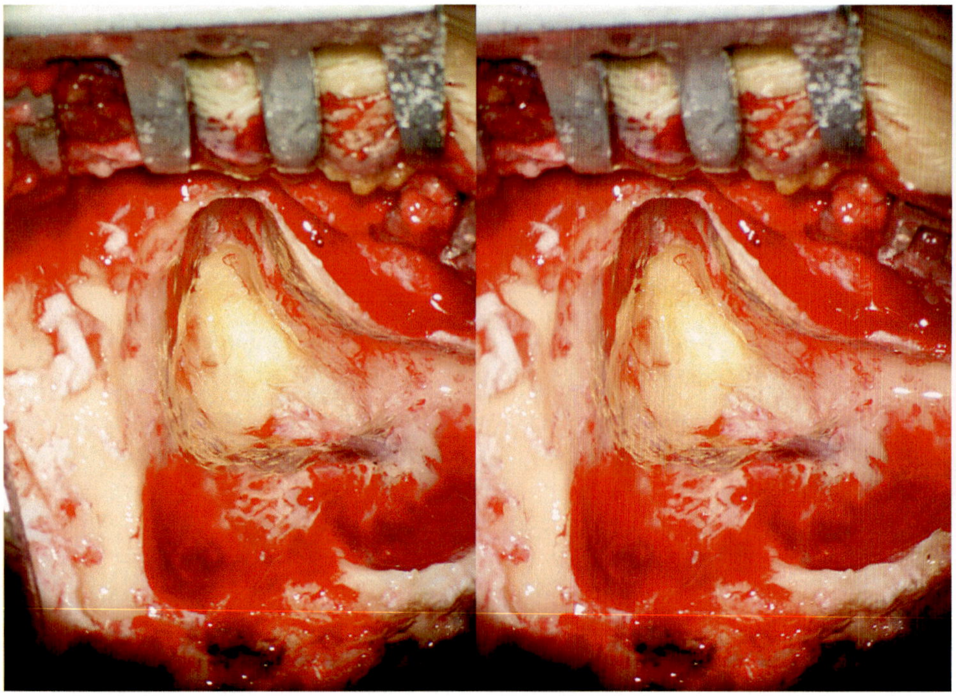

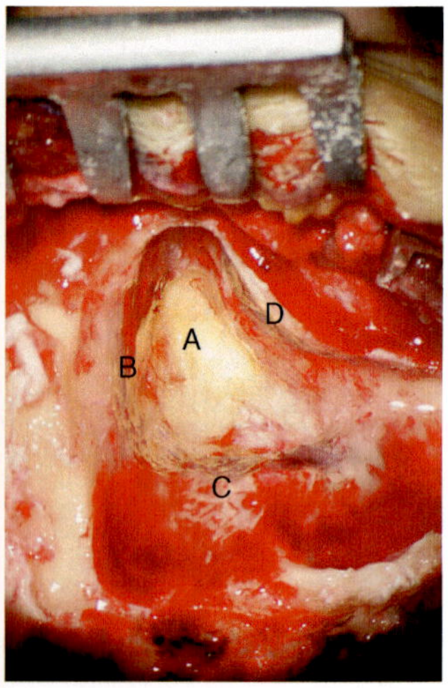

A. Vestibule opened
B. Tegmen of mastoid
C. Sigmoid sinus
D. Posterior wall of external ear canal

Fig. 4.52 Enlarging and opening the vestibule
Remove the bone over the vestibule by connecting the three ampullated ends. Once this is done, the ampullae of each semicircular canal, the utricle, and the saccule are all identified

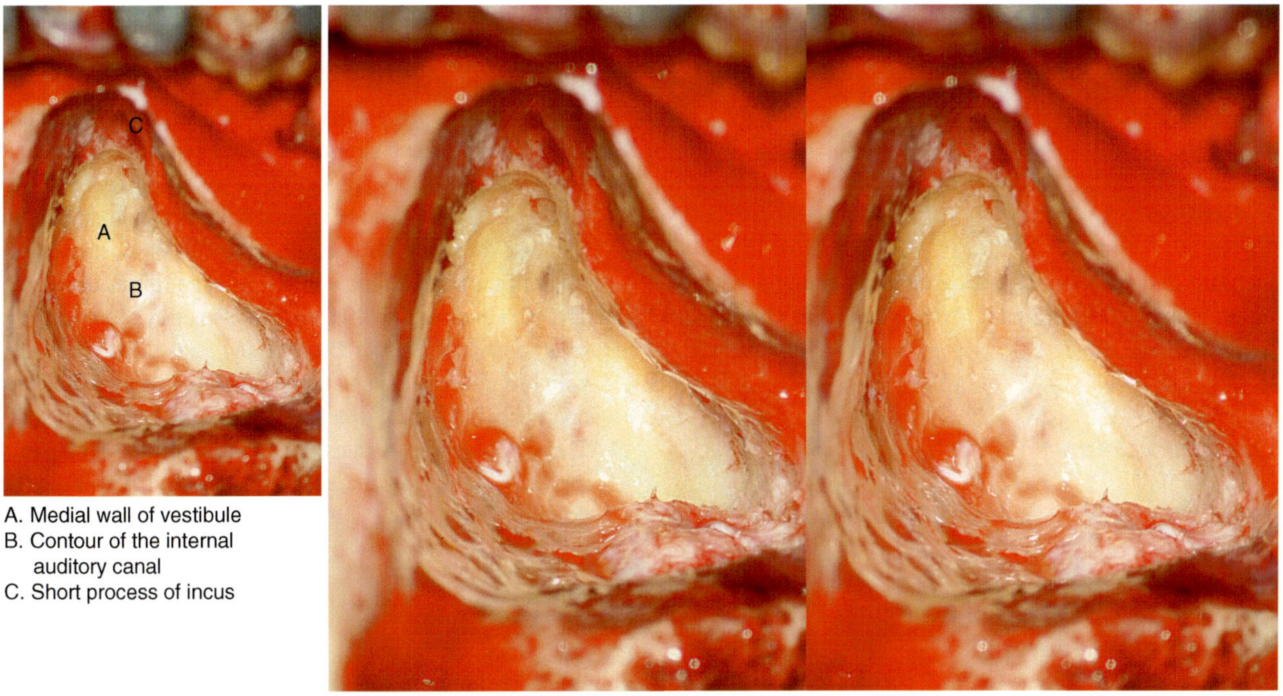

Fig. 4.53 Complete the labyrinthectomy
The neuroepithelium of the ampullae, the saccule and the utricule is all removed with a hook and suction tip. The medial wall of labyrinth is thinned and the outline of the internal auditory canal is seen

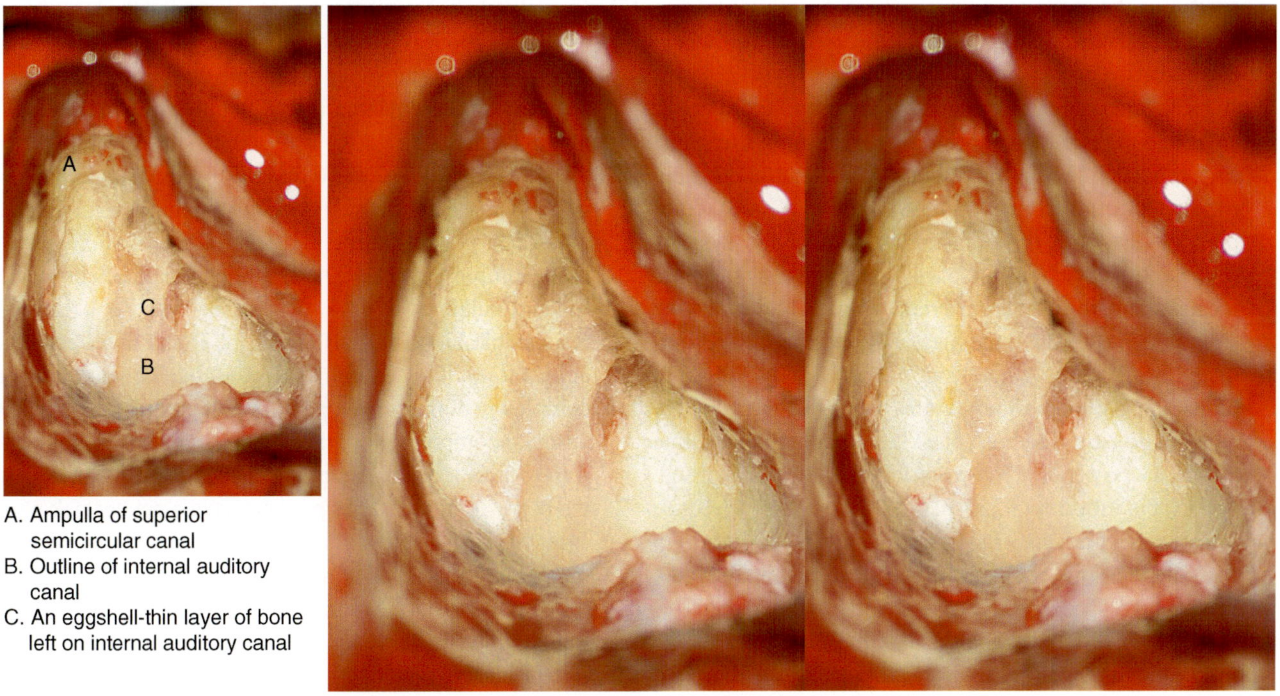

Fig. 4.54 Blue-lining of the internal auditory canal
Labyrinthectomy is used in refractory vertigo, but it is also the first step in the approach to the internal auditory canal. The medial wall of the vestibule is also the lateral wall of IAC. Care should be taken to not perforate the thin bone at the lateral end of the internal auditory canal while removing the neuroepithelium. The labyrinthine portion of the facial nerve is located just under the ampulla of the superior semicircular canal. Preserve the medial wall of the ampullated end of superior canal to prevent the injury to the facial nerve at the fundus of the internal auditory canal

Glossopharyngeal Neurotomy via Retrosigmoid Approach

Jian-dong Zhao and Pu Dai

Indication

Definite diagnosis of glossopharyngeal neuralgia with frequent attacks of severe pain not responsive to conservative treatment.

Contraindication

Patients with poor general condition and unable to tolerate surgery.

Operative Procedures

1. A "U"-shaped post-auricular incision is made with the flap based in the sulcus. It extends for 4 cm posteriorly and extends from the top of the pinna above to the mastoid process below.

   The scalp, subcutaneous tissue and periosteum are elevated forward and held in place, exposing the whole mastoid.
2. A 3 × 3.5 cm craniotomy is made posterior to the sigmoid sinus and inferior to the transverse sinus, using a trephine and rongeur. The surface anatomical landmarks help localize the underlying transverse-sigmoid sinus complex. A line from the inion to the root of the zygoma (essentially an extension of the superior nuchal line) locates the level of the transverse sinus. The axis of the sigmoid sinus through the mastoid bone can be approximated by dropping a line from the junction of the squamous and parietomastoid sutures through the tip of the mastoid process. The bone plate is stored in normal saline during the procedure. The posterior fossa dura is exposed.
3. After rapid infusion of 250 ml of 20 % mannitol to reduce intracranial pressure, the dura mater is incised in a "V"-shape behind the sigmoid sinus and below the transverse sinus. The flap is based anteriorly and reflected forwards and fixed in place with a suture.
4. Cottonoids and gelatin sponge are placed over the cerebellum and it is then retracted posteriorly with a brain spatula. Arachnoid is divided to allow outflow of cerebrospinal fluid, and the cerebellopontine angle is exposed.
5. The trigeminal nerve is seen superiorly, the lower cranial nerves are seen below with the VIIth and VIIth cranial nerve in the middle. The cerebellopontine angle is explored to identify and manage the relevant pathology which may include dealing with a space-occupying lesion, vascular compression or arachnoid adhesions.
6. The glossopharyngeal nerve is composed of a number of rootlets. The upper 1–2 rootlets of the vagus are sectioned as well. A 2 mm segment of the glossopharyngeal nerves is removed. In order to prevent nerve regeneration, the distal stump of the nerve can be treated with bipolar coagulation.
7. Remove the cottonoids and ensure full hemostasis; irrigate with normal saline in order to expel intracranial gas.
8. The dura is closed with a continuous suture incorporating small pieces of muscle to cover any gaps. This is covered with bioprotein glue and the bone plate is reinserted. Any open mastoid air cells can be sealed with bone wax.
9. The subcutaneous tissues and skin are closed with interrupted sutures, and the wound is covered with a sterile dressing.

Special Comments

1. When opening the dura mater, care should be taken to not damage the sigmoid and transverse sinuses and avoid consequent bleeding. Gelatin sponge can be used to cover any injured area for hemostasis, and bipolar coagulation may be used to seal small defects.
2. Care should be taken when working around the lower cranial nerve rootlets, whether dealing with tumors, vascular compression or thickened arachnoid adhesions. The latter two may be present even with a negative preoperative CT or MRI scan.
3. At the present time, the otoneurosurgical treatments for glossopharyngeal neuralgia mainly include retrosigmoid glossopharyngeal neurotomy (GN) or neural microvascular decompression (MVD). The selection of GN or MVD has not achieved a uniform standard yet. As causative responsible blood vessels cannot be found in all patients at operation, it is generally believed that the latter cannot completely eliminate the pain. In patients with significant vascular compression of the vagus nerve, and particularly if they have a contralateral vocal cord paralysis, MVD is the better option. Elderly patients have a greater risk with surgical release and padding due to factors such as angiosclerosis, and GN is a more sensible choice. We have found fewer complications when reviewing our GN experience, so we generally prefer to use this technique.
4. In considering whether to divide the upper rootlets of the vagus nerve at the same time, it is believed that there is communication between the vagus and glossopharyngeal nerves, so 1or 2 rootlets of vagus should be severed as well. In theory one might expect temporary or persistent dysphagia and vocal cord paralysis to occur in 10–20 % of cases when dividing part of the vagus. In practice, this is seen much less often.

Complications

1. Aseptic or purulent meningitis.
2. Cerebrospinal fluid leakage.
3. Lower cranial nerve dysfunction in about 10–20 %, such as: numbness and dry sensation in the posterior 1/3 of the tongue, difficulty swallowing, fluid aspiration, hoarseness, etc. Most are temporary but may persist although mostly at a mild level as compensation takes place.
4. The operation fails. Pain immediately disappears in the vast majority of patients after operation, but it has been reported to persist in nearly 10 % of the patients.
5. Recurrence or relapse in a small number of cases. The recurrence rate is about 0.5–1.5 %.
6. Death. Mortality is very low.

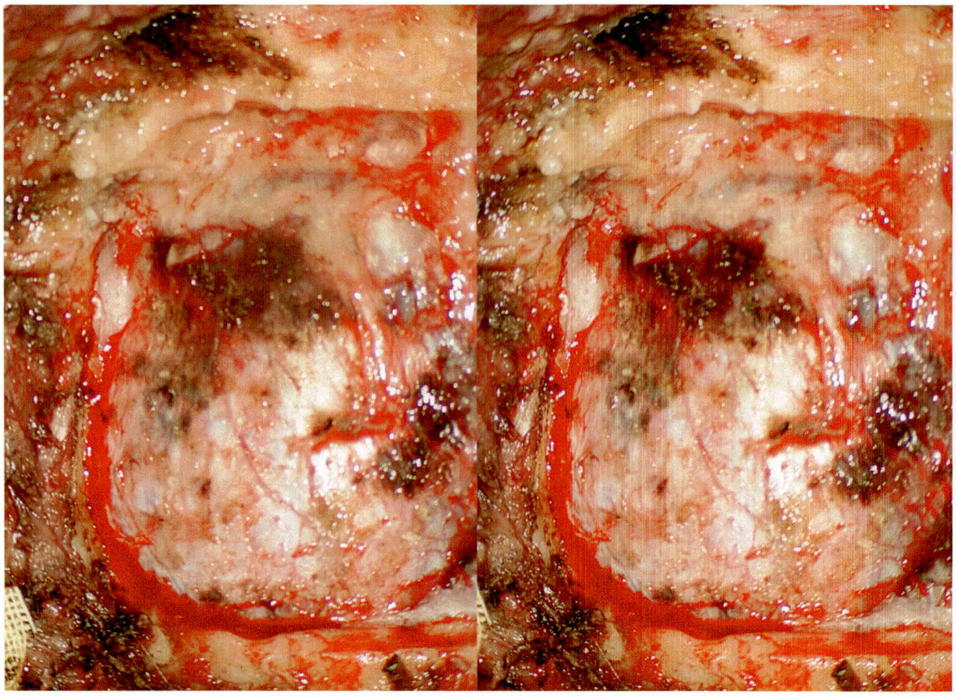

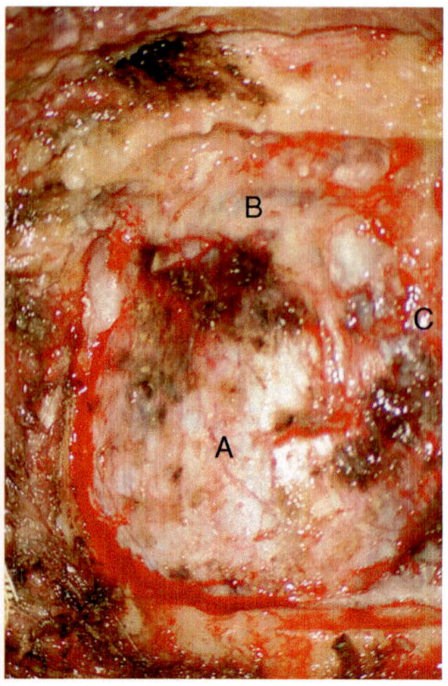

A. Posterior fossa dura
B. Sigmoid sinus
C. Transverse sinus

Fig. 4.55 Exposure of the posterior cranial fossa dura (*left*)
"U"-shaped post-auricular incision, extending 4 cm posteriorly from the sulcus to expose the mastoid. The scalp is elevated from the periosteum and reflected forward. The subcutaneous tissues and periosteum are then elevated to expose the skull from the parietal bone above to the mastoid tip below. A 3 × 3.5 cm craniotomy is made with its upper limit at the level of the temporal line. The posterior fossa dura is then exposed

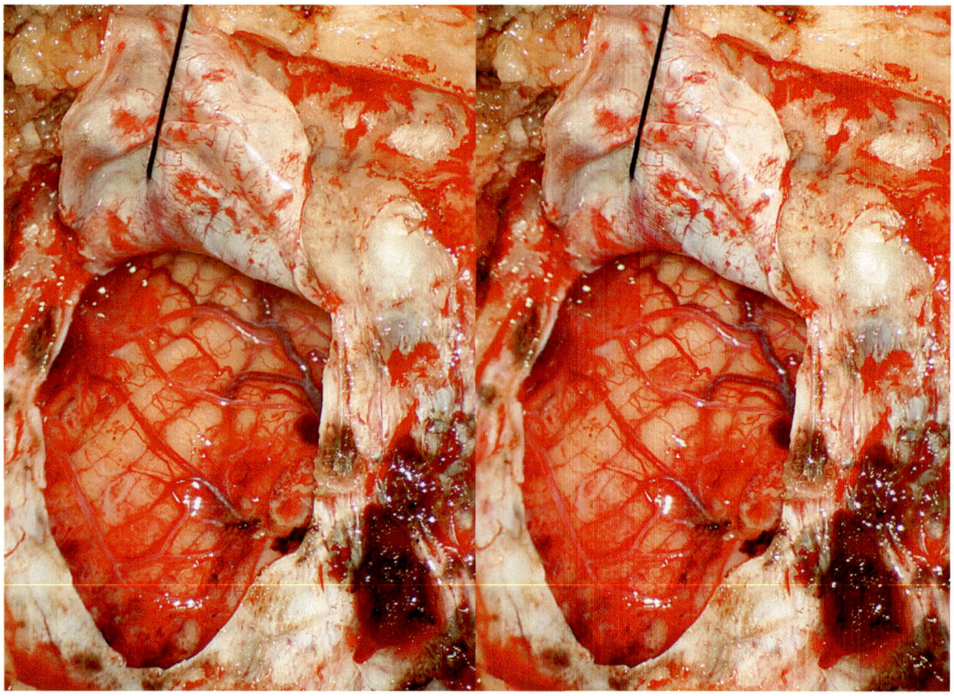

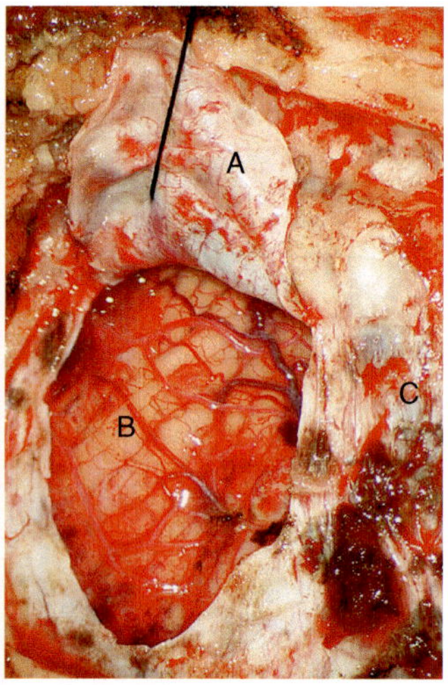

A. V-shaped flap of posterior fossa dura
B. Cerebellar surface
C. Transverse sinus

Fig. 4.56 Incision of posterior fossa dura
After rapid infusion of 250 ml of 20 % mannitol to reduce intracranial pressure, the dura is opened with V or U-shaped incision behind the sigmoid sinus and below the transverse sinus. The dural flap is reflected forwards and held in place with a suture to expose the cerebellar surface

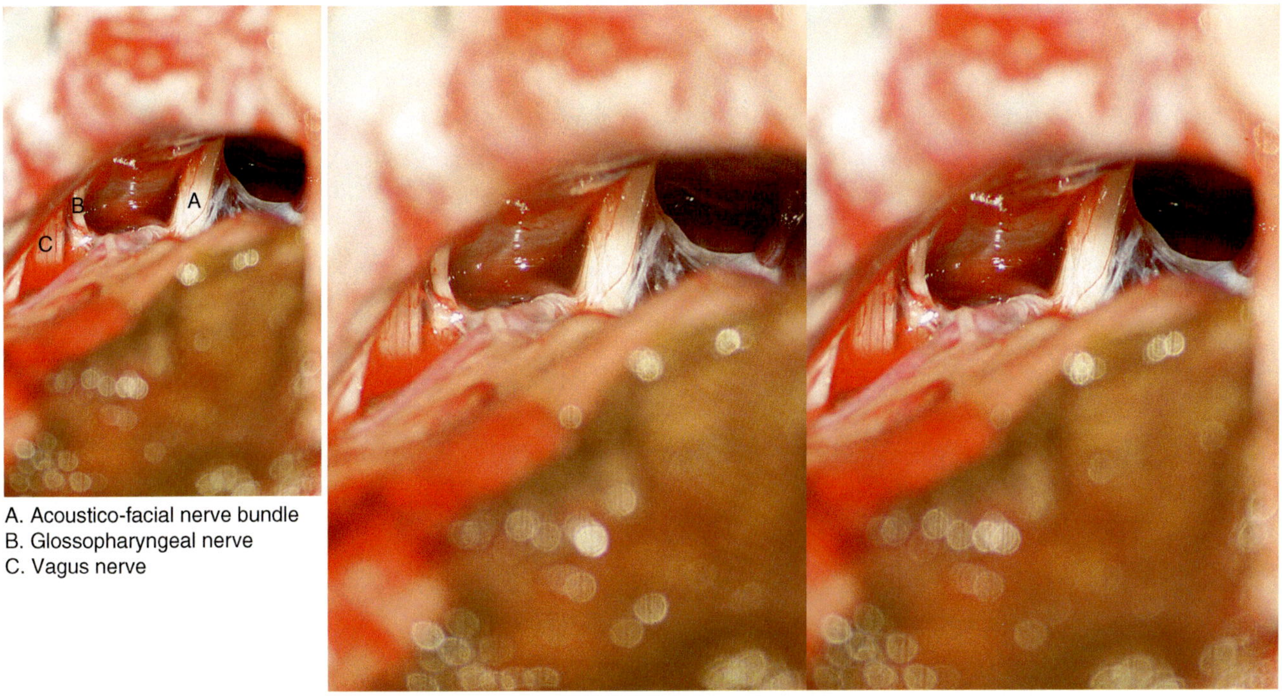

A. Acoustico-facial nerve bundle
B. Glossopharyngeal nerve
C. Vagus nerve

Fig. 4.57 Exposure of the cerebellopontine angle
Cottonoids are used to cover the cerebellum and the cerebellum is gently retracted using a brain spatula. Cerebrospinal fluid is removed to expose the nerves and blood vessels of the cerebellopontine angle. Identify the VII – XI cranial nerves under the microscope and carefully explore the area to assess whether or not there is a tumor, vascular compression, arachnoid adhesive disease or other pathology. Any such lesions when present should be treated at the same time. The acoustico-facial nerve bundle can be seen at the middle of the field of vision shown. The lower cranial nerves are seen inferiorly, with glossopharyngeal, vagus and accessory nerve from above down

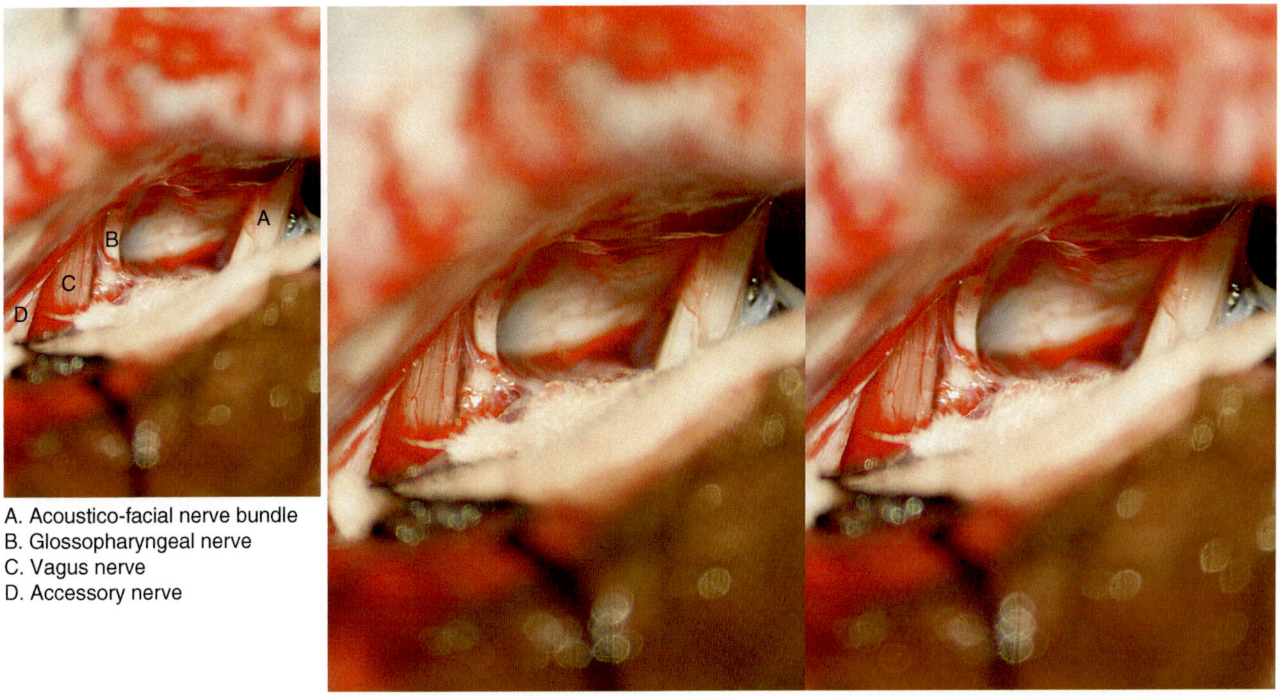

A. Acoustico-facial nerve bundle
B. Glossopharyngeal nerve
C. Vagus nerve
D. Accessory nerve

Fig. 4.58 Exposure of lower cranial nerves
The VII and VIII cranial nerves are located in the upper part of the cerebellopontine angle. The jugular foramen is more inferior, and contains the glossopharyngeal, vagus and accessory nerves from the front to the back. The figure shows a clear interval between the glossopharyngeal and vagus nerves

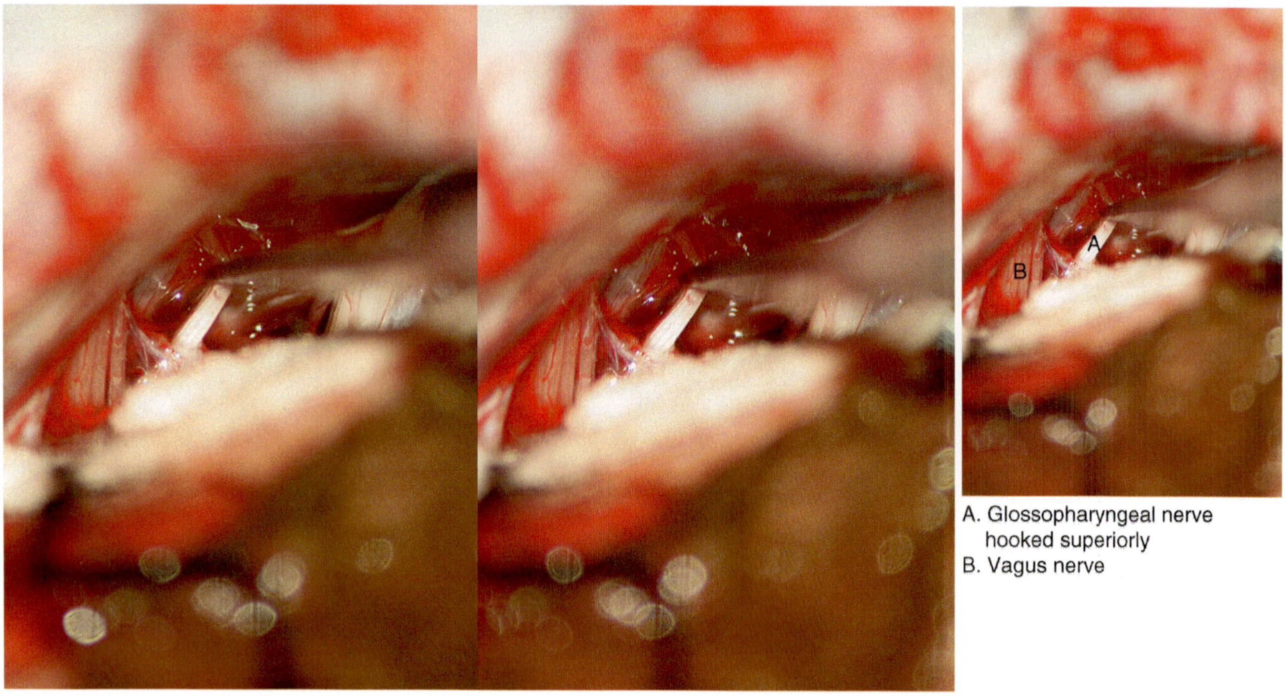

Fig. 4.59 Identification of glossopharyngeal nerve
The glossopharyngeal nerve is the upper of the lower group of cranial nerves, and composed of one or more nerve trunks, usually branching to 4–6 rootlets. It must be carefully identified during operation. The glossopharyngeal nerve in this case is composed of a single nerve bundle

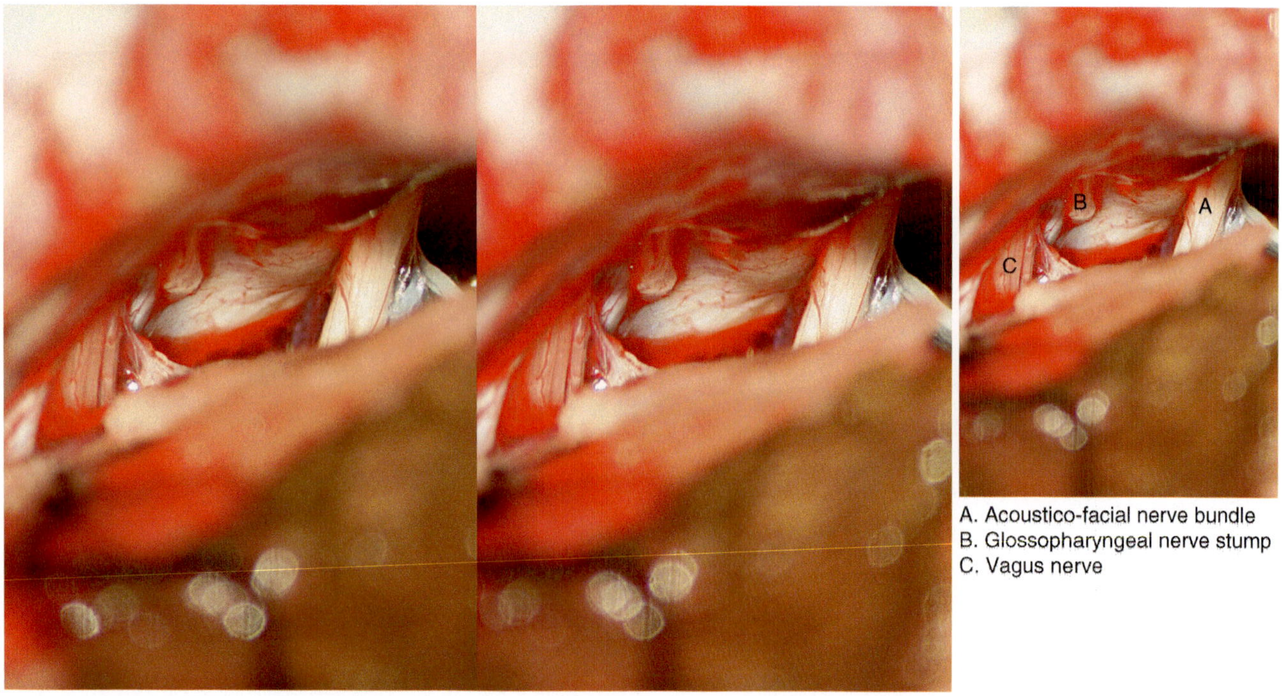

Fig. 4.60 Division of glossopharyngeal nerve
After correct identification of the glossopharyngeal nerve it is cut with microsurgical scissors. In order to prevent recurrence of symptoms due to nerve re-anastomosis, it is the best to resect a segment of the nerve. Some authors cauterize distal nerve with bipolar electro-coagulation for the same purpose

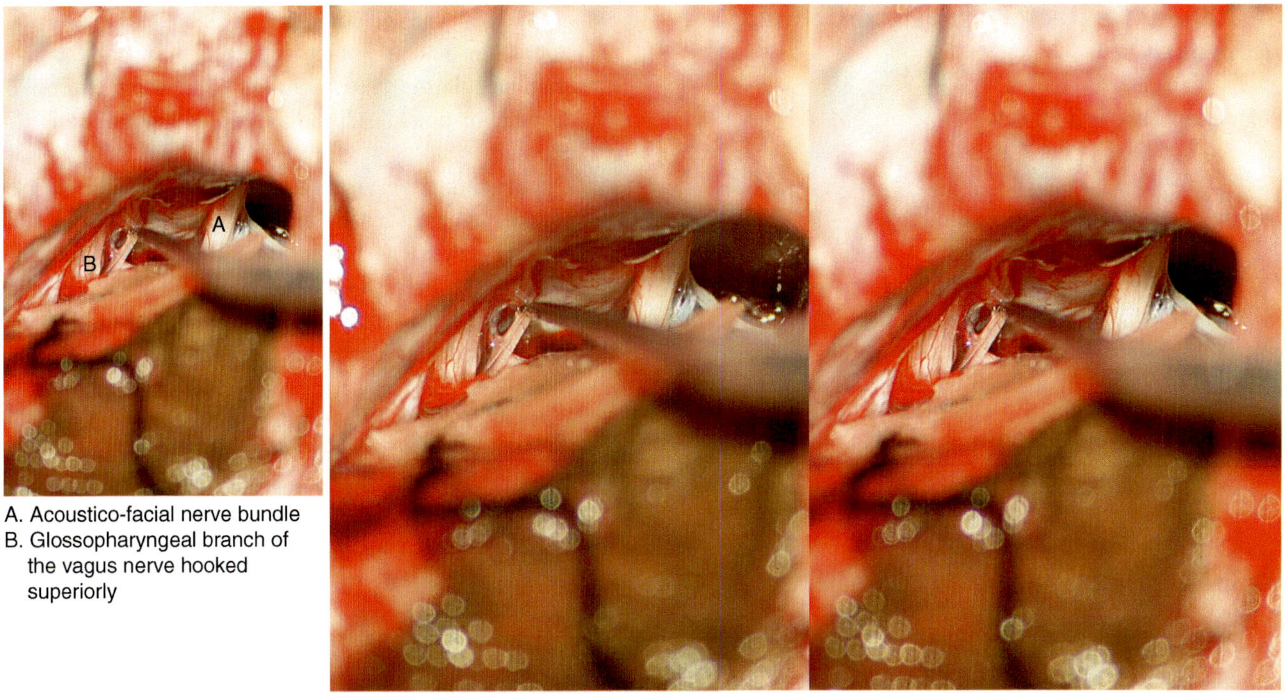

A. Acoustico-facial nerve bundle
B. Glossopharyngeal branch of the vagus nerve hooked superiorly

Fig. 4.61 Identification of the upper fibers of the vagus nerve
Identify the upper vagal nerve fibers (vagal glossopharyngeal branch) carefully and then section it. Clinically, it cannot be determined how much of the vagus nerve fibers to cut off. Only a small component should be sectioned

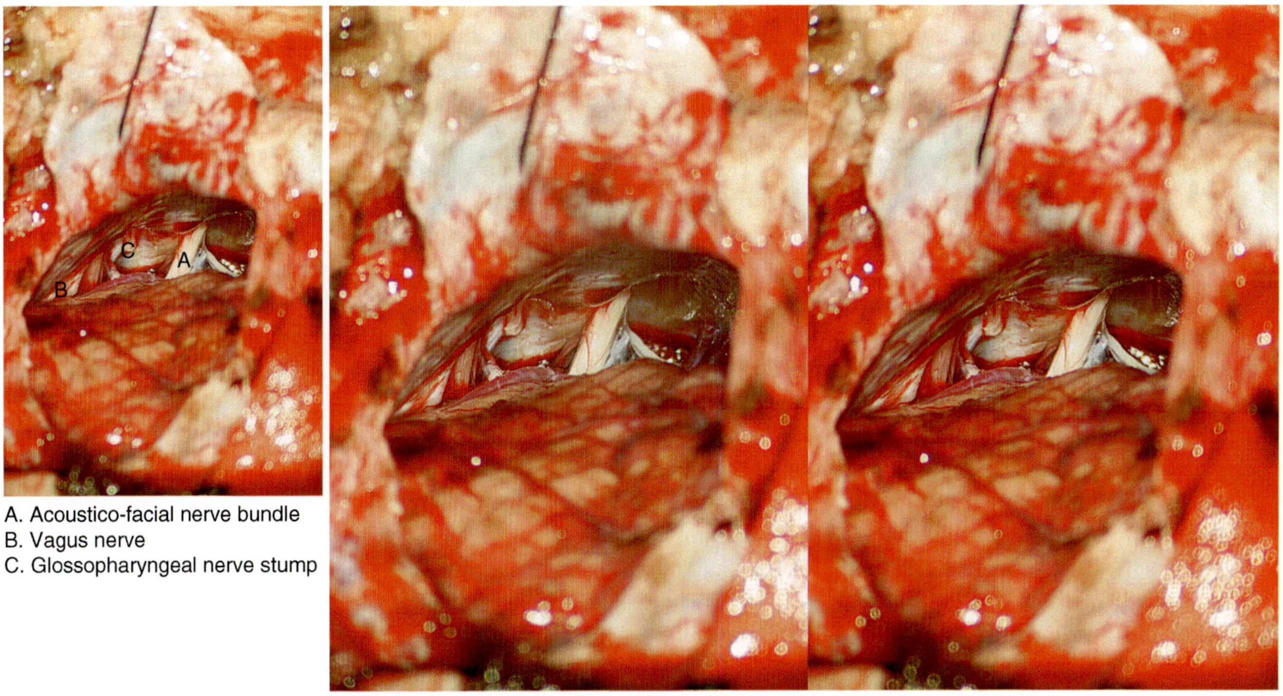

A. Acoustico-facial nerve bundle
B. Vagus nerve
C. Glossopharyngeal nerve stump

Fig. 4.62 Section the upper fibers of vagus nerve
Cut a certain way into the glossopharyngeal branch of the vagus nerve with micro-scissors. Irrigate the cavity, carefully ensure hemostasis and close the dura with a continuous nylon suture. Reinsert the bone flap, suture the muscle, subcutaneous tissue and skin layer by layer

Vestibular Neurectomy via Retrosigmoid Approach

Jian-dong Zhao and Pu Dai

Indications

1. Refractory, progressive vestibular vertigo or Meniere's disease with severe vertigo and failed, conservative medical treatment;
2. Recurrence of vertigo after endolymphatic sac decompression
3. Desire to preserve the hearing in the affected ear such as in patients not accepting effects of chemical labyrinthectomy

Contraindication

Patients with poor general condition unable to tolerate surgery.

Operative Procedures

1. A "U"-shaped post-auricular incision is made with the flap based in the sulcus. It extends for 4 cm posteriorly and extends from the top of the pinna above to the mastoid process below.

   The scalp, subcutaneous tissue and periosteum are elevated forward and held in place, exposing the whole mastoid.
2. A 3 × 3.5 cm craniotomy is made posterior to the sigmoid sinus and inferior to the transverse sinus, using a trephine and rongeur. The surface anatomical landmarks help localize the underlying transverse-sigmoid sinus complex. A line from the inion to the root of the zygoma (essentially an extension of the superior nuchal line) locates the level of the transverse sinus. The axis of the sigmoid sinus through the mastoid bone can be approximated by dropping a line from the junction of the squamous and parietomastoid sutures through the tip of the mastoid process. The bone plate is stored in normal saline during the procedure. The posterior fossa dura is exposed.
3. After rapid infusion of 250 ml of 20 % mannitol to reduce intracranial pressure, the dura mater is incised in a "V"-shape behind the sigmoid sinus and below the transverse sinus. The flap is based anteriorly and reflected forwards and fixed in place with a suture.
4. Cottonoids and gelatin sponge are placed over the cerebellum and it is then retracted posteriorly with a brain spatula. Arachnoid is divided to allow outflow of the cerebrospinal fluid, and the cerebellopontine angle is exposed.
5. The trigeminal nerve is seen superiorly, the lower cranial nerves are seen below with the VIIth and VIIIth cranial nerves in the middle. The cerebellopontine angle is explored to identify and manage the relevant pathology which may include dealing with a space-occupying lesion, vascular compression or arachnoid adhesions.
6. Carefully identify the vestibular nerve in the cerebellopontine. The VII is clearly identified as separate from the VIIIth. The vestibular nerve is the upper gray part of the nerve, while the cochlear nerve is the lower whiter segment. We have noted an identifiable minor groove between the two VIIIth nerve components in the majority of cases, and some microscopic blood vessels along the line of fusion.
7. After confirmation, the vestibular nerve is isolated from the lower cochlear nerve using a needle to separate the two. The facial nerve is more anterior. Care is taken to not damage cochlear nerve fibers during the operation, and not unnecessarily manipulate the internal auditory artery to avoid injury and spasm. A 3 mm segment of the vestibular nerve is resected with a nerve hook and knife or microsurgical scissors.
8. Remove the cottonoids and ensure full hemostasis; irrigate with normal saline in order to expel intracranial gas.
9. The dura is closed with a continuous suture incorporating small pieces of muscle to cover any gaps. This is covered with bioprotein glue and the bone plate is reinserted. Any open mastoid air cells can be sealed with bone wax.
10. The subcutaneous tissues and skin are closed with interrupted sutures, and the wound is covered with a sterile dressing.

Special Comments

1. The special points of note for posterior cranial fossa surgery are the same as for glossopharyngeal neurectomy.
2. Other surgical treatment of intractable vertigo includes vestibular neurectomy via a translabyrinthine approach, but any residual hearing in the operated ear is sacrificed. Vestibular neurectomy via a retrosigmoid approach

allows preservation of hearing in the affected ear which is a particular advantage if there is significant sensorineural hearing loss on the contralateral side.

3. Vestibular neurectomy via either approach has a much better vertigo control rate than an endolymphatic sac decompression.
4. In order to ensure cutting the vestibular nerve completely, carefully identify the junction of the vestibular and cochlear nerves. The nerves are separated up to 0.5 mm from the line of fusion to preserve most on the cochlear nerve fibres.

Complications

1. Deafness or severe hearing loss. The vestibular and cochlear nerves need to be clearly identified in order to avoid cochlear nerve injury.
2. Facial paralysis. It is best to use facial nerve monitoring to clearly identify the nerve and avoid injury to it.
3. Cerebrospinal fluid leakage.
4. Meningitis. Its prevention requires strict adherence to the principles of asepsis and the use of antibiotics to prevent infection after operation.

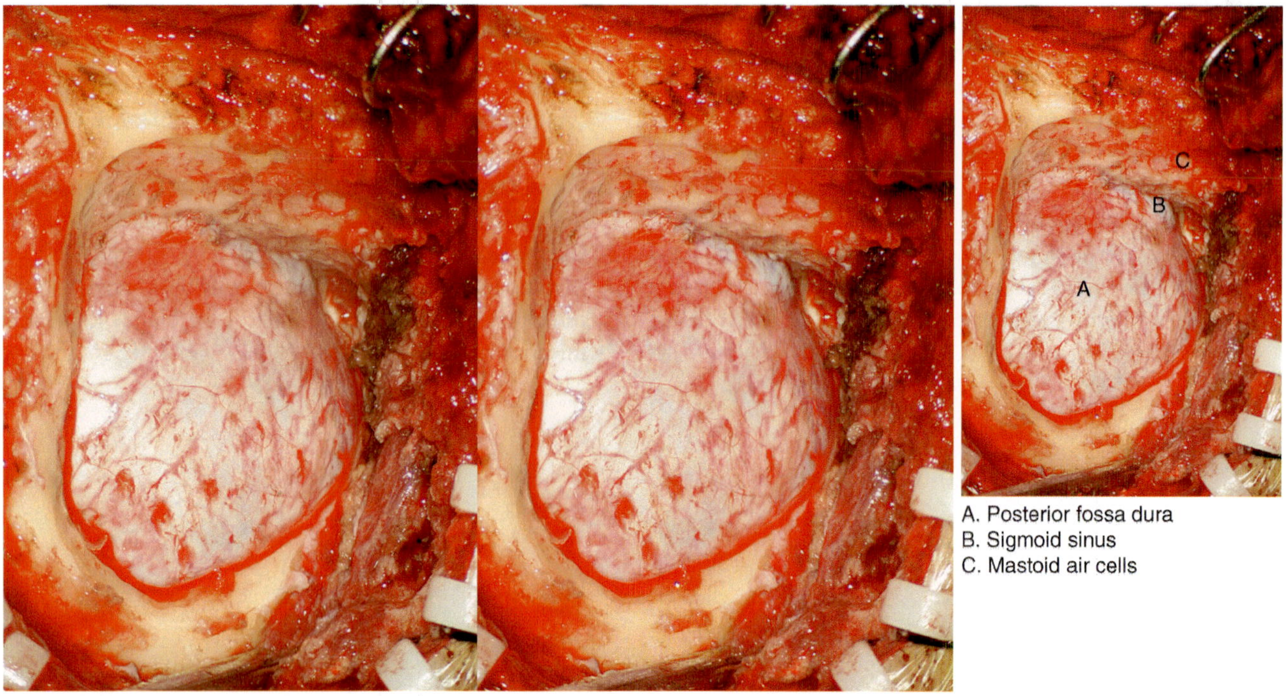

Fig. 4.63 Exposure of posterior cranial fossa dura (right)
(For the incision - see glossopharyngeal neurectomy) The posterior border of the sigmoid sinus should be exposed at the front of the field, and the transverse sinus superiorly

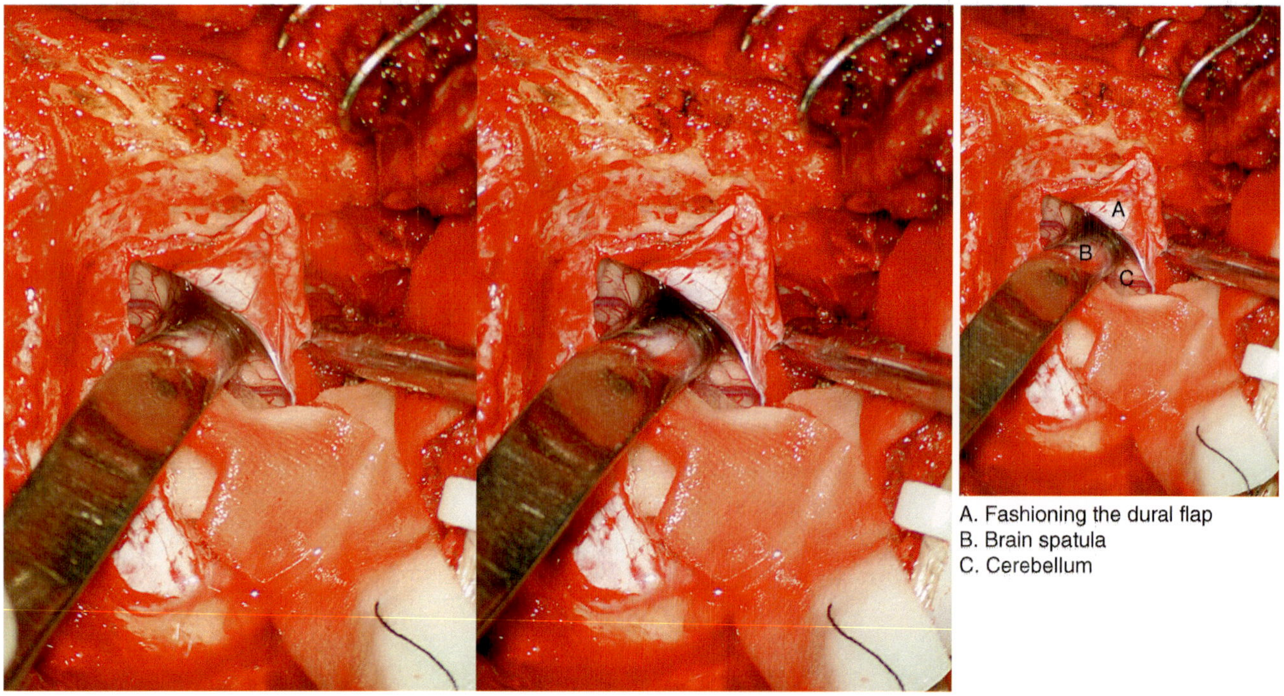

Fig. 4.64 Incision of posterior fossa dura, slight retraction of cerebellum
The dura is incised in a "V" shaped posterior to the sigmoid sinus and inferior to the transverse sinus. The dural flap is reflected forward and fixed with a silk thread to expose the cerebellum. The cerebellum is gently retracted with a brain spatula and cottonoids are placed over the cerebellum for protection

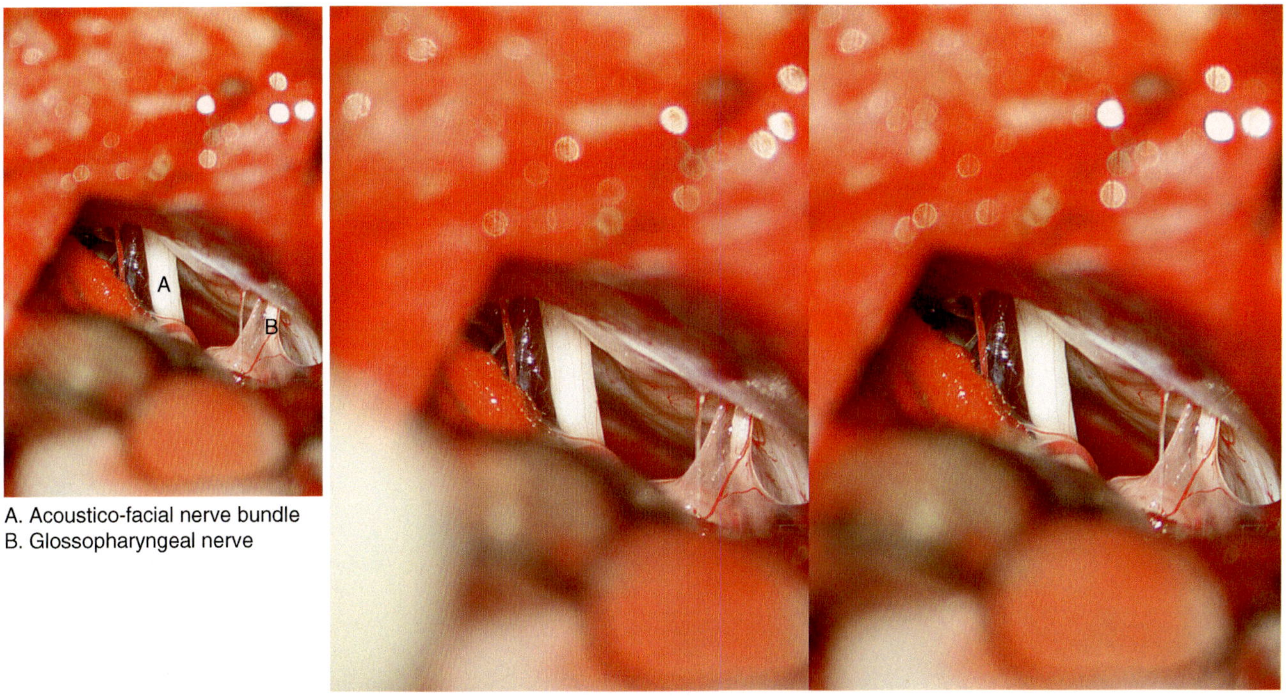

A. Acoustico-facial nerve bundle
B. Glossopharyngeal nerve

Fig. 4.65 Exposure of the cerebellopontine angle
After aspiration of cerebrospinal fluid, the nerves and blood vessels of the cerebellopontine angle are exposed. Carefully identify the VIIth and VIIIth cranial nerves under the microscope. The glossopharyngeal nerve can be seen below

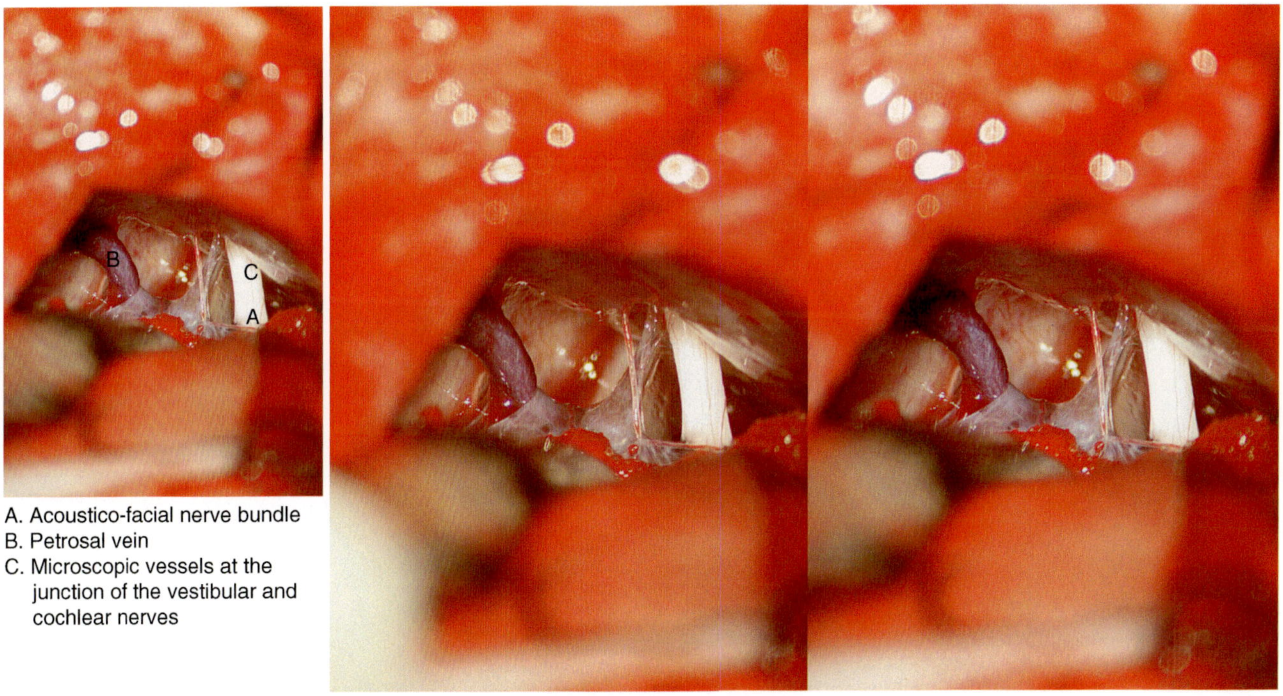

A. Acoustico-facial nerve bundle
B. Petrosal vein
C. Microscopic vessels at the junction of the vestibular and cochlear nerves

Fig. 4.66 Exposure the nerve bundle in the internal acoustic meatus
The figure shows that the vestibular nerve as the upper part of the VIIIth nerve with a small blood vessel marking its junction with the lower cochlear nerve. The petrosal vein can be seen more superiorly. Care is taken to not damage it

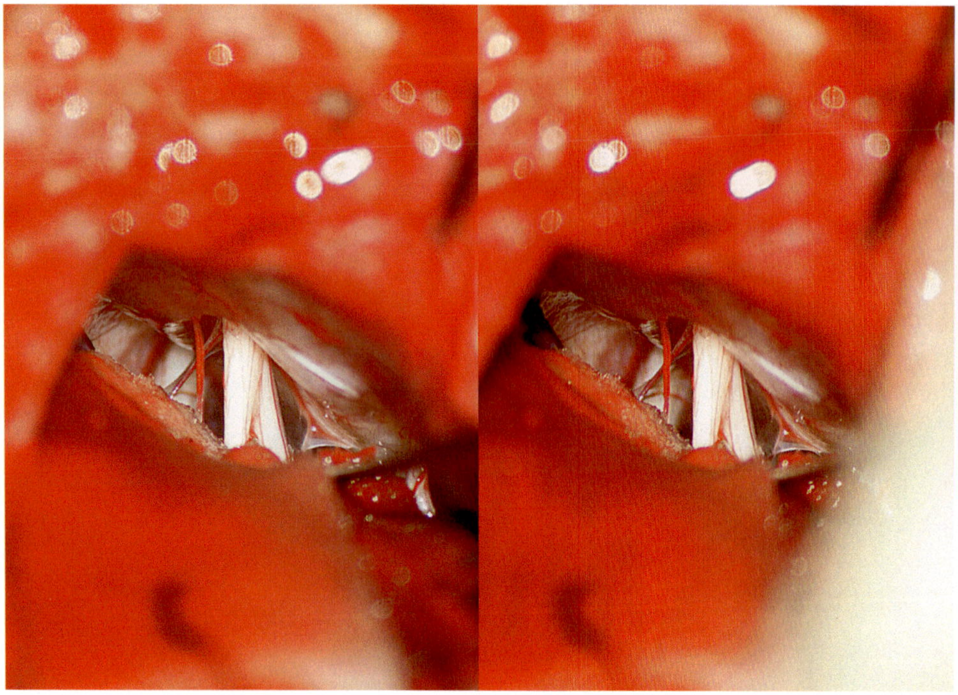

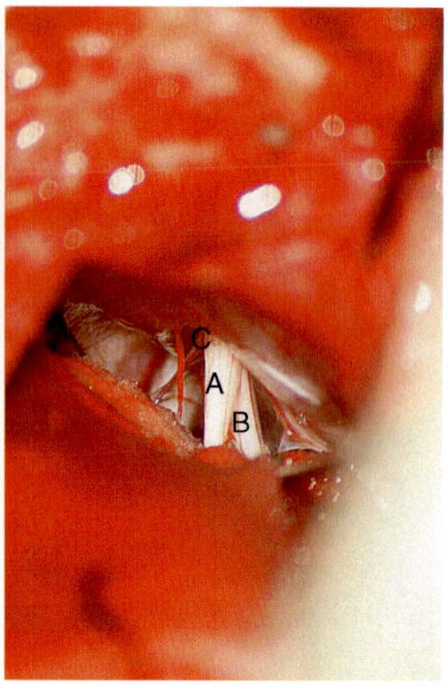

A. Vestibulocochlear nerve bundle
B. Facial nerve
C. Porus of the internal acoustic meatus

Fig. 4.67 Exposure of the facial nerve
Using gentle upward retraction of the Vestibulocochlear nerve, the facial nerve can be seen more anteriorly. A leash of small blood vessels is seen around the facial nerve at the porus of the internal acoustic meatus. This is likely to be the internal auditory artery

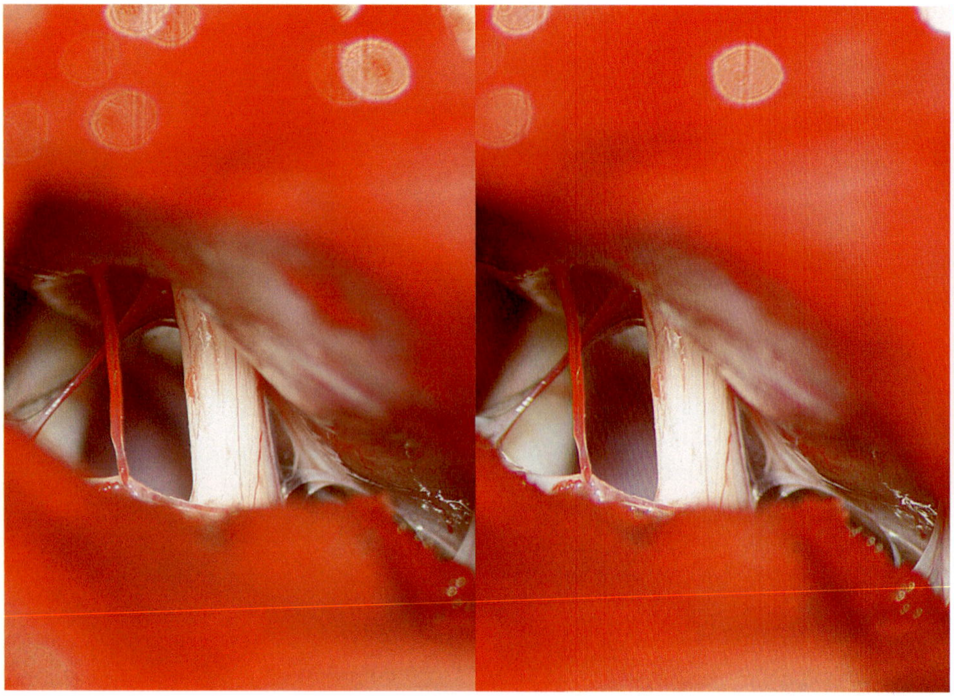

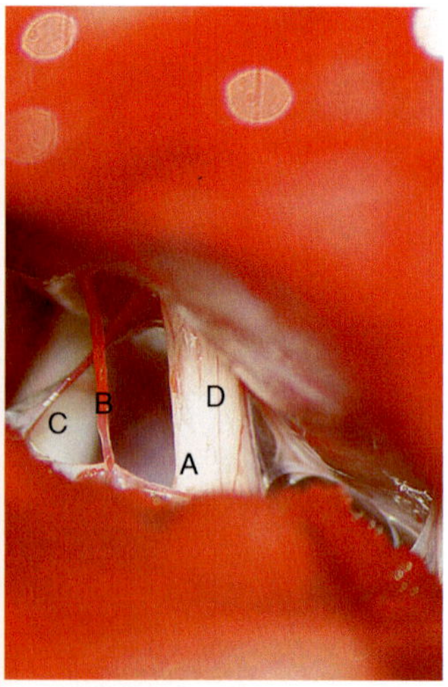

A. Acoustico-facial nerve bundle
B. Labyrinthine artery
C. Trigeminal nerve
D. Microscopic vessels at the junction of the vestibular and cochlear nerves

Fig. 4.68 Identification of the vestibular and cochlear nerves
The figure shows more clearly the upper part of the VIIIth nerve, the vestibular nerve. There is a small blood vessel at the junction between it and the lower cochlear nerve. The trigeminal nerve can be seen at the depths, antero-superior to the acoustico-facial nerve bundle

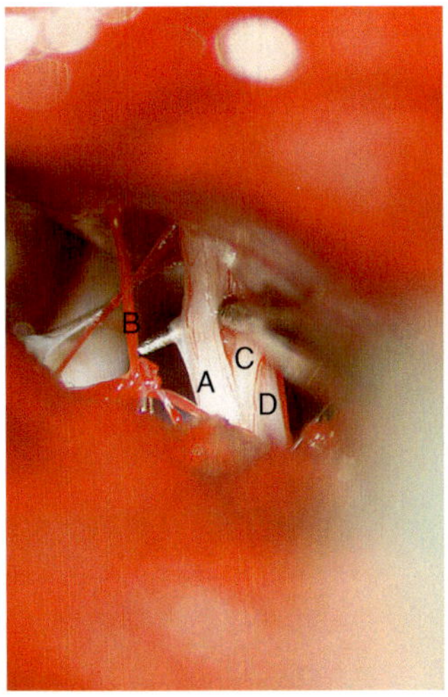

A. Vestibular nerve
B. Internal auditory artery
C. Cochlear nerve
D. Facial nerve

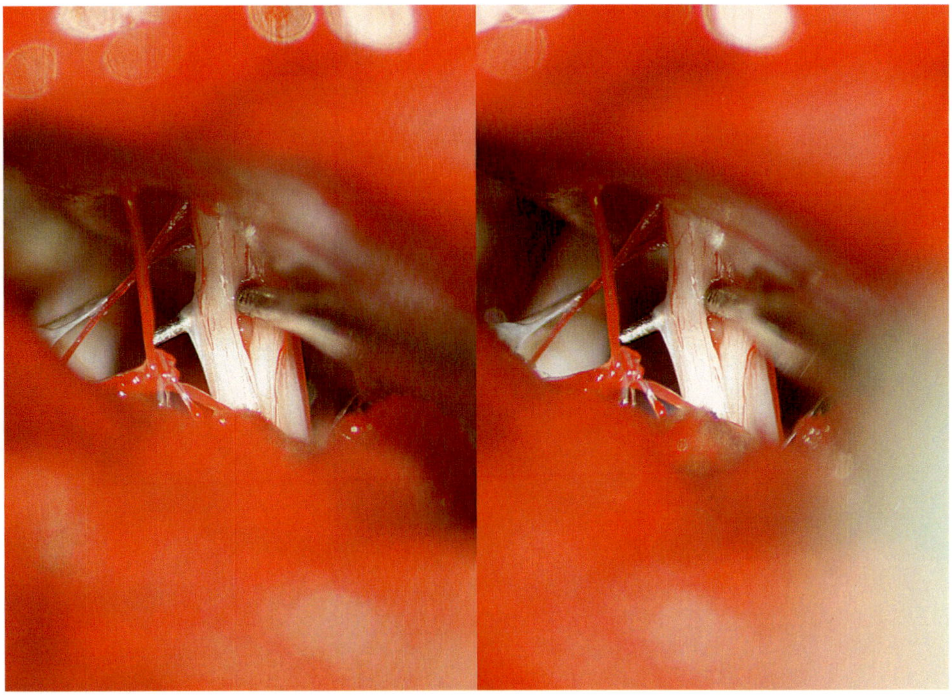

Fig. 4.69 Separation of the vestibular nerve
Once each of the nerves is clearly identified, the vestibular nerve is gently separated from the cochlear nerve under the microscope. The lower part of the nerve is the cochlear nerve and the facial nerve is seen more deeply. Care is taken to not damage cochlear nerve fibers during the operation, and to not unnecessarily manipulate the internal auditory artery to avoid injury and spasm

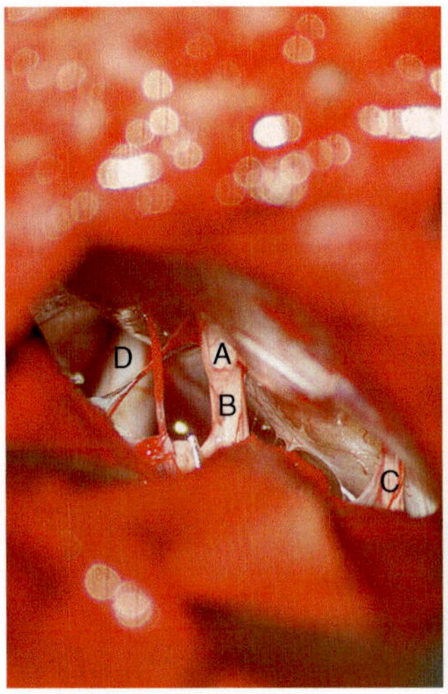

A. Vestibular nerve stump
B. Cochlear nerve
C. Glossopharyngeal nerve
D. Trigeminal nerve

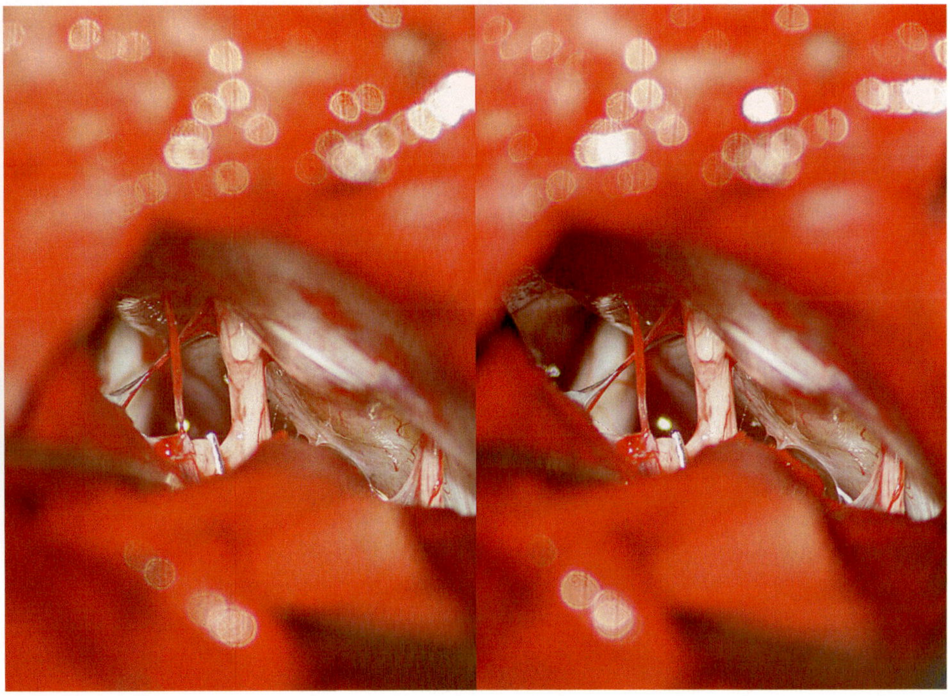

Fig. 4.70 Sectioning the Vestibular nerve
A 3 mm segment of the vestibular nerve is resected with a nerve hook and a knife or microsurgical scissors. The distal nerve stump can also be treated with bipolar coagulation to prevent nerve re-anastomosis

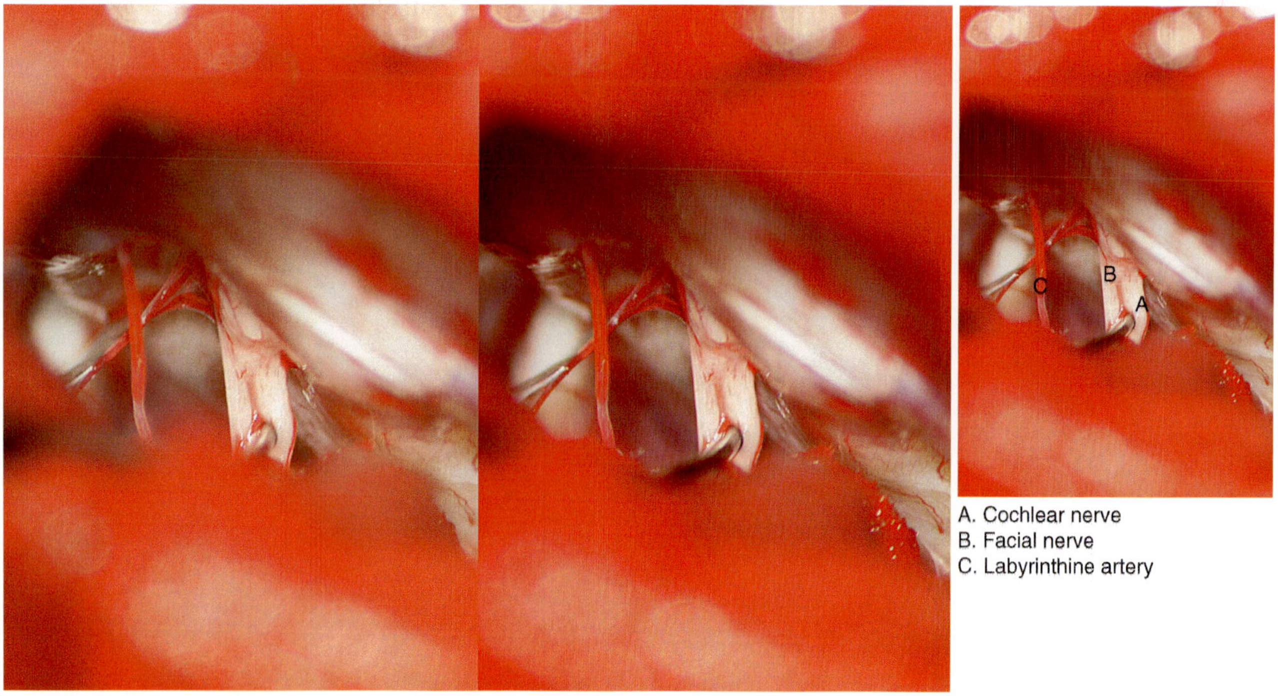

Fig. 4.71 Identification of facial nerve after section of the vestibular nerve
After resecting a segment of the vestibular nerve, the cochlear nerve can be gently retracted to expose the facial nerve more deeply. A facial nerve monitor can be used to help to identify the facial nerve

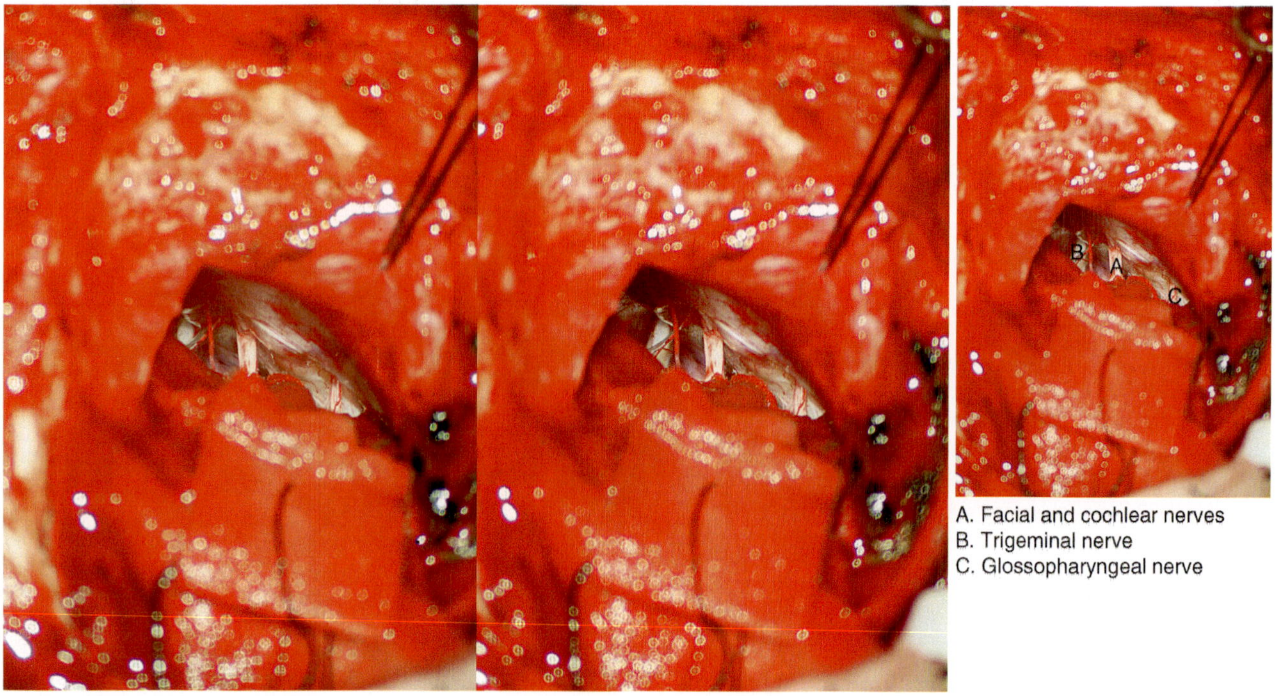

Fig. 4.72 Surgical field (cerebellopontine angle)
The cerebellopontine angle is inspected under lower magnification and the integrity of cochlear and facial nerves is confirmed. The trigeminal nerve can be seen at the depths superiorly and the glossopharyngeal nerve at the bottom of cerebellopontine angle

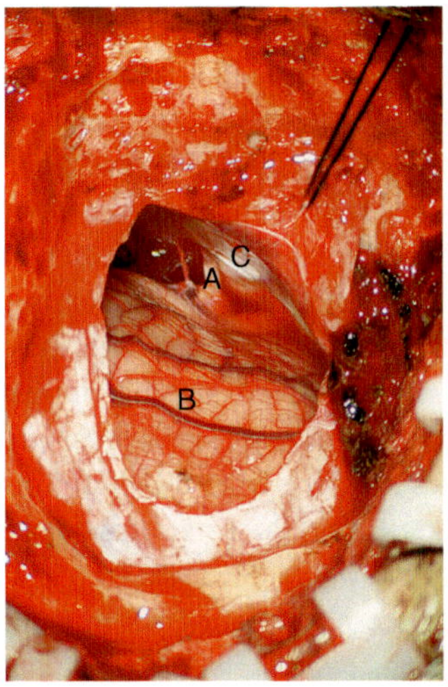

A. Facial and cochlear nerves
B. Cerebellum
C. Petrous bone

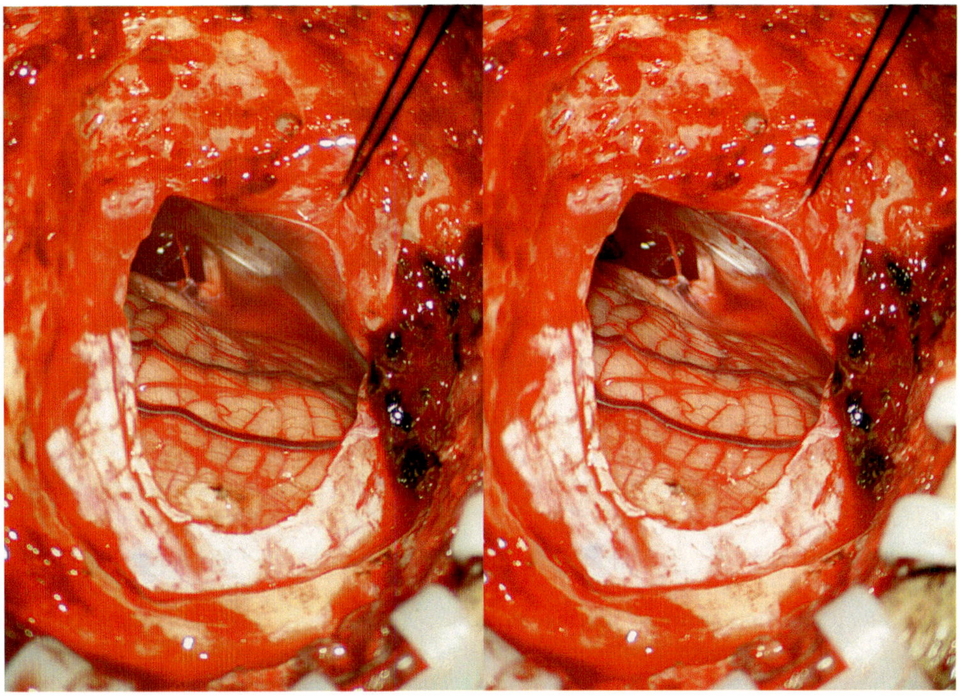

Fig. 4.73 Repeat irrigation and inspection before closure
Cottonoids are removed and the cavity is liberally irrigated to ensure active bleeding is identified and dealt with before closure

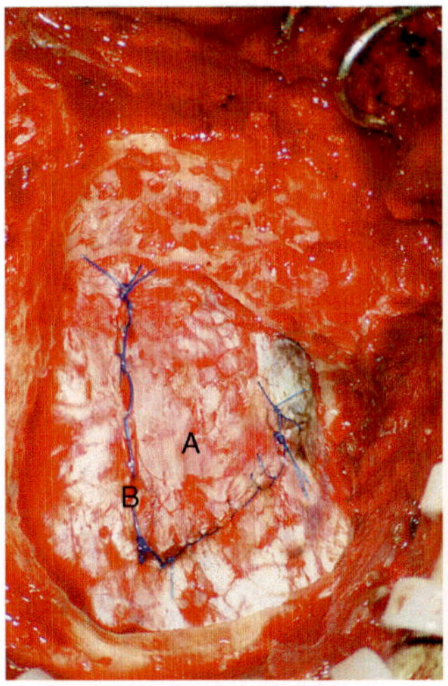

A. Posterior cranial fossa dura
B. Continuous dural suture

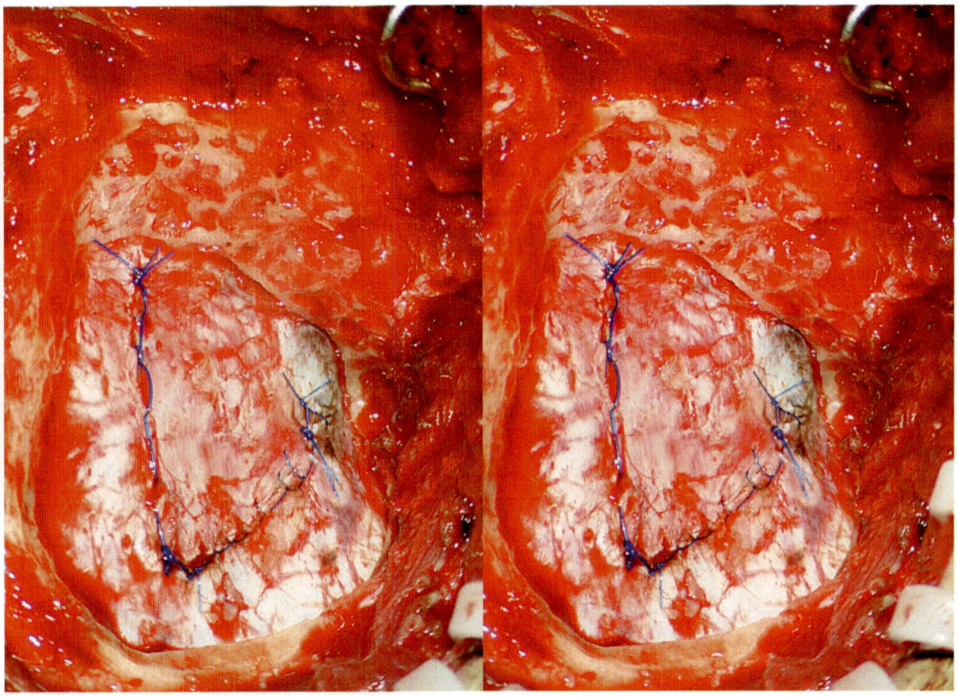

Fig. 4.74 Dural closure
A continuous dural suture is made with nylon. Any dural defects can be repaired with small pieces of muscle and sealed with biogel

Cochlear Implantation

Sha-sha Huang and Pu Dai

Indications

Children under 18 years of age

1. bilateral severe-to-profound hearing impairment
2. lack of development of auditory ability and minimal hearing aid benefit
3. enrolment in an education program emphasizing auditory development
4. no surgical contraindication

Adults over 18 years of age

1. bilateral severe-to-profound hearing impairment
2. no or minimal benefit from conventional hearing aids (typically defined as sentence recognition rates under 50–60 % in the best aided condition)
3. no surgical contraindication

Contraindications

1. Sensorineural hearing loss caused by retro-cochlear lesions such as the hearing loss after removal of an acoustic neuroma.
2. Cochlear aplasia or severe cochlear ossification that limits electrode insertion, and cochlear auditory nerve damage such as that caused by fractures
3. Psychiatric history. There is a contraindication to cochlear implantation in patients with psychosis, as electrical stimulation may stimulate the cerebral cortex.
4. Middle ear infection. Active acute or chronic otitis media will predispose to inner ear infections in this surgery.

Operative Procedures

1. A post auricular skin incision is made and extended postero-superiorly to the temporal scalp according to the requirements of the specific cochlear implant being used, and ensuring the incision as far as possible away from the cochlear receiver stimulator.
2. The muscle and periosteum are incised away from the skin incision in order to provide coverage of the cochlear receiver stimulator. The musculo-periosteal flap is elevated from the mastoid cortex.
3. A mastoidectomy is performed, with drilling starting in the cribriform area.
4. The mastoid air cells are gradually removed to expose the antrum, tegmen mastoideum and sigmoid sinus and preserving the bony wall of the external auditory meatus.
5. After exposing the lateral semicircular canal and short process of the incus, the bone is gradually lowered along the posterior wall of the external auditory meatus to locate the facial recess. The facial recess lies deep to a triangle formed by the chorda tympani antero-inferiorly, the facial nerve canal postero-inferiorly and the buttress of bone above that covers the short process of the incus. The facial nerve canal lies in a line from the mid-point of the lateral semicircular canal to the front of the mastoid tip.
6. After locating the facial recess, the facial nerve canal and chorda tympani are skeletonized.
7. Opening the facial recess. The bone is removed in the angle between the vertical segment of facial nerve and the chorda tympani with a small drill or a diamond bur to expose the pyramidal eminence, stapedius tendon and stapes.
8. Exposing of round window niche. Further opening of the facial recess with a diamond bur enables exposure of the round window niche.
9. The bone of the promontory anterior to the round window niche is gently drilled to show the blue line of the endosteum of the scala tympani. A circular fenestrum is made slightly larger than the electrode array, and the endosteum is initially kept intact.
10. The temporalis muscle and periosteum are incised along the superior edge of incision and elevated to expose the cortex of the mastoid. The bone well for the receiver stimulator is drilled using the appropriate template for the implant being used. A circular well is generally made for the Nucleus CI24M (Australian) and Clarion implant (American), but square one with one rounded end is made for the Med-E1 implant (Austrian).
11. A groove is created between the facial recess and mastoid well to hold the electrode. There is a multichannel cochlear insertion electrode and a ground electrode for the Nucleus and Med-E1 implants, but only the insertion electrode with the Clarion. There must be sufficient space in the bony groove to place the electrode, otherwise bone regrowth may compress the electrode array.
12. The Med-E1 implant body needs to be fixed to bone well using nylon tie over sutures. The Nucleus CI24M and Clarion do not.
13. The endosteal membrane seen through the cochleostomy is opened to expose the scala tympani, taking care not to suction perilymph.
14. The cochlear electrode array is inserted into the scala tympani via the cochleostomy area with a specialized claw and electrode forceps. There is stylet inside the

curved electrode of the Nucleus Contour Advance. After the electrode is inserted, it is held with the claw while removing the stylet with otologic forceps.

15. After insertion of the electrode, the cochleostomy is sealed with small pieces of muscle or fascia.
16. After stabilizing the electrode under the overhanging margins of the mastoidectomy, the facial recess is packed with gelatin sponge or fascia to separate the bony facial canal and the electrode.
17. The temporalis fascia and periosteum are sutured to secure the implant. The skin incision is closed. In children, interrupted absorbable subcutaneous and continuous intradermal sutures are used.

Special Comments

1. Care is taken not to damage the posterior wall of the external auditory meatus anteriorly and the vertical segment of facial nerve posteriorly whilst opening the facial recess into the middle ear cavity.
2. Care is taken not to damage the dura whilst drilling the well for the receiver-stimulator which may lead to a cerebrospinal fluid leak.
3. Attention needs to be paid to the direction and depth of insertion of the electrode into the cochlea, and to not damaging the electrode array when handling it with forceps.
4. Hemostasis must be ensured during operation, the scalp wound closed in layers, and a compression dressing applied to prevent hematoma formation.

Complications

1. Hematoma and infection. A strict aseptic operative technique, complete hemostasis and the use of perioperative antibiotics will prevent hematoma and infection.
2. Facial nerve injury. Care must be taken with the facial nerve whilst opening the facial recess. If it is injured or a severe paralysis appears postoperatively, a decompression of the facial nerve should be performed immediately.
3. Cerebrospinal fluid leak. If the dura is breached whilst drilling the recipient bed, it is necessary to pack and repair it with muscle. A cerebrospinal fluid gusher may be seen in patients with inner ear malformations when performing the cochleostomy. This will be packed tightly with muscle or fascia.
4. Wound dehiscence. Sufficient space must be made under the skin and muscle flap for the implant and the wound sutured in layers.
5. Implant migration. The risk of implant migration is associated with hypersensitivity or infection. Attention is paid to prevention of hematoma and infection. Allergic patients will require specific treatment.

Surgery 1: Cochlear Implantation (American AB products)

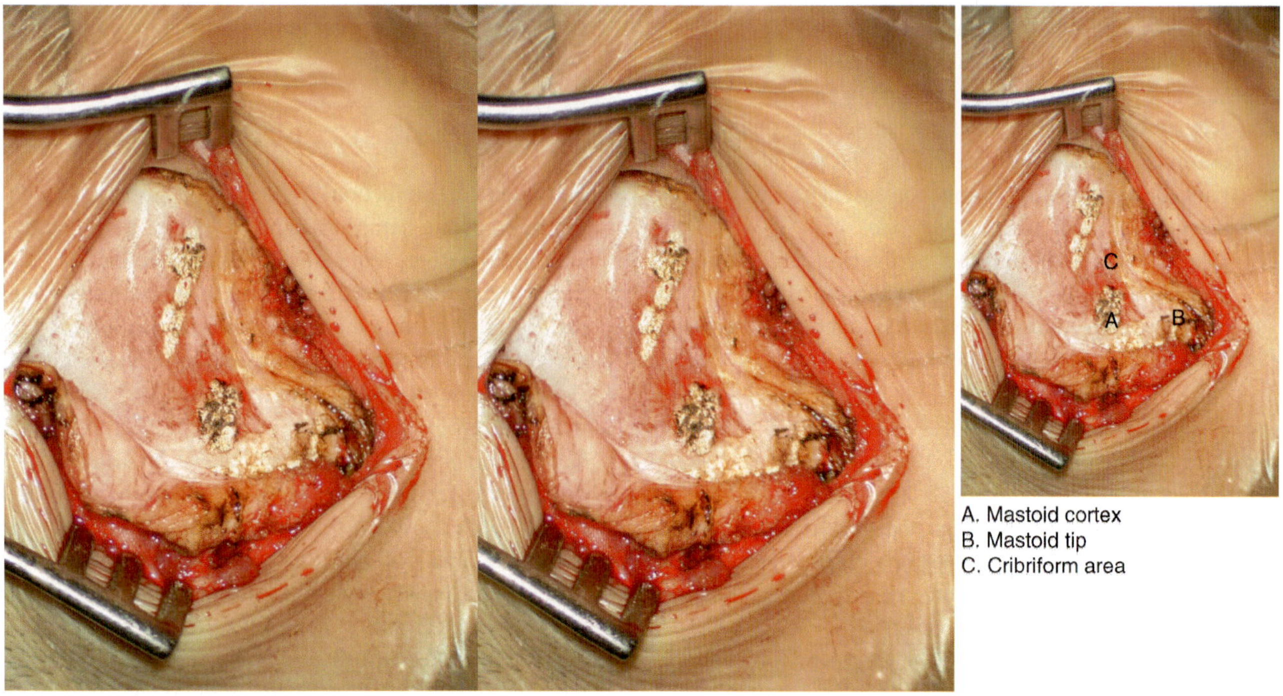

Fig. 4.75 Exposure of mastoid
Post auricular skin incision. Incise the skin and subcutaneous tissues and elevate the muscle and periosteum from the mastoid cortex. Identify the suprameatal spine and posterior wall of the external auditory meatus anteriorly, the anterior surface of the mastoid tip inferiorly, the mastoid posteriorly and the temporal line and squamous skull surface superiorly

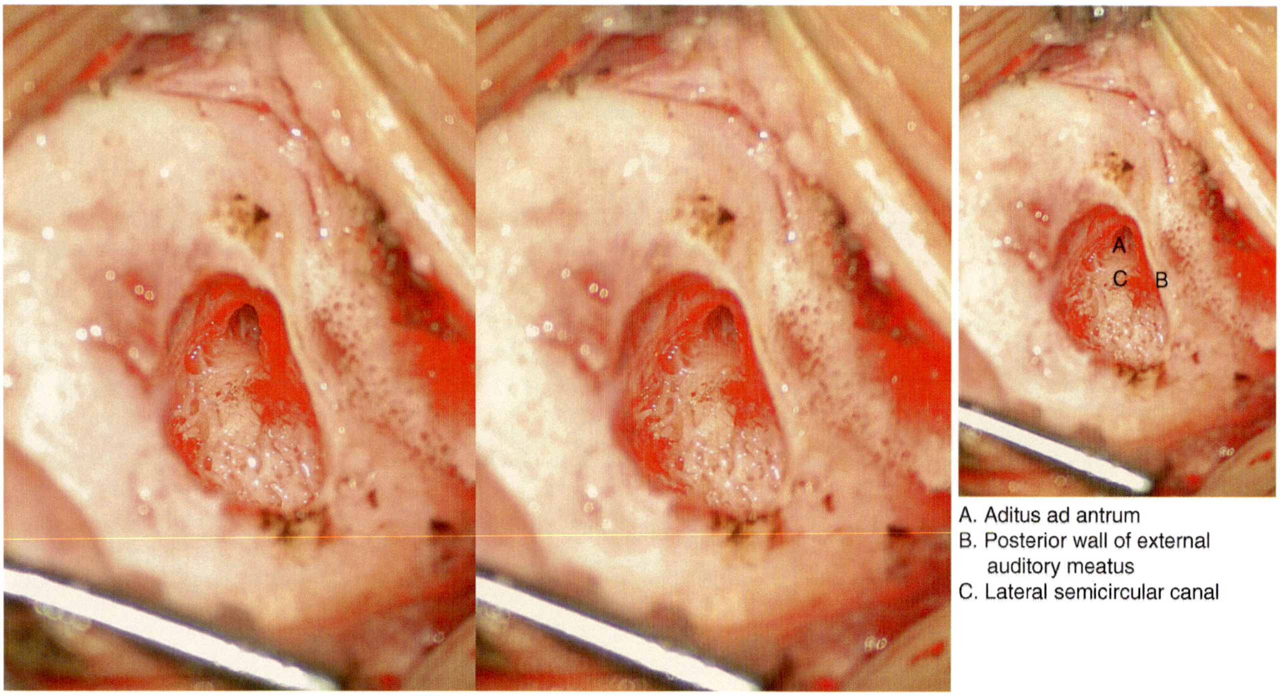

Fig. 4.76 Exposure of tympanic antrum
After drilling the mastoid cortex from the cribriform area with a cutting bur, the tympanic antrum is exposed to begin a cortical mastoidectomy. Overhangs of the mastoid cortex can be created posteriorly and inferiorly. The posterior bony external auditory canal wall is thinned but not breached to avoid soft tissue prolapsing into the operative cavity

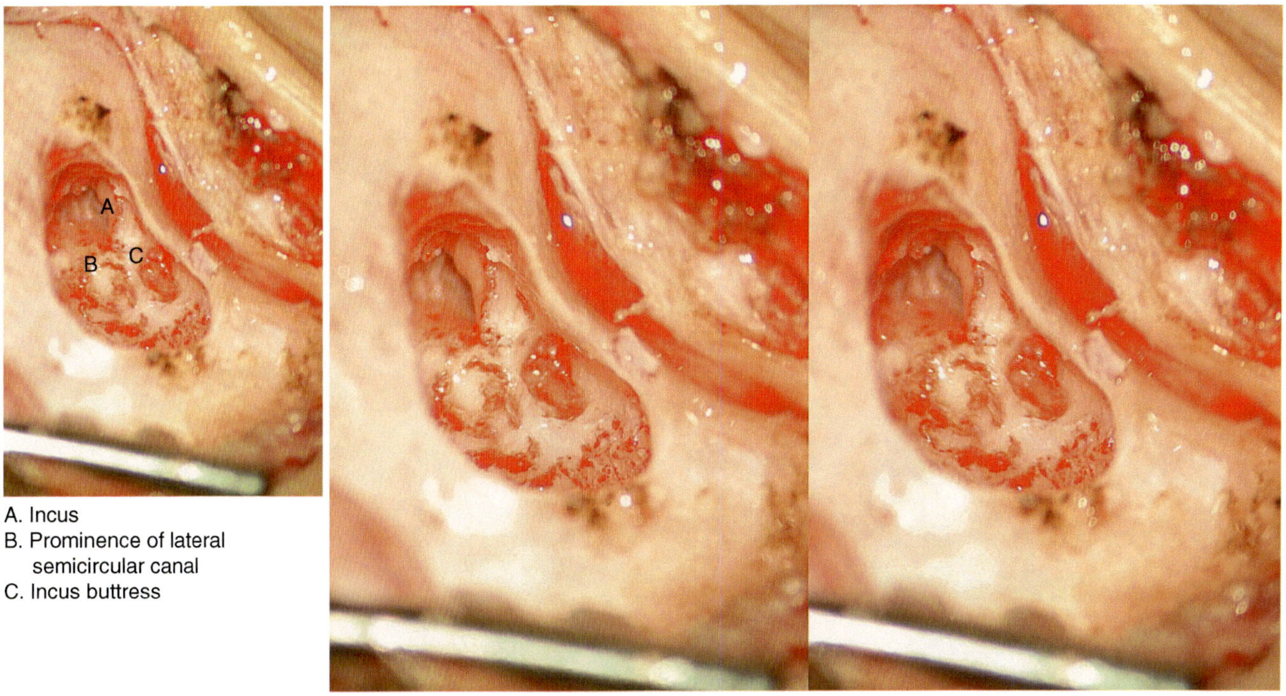

Fig. 4.77 Location of facial recess
After exposure of the lateral semicircular canal and incus short process, the posterior wall of external auditory canal is thinned to allow location of the facial recess. The facial recess is bound by the posterior arch (incus buttress) under the incus short process superiorly, the chorda tympani anteriorly and the vertical segment of the facial nerve posteriorly. Care is taken to not damage the chorda tympani or facial nerves. The facial recess approach connects the tympanic cavity to the mastoid cavity

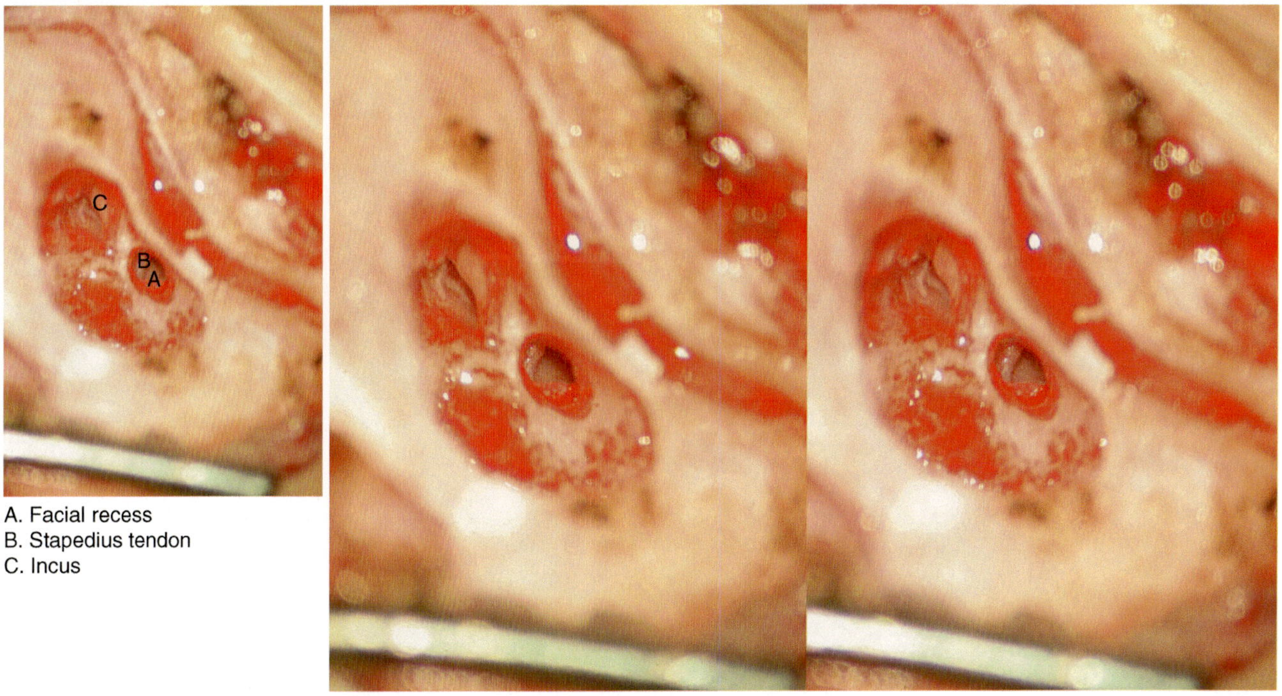

Fig. 4.78 Opening the facial recess
After locating the facial recess, the vertical canal of facial nerve and the chorda tympani are identified. Bone is removed between these two structures with small cutting or diamond burs to expose the pyramidal eminence, stapedius tendon and stapes

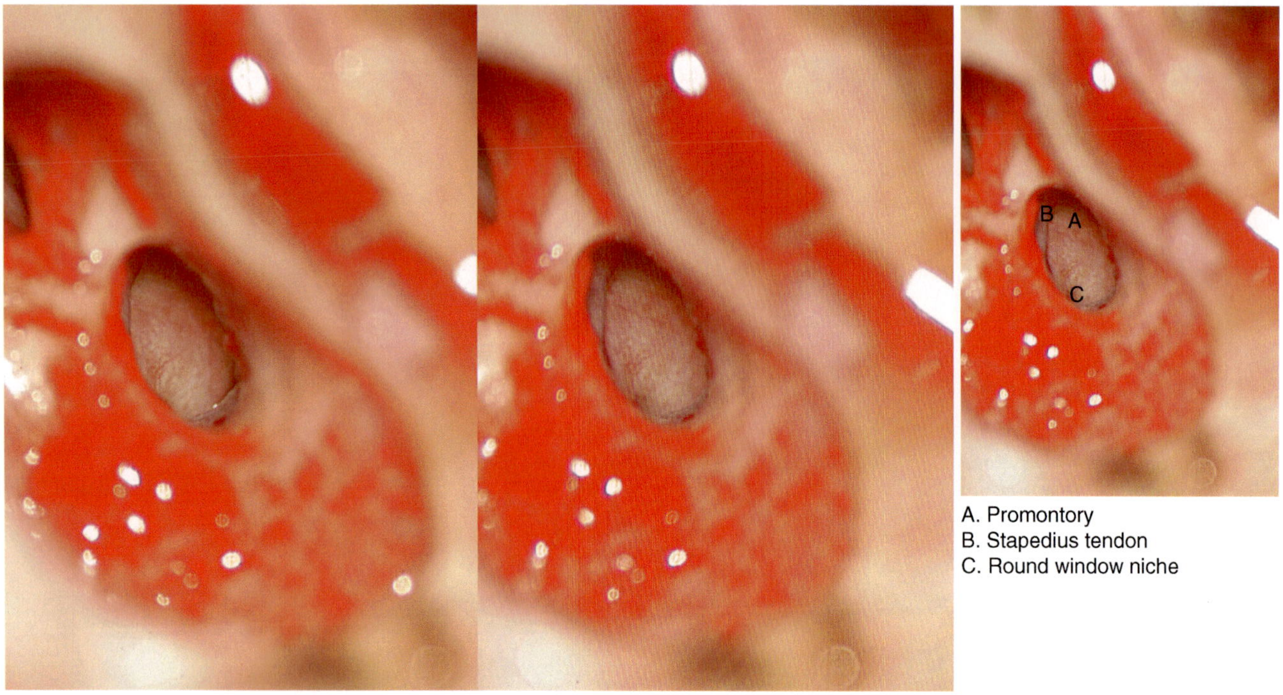

Fig. 4.79 Fully opening the facial recess
After locating the facial nerve, maximize the size of the facial recess superiorly and inferiorly to visualize the stapes, stapedius tendon, the promontory, the round window niche and the site of the cochleostomy

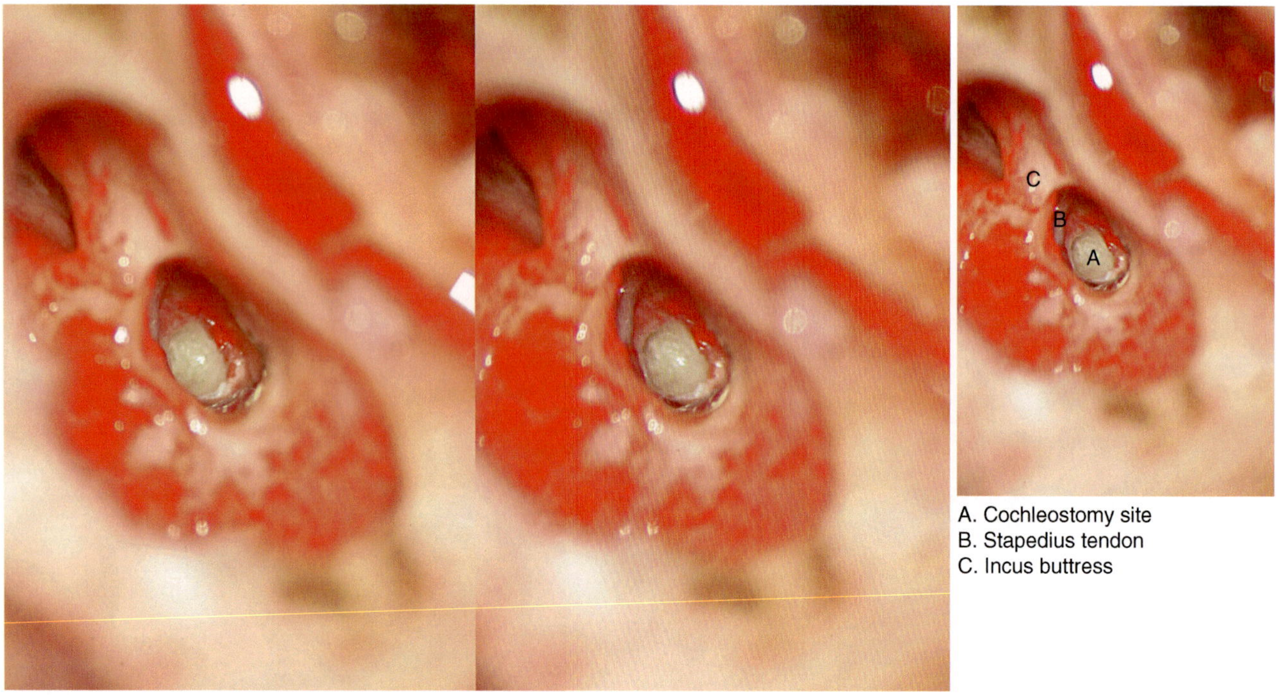

Fig. 4.80 (**a**) Fenestrating the scala tympani
After maximizing the size of the facial recess, use a 1.5 mm bur to saucerize the promontory anterior to the round window niche until the blue line the endosteum of scala tympani is exposed. The cochleostomy opening is made slightly larger than the electrode to be inserted, and the endosteum initially kept intact

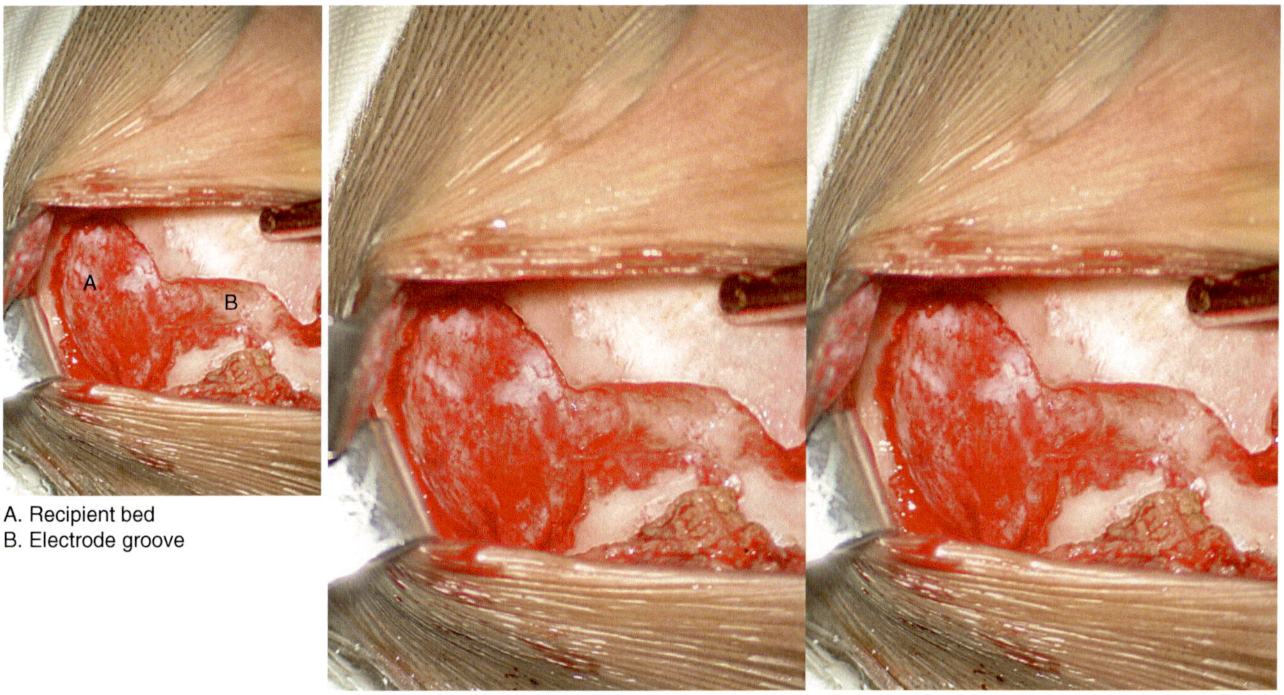

Fig. 4.81 Fashioning the recipient bed
Incise the temporalis muscle and periosteum posteriorly along the superior edge of the incision and elevate the musculo-periosteal flap to expose the bony surface of the skull. Drill the bone well using the guide supplied with implant being used. A groove is created between the bony well and the mastoid cavity to hold the electrode

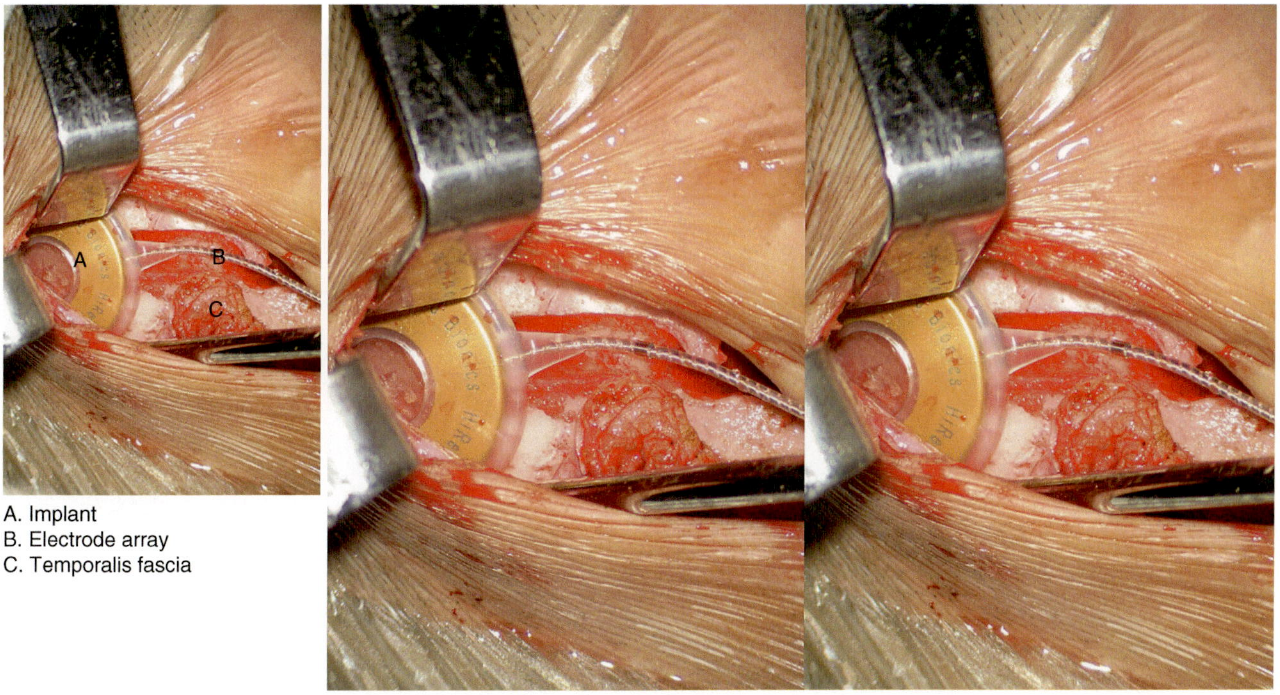

Fig. 4.82 Placement of the implant
After drilling the bony well, seat the implant in it and confirm that it fits appropriately. Attention: Suture the temporalis fascia and periosteum to secure the implant, covering it and separating it from the skin incision

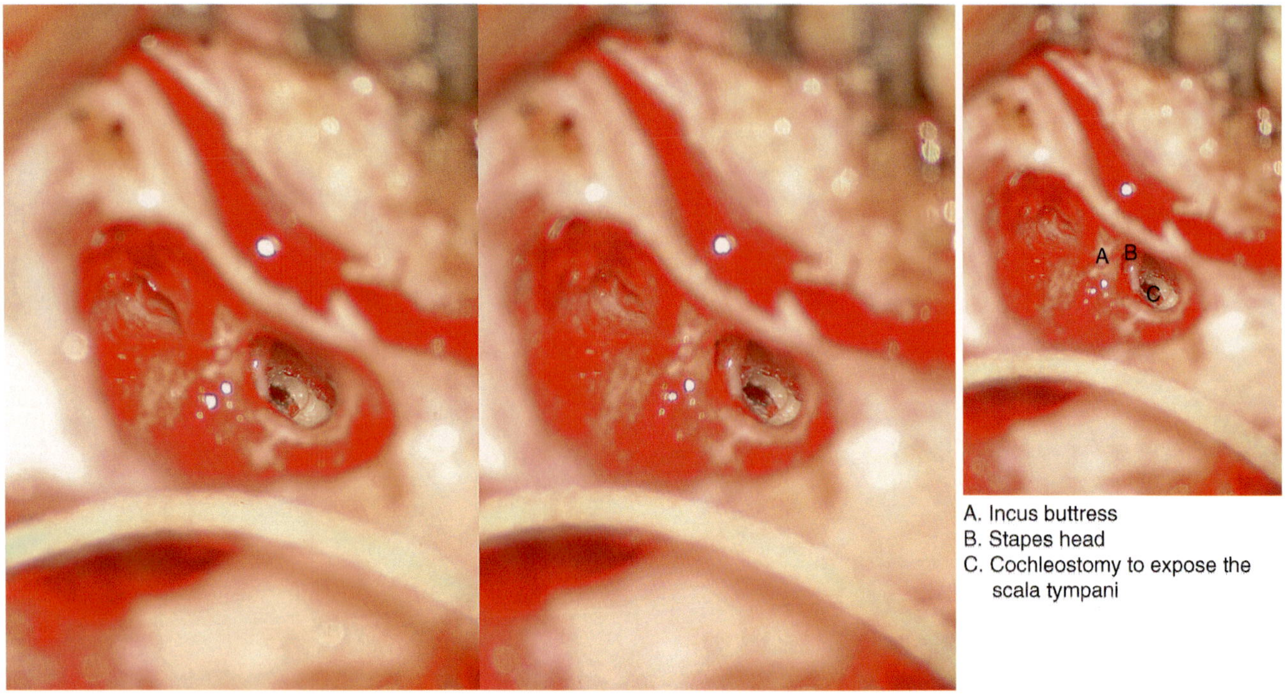

A. Incus buttress
B. Stapes head
C. Cochleostomy to expose the scala tympani

Fig. 4.83 Exposure of scala tympani
The endosteal membrane of the cochleostomy is opened to expose scala tympani with a small hooked needle. Take care to not suction perilymph. The size of cochleostomy should be suitable for the electrode array being used to allow easy insertion and avoid damaging it and the inner ear

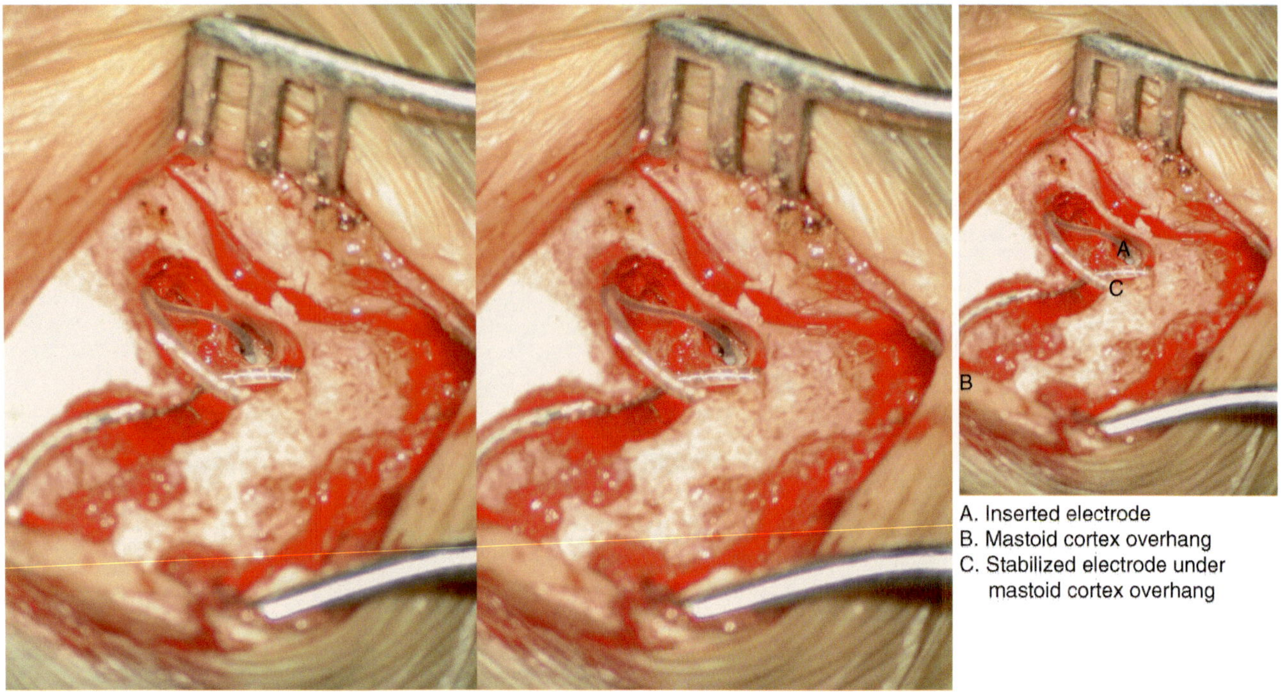

A. Inserted electrode
B. Mastoid cortex overhang
C. Stabilized electrode under mastoid cortex overhang

Fig. 4.84 Electrode insertion
The cochlear electrode is inserted into the scala tympani via the cochleostomy with a specialized electrode claw and forceps. Grip the electrode carefully to avoid damage to it. This picture shows the American AB cochlear implant which has no reference electrode

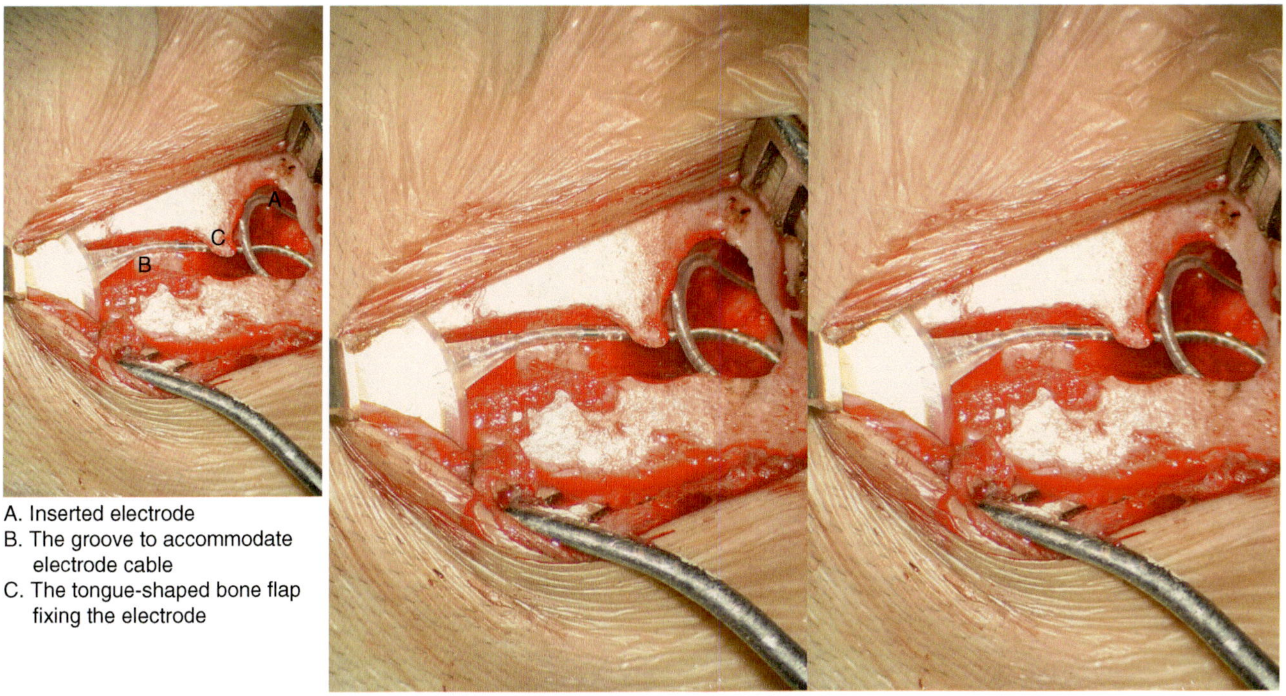

A. Inserted electrode
B. The groove to accommodate electrode cable
C. The tongue-shaped bone flap fixing the electrode

Fig. 4.85 Stabilize the electrode under the overhangs of the mastoid cortex
After insertion of the electrode, the cochleostomy is sealed with small pieces of muscle or fascia. It is important to stabilize the electrode under the overhangs in mastoidectomy, otherwise the electrode may extrude form the cochlea

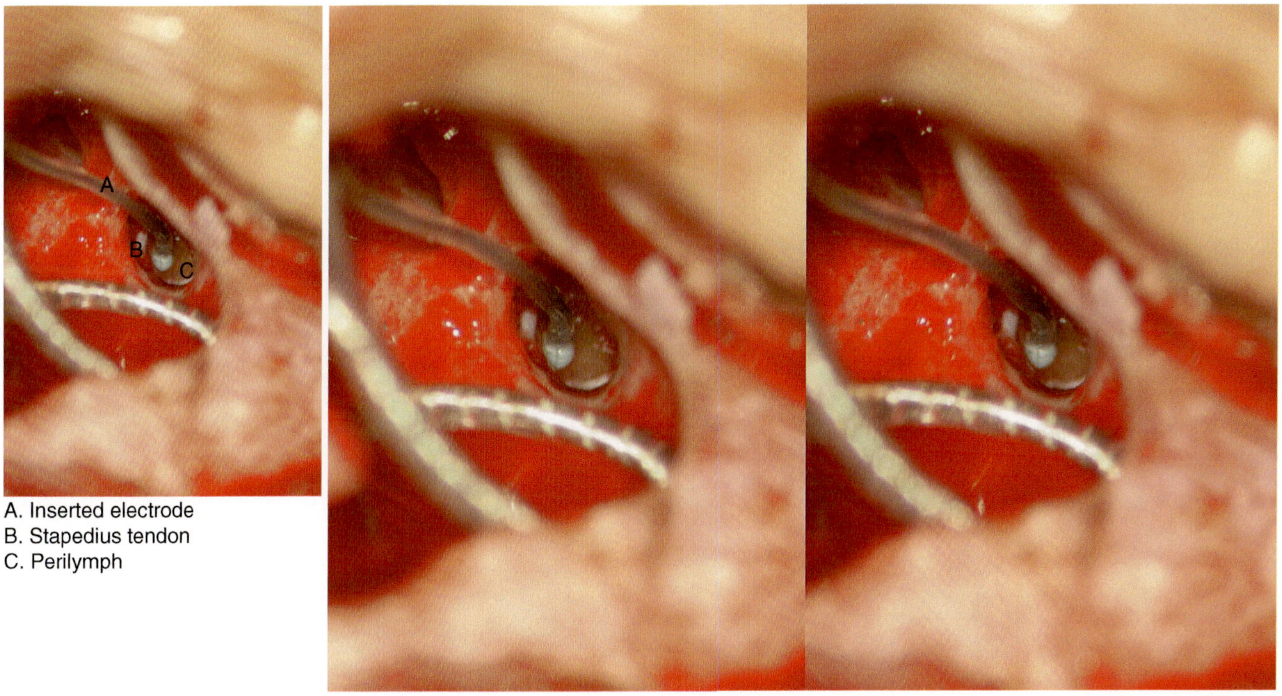

A. Inserted electrode
B. Stapedius tendon
C. Perilymph

Fig. 4.86 Verify the position of the electrode
After stabilizing the electrode, its position should be verified. This picture shows that the electrode has been inserted completely, noting the position of the white marker on it. The stapes and its tendon are seen superior to the electrode

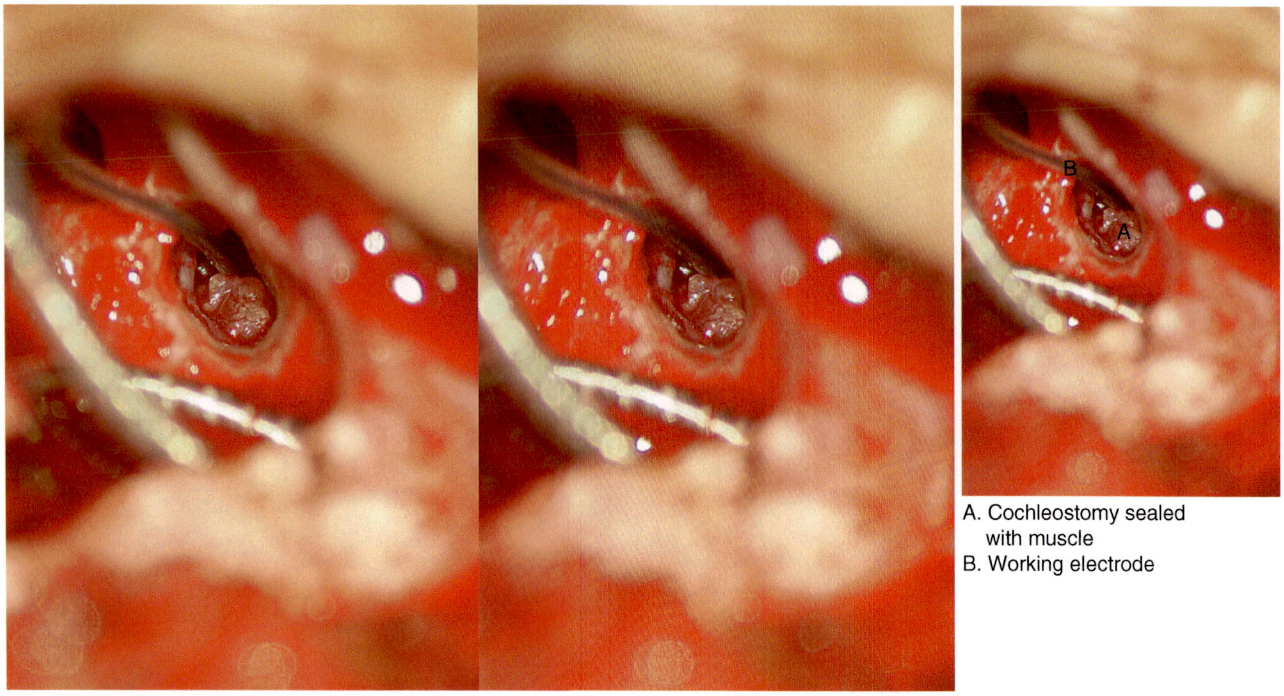

Fig. 4.87 Seal cochleostomy
After inserting the working electrode completely, pack the cochleostomy with small pieces of muscle or fascia. The picture shows the cochleostomy sealed with a small piece of muscle. If a cerebrospinal fluid gusher occurs, the primary means of closure is to pack the cochleostomy firmly

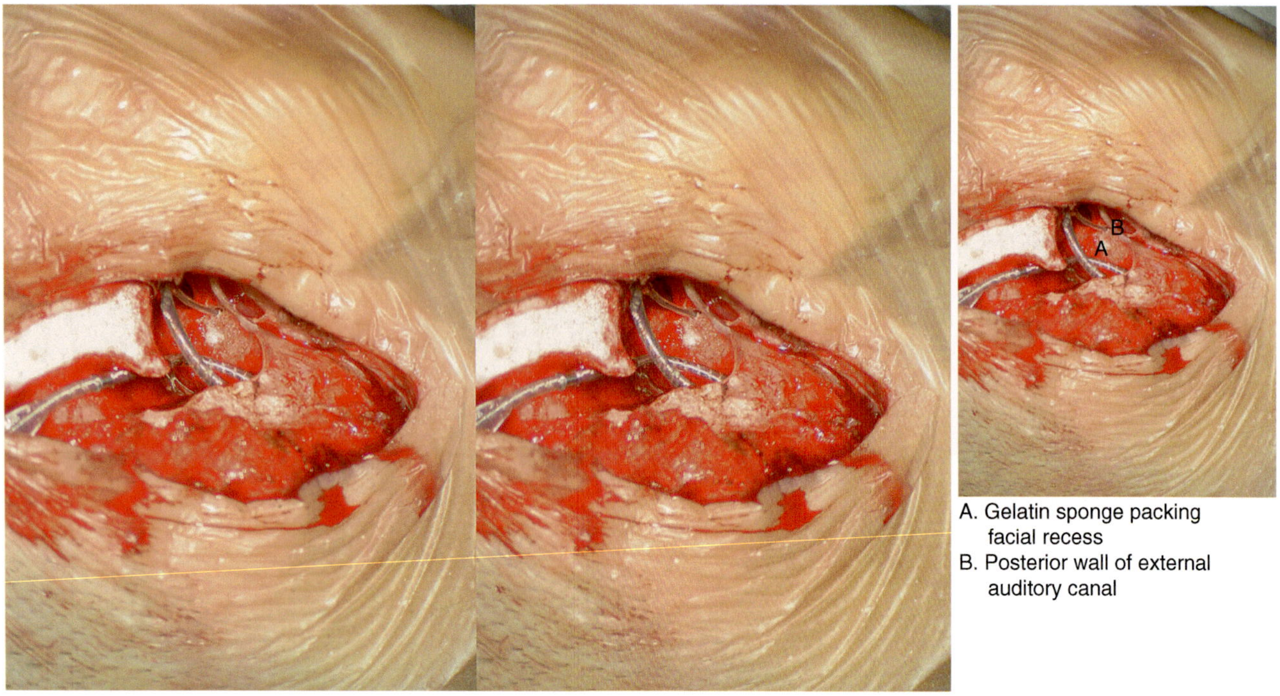

Fig. 4.88 Seal the facial recess
After insertion of the electrode, stabilize the lead under the overhangs of the mastoid cortex and pack the facial recess with gelatin sponge or fascia to separate the electrode from the facial canal

Surgery 2: Cochlear Implantation (Australia Contour Advance products)

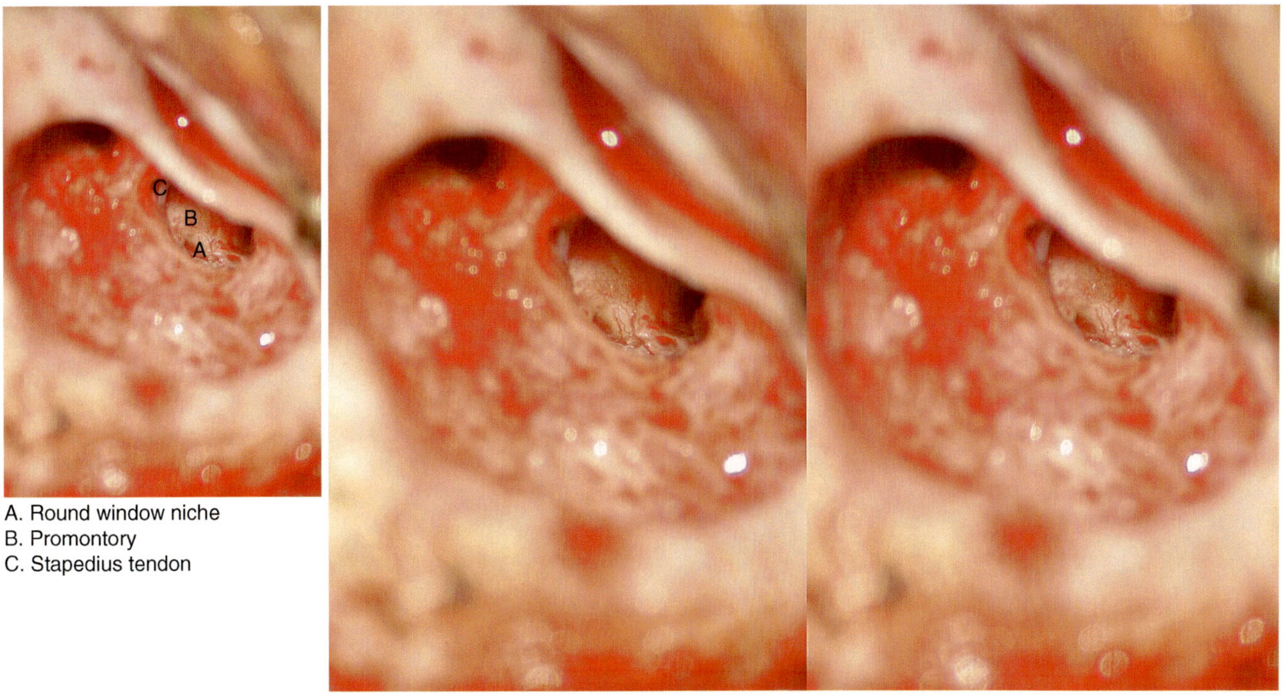

Fig. 4.89 Maximize the size of the facial recess
After opening the facial recess, carefully maximize its size inferiorly with micro diamond bur to better expose the inferior edge of the round window niche. Carefully remove the round window mucosal folds with a small pick to identify the margins of the window, especially its inferior edge

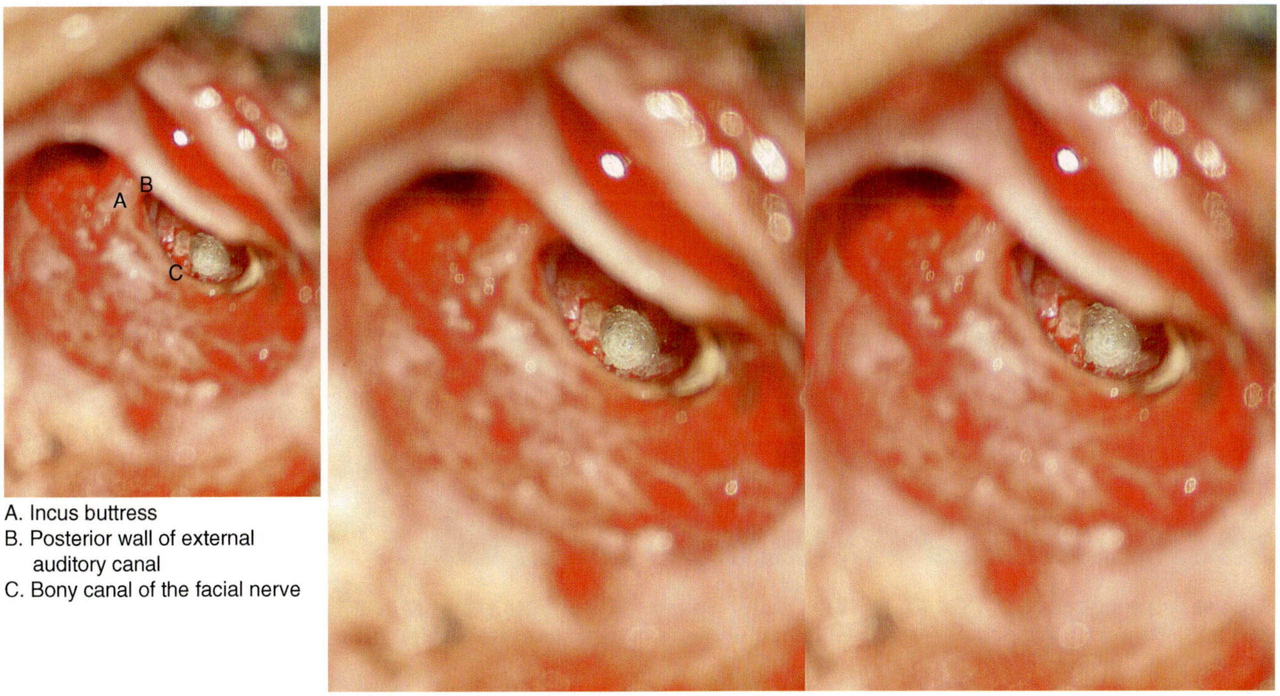

Fig. 4.90 Cochleostomy inferior to round window
Remove the round window overhang to exposure the round window membrane. Saucerize the promontory with a diamond bur 1 mm inferior to the niche until the blue line of the scala tympani is seen

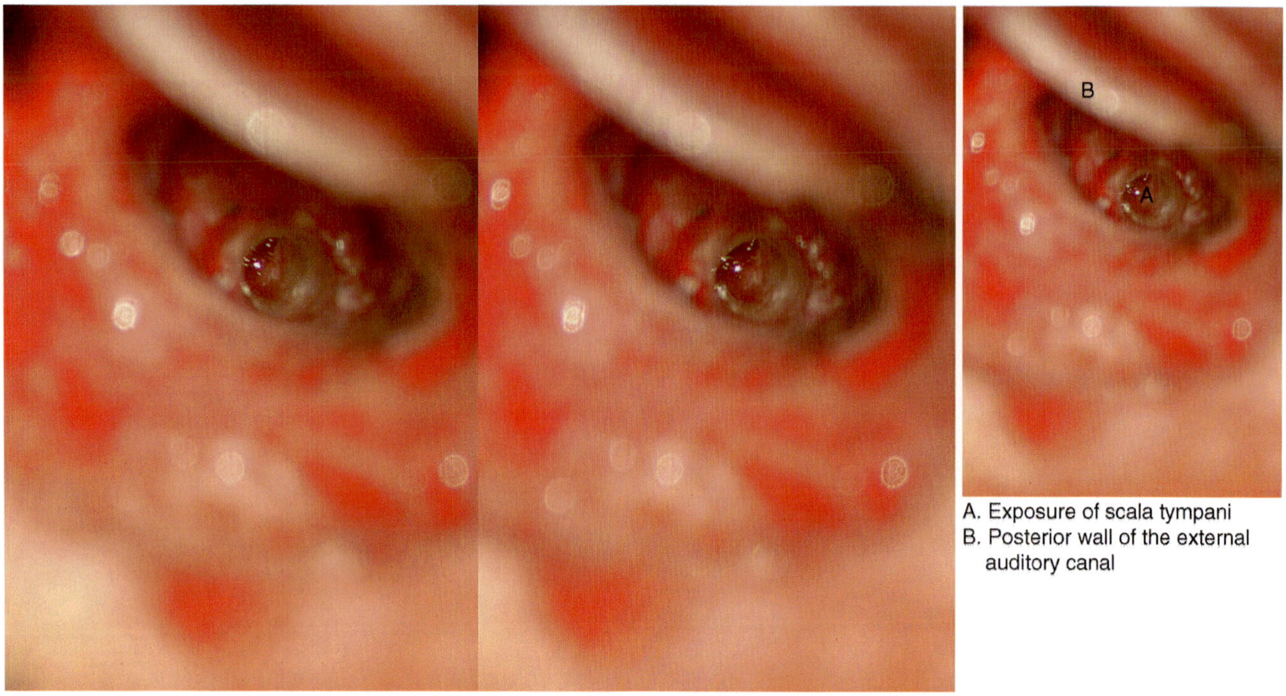

Fig. 4.91 Exposure of scala tympani
Using a 0.6 mm micro diamond bur, a fenestra is created into the basal scala tympani, and then the endosteum is removed to expose the scala tympani. Take care to not suction the cochleostomy area

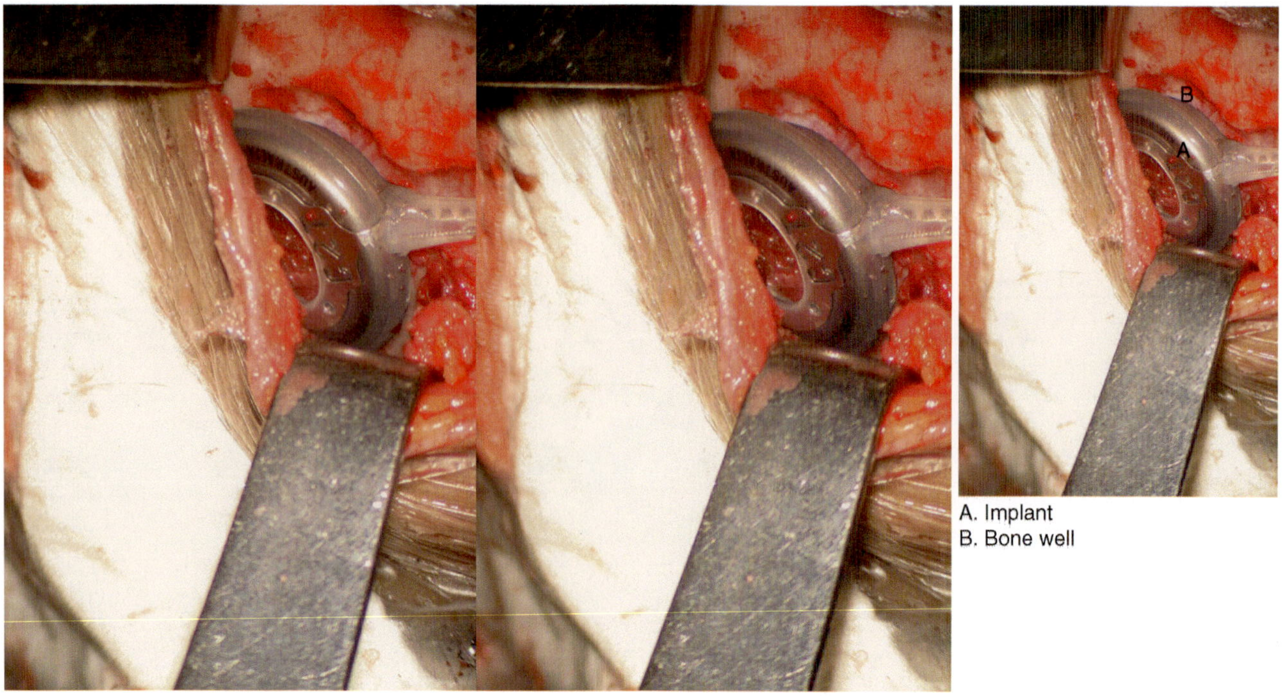

Fig. 4.92 Place implant
Seat the implant in its well. It does not require tie-down sutures as the periosteum and the pocket created in skull surface will stabilize its position

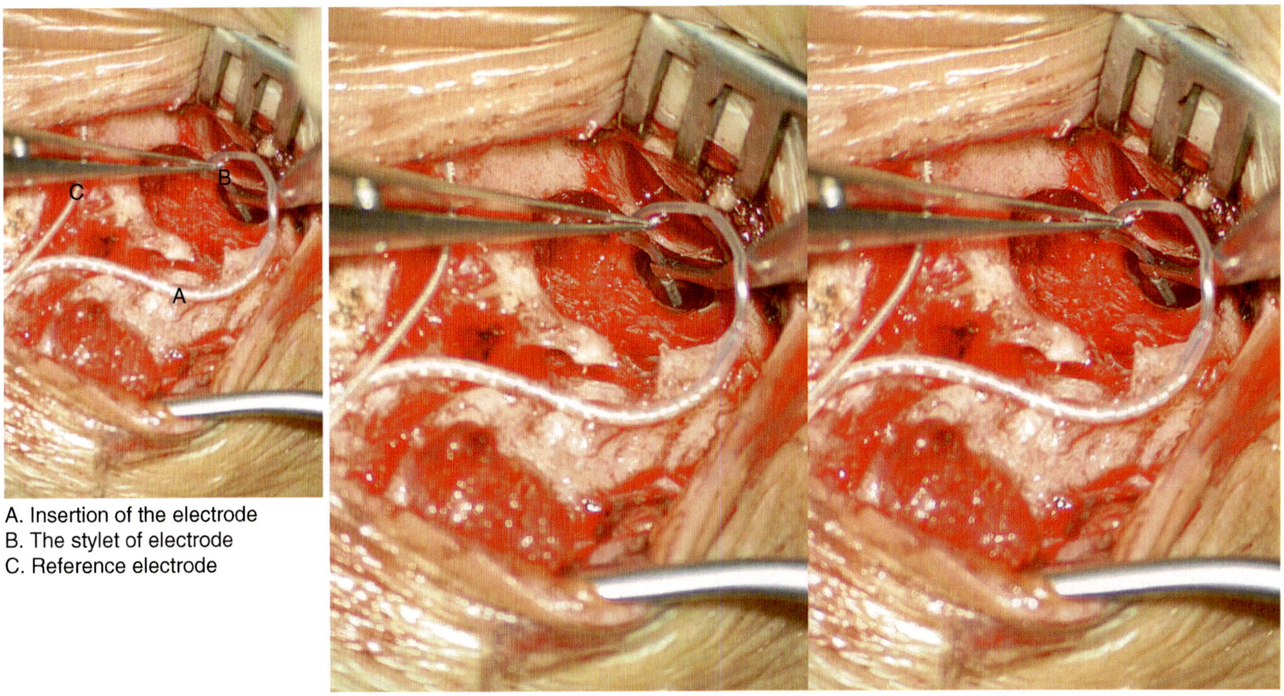

A. Insertion of the electrode
B. The stylet of electrode
C. Reference electrode

Fig. 4.93 Electrode insertion
Place the reference electrode under the temporalis muscle. The electrode is inserted using a specialized claw and electrode forceps. There is a white marker on the electrode 1 cm from its end. When white maker is just at the cochleostomy, the stylet is gripped with forceps whilst the electrode is fully inserted using the claw. This implantation technique is aimed at prevention of damage to the inner ear during electrode insertion

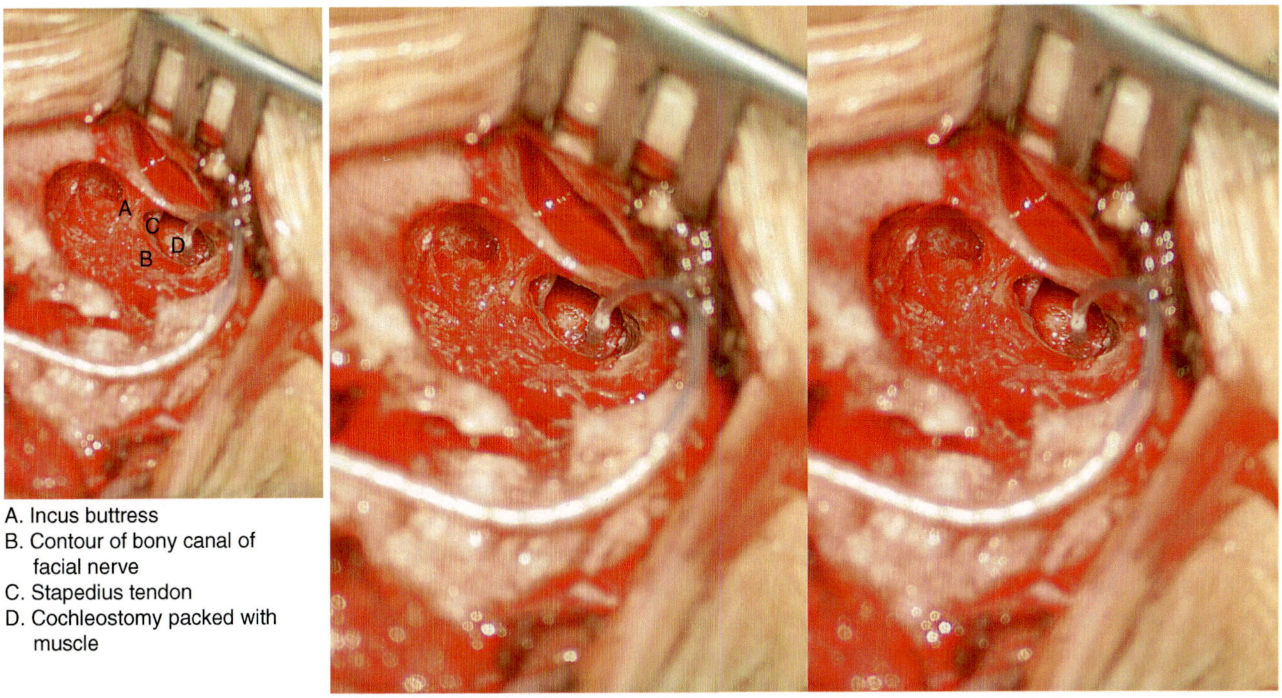

A. Incus buttress
B. Contour of bony canal of facial nerve
C. Stapedius tendon
D. Cochleostomy packed with muscle

Fig. 4.94 Electrode insertion
After insertion of the electrode, packs the cochleostomy with small pieces of muscle or fascia, then stabilizes the electrode under the overhangs of the mastoid cortex. Pack the facial recess with gelatin sponge, suture the muscle and subcutaneous tissues and close the skin in layers

Fenestration of Inner Ear

Yi-hui Zou and Pu Dai

Indications

1. Congenital atresia or absence of the vestibular window, extensive sclerosis and obliteration of the stapes footplate associated with good bone conduction where the hearing loss is conductive or mixed with predominance of the conductive component.
2. Oval window niche is totally obstructed by prolapse of the facial nerve or a large remnant of the stapedial artery covers the vestibular window.

Contraindications

1. Infective conditions such as otitis or furuncle of the external auditory canal, otitis media, perforation of the tympanic membrane, acute or chronic inflammation of the nasal or nasopharyngeal cavity. This procedure should be done only after recovery of any otitis media caused by dysfunction of Eustachian tube.
2. Little or no hearing improvement is likely due to significant pre-existing sensorineural hearing loss.
3. The patient's general health is too poor for surgery to be performed. Chronic infectious diseases such as hepatitis and tuberculosis should be cured or stable before the operation to be performed.
4. Bleeding and clotting disorders. Long term aspirin usage and active menstruation are conditions that may interfere with surgery by causing excessive bleeding. Sensorineural hearing loss may result from blood entering the inner ear.
5. Very young or very old patients. Informed consent needs to obtained from the patient who also needs to be able to cope with the early post- operative effects of surgery including dizziness, nausea and vomiting.

Operative Procedures

1. Anaesthesia: This operation is usually performed under general anesthesia as this ensures the patient remains still, avoiding intra-operative problems with the ossicles or blood entering the inner ear, and making it less likely that the procedure would need to be abandoned.
2. First incision: Incise the skin, subcutaneous tissue, and periosteum of the external auditory canal (EAC) anterior to the root of the helix and extend the incision medially to the junction of cartilage and bone.
3. Second incision: Start at the 6 o'clock position, 5–8 mm lateral to the fibrous annulus, along the posterior meatal wall in an ascending spiral fashion, to meet the first incision at its medial end. The distance from the second incision to the tympanic ring can vary depending on the shape of the canal and position of the tympanic membrane.
4. Elevate the tympanomeatal flap: The meatal flap is elevated to the tympanic ring with a blunt elevator and the fibrous annulus is then elevated from the sulcus. The tympanomeatal flap is reflected forward. Special care should be taken to avoid tearing the flap. In some atresia cases, the external auditory canal may need to be widened by removing bone from the posterior and superior walls.
5. To gain adequate exposure of the oval window niche, part of postero-superior bony canal rim must be removed with an angled middle ear curette or chisel, taking care not to injure the facial nerve or ossicular chain. Bone should be removed until the facial nerve canal, the whole oval window niche and the pyramidal eminence can be seen.
6. Assessment of the tympanic cavity. Examine the malleus, incus, stapes, round window, oval window niche and tympanic segment of the facial nerve. Assess whether the oval window is absent or blocked by an overhanging facial nerve. Evaluate the condition of the ossicular chain and prepare for the fenestration of the inner ear insertion of the prosthesis.
7. Make a fenestration at the oval window niche or at the site of promontory just inferior to the oval window niche or overhang facial nerve.
8. Cut the stapedius tendon if it is present. Separate the incudostapedial joint.
9. Remove of the stapes or stapes remnant.
10. Open a window at the area of vestibular window or near the promontory with a micro-drill.
11. Implantation of ossicular prosthesis. Either a piston or a TORP is used according to the situation and whether the incus and/or malleus are present. When using a TORP, we place a piece of fascia over the open window into the vestibule, then position the TORP between the fascia and tympanic membrane.
12. The vestibular window is sealed by a small piece of fat after the piston or prosthesis in implanted. The prosthesis is checked to ensure its mobility.
13. The tympanomeatal flap is returned to its original position.
14. The EAC is packed with gelatin sponge and iodoform gauze. The first incision is sutured.

Special Comments

1. Avoid injury to the inner ear. The procedure is performed with a delicate technique. Avoid foreign body or prosthesis falling into the open vestibule. Suction must not be applied to the open window of the vestibule.
2. Ensure complete hemostasis before making the fenestration to avoid blood entering the inner ear which may cause sensorineural hearing loss.
3. The patient is rested in bed for 3 days after the operation and instructed to avoid straining and nose blowing.
4. Prevent infection. A strict sterile operative technique is used and antibiotics are administered during and after operation.

Complications

1. Total deafness due to inner ear injury or infection.
2. Dizziness, nausea and vomiting can occur to a variable degree, but usually resolve within 3–7days.
3. Facial paralysis after the facial nerve is manipulated or injured. A further operation may be needed to explore the condition of facial nerve.
4. Perilymph fistula resulting from a failure to seal the oval window or fenestration. The mucosa of the oval window niche should be removed before sealing the window with fat or fascia.
5. Tympanic membrane perforation: due to failure to repair a torn tympanic membrane. Special care should be taken not to tear the tympanic membrane when elevating the annulus. If a tear does occur, it should be repaired with a piece of fascia or fat effectively.
6. Taste disturbance is common and due to dissection and stretching of the chorda tympani during surgery. The symptom usually recovers within a month.
7. Perilymph gusher. This usually occurs in the case of severe inner ear malformation and may need further surgical intervention.

Surgery 1: Absence of oval window, fenestration of inner ear and ossicular reconstruction (piston)

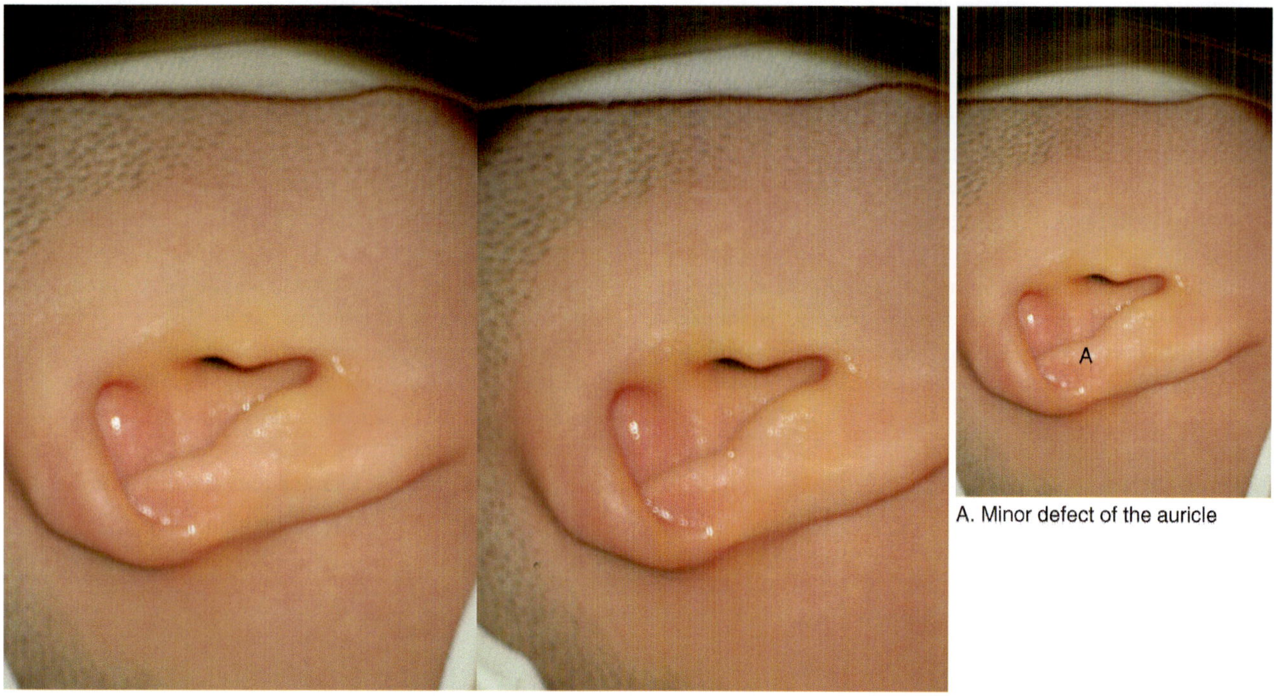

Fig. 4.95 Congenital defect of middle and external ear. It is common that congenital microtia occurs with atresia or stenosis of external auditory meatus (EAM). The degree of outer ear defect may predict the degree of middle ear defect to some extent. The picture shows this patient's auricle has developed, but without some features including the triangular and vestibular fossae

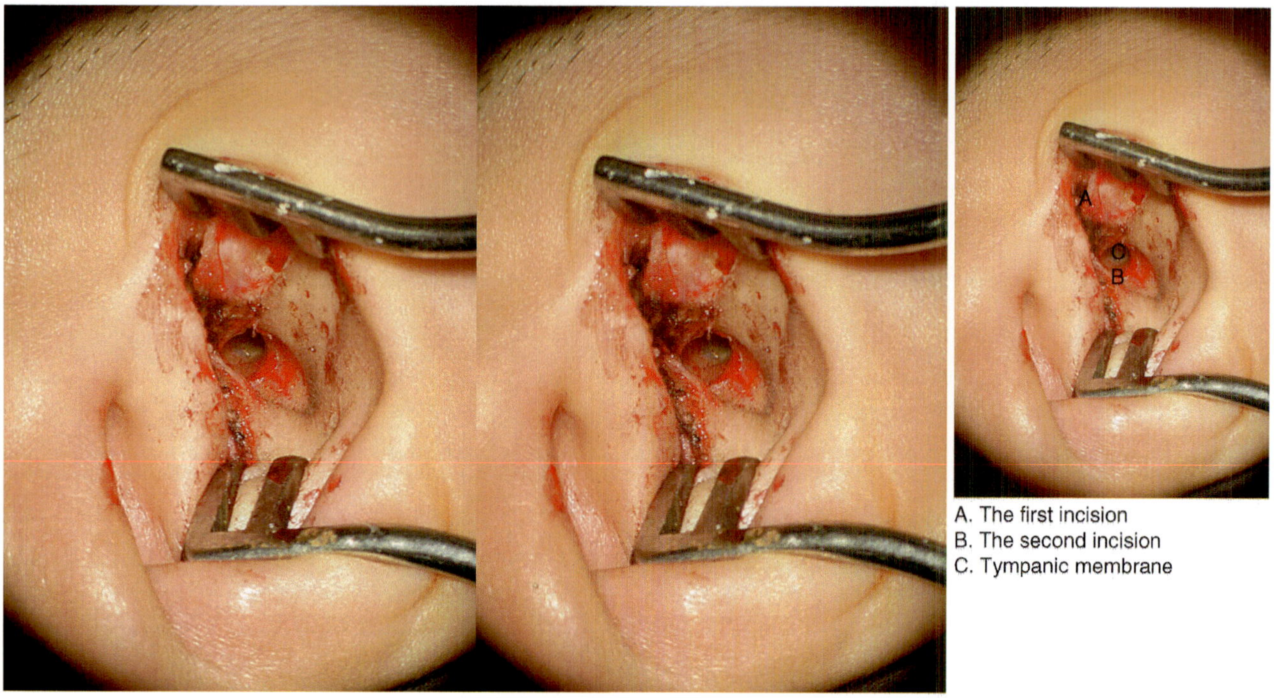

Fig. 4.96 Endaural incision
The first skin incision starts from the 12 o'clock position of EAC and is carried down to the bone. It is extended laterally between the tragus and the root of helix for about 0.5–1.0 cm and medially to a point 8 mm lateral to the tympanic membrane. Make the second incision starting at the 6 o'clock point, running 6–8 mm lateral to the annulus, and meet the medial end of the first incision. Remove the overhanging suprameatal spine to make a wider EAC to get better exposure using a diamond burr or chisel if necessary

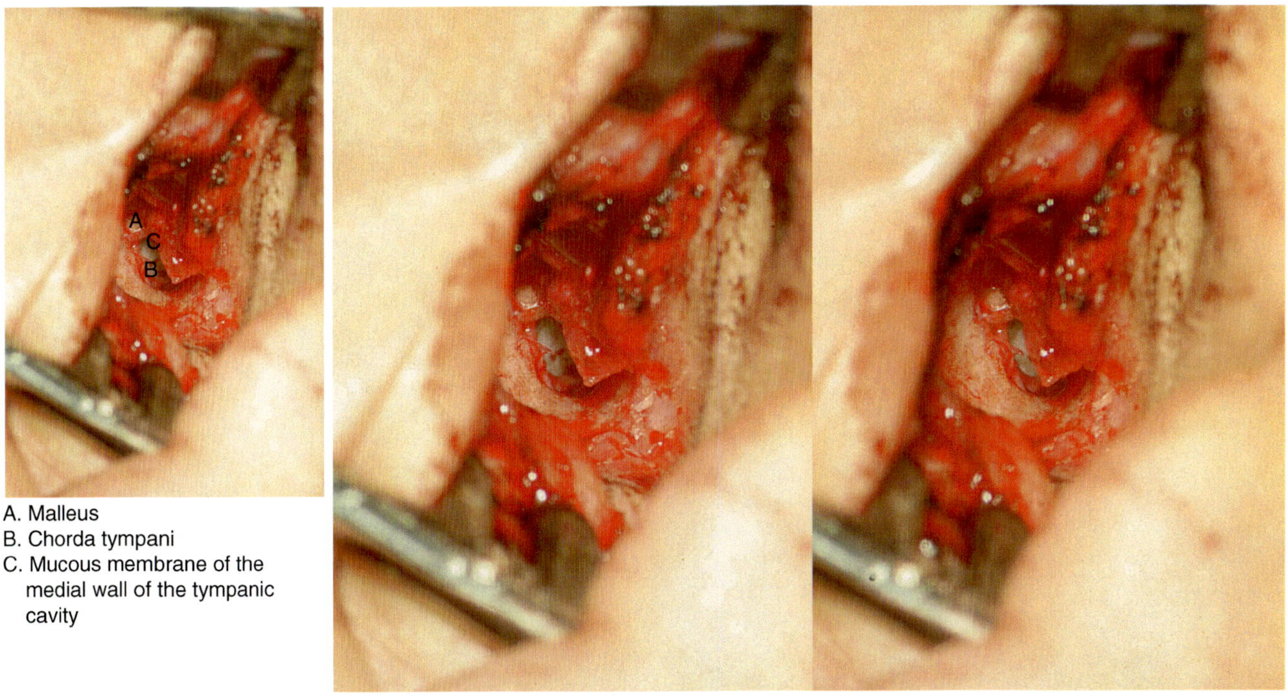

A. Malleus
B. Chorda tympani
C. Mucous membrane of the medial wall of the tympanic cavity

Fig. 4.97 Expose the tympanic cavity
Elevate the EAC skin and tympanic membrane flap from the second incision along posterior wall of the canal. Elevate the fibrous annulus from posterior, reflecting the tympanomeatal flap in an anterior-inferior direction to expose the tympanic cavity. The malleus, incus and chorda tympani passing between them in a posterior-inferior to antero-superior direction can be seen

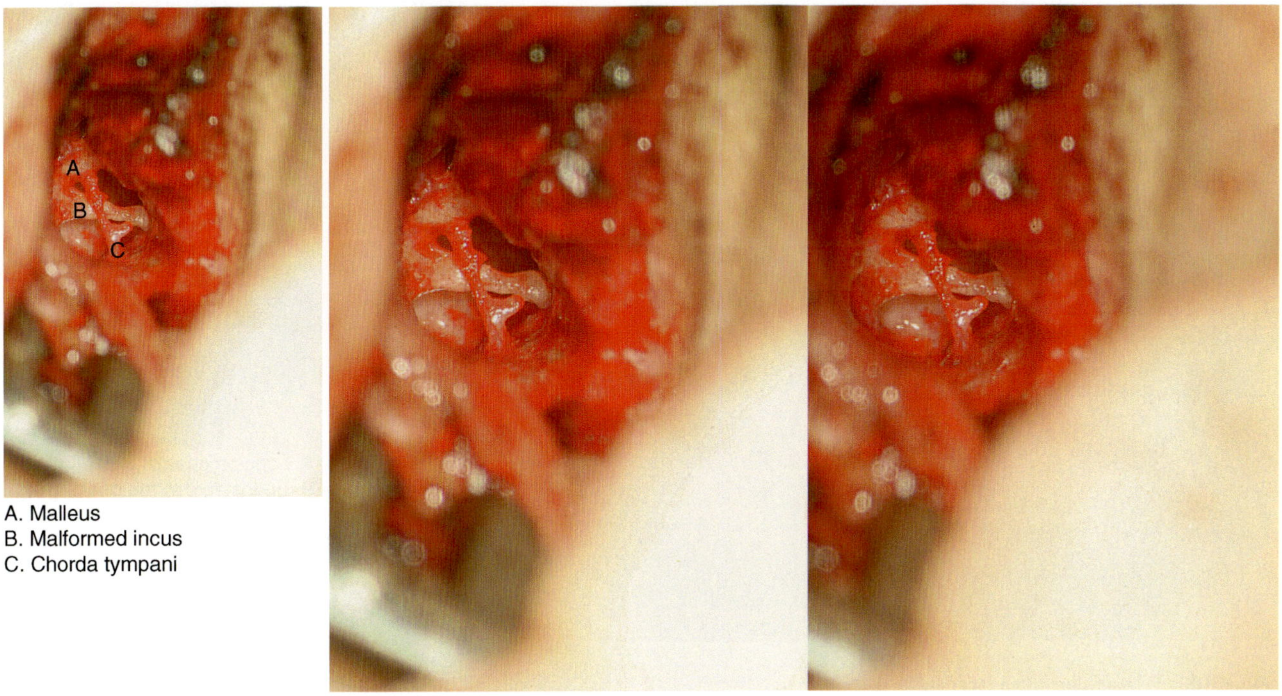

A. Malleus
B. Malformed incus
C. Chorda tympani

Fig. 4.98 Assess the ossicles
Curette or chisel part of the postero-superior wall of the bony EAC to provide a better view of the structures in the tympanic cavity. In this case, the long process of the incus was significantly longer than normal and fixed to the inferior wall of the tympanic cavity. The whole incus is fixed. The stapes and oval window were underdeveloped. The malleus and incus had little mobility

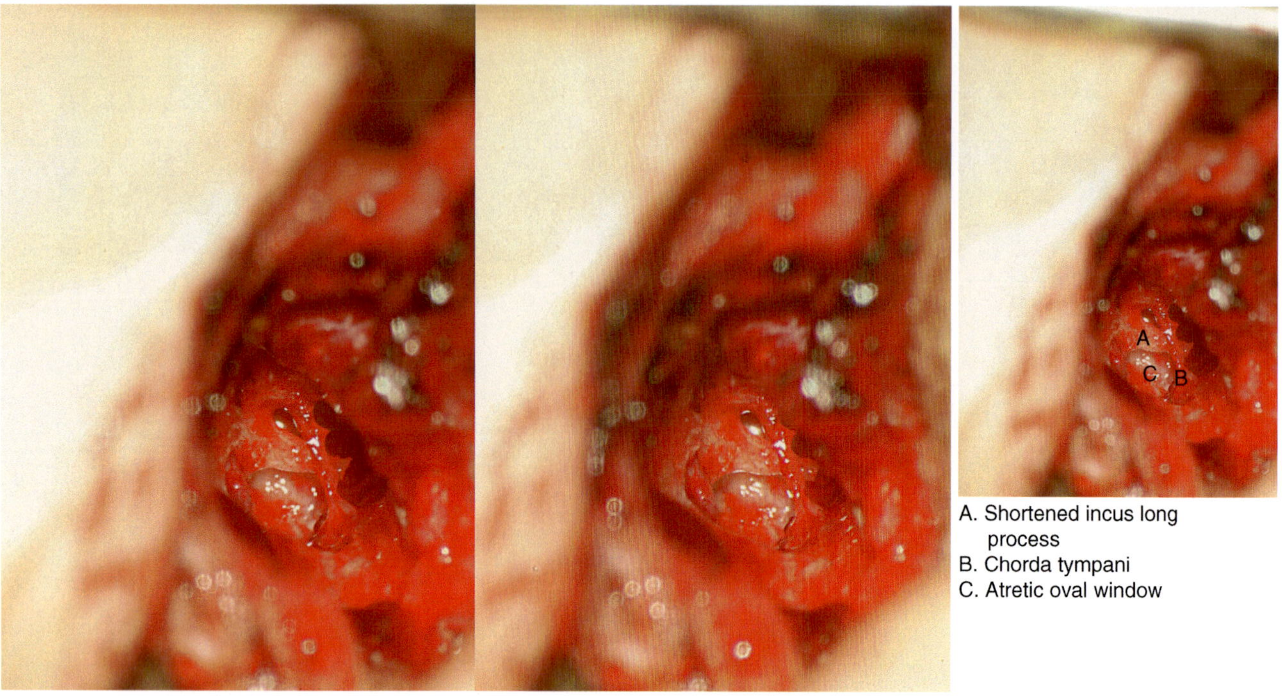

A. Shortened incus long process
B. Chorda tympani
C. Atretic oval window

Fig. 4.99 Shorten the long process of the incus
Cut the fixed tip of the incus long process. The movement of malleus and incus improved dramatically

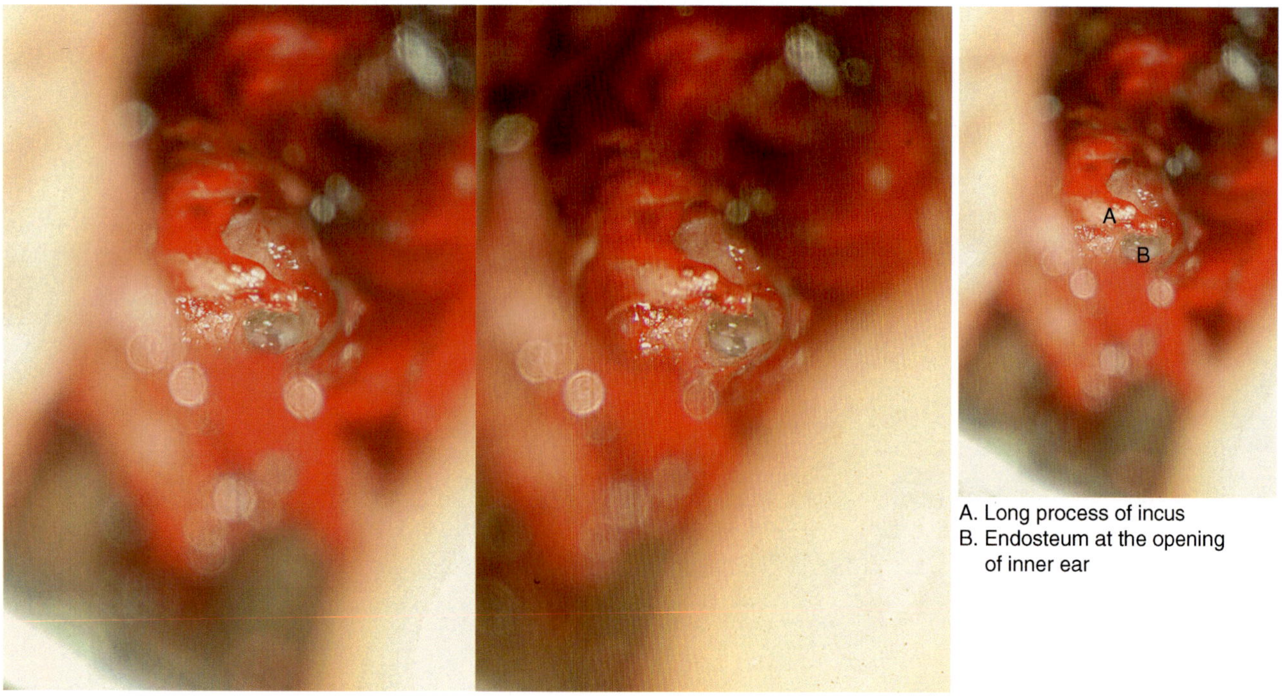

A. Long process of incus
B. Endosteum at the opening of inner ear

Fig. 4.100 Fenestration of the inner ear
Cut the chorda tympani in advance to avoid its damage with the drill. Open window with micro-drill in the area of the promontory inferior to the vestibular window niche or overhanging facial nerve

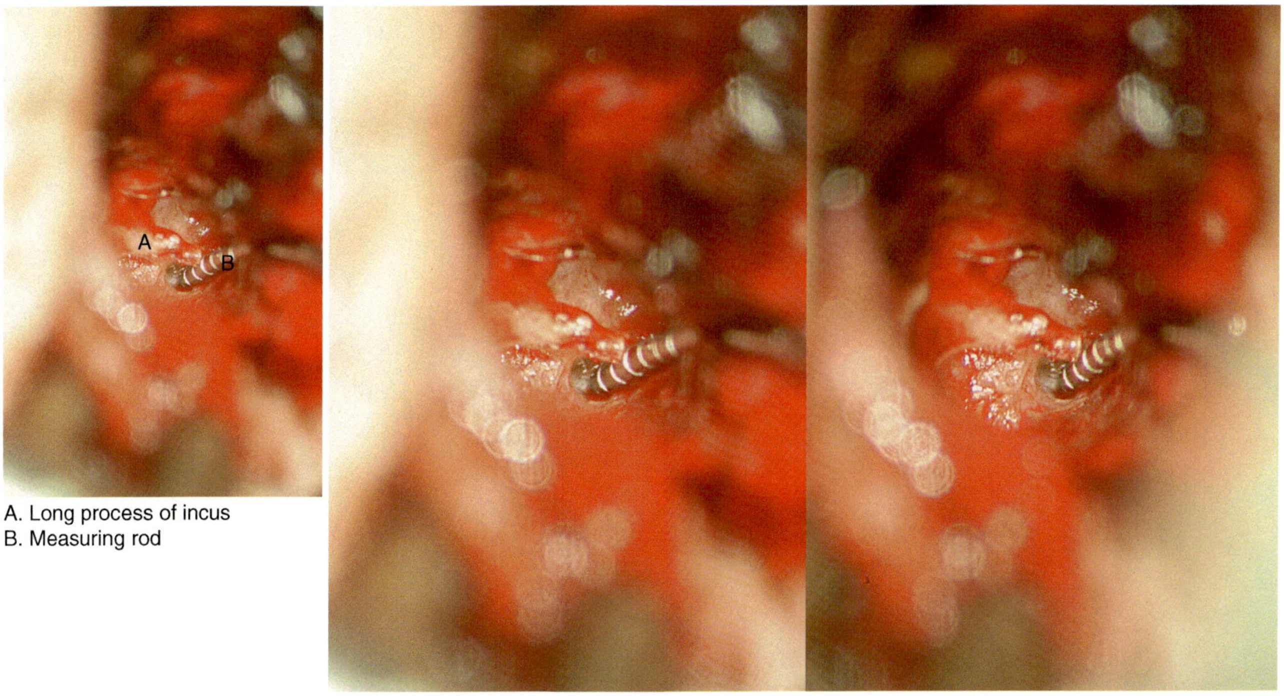

Fig. 4.101 Measure the distance between the incus and the inner ear window
Measure the distance from the center of the inner ear window to the medial aspect of incus long process with a measuring rod, then trim the prosthesis to the appropriate length

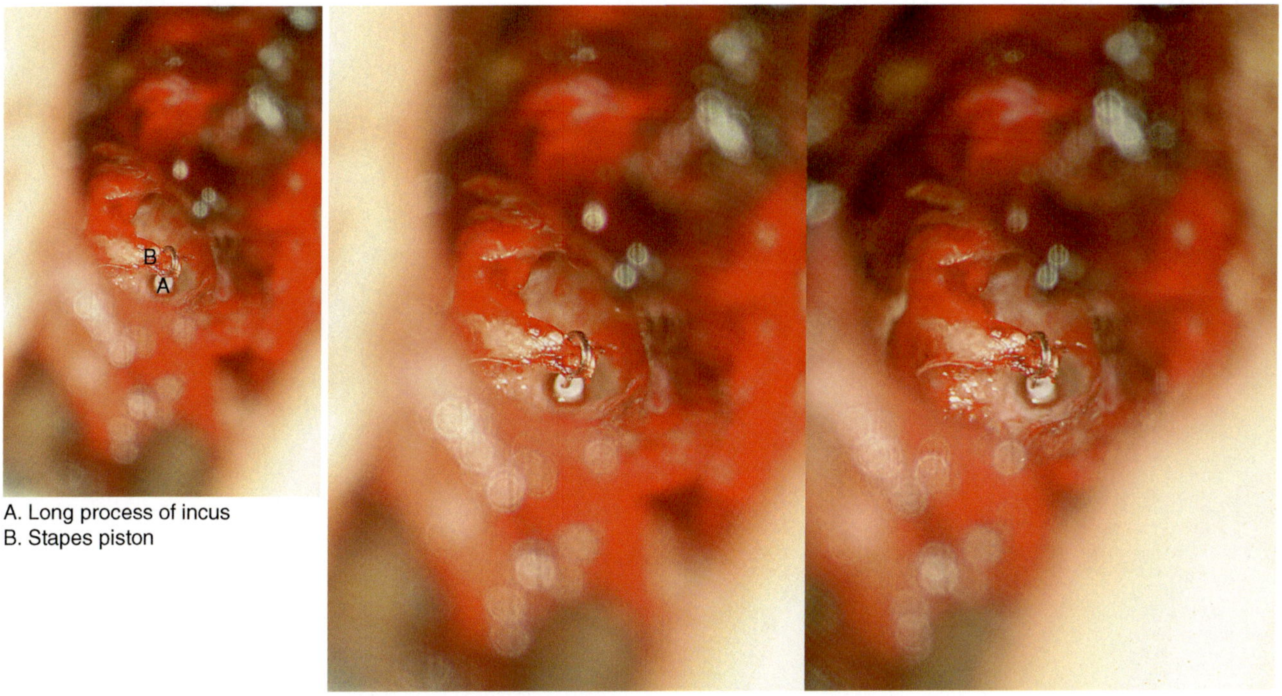

Fig. 4.102 Implantation of the prosthesis
Cut prosthesis (Piston) to the measured length between the center of the open window and the medial aspect of incus long process. Place the hook of the piston on the long process of the incus, move the tip of the prosthesis into the open window and crimp the hook

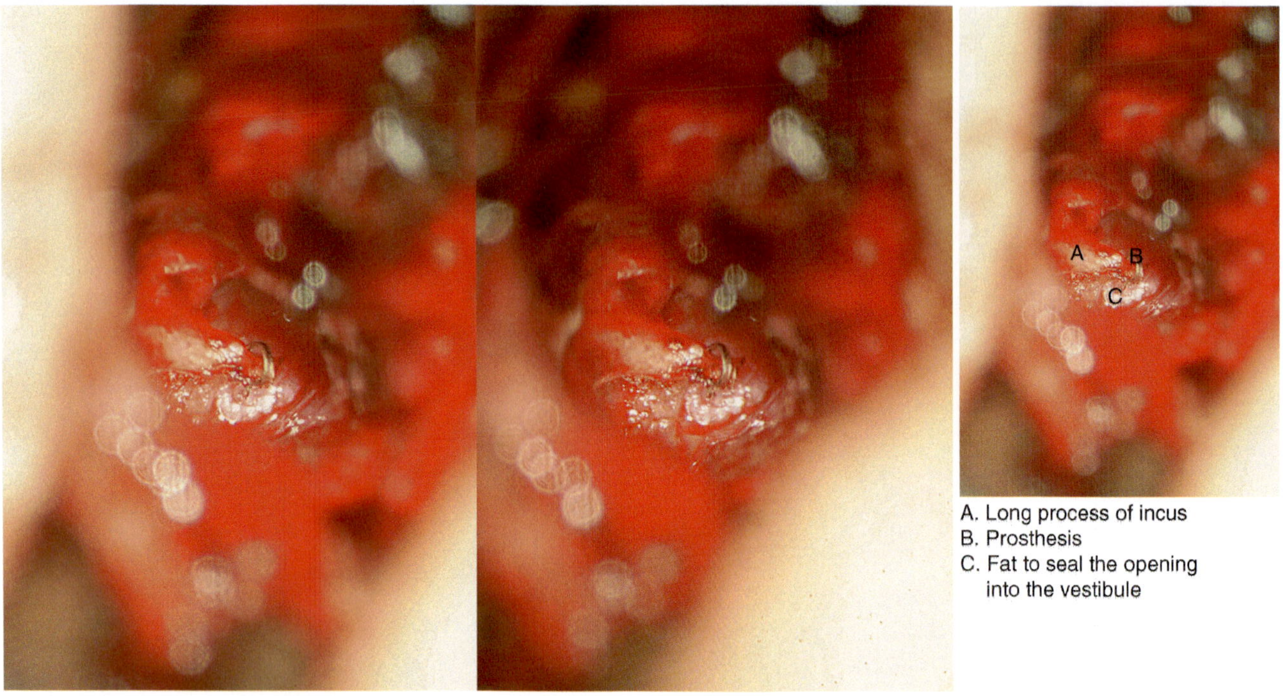

Fig. 4.103 Seal the open window of the inner ear
Use a small piece of fat to cover the edge of the open window, surrounding the shaft of the piston to prevent a perilymph leak

Surgery 2: Absence of oval window, fenestration of inner ear and ossicular reconstruction (TORP)

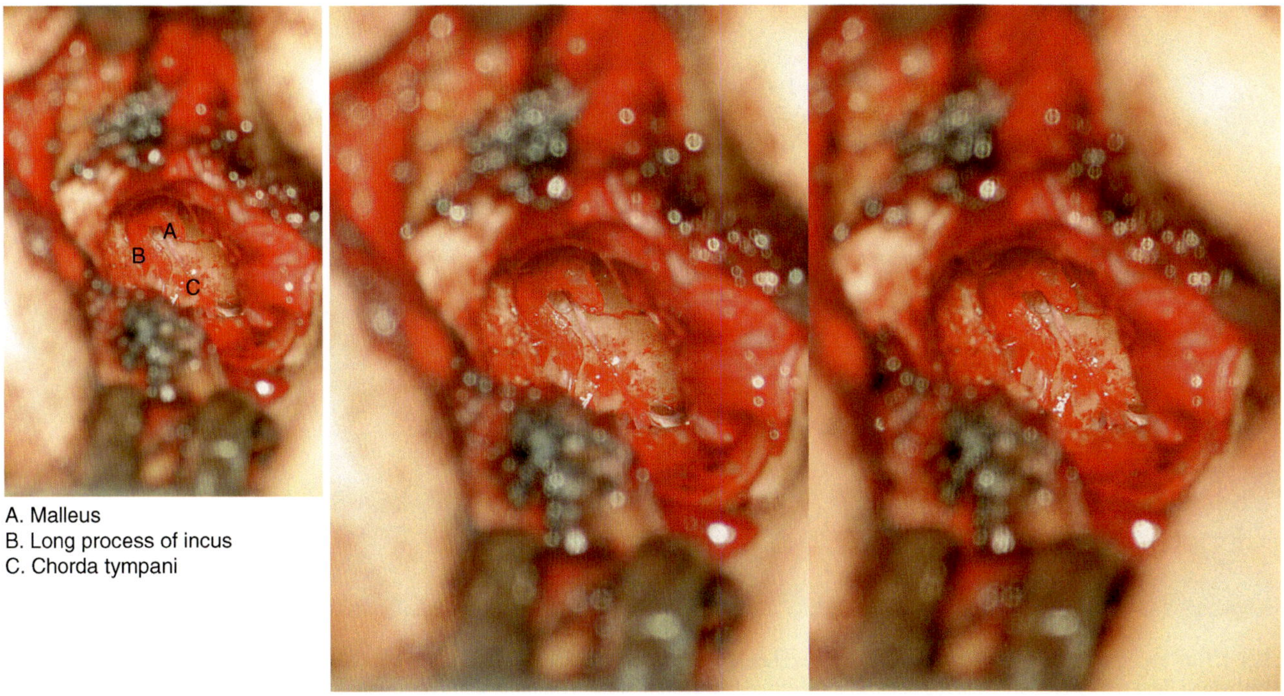

Fig. 4.104 Assess the tympanic cavity
There is an abnormal malleus and incus with normal chorda tympani. There is a stapedius tendon-like structure at the tip of incus long process and part of the round widow niche is seen postero-inferiorly on the medial wall

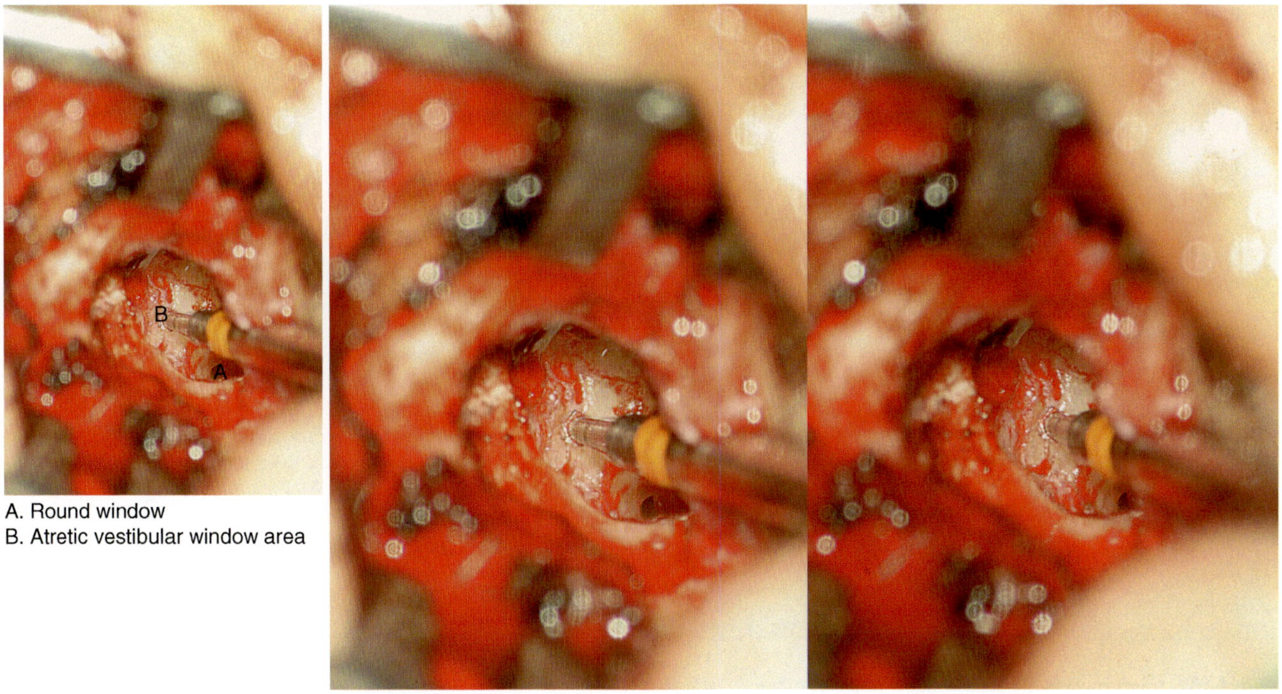

Fig. 4.105 Opening a window into the inner ear
Remove the malformed incus and malleus and the superstructures of the stapes. The vestibular window is absent. The wall of the vestibule is thick. A window is opened in to the vestibule with a micro-drill

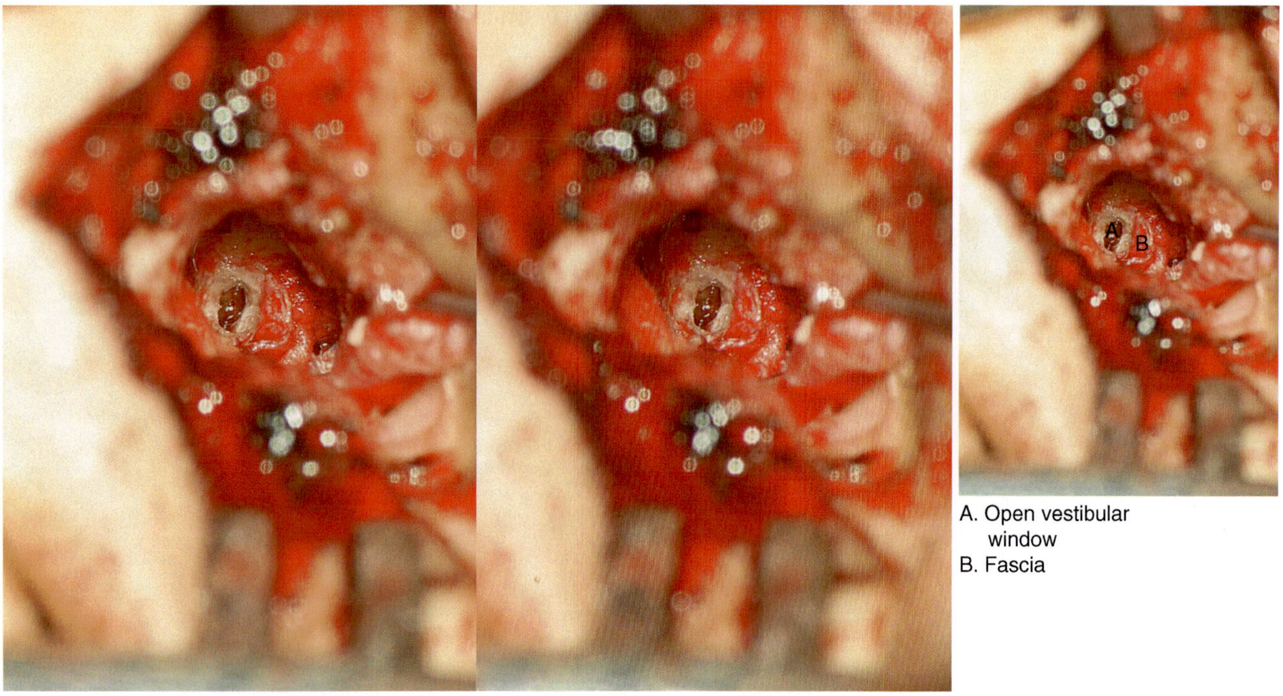

Fig. 4.106 Open a window in the lateral wall of the vestibule
Perilymph fluid can be seen through the open window in the lateral wall of the vestibule. Use a small piece of fascia to seal the open window

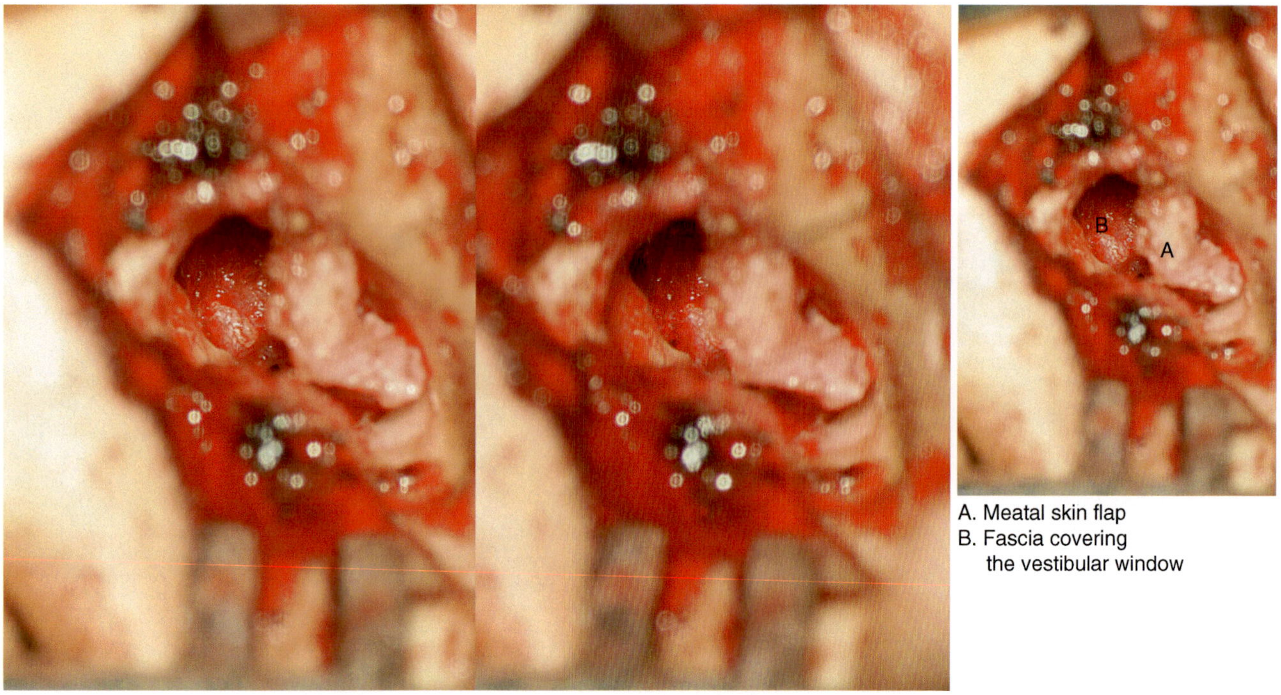

Fig. 4.107 Fascia covers the open window of the vestibule
Cover the open window of vestibule with the prepared fascia

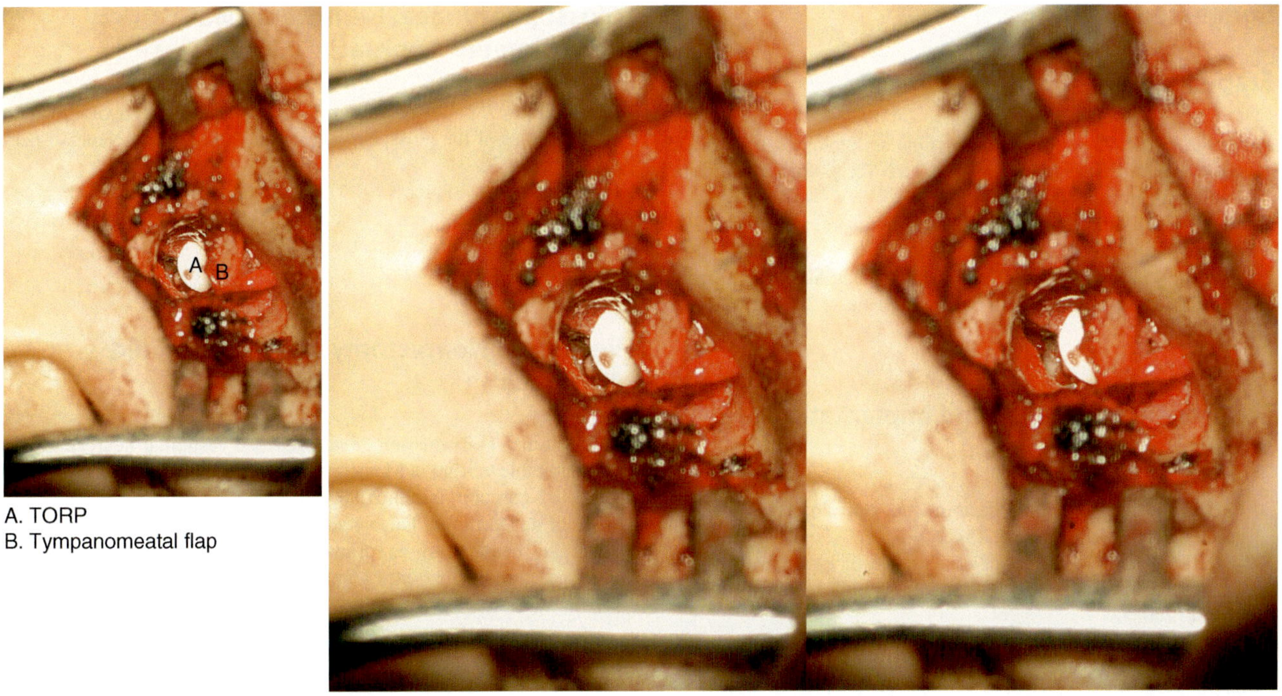

A. TORP
B. Tympanomeatal flap

Fig. 4.108 Implantation of artificial ossicle (TORP)
An artificial ossicle (TORP) is implanted into the tympanic cavity. The inner end of the stem is positioned on to the center of the fascia sealing the open window of the vestibule. The plate-like outer end will sit under the tympanic membrane

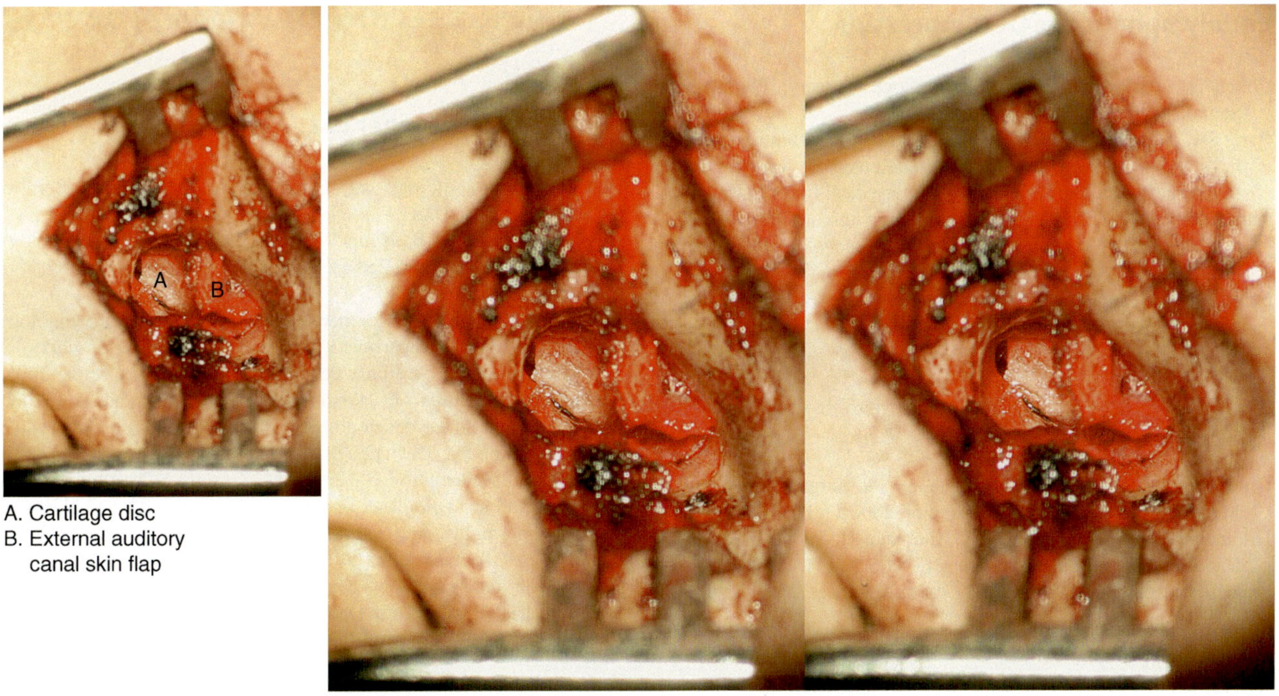

A. Cartilage disc
B. External auditory canal skin flap

Fig. 4.109 Implantation of artificial ossicle (TORP)
The plate-like end of artificial ossicle (TORP) connects with the tympanic membrane with the protection of a cartilage disc between them. The cartilage is important to prevent extrusion of the prosthesis

Suggested Reading

Stapedectomy

Jiang S-C, Gu R, Zheng-Min W. Otorhinolaryngology – otology. 2nd ed. Shanghai: Shanghai Scientific and Technological Education Publishing House; 2002a. p. 777–59.
Sanna M, et al. Middle Ear and Mastoid Microsurgery. Thieme; 2003. p. 335–416.
Zheng-Min W. Microsurgery of the ear. Shanghai: Shanghai Scientific and Technological Education Publishing House; 2004. p. 141–9.

Fenestration of Stapes and Implantation of Stapes Prosthesis

Al-Qahtani M, Hagr A. Stapedectomy in tympanosclerosis, hearing results. Saudi Med J. 2008;29(5):760–2.
Huang X-Z, Wang J-B, Kong W-J. Practice of otorhinolaryngology head and neck surgery. 2nd ed. Beijing: People's Medical Publishing House; 2008a.
Jiang S-C, Yang W-Y, Gu R. Operative surgery of otorhinolaryngology head and neck Department. 2nd ed. The complete works of operative surgery. Beijing: People's Military Medical Press; 2005.
Parrilla C, Galli J, Fetoni AR, et al. Erbium: yttrium-aluminum-garnet laser stapedotomy a safe technique. Otolaryngol Head Neck Surg. 2008;138(4):507–12.

Endolymphatic Sac Decompression

Coker NJ, Jenkins HA. Atlas of otologic surgery. Philadelphia: Saunders; 2001.
Jiang S-C, Yang W-J, Gu R. Operative surgery of otorhinolaryngology head and neck Department. 2nd ed. The complete works of operative surgery. Beijing: People's Military Medical Press; 2005.
Jiang S-C, Gu R, Zheng-Min W. Otorhinolaryngology – otology. 2nd ed. Shanghai: Shanghai Scientific and Technological Education Publishing House; 2002b.
Sanna M, et al. The temporal bone a maunal for dissection and surgical apporaches. New York: Thieme; 2005.

Transmastoid Labyrinthectomy

Ghossaini SN, Wazen JJ. An update on the surgical treatment of Meniere's diseases. J Am Acad Audiol. 2006;17(1):38–44.
Hildmann H. Labyrinthectomy. In: Hildmann H, Sudhoff H, editors. Middle ear surgery. Berlin: Springer; 2006. p. 156–7.
Sajjadi H, Paparella MM. Meniere's disease. Lancet. 2008;372(9636): 406–14.

Glossopharyngeal Neurotomy via Retrosigmoid Approach

Taha JM, Tew JM. Long-term results of surgical treatment of idiopathic neuralgias of the glosspharyngeal and vagal nerves. Neurosurgery. 1995;36:926–31.
Teixeira MJ, de Siqueira SRDT, Bor-Seng-Shu E. Glossopharygeal neuralgia: neurosurgical treatment and differential diagnosis. Acta Neurochir(Wien). 2008;150:471–47.

Vestibular Neurectomy via Retrosigmoid Approach

Li C-S, Lai J-T. Evaluation of retrosigmoid vestibular neurectomy for intractable vertigo in Meniere's disease: an interdisciplinary review. Acta Neurochir(Wien). 2008;150:655–61.
Pareschi R, Destito D, Falco Raucci A, Righini S. Posterior fossa vestibular neurectomy as primary surgical treatment of Meniere's disease:are-evaluation. J Larynngol Otol. 2002;116:593–69.

Cochlear Implantation

Han D-M. Cochlear implant. Beijing: People's Medical Publishing House; 2003.
Jackler RK, Brackmann DE. Neurotology. 2nd ed. Philadelphia: C.V. Mosby; 2005. p. 1301–22.
Papsin BC, Gordon KA. Cochlear implants for children with severe-to-profound hearing loss. N Engl J Med. 2007;357(23):2380–7.

Fenestration of Inner Ear

Han D-Y. Nerve otology and Lateral skull base surgery. Beijing: Science Press; 2008.
Huang X-Z, Wang J-B, Kong W-J. Practice of otorhinolaryngology head and neck surgery. 2nd ed. Beijing: People's Medical Publishing House; 2008b.
Jiang S-C, Yang W-Y, Gu R. Operative surgery of otorhinolaryngology head and neck Department. 2nd ed. The complete works of Operative Surgery. Beijing: People's Military Medical Press; 2005.
Kountakis SE, Helidonis E, Jahrsdoerfer RA. Microtia grade as an indicator of middle ear development in aural atresia. Arch Otolaryngol Head Neck Surg. 1995;121(8):885–6.
Morimitsu T, Matsumoto I, Takahashi M, Komune S. Vestibular fenestration and stapedioplasty in congenital stapes and vestibular window abnormality. Arch Otorhinolaryngol. 1980;226(1–2):27–33.
Pau HW, Just T, Dommerich S, Behrend D. Temporal bone investigations on landmarks for conventional or endosteal insertion of cochlear electrodes. Acta Otolaryngol. 2007;127(9):920–6.

Lateral Skull Base Surgery

5

Dong-yi Han, Vincent C Cousins, Guo-jian Wang, Wei-dong Shen, Yi-hui Zou, Jun Liu, Shi-ming Yang, Jia-nan Li, Wei-ju Han, and Pu Dai

Removal of Facial Nerve Tumor and Hypoglossal-Facial Anastomosis

Guo-jian Wang and Dong-yi Han

Indications

Facial nerve trunk defect from the facial nerve tumor removal with distal stump available

Contraindications

1. The facial muscle has lost its tension due to atrophy and fibrosis; fibrillation potential disappears in the electromyogram (EMG).
2. Patient unable to undergo surgery.
3. Professional voice users who need flexible tongue movement.

Operative Procedures

Body position: Supine position, affected ear side up.

1. Exposure and resection of the facial nerve lesion – different approaches will be required depending on the location of lesions.
2. A post-auricular incision is performed and is extended inferiorly from the mastoid tip to the level of the superior margin of thyroid cartilage along the anterior border of the sternocleidomastoid muscle, keeping the greater auricular nerve intact.
3. Separate the sternocleidomastoid and parotid, expose the mastoid tip, and then use blunt dissection technique to separate the soft tissue in front of the mastoid tip to find the trunk of facial nerve. Divide and cut the trunk as close to the stylomastoid foramen as possible.
4. The sternocleidomastoid is retracted backwards, to expose the facial vein which will be found at the level of hyoid, and then the vein is ligated. The posterior belly of the digastric muscle is retracted upwards to expose the internal and external carotid arteries and the jugular vein. The hypoglossal nerve passes between the arteries and the vein.
5. Divide the trunk of the hypoglossal nerve and its descending limb. Cut the trunk as far distal as possible.
6. An end-to-end anastomosis of the hypoglossal nerve and facial nerve is performed under the microscope. A 9–0 monofilament suture is used to join the nerve sheaths with 4–6 stitches around the circumference. The proximal end of the hypoglossal nerve trunk is anastomosed to the distal end of the facial nerve. The proximal end of the descending branch of the hypoglossal nerve is anastomosed to the distal end of its trunk.
7. Prior to the anastomosis of the main nerves, a short segment of intact vein is placed over the hypoglossal nerve to later slide over the joined nerves to support the anastomosis and prevent the growth of the granulation tissue into it. The vein must have a greater diameter than the nerves to allow for swelling and avoid compression.
8. The cavity is liberally irrigated, any bleeding is controlled. A drain is inserted, the wound is closed and a dressing is applied.

D.-y. Han, MD (✉) • G.-j. Wang, MD • W.-d. Shen, MD
Y.-h. Zou, MD • J. Liu, MD • S.-m. Yang, MD • J.-n. Li, MD
W.-j. Han, MD • P. Dai, MD (✉)
Department of Otolaryngology Head and Neck Surgery, Chinese PLA General Hospital, Beijing 100853, China
e-mail: hdy301@263.net; daipu301@vip.sina.com

V.C Cousins, MBBS, FRACS (✉)
Department of Ear Nose and Throat Surgery, Alfred Hospital, Melbourne, Australia
e-mail: vccousins@iinet.net.au

P. Dai et al. (eds.), *Stereo Operative Atlas of Micro Ear Surgery*, DOI 10.1007/978-981-10-2089-6_5

Special Comments

1. The nerves should not be compressed with forceps or traumatized directly with suction.
2. There are three forms of anastomosis of the hypoglossal nerve and facial nerve: ① the trunk of the hypoglossal nerve is cut, and the proximal end of the hypoglossal nerve trunk is joined with distal end of the facial nerve, and the proximal end of the hypoglossal nerve's descending limb joined with the distal end of its trunk. This is the commonest procedure; ② the descending limb of the hypoglossal nerve is cut, and its proximal end is joined to the distal end of the facial nerve; ③ 1/3–1/2 of the trunk of the hypoglossal nerve is cut diagonally and joined to the distal end of the facial nerve.
3. There are three methods to locate the facial nerve trunk near the stylomastoid foramen: ① the stylomastoid foramen can be found in front of the site where the posterior belly of the digastric muscle attaches to the mastoid; ② the trunk can be found passing forwards about 1 cm deep to the tympanomastoid suture; ③ the trunk of facial nerve runs along the line passing vertically through the middle point between the mastoid tip and inner edge of tragus cartilage.
4. The hypoglossal nerve is located beneath the common facial vein and posterior belly of digastric muscle and it always runs along the lingual artery. These are the three reliable landmarks for identifying the hypoglossal nerve.
5. It is very important to keep the nerve anastomosis free of any tension for the best nerve regrowth. If necessary, the mastoid tip can be drilled off to expose more of the facial nerve and give adequate length.
6. The hypoglossal and facial nerves should be sectioned in such a way that the cut ends have a similar size for better anastomosis.
7. The nerve sutures should be through the sheath only, and not through nerve bundles to avoid scar formation inside the nerve. If the nerve is too thin, the peripheral connective tissue can be sutured loosely and fibrin glue can be used to support the anastomosis.

Complications

1. Conductive deafness due to the direct injury of the tympanic membrane and/or the ossicular chain.
2. Sensorineural hearing impairment due to direct injury to the inner ear or drill contact with the incus transmitting intense vibration to the inner ear.
3. Vertigo due to injury of the semicircular canals or vestibule.
4. Synkinetic movements of the face where unintentional movement of one group of facial muscles occurs with voluntary movement of another group. This is one of the complications of nerve regeneration but can be reduced with effective physical therapy.
5. Facial spasm due to the re-innervation of facial muscle. It may vary from mild flickering of the eyelid to severe spasm and is often permanent.
6. Crocodile tears syndrome due to the lacrimal gland (normally innervated by the greater superficial petrosal nerve) being reinnervated by the salivary gland secretomotor nerve.
7. Permanent facial paralysis due to irreversible nerve degeneration. This may require other facial reanimation or suspension techniques.
8. Unilateral atrophy of tongue due to sacrifice of the hypoglossal nerve.
9. Dysmasesia (Chewing difficulty) and dysphagia in a small number of patients and can be successfully treated with rehabilitation training.

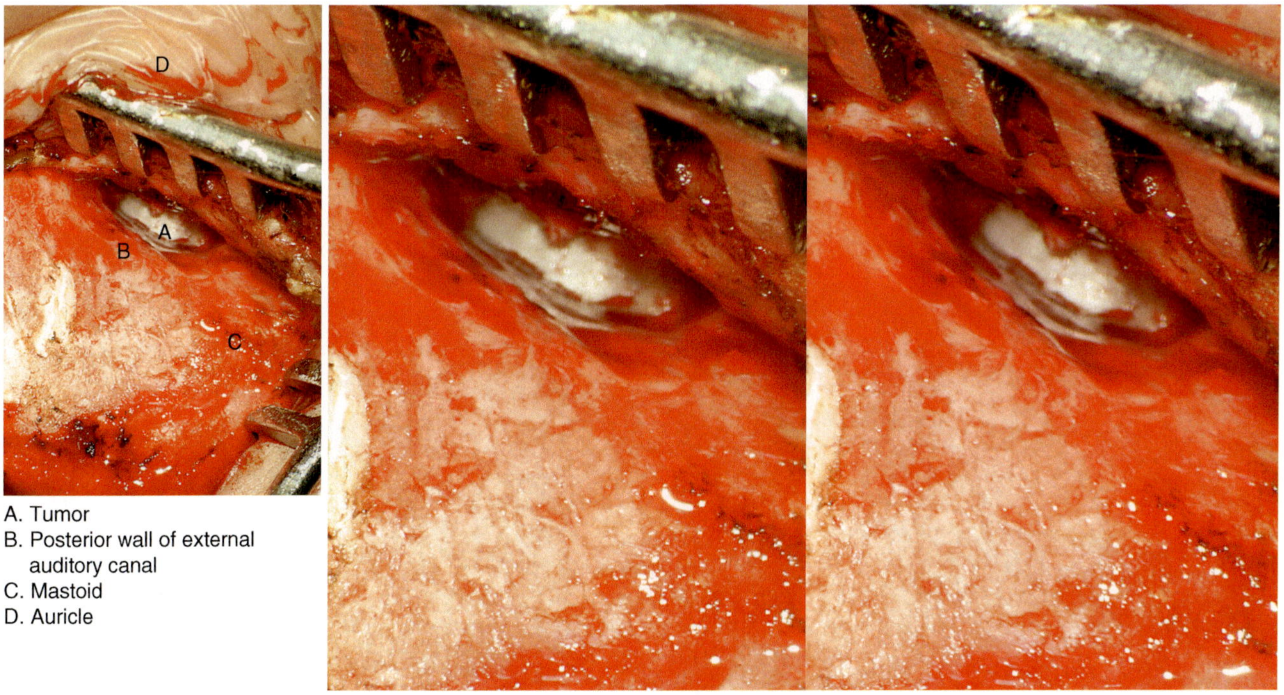

A. Tumor
B. Posterior wall of external auditory canal
C. Mastoid
D. Auricle

Fig. 5.1 Post-auricular incision, elevate the tympano- meatal flaps forward and expose the tumor
A C-shaped incision, 0.5 cm behind the post-auricular sulcus is performed; skin and subcutaneous tissue are separated to expose the cortex of the mastoid, root of zygoma and posterior and inferior walls of the external auditory canal. The bone of the external auditory canal is eroded, and its inner part is occupied by a tumor whose envelope is intact

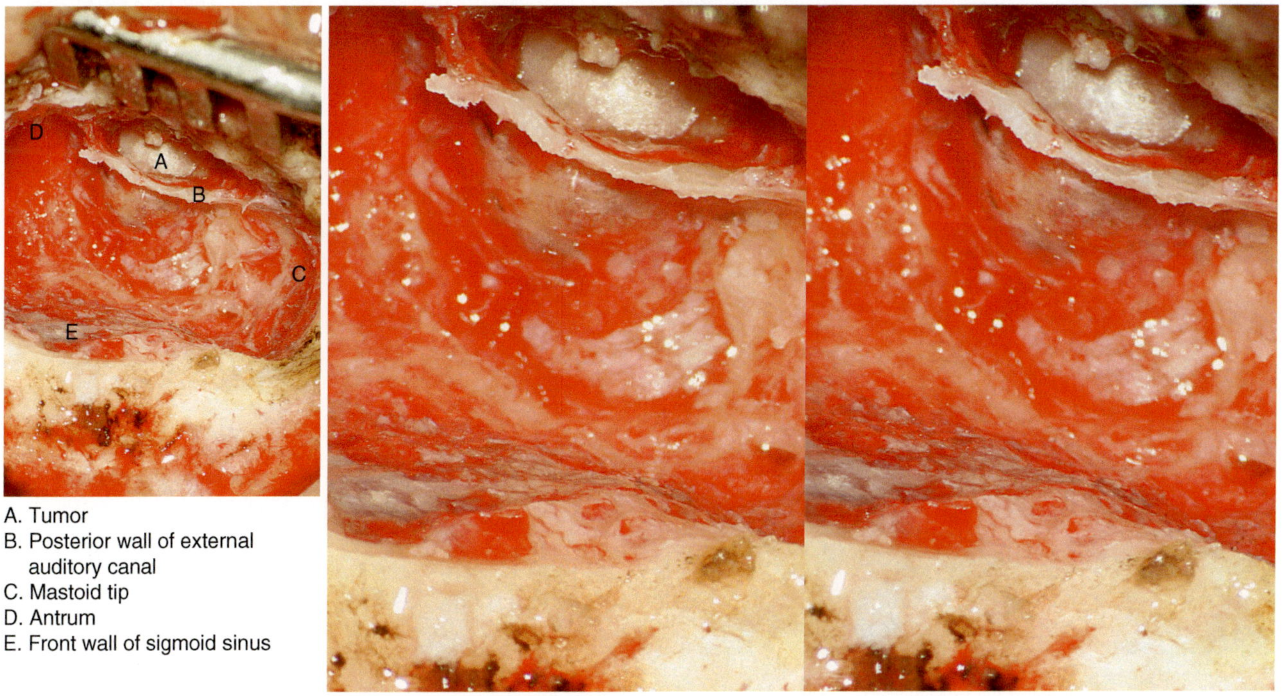

A. Tumor
B. Posterior wall of external auditory canal
C. Mastoid tip
D. Antrum
E. Front wall of sigmoid sinus

Fig. 5.2 Exposure of the antrum and mastoid cavity
Remove the cortex and cells of the mastoid and expose the tympanic sinus and mastoid cavity. The front of the mastoid cavity has been damaged by tumor. After being separated, the tumor is found to penetrate the back wall of external auditory canal and reach the back margin of the parotid

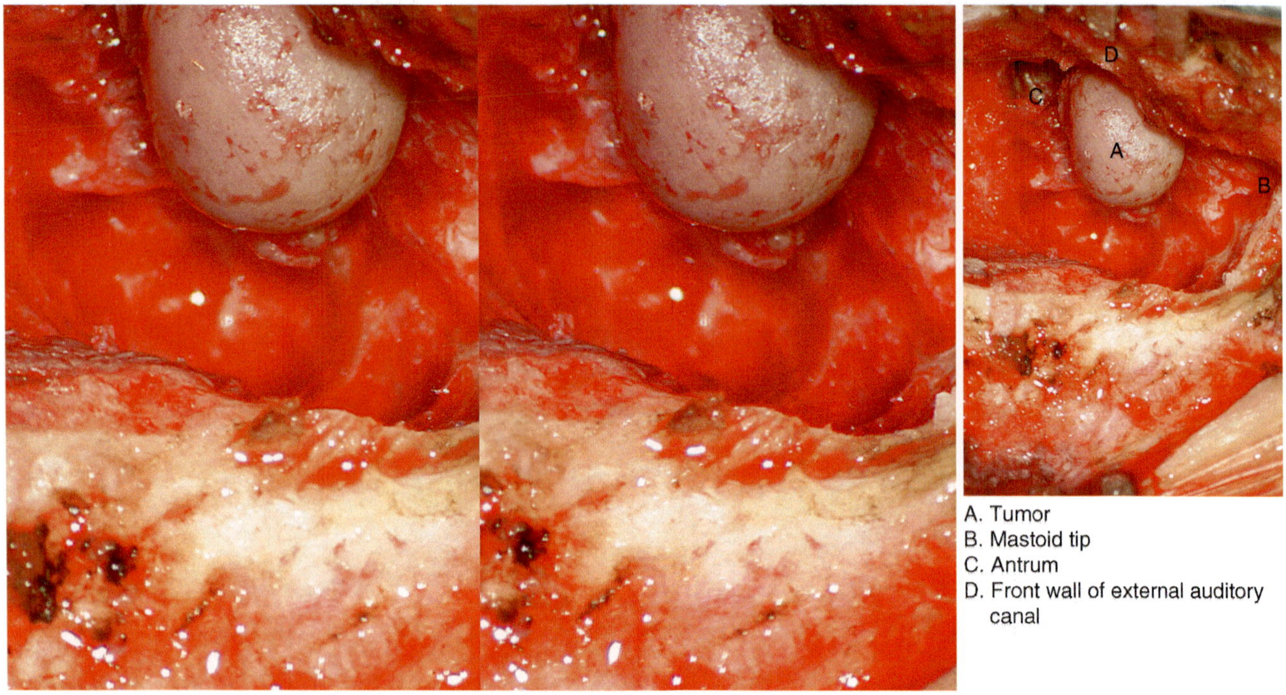

A. Tumor
B. Mastoid tip
C. Antrum
D. Front wall of external auditory canal

Fig. 5.3 Remove the posterior wall of the external auditory canal, and expose the back margin of tumor
Using an electronic drill, the superior, inferior and posterior margins of the tumor are exposed. The tumor is large and occupies the inner part of external auditory canal and erodes into the mastoid

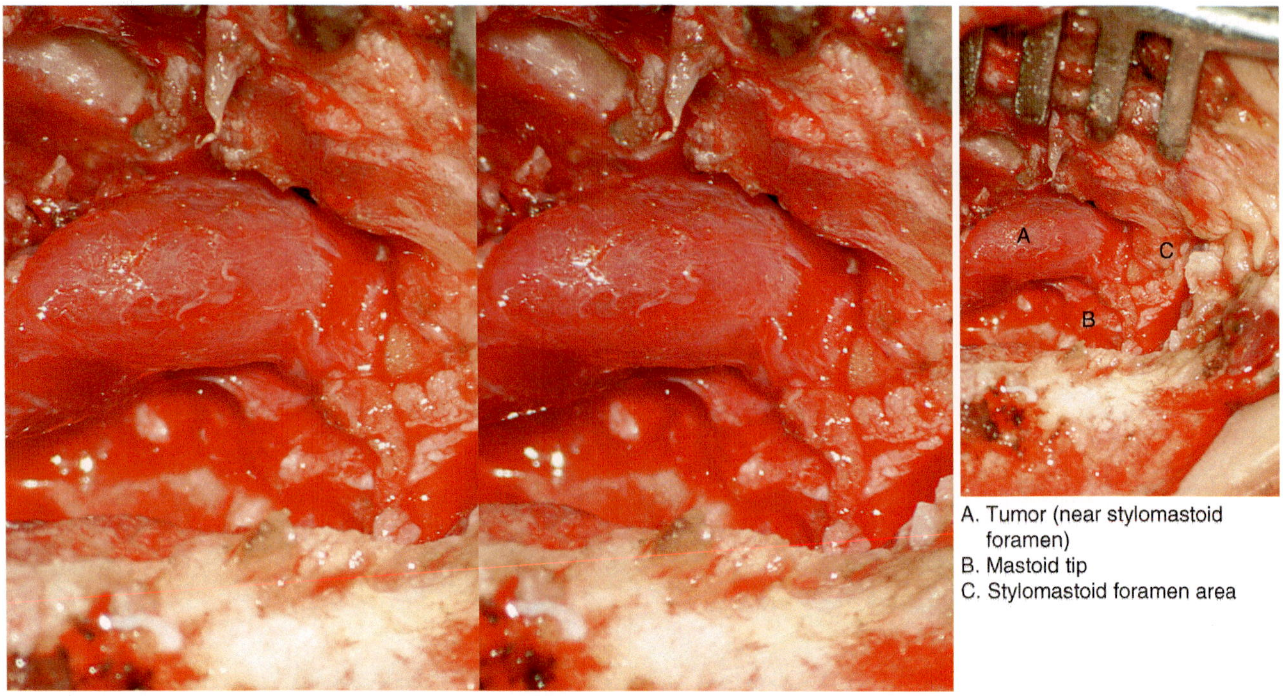

A. Tumor (near stylomastoid foramen)
B. Mastoid tip
C. Stylomastoid foramen area

Fig. 5.4 Remove the bone of the inferior wall of external auditory canal and the mastoid tip
Remove the bone of the inferior wall of external auditory canal and the mastoid tip to identify the lower part of the tumor which has reached the parotid through the stylomastoid foramen

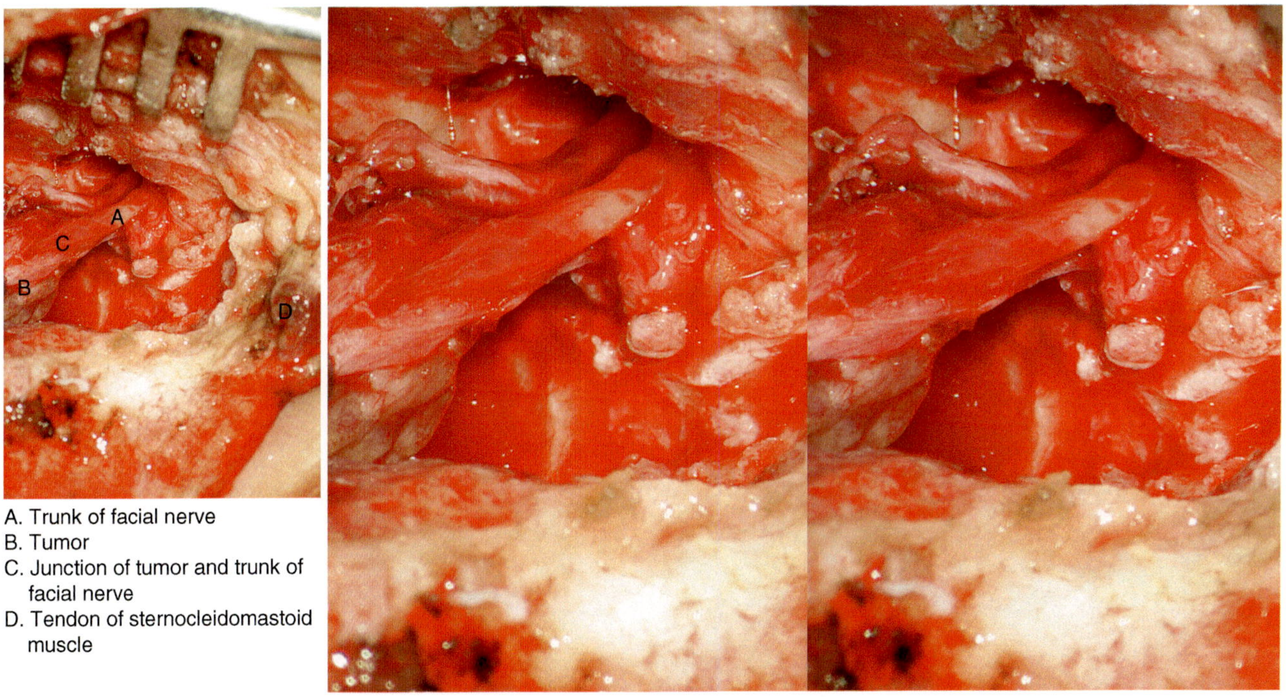

Fig. 5.5 Exposure of the inferior margin of tumor
Remove the bone near the stylomastoid foramen, and expose the inferior margin of the tumor, which is found to originate from the facial nerve. The normal facial nerve is identified just outside the stylomastoid foramen

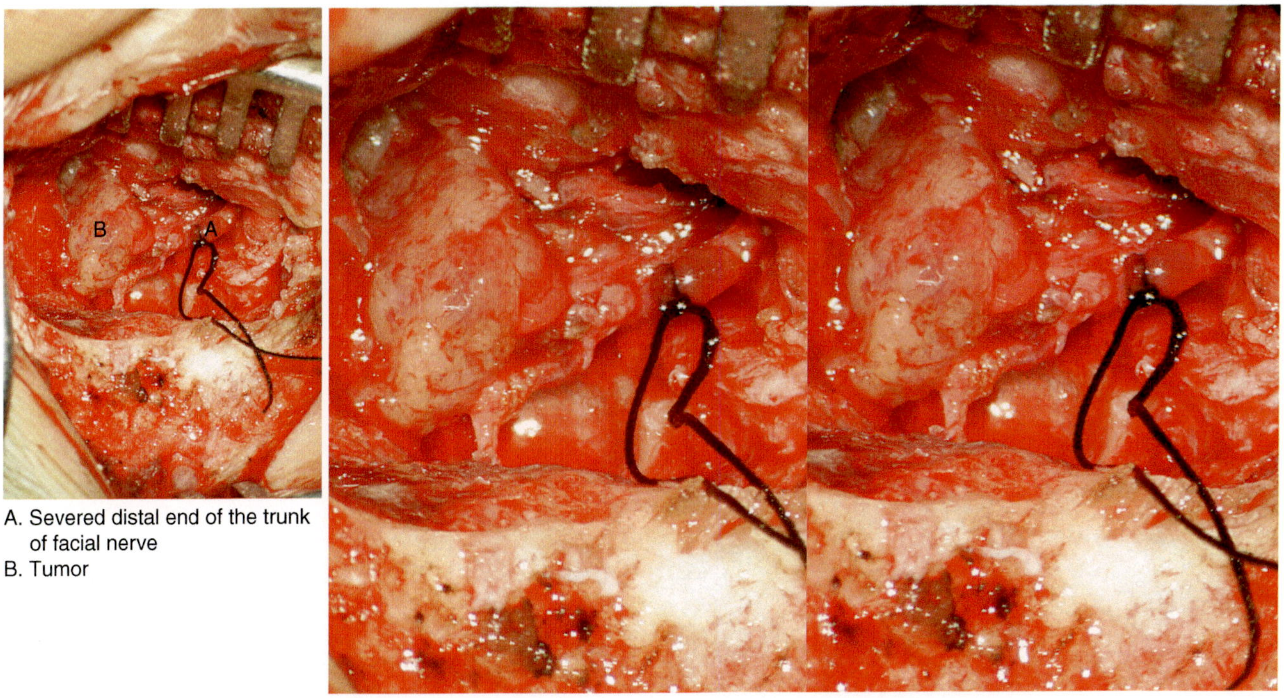

Fig. 5.6 Cut the distal end facial nerve trunk beyond the tumor
As the facial nerve cannot be preserved, the distal trunk is severed well beyond its junction with the tumor. The end is marked with thread

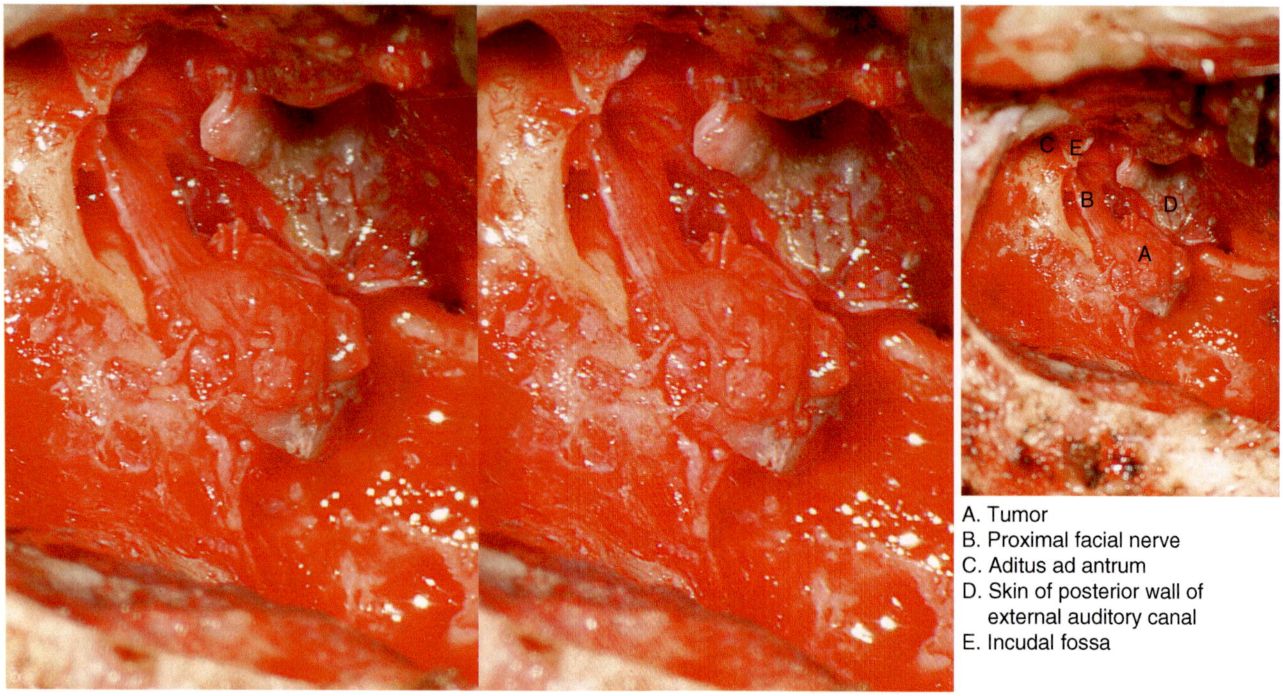

Fig. 5.7 Expose the superior margin of the tumor
Separate the soft tissue along the tumor, and expose its superior margin. The junction of the tumour and normal facial nerve is located between the horizontal and pyramidal segments

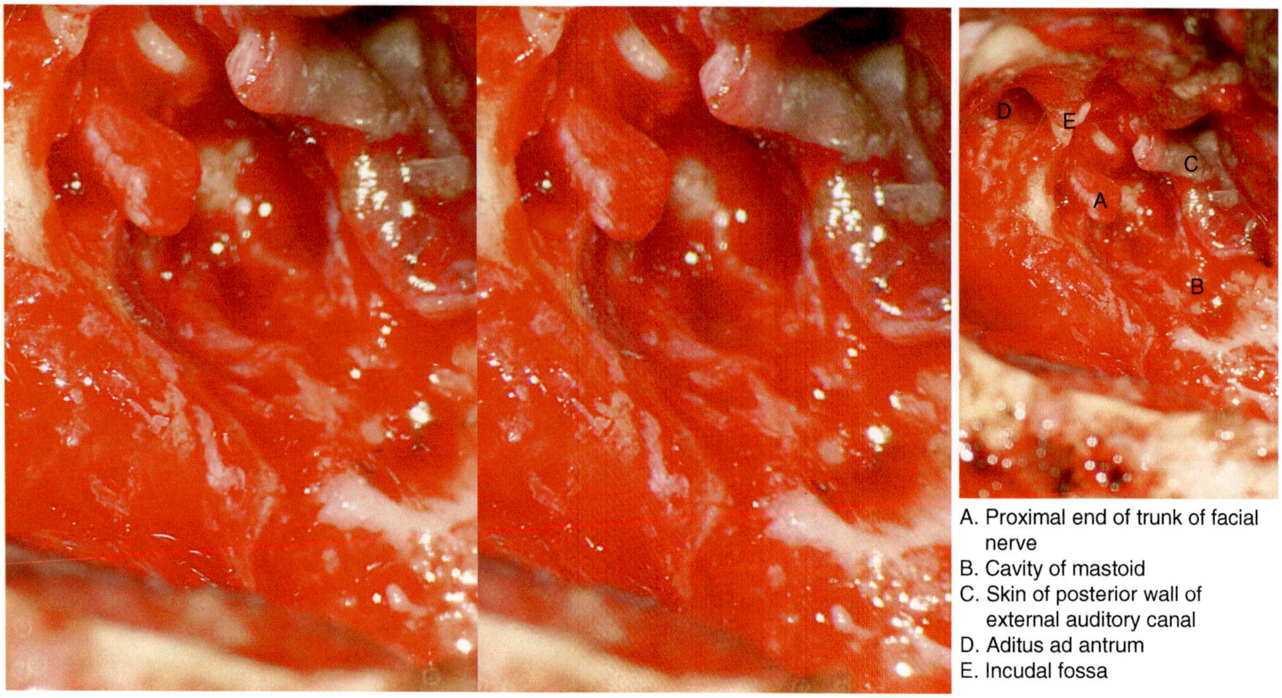

Fig. 5.8 Excise the affected proximal facial nerve and tumor
Cut the facial nerve, a little proximal to its junction with the tumor. The severed end of the horizontal segment should be diathermied or ligated unless nerve transplanting is performed. After removal of the inferior wall of external auditory canal, there is a large cavity, but the tympanic membrane and ossicles can be left intact

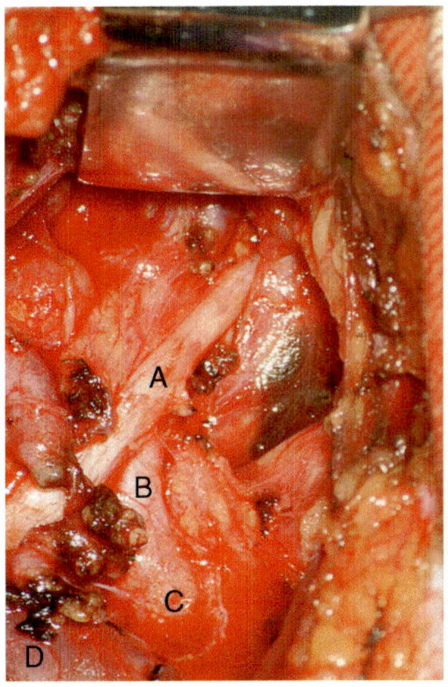

A. Hypoglossal nerve
B. Lingual artery
C. External carotid artery
D. Jugular vein

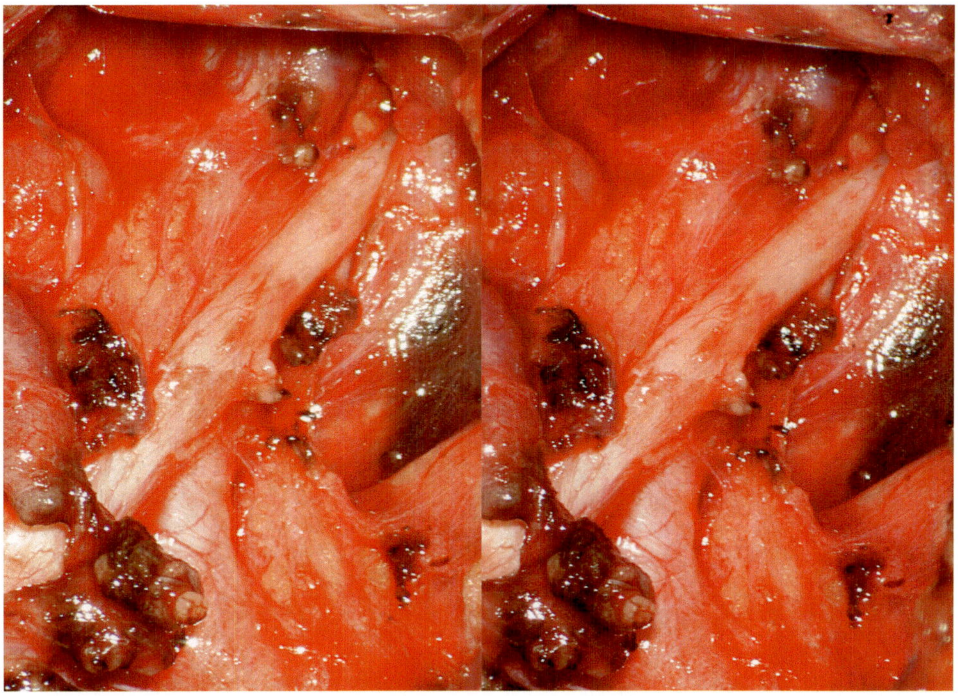

Fig. 5.9 Extend the incision, separate the trunk of hypoglossal nerve
Extend the incision inferiorly along the anterior margin of sternocleidomastoid muscle, expose and ligate the facial vein. Retract the sternocleidomastoid and posterior belly of digastric muscles, beneath which there is the hypoglossal nerve passing forwards and downwards near the lingual artery

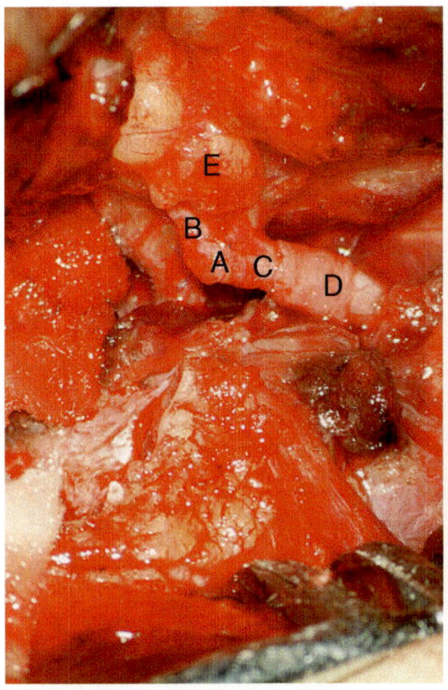

A. Anastomosis of hypoglossal nerve and facial nerve
B. Distal end of facial nerve
C. Proximal end of hypoglossal nerve
D. Segment of vein
E. Parotid

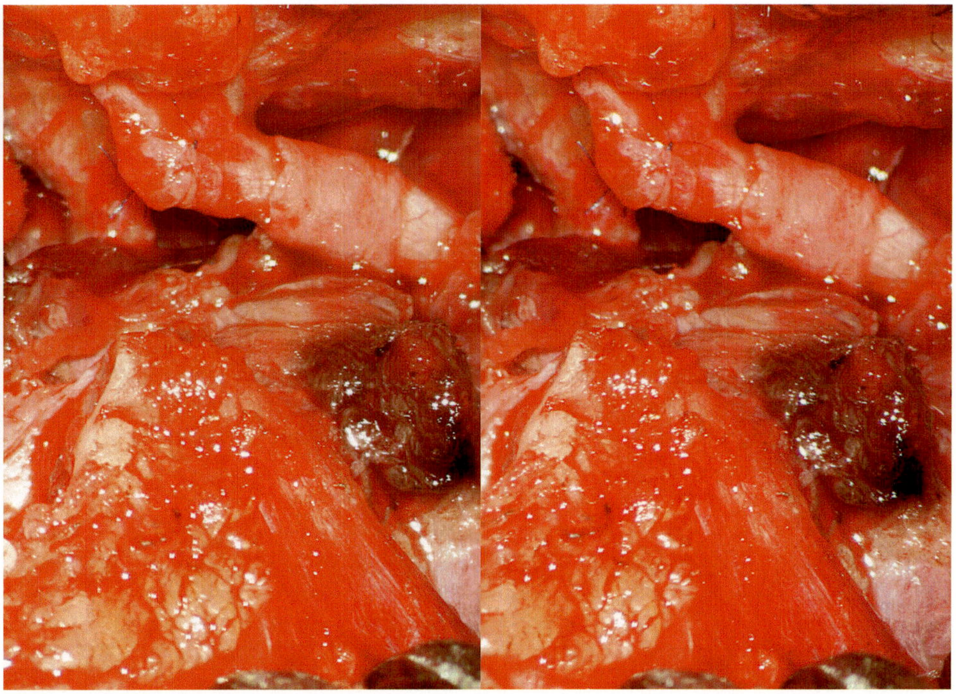

Fig. 5.10 Anastomosis of hypoglossal nerve and facial nerve
Separate the trunk of the hypoglossal nerve and its descending limb. Cut the trunk as far distal as possible. The proximal end of hypoglossal nerve trunk is anastomosed to the distal end of facial nerve under the microscope. A 9–0 monofilament suture is used to join the nerve sheaths using 4–6 stitches. A segment of intact vein is placed over the proximal hypoglossal nerve before the anastomosis

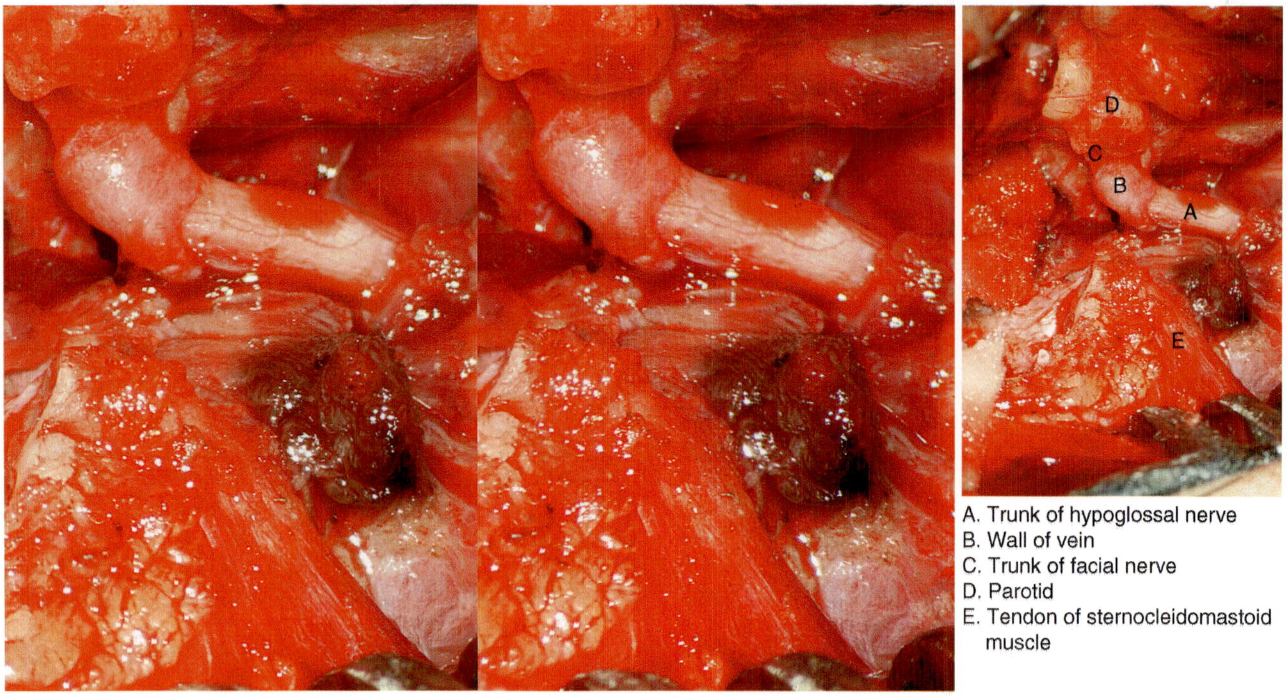

Fig. 5.11 Covering the nerve anastomosis with a segment of intact vein
After suturing, the anastomosis is surrounded with a segment of intact vein with intact wall. The aditus ad antrum and the floor of the external auditory canal are covered with a temporalis musculofascial flap. Suture the post-auricular incision in layers. Pack the mastoid cavity with gelatin sponge and iodoform gauze, and apply a dressing

CPA Microvascular Decompression (MVD) of Facial Nerve by Retrosigmoid Approach

Wei-dong Shen and Dong-yi Han

Indications

Microvascular decompression (MVD) via a retrosigmoid approach is used to elevate a compressing vascular loop from the affected facial nerve in hemifacial spasm (HFS) and Convulsive Tic Syndrome when medical control is ineffective, or the patients prepared to undergo early surgery. A primary lesion in the CPA must be excluded in all cases, such as facial muscle spasm secondary to trauma, Bell's palsy and, in rare cases, otitis media with effusion.

Contraindications

Patients unable to tolerate general anesthesia or craniotomy due to poor general health.

Operative Procedures

Microvascular decompression surgery is performed via a Retrosigmoid Approach.

1. Anesthesia and position: All MVD operations are performed under endotracheal general anesthesia. The patient is positioned supine. The head is rotated away from the side of operation.
2. Surgical incision: An anteriorly based U-shaped incision is made over the retroauricular and suboccipital region.
3. Posterior fossa craniotomy: A posterior fossa craniotomy of 4–5 cm diameter is completed in the angle between the posterior border of the sigmoid sinus and the inferior border of the transverse sinus.
4. Exposure to the cerebellopontine angle (CPA): After the bone flap is removed, the dura is incised in a curvilinear, cruciform or T-shaped fashion. Once CSF is drained from the cerebellomedullary cistern, the cerebellum should begin to retract and fall away from the petrous bone and tentorium.
   - 4.1. The most important vascular structure within the CPA is the anterior inferior cerebellar artery (AICA). It arises most commonly as a single trunk from the basilar artery. It courses posteriorly, ventromedial to the facial and vestibulocochlear nerve and takes a long loop laterally to the porus acousticus. In 15–20 % of cases, the AICA actually passes into the lumen of the internal auditory canal before turning back to the brainstem. The AICA can thus be divided into the premeatal, meatal, and postmeatal segments in its course. The main branch of the AICA passes over cranial nerves VII and VIII in only 10 % of cases. The remainder of the cases, it either passes below the VII and VIII cranial nerves or, in 25–50 % of individuals, actually passes between them. Three branches that regularly arise from the meatal segment of the AICA can be identified. Small perforating arteries supply blood to the brainstem. The subarcuate artery passes through the subarcuate fossa into the posterior surface of the temporal bone, and the third regular branch is the internal auditory artery (labyrinthine artery). Cranial nerves VII and VIII receive their blood supply from small braches of AICA.
   - 4.2. The petrosal vein (Dandy vein) drains large parts of the anterior portion of the cerebellar hemisphere and sizeable anterolateral areas of the pons and medulla oblongata to the superior or inferior petrosal sinus. It is closely related to the internal acoustic meatus and may be encountered in the area of the trigeminal nerve anterior to the porus acousticus. Obstruction of the petrosal vein can lead to bleeding, or venous infarction and cerebellar edema.
   - 4.3. The vestibulocochlear nerve root arises from the brainstem at the lateral end of the pontomedullary sulcus, immediately in front of the foramen of Luschka and the lateral recess of the fourth ventricle. The facial nerve arises in the pontomedullary sulcus 1–2 mm anterior to the point at which the vestibulocochlear nerve joins the brainstem. The vestibulocochlear and facial nerves are in close approximation at the porus. The facial nerve enters the facial canal at the anterior-superior quadrant of the lateral end of the meatus.
   - 4.4. As it leaves the brainstem, the facial nerve fibers are sheathed in oligodendroglia derived from the central nervous system. The nerve loses this covering within a few millimeters lateral to the brainstem and becomes ensheathed instead by Schwann cells. The vestibulocochlear nerve sheath is derived from oligodendroglia and extends further lateral than that of the facial nerve (about 15 mm). The junction of the oligodendroglia and Schwann cells (i.e., the Obersteiner-Redlich zone) occurs just medial to the porus acousticus. Most acoustics neuromas arise from Schwann cells in this region.
   - 4.5. The trigeminal nerve root is located superior (approx. 8 mm) to the acoustic-facial bundle and passes through the anterior superior part of CPA to reach the trigeminal ganglion on the petrous apex. The abducens nerve is located in the medial part of the CPA. It leaves the brainstem anterior-inferiorly to the facial nerve and courses along the brainstem in an anterior direction. The lower cranial nerves (the glossopharyngeal, vagus and accessory nerves) are

located inferiorly to the acoustic-facial bundle. The upper rootlets of the glossopharyngeal make contact with the vestibulocochlear nerve bundle.

5. Microvascular decompression: It is most important for a successful microvascular decompression to accurately-identify the compressing artery (offending vessel). The nerve-vessel contact area is generally located at the root exit zone (REZ) of the facial nerve in nearly all cases. This zone needs to be systematically inspected for nerve compression; paying particular attention to the PICA compression of the facial nerve inferiorly. The offending vessel may not always be seen in contact with the facial nerve as retraction of several millimeters may have occurred after the dura matter incision and drainage of CSF. A depression on the surface of the facial nerve may be a sign of nerve compression. Careful separation of the vessels, including small veins and arteries, and adherent arachnoid membrane is carried out to free the facial nerve. After identification and separation of the offending vessel, small pieces of temporalis muscle, or Teflon sponge are placed between the vessel and the REZ to prevent any further contacts.
6. Closing technique: Once hemostasis is assured, the operative field is filled with saline using a bulb syringe. Closure is performed with a running suture to the dura and the bone flap is fixed with titanium fixing rivets. The skin sutured in two layers over a subcutaneous drain.

Special Comments

1. Intraoperative monitoring of facial nerve function and of hearing with ABR improve the safety of the CPA Microvascular Decompression.
2. Correct preoperative positioning of the patient greatly assists this procedure. A block is placed under the shoulder and neck is minimally stretched with mild flexion and rotation toward the unaffected side. The table should be rotated laterally. Excess tension on the neck is avoided. The head is secured in a Mayfield headrest system.
3. To reduce the bleeding from the wound, the incision site is injected with a mixture of 2 % lidocaine with 1:1000 epinephrine and scalp clips are applied to its edges during the operation.
4. At the beginning of the bony exposure, intravenous mannitol (1.0 g/kg body weight) is administrated to achieve a rapid diuresis and brain relaxation.
5. A craniotomy (4–5 cm in diameter) is required in the posterior fossa.
6. Dural vessels are avoided or sealed with bipolar coagulation before making the incision.
7. The dural incision should be kept 0.5 cm away from the venous sinuses. Care is taken to avoid damage to the transverse and sigmoid sinus and cerebellum when incising the dura.
8. The dura is retracted with 5–0 silk thread to improve exposure.
9. Formal opening of the cisterna magna and drainage of cerebrospinal fluid (CSF) allows for gentle cerebellar-retraction and exposure of the CPA. Excessive cerebellar retraction can result in postoperative edema and should be avoided.
10. At the end of the procedure, the dura is closed in a water-tight manner. Muscle with fibrin glue is carefully interposed between the interrupted sutures and any open air cells are packed with bone wax, to avoid CSF leakage.
11. After surgery the patient should stay in the intensive care unit (ICU) overnight for close observation.

Complications

1. Hearing loss
2. Intracranial hemorrhage
3. Postoperative brain edema
4. Facial weakness or Facial palsy
5. Cerebrospinal fluid otorrhea
6. Meningitis
7. Post-operative dizziness or headache

Note: It has been reported that there is an 80–85 % effective rate with MVD for HFS. The reported complications related to MVD are low, with partial or complete loss of hearing as the most common. Other complications, such as brainstem infarction or CSF leak are rare. In a retrospective study of 782 MDV for hemifacial spasm, Barker et al. reported complications after the first microvascular decompression for hemifacial spasm included hearing loss in 2.6 % cases and irreversible severe facial weakness in 0.9 % of patients at the operating side. In all 782 microvascular decompression procedures for hemifacial spasm in 703 patients (705 sides, 57 patients underwent more than one procedures), one operative death (0.1 %) and two brainstem infarctions (0.3 %) occurred. The same author also noted that complications were more frequent in reoperated patients.

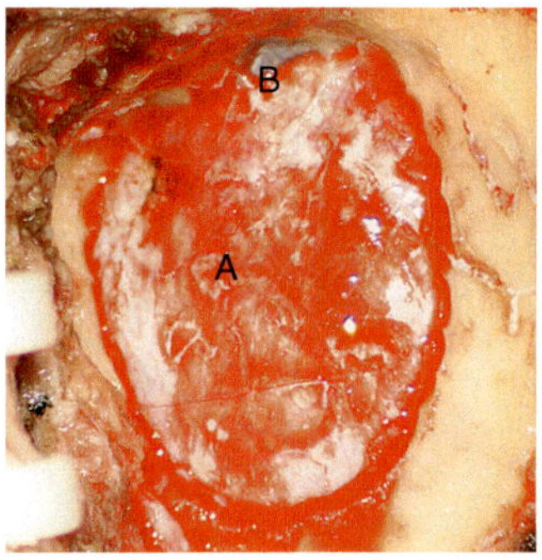

A. Dura matter of posterior cranial fossa
B. Posterior edge of sigmoid sinus

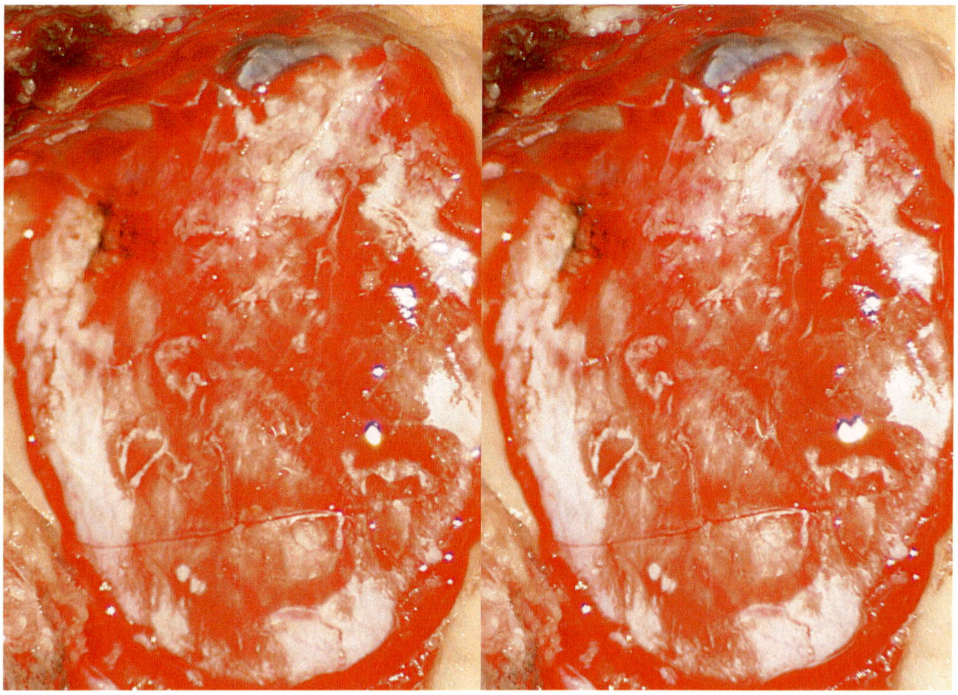

Fig. 5.12 Posterior Fossa Craniotomy
A U-shaped incision is made over retroauricular and suboccipital region. The bone flap is approximately 4 cm in diameter. The bony opening is placed behind the sigmoid sinus and inferior to the transverse sinus

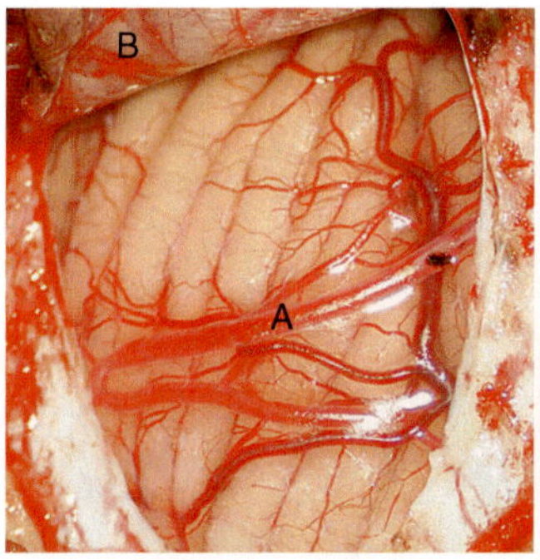

A. Vessels and pia mater on the surface of the cerebellum
B. Dura retracted forward.

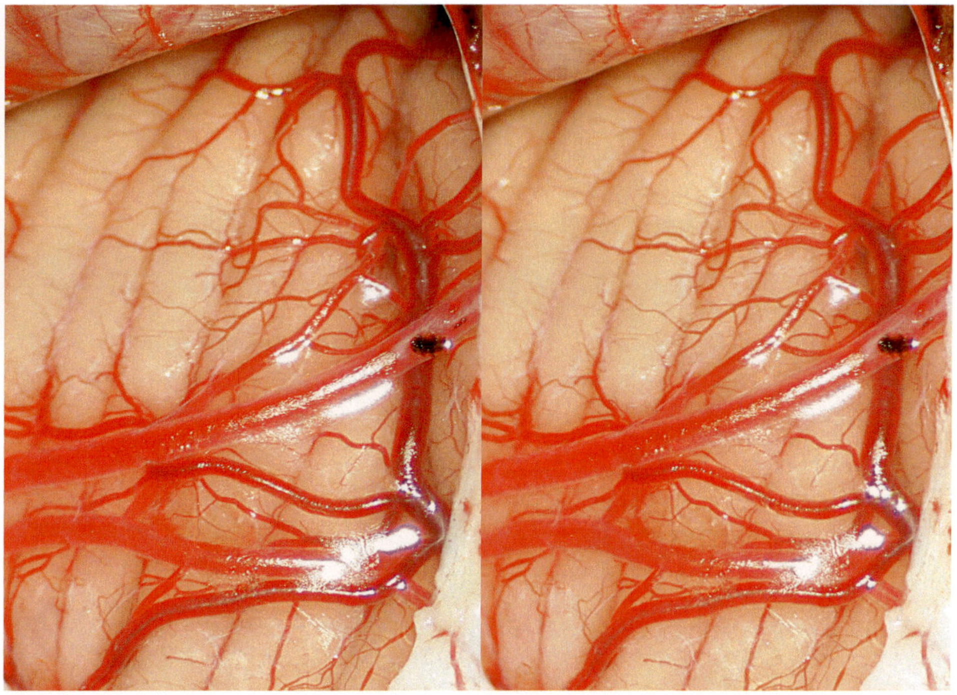

Fig. 5.13 Incision of Dura Mater
A curvilinear incision is made in the dura and the anterior flap, based on the sigmoid sinus, is tacked forwards. Cottonoids are placed along the incision edges of dura matter to protect the cerebellum

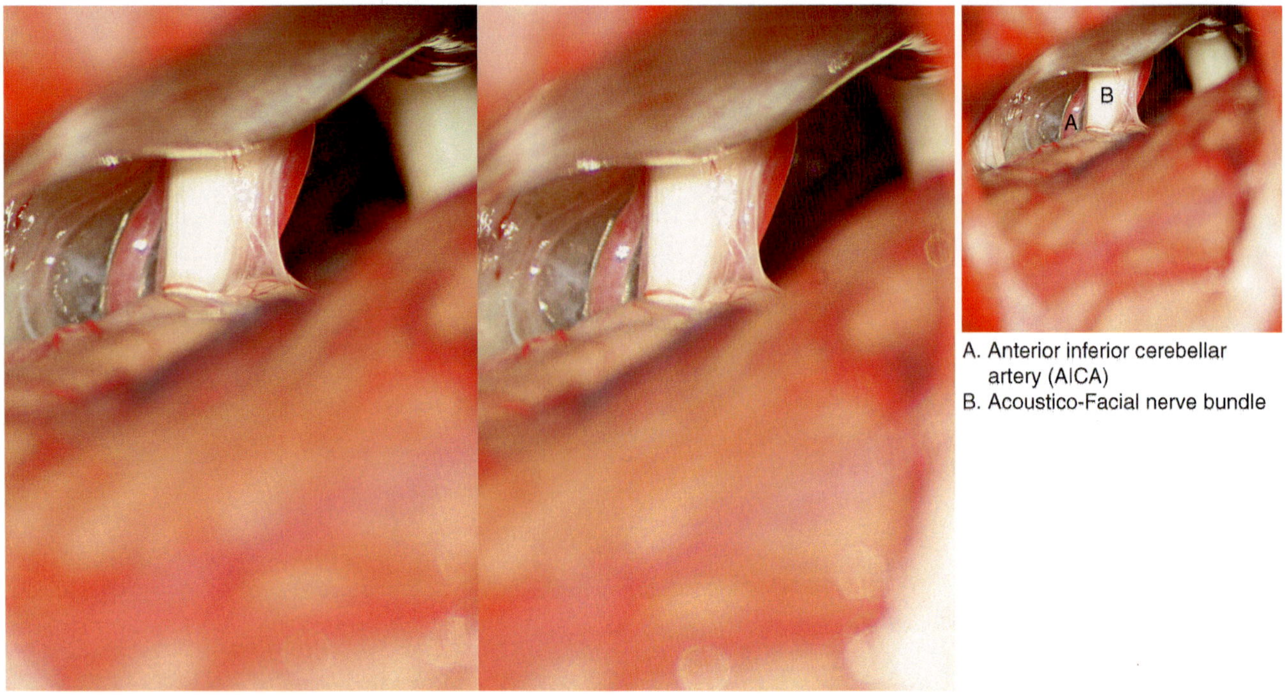

Fig. 5.14 Exposure of the structures in left cerebellopontine angle
Open the arachnoid of the cerebellomedullary cistern to allow drainage of the cerebrospinal fluid and obtain a relaxed cerebellum. At this point, cranial nerves VII and VIII are visualized. Cranial nerve V is also in view in the superior part of the field

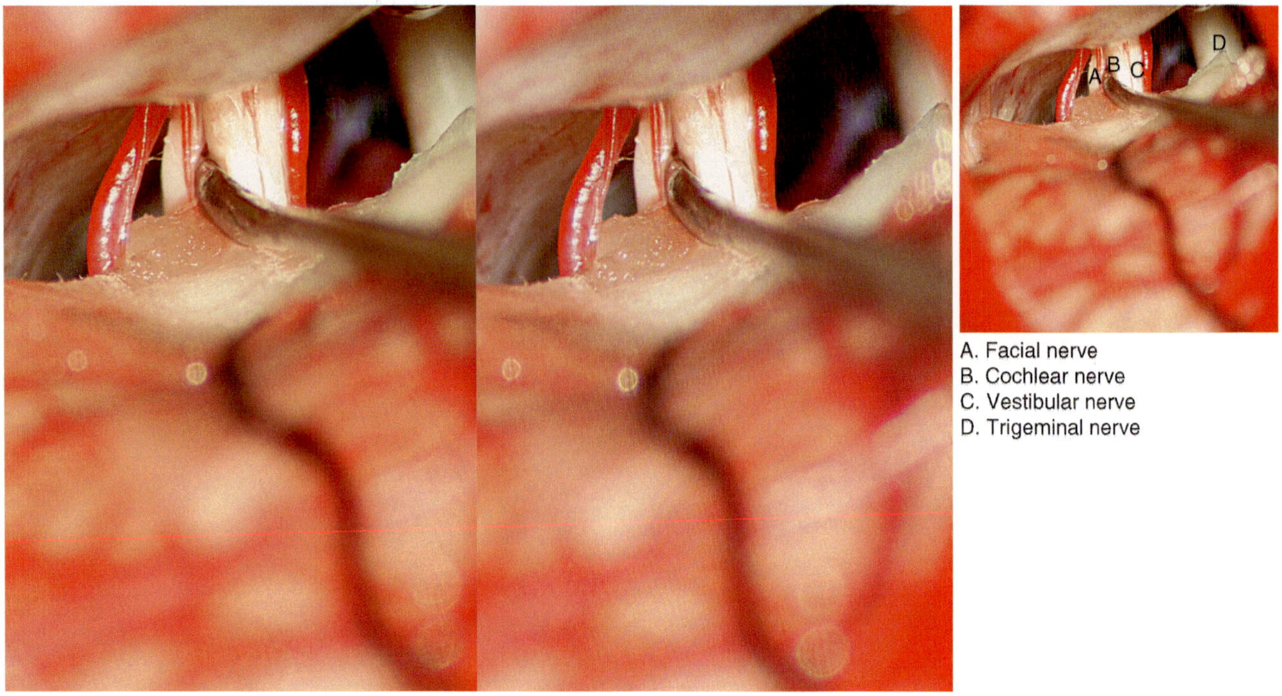

Fig. 5.15 Identify and separate offending vessels from the facial nerve
Free up the facial nerve which is located inferior and deep to the auditory nerve using an elevator or hook

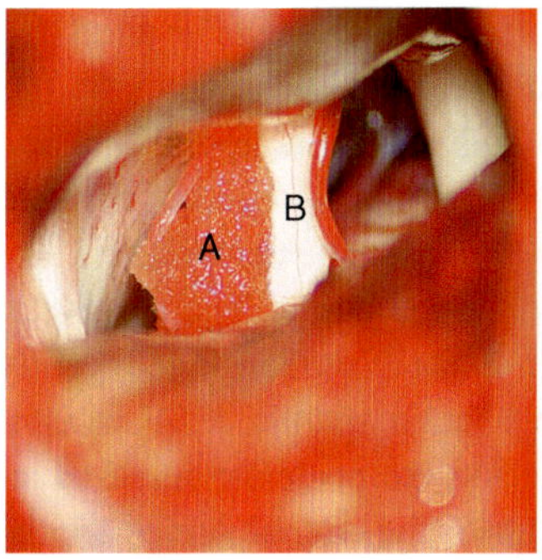

A. A block of gelatin sponge
B. The acoustico-facial bundle

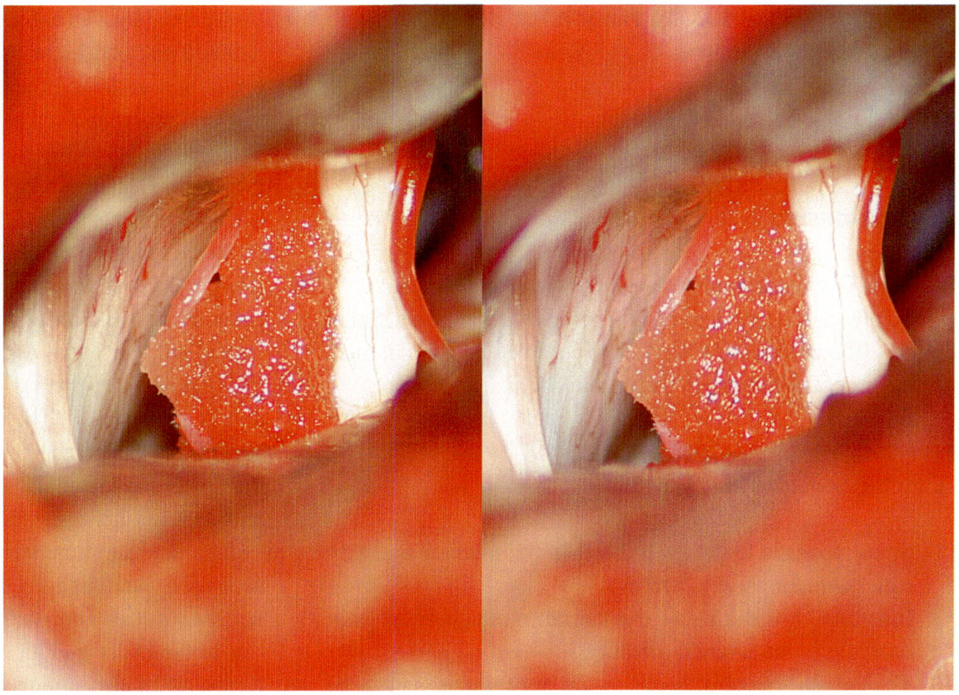

Fig. 5.16 Separate the AICA and the acoustico-facial bundle
Separate the AICA and the acoustico-facial bundle using a block of gelatin sponge

Retrosigmoid Sinus Approach for Removal of Acoustic Neuroma

Yi-hui Zou and Vincent C Cousins

Indications

1. Tumors located mainly in cerebellopontine angle area.
2. To preserve hearing and facial nerve function when it may be difficult to remove the tumor completely through middle cranial fossa or via a translabyrinthine approach.

Contraindications

1. Small acoustic neuroma located in the internal auditory canal without useable hearing
2. Infection in the area of the operation, such as a scalp furuncle or intracranial infection.
3. The patient's general health is too poor for surgery to be performed. Chronic infectious diseases such as hepatitis and tuberculosis should be cured or stable before the operation to be performed.
4. Bleeding and clotting disorders. Long term aspirin usage and active menstruation are conditions that may interfere with surgery by causing excessive bleeding or lead to intracranial hemorrhage.
5. In older patients, it may be better not to operate. Tumors such as acoustic neuromas are benign and patients can live for long time with tumors which may not show further growth. The effects of age may add risk to the surgery. Large tumors with brainstem compression will usually require surgery. Careful consideration needs to be given to the relative risks and benefits of this surgery.

Operative Procedures

1. Anaesthesia: This surgery is always performed under general anaesthesia with appropriate monitoring.
2. Incision. A C-shaped post-auricular incision is made from the upper attachment of the auricle to the mastoid, passing 4–5 cm posterior to the sulcus and extending 1–2 cm below the tip on the mastoid process. The flap is elevated anteriorly to expose the skull.
3. Opening the bone window. The upper boundary is the temporal line. The anterior limit is a line joining the parietal notch and the tip of mastoid (the surface projection of the sigmoid sinus). A bone window of about 3×4 cm is made in the area where parietal, temporal and occipital bones have a common boundary. The posterior fossa dura is exposed.
4. Incise the dura. An anteriorly based rectangular dural flap is made just inside the margins of the bone window. The upper and anterior boundaries are the temporal line and sigmoid sinus respectively. The flap is reflected forward and held with stay sutures to expose the cerebellum.
5. Exposure of the cerebellopontine angle. The cerebellar surface is protected with moist cottonoids and gently retracted posteriorly with a brain spatula. CSF is aspirated to expose the tumor and the posterior fossa structures. From superior to inferior the cranial nerves are the trigeminal, the facial and acoustic nerve bundle, and the IX (glossopharyngeal), X (vagus) and XI (accessory) nerves inferiorly. The vestibulo-cochlear nerve lies behind the facial nerve at the brainstem. More laterally the upper and lower vestibular nerves lie behind the facial and cochlear nerves respectively.

   The abducent nerve (VI) lies well anterior to the acoustico-facial bundle. The hypoglossal nerve is usually not seen in this approach, but lies well anterior and inferior to the IX, X and XI nerves
6. Removal of the tumor. Big acoustic neuromas have a pseudo capsule which can be opened posteriorly and tumor can be gradually removed from within. Once the tumor has been debulked, the capsule can be reflected off the facial and cochlear nerves and complete removal achieved. For small tumors, the involved nerve can be separated from the facial and cochlear nerves and resected directly. Real-time monitoring of facial nerve and hearing (brainstem evoked potential) is used in all cases to assist with their preservation. Acoustic neuromas usually originate from one of the vestibular nerves but always have some attachment to the facial and cochlear nerves and must be clearly separated from them before resection.
7. Opening internal auditory canal. The posterior wall of the internal auditory canal has to be drilled away to expose tumor extending into the canal to remove it completely.
8. Hemostasis. Hemostasis is achieved with use of bipolar electrocoagulation or application of hemostatic gauze. The latter is better for bleeding on the brain surface.
9. Closure of the operative cavity. Suture the dura closed. Reinsert the bone flap and fix it with craniotomy rivets. Suture the scalp in layers and apply a compression dressing.

Special Comments

1. Minimal retraction is used on the cerebellum and brainstem to prevent brain edema and brain herniation. Intracranial pressure can be controlled at the start of the procedure using an agent such as 20% mannitol. 250 ml is given by rapid intravenous injection.

2. Avoid injury to the main blood vessels and dural venous sinuses. The mastoid emissary and petrosal veins, the anterior inferior cerebellar artery and the sigmoid and transverse sinuses can all cause significant bleeding. Complete hemostasis must be achieved before closing the operative cavity to prevent post-operative intracranial hematoma
3. Protect the facial and cochlear nerves using intra-operative monitoring.
4. Prevent leakage of cerebrospinal fluid. Repair the dura in a watertight fashion. Maintain normal intracranial pressure post-operatively to avoid leakage of cerebrospinal fluid.

Complications

1. Intracranial hemorrhage and hematoma. As mentioned above.
2. Injury of the cerebellum and brainstem, brain edema. Excessive retraction and injury to the cerebellum and brainstem during operation can cause brain edema and permanent neural dysfunction.
3. Injury of facial and acoustic nerves. The nerves are easily damaged when separating and resecting the tumor, leading to facial paralysis, hearing loss and tinnitus. Injury to the facial nerve may necessitate further surgery for repair and partial restoration of function.
4. Damage of the other cranial nerves. Cranial nerves V, IX, X, XI can be damaged with permanent loss of function. Cranial nerves VI and XII are generally not involved as they are located deeply.
5. Leakage of cerebrospinal fluid. Leakage of cerebrospinal fluid can occur when the dural repair is inadequate or postoperative intracranial pressure increases. A compression dressing will help stop a leak of fluid via the wound. Intracranial pressure should be maintained at normal levels.
6. Intracranial infection and meningitis. A strict sterile operation technique and antibiotic administration during and after operation will mostly prevent infection.
7. Brain hernia. Intracranial hemorrhage, hematoma, excessive brain edema and increased intracranial pressure can cause brain herniation. This is likely to be life-threatening and must be recognized early and appropriate action taken.

Surgery 1: Retro-Sigmoid sinus approach for removal of acoustic neuroma

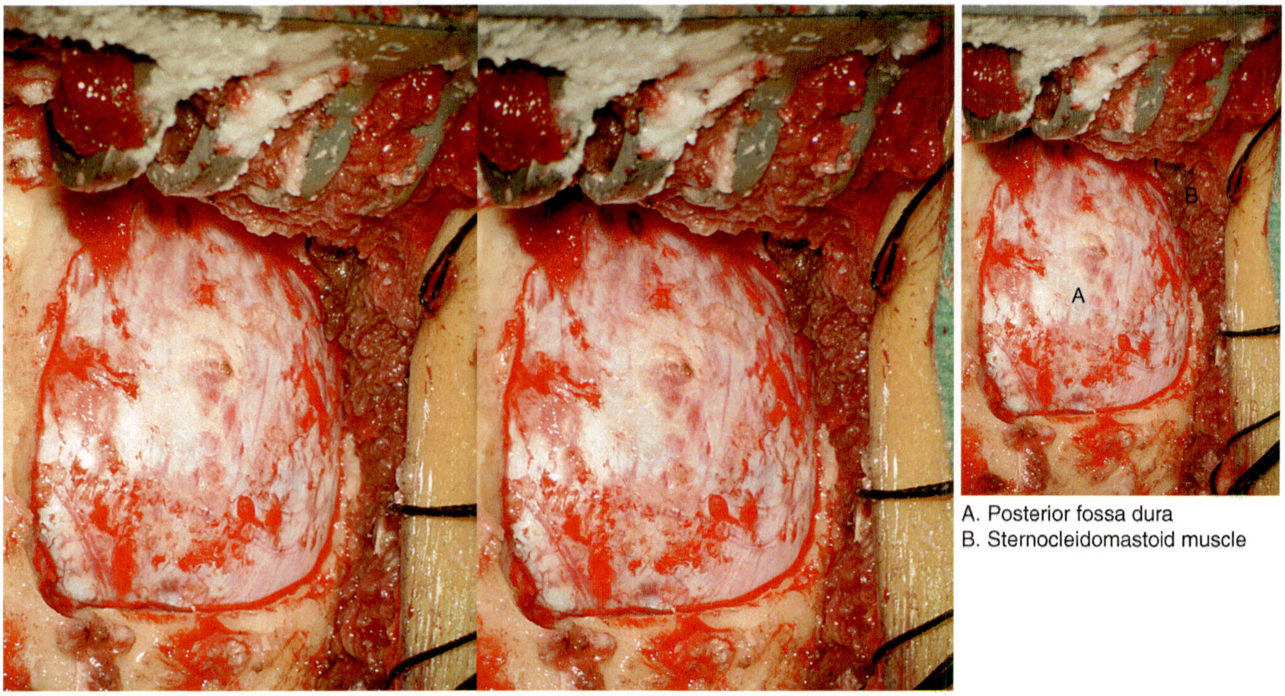

A. Posterior fossa dura
B. Sternocleidomastoid muscle

Fig. 5.17 Craniotomy
An anteriorly based C-shaped post-auricular flap is raised with a size of about 5×4 cm, to expose the cranial bone and open a bone window. The upper boundary is the temporal line, and the anterior limit is a line between the parietal notch and the tip of the mastoid process. A bone flap of approximately 3×4 cm bone is removed from the area where parietal, temporal and occipital bone share a common boundary, behind the sigmoid sinus

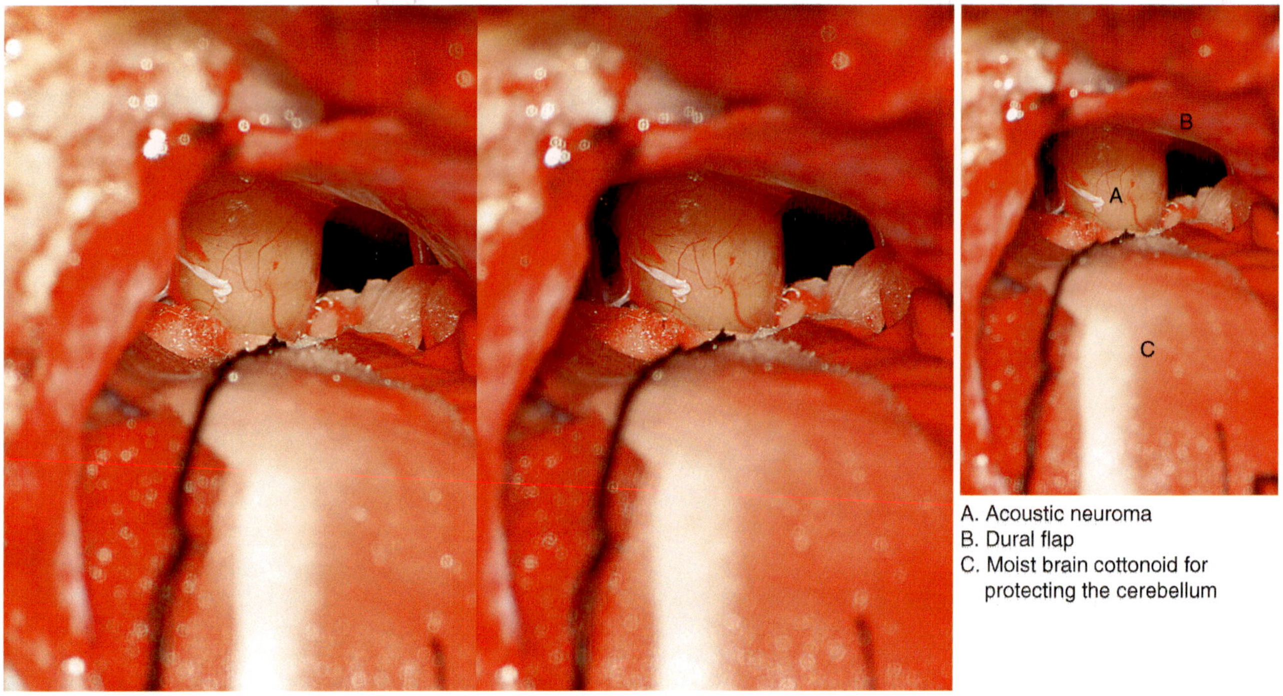

A. Acoustic neuroma
B. Dural flap
C. Moist brain cottonoid for protecting the cerebellum

Fig. 5.18 Expose tumor in the cerebellopontine angle
A U-shaped dural flap is raised. It is based anteriorly behind the sigmoid sinus and below the transverse sinus. The flap is reflected forwards to expose the cerebellum. The cerebellum is protected with moist cottonoids and gently retracted posteriorly with a brain spatula to expose the tumor in the cerebellopontine angle

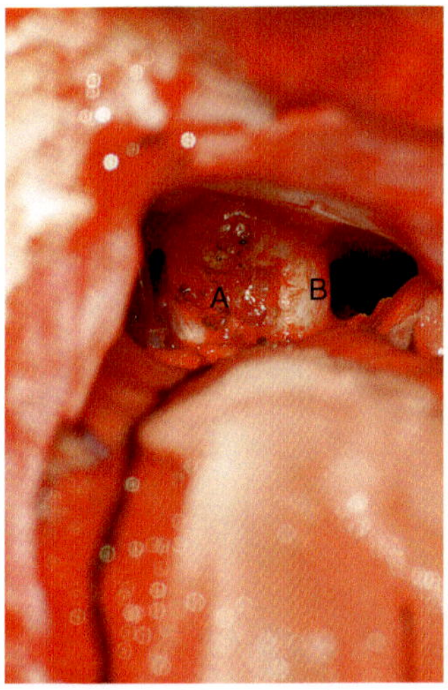

A. Removal of the acoustic neuroma inside its capsule
B. The lower boundary of the acoustic neuroma

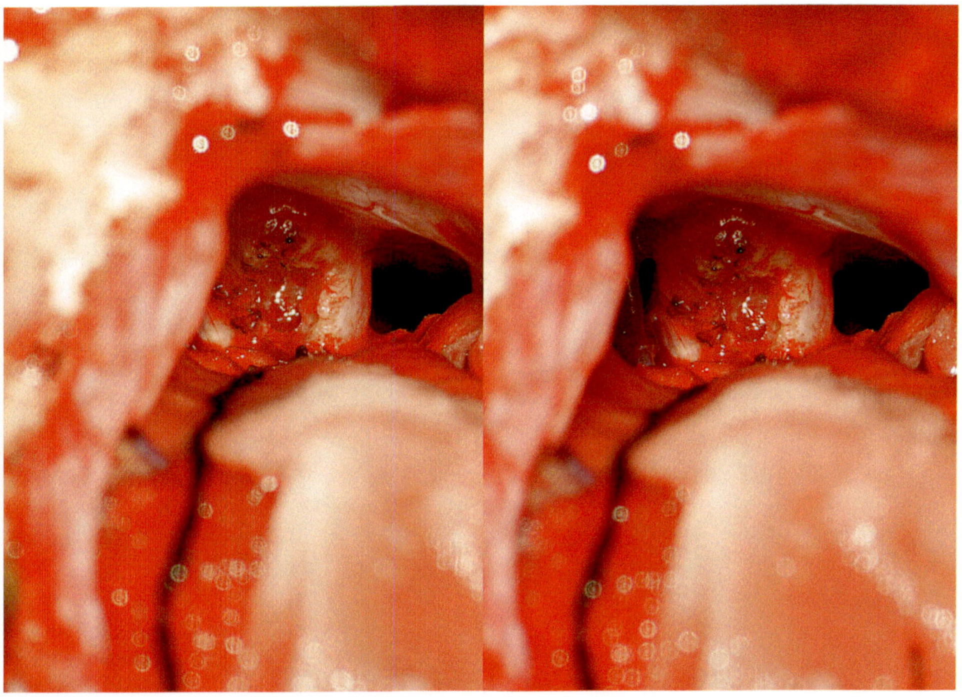

Fig. 5.19 Removal of the tumor
First ensure that the facial nerve is not lying on the posterior surface of the tumor using the nerve monitor probe. If not, coagulate the tumor surface, open the capsule and remove the tumor from inside the capsule preserving the facial and cochlear nerves located outside the tumor capsule

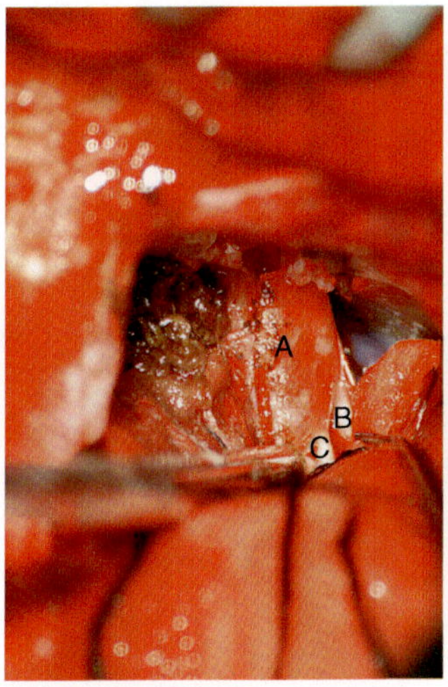

A. Acoustic neuroma
B. Facial nerve
C. Vestibular nerve

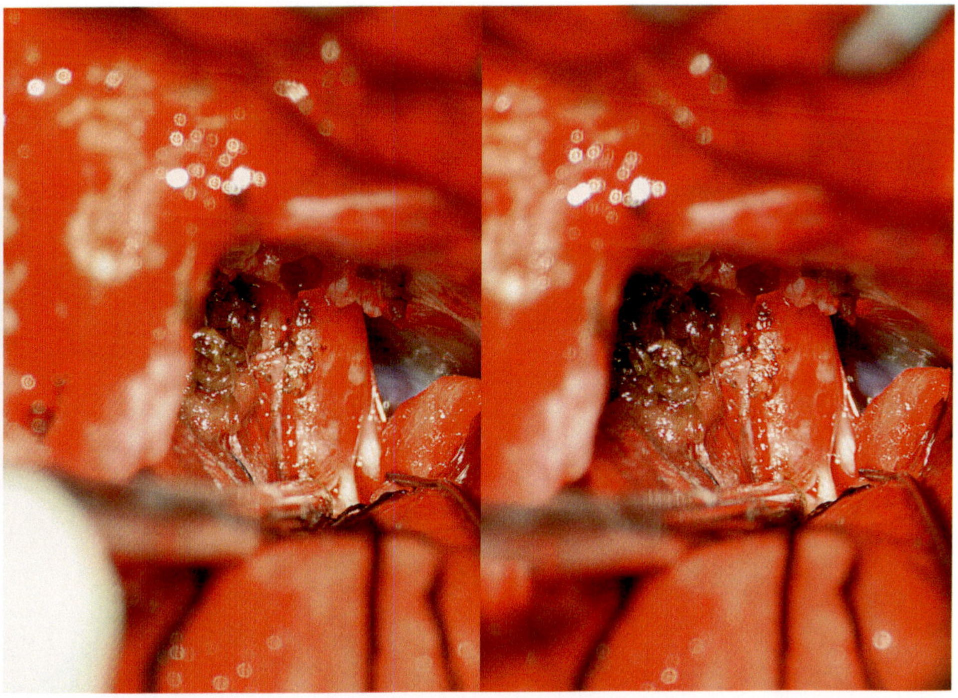

Fig. 5.20 Removal of the tumor
Open the posterior wall of the internal auditory canal to expose its contents. Isolate the tumor and remove it completely. The vestibular nerves and tumor are usually posterior to the facial nerve

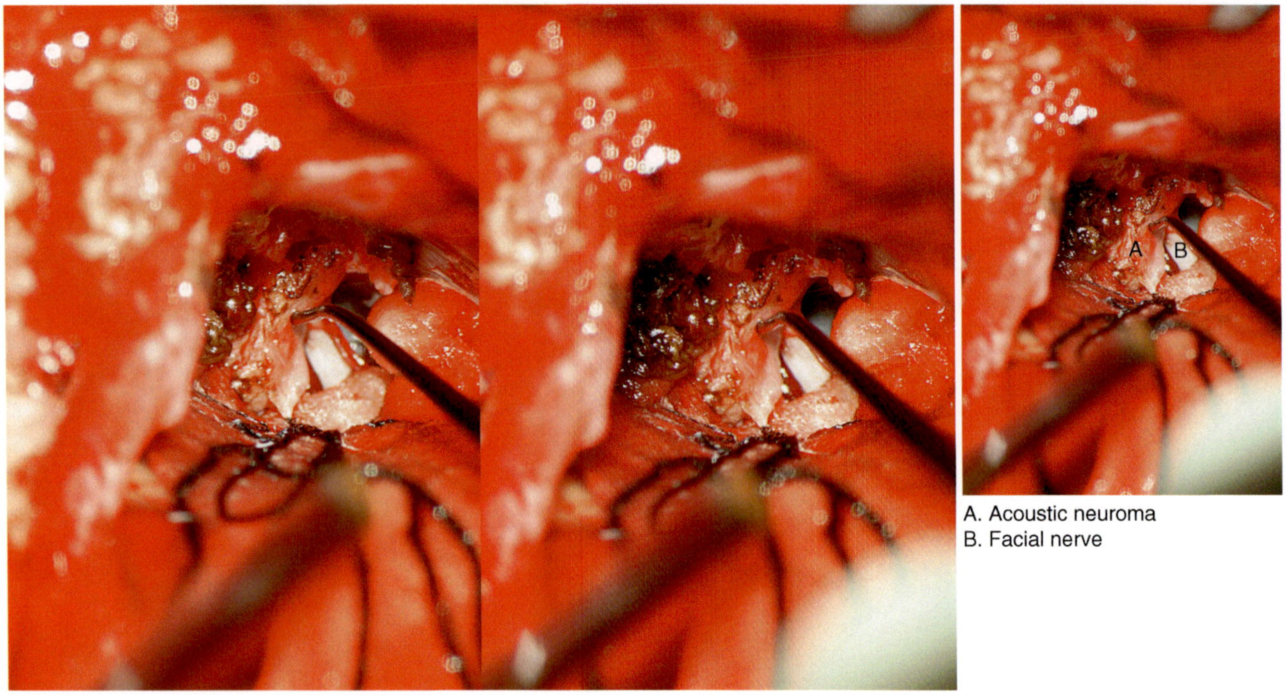

A. Acoustic neuroma
B. Facial nerve

Fig. 5.21 Separate and protect the facial nerve
Elevate the superficial involved nerves and tumor, to identify the facial nerve more anterior and deep. Separate and resect the tumor progressively under facial nerve monitoring

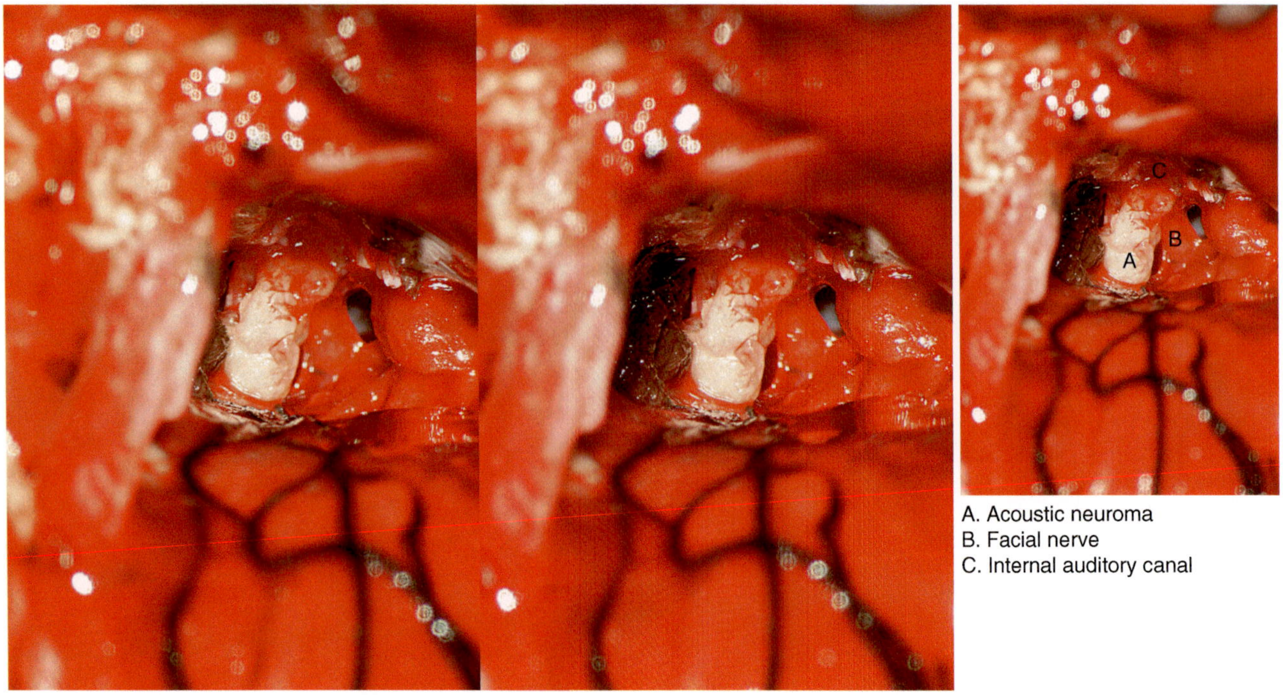

A. Acoustic neuroma
B. Facial nerve
C. Internal auditory canal

Fig. 5.22 Protect facial nerve and remove the remaining tumor
Separate and resect tumor progressively under facial nerve monitoring. The remaining tumor can be seen and separated from the intact facial nerve which is seen deeper. The tumor in the internal auditory canal has been removed completely

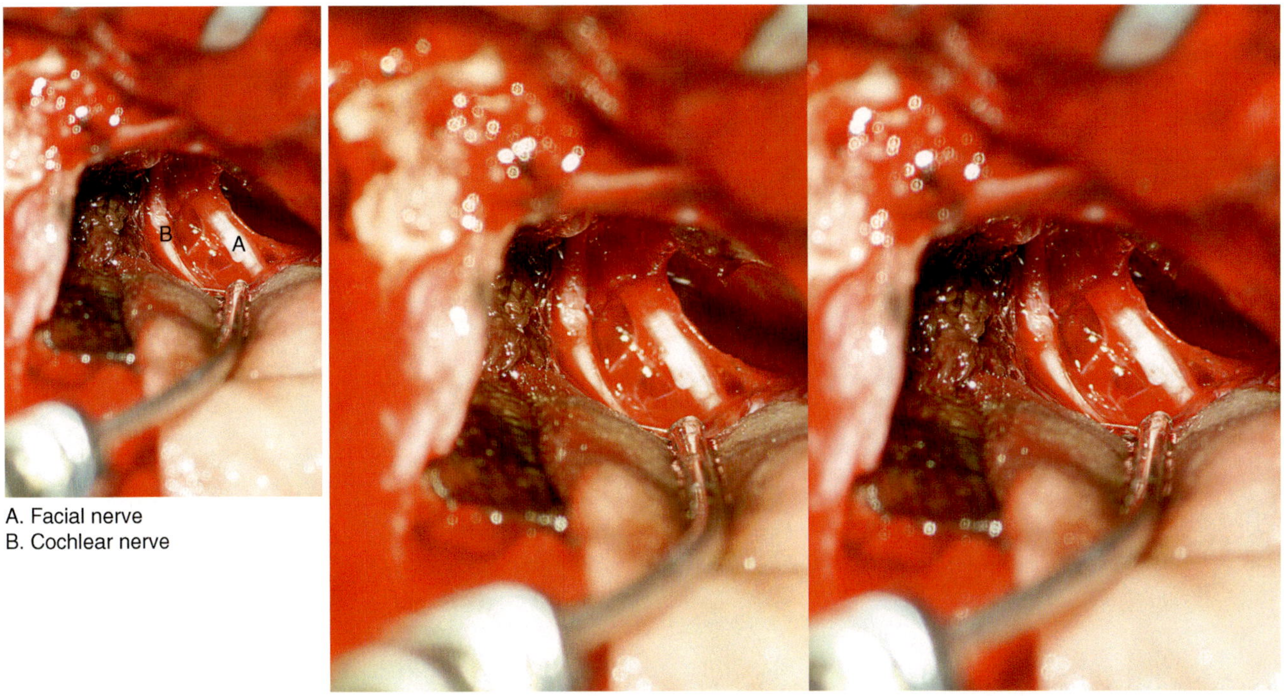

Fig. 5.23 Preserve the facial and cochlear nerves
Showing the preserved facial and cochlear nerve after the tumor was removed completely

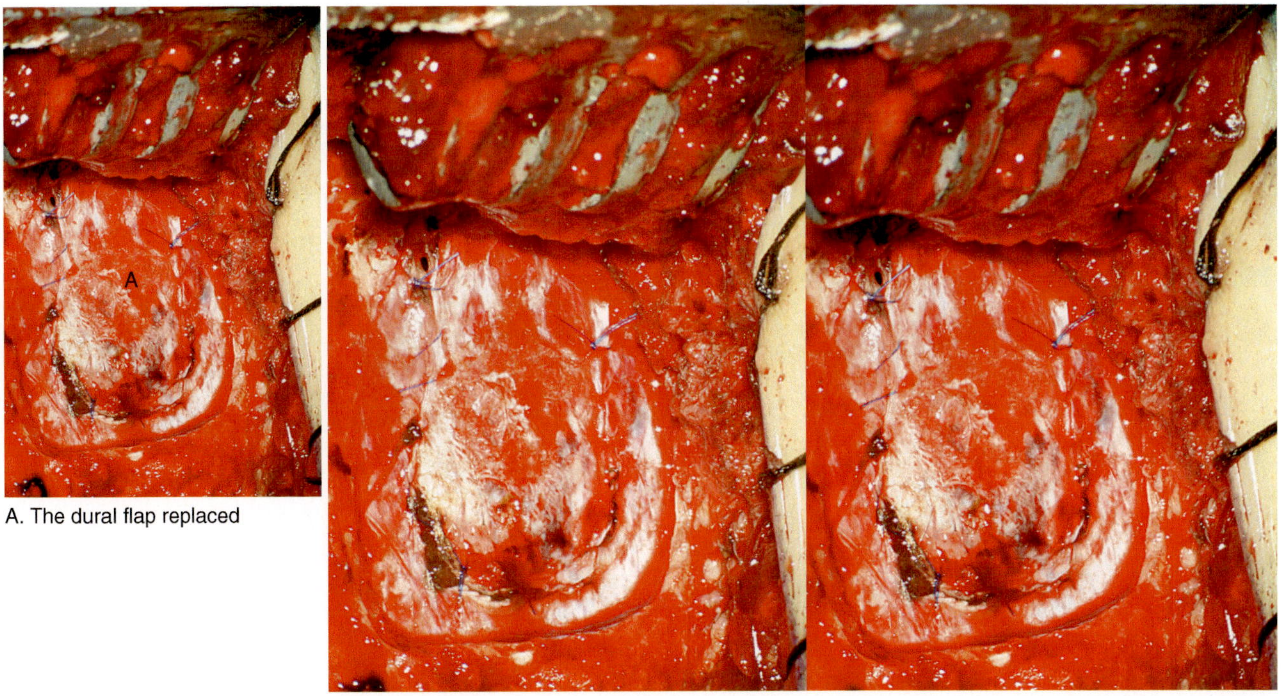

Fig. 5.24 Closure of the operative cavity
Reposition the dural flap after complete hemostasis is assured and suture it with a continuous nylon thread in a watertight fashion

Surgery 2: Retro-Sigmoid sinus approach for removal of acoustic neuroma

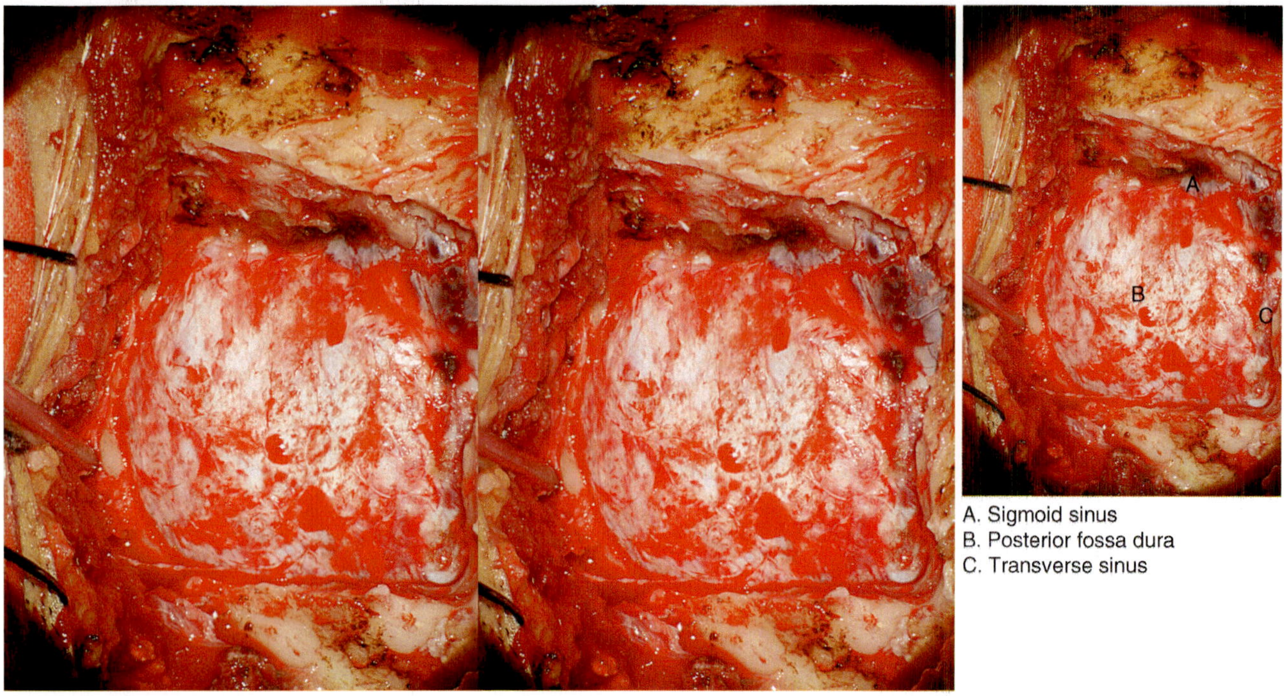

Fig. 5.25 Craniotomy
Make an anteriorly based C-shaped post-auricular flap to expose the cranial bone and create a bone window about 3 × 4 cm with its upper boundary at the temporal line, and the anterior limit is a line between the parietal notch and the tip of the mastoid process. Drill holes with a trephine at the four angles or drill along the four borders with a milling cutter or electric drill. Take care not to damage the dura. Any bleeding from the emissary vein or sigmoid sinus should be controlled completely

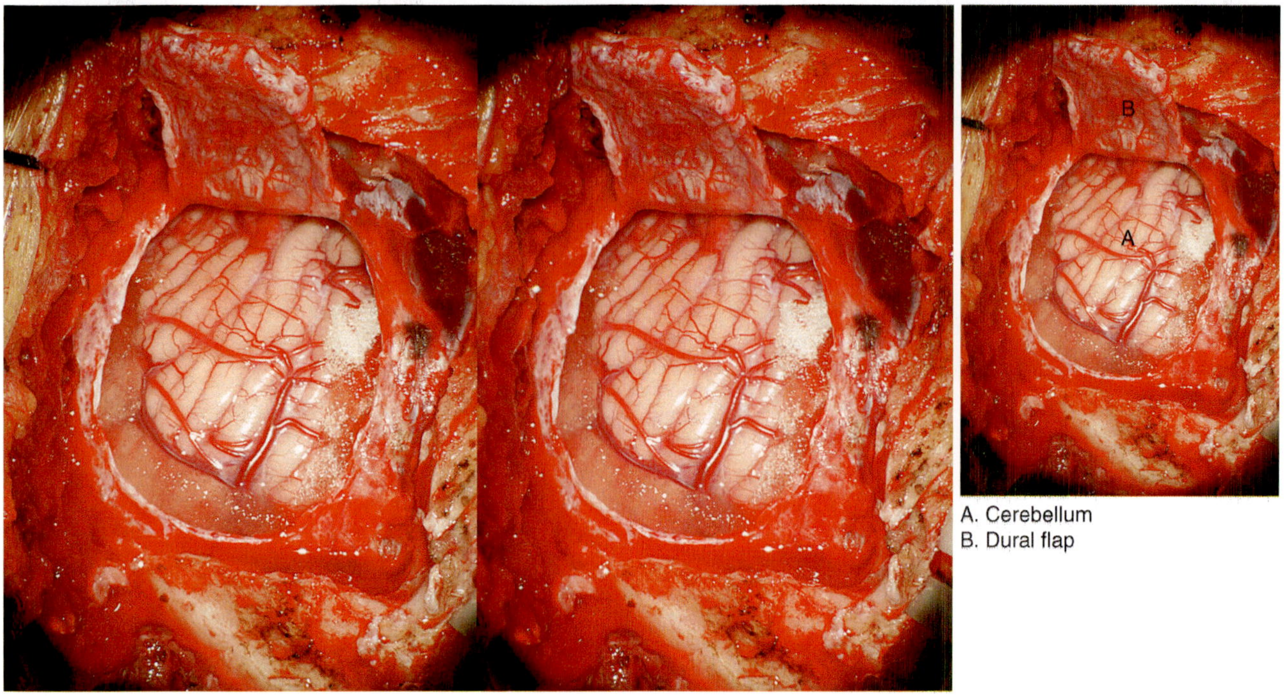

Fig. 5.26 Exposure of the cerebellum
Make a U-shaped dural flap with an anterior pedicle along the edge of the bone window. Reflect it forward to expose the cerebellum. Protect the dural edges promptly with gelatin sponge and brain cottonoids. The cerebellum is gently retracted posteriorly with brain spatula and brain cottonoids. Aspirate cerebrospinal fluid to reduce the intra-cranial pressure and expose the tumor in the cerebellopontine angle

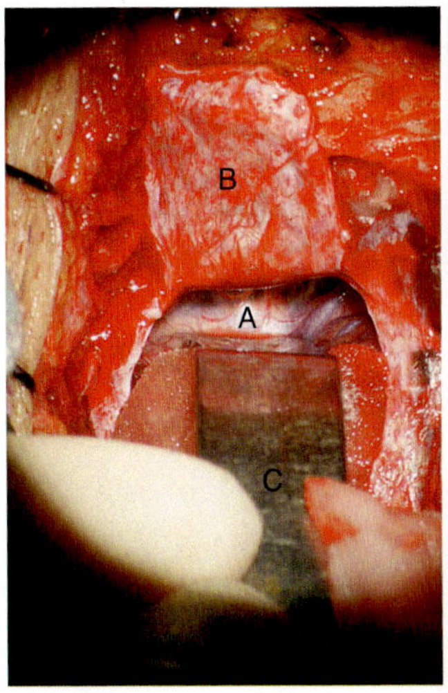

A. Arachnoid folds in cerebellopontine angle
B. Dural flap
C. Brain spatula

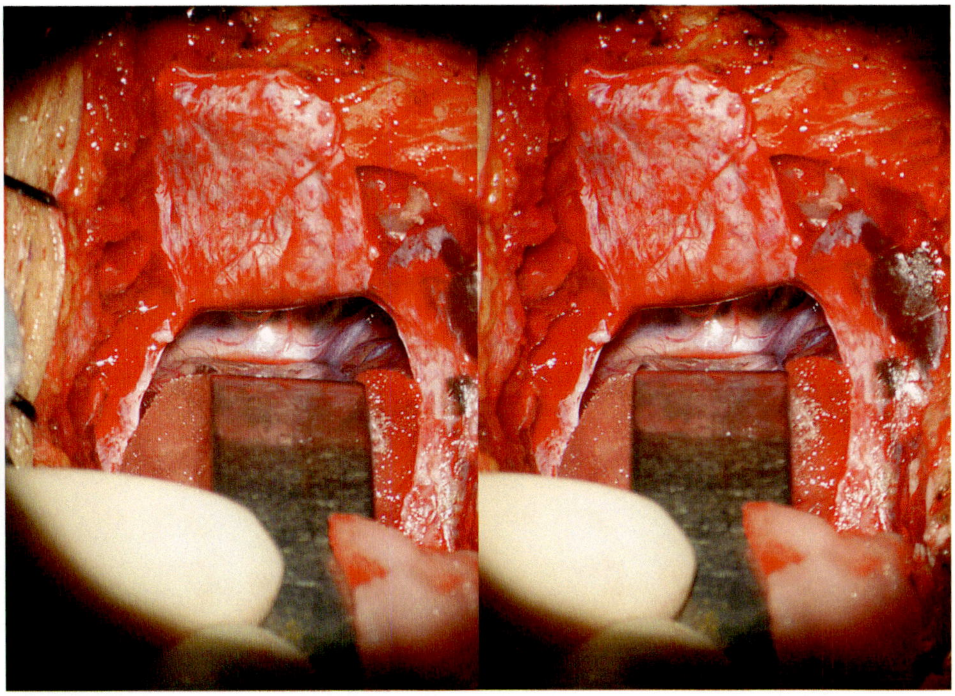

Fig. 5.27 Expose the cerebellopontine angle
Beginning of exposure of the cerebellopontine angle. The arachnoid is still wrapped around the nerves and blood vessels. The petrosal vein can be seen in the upper part of the operation field

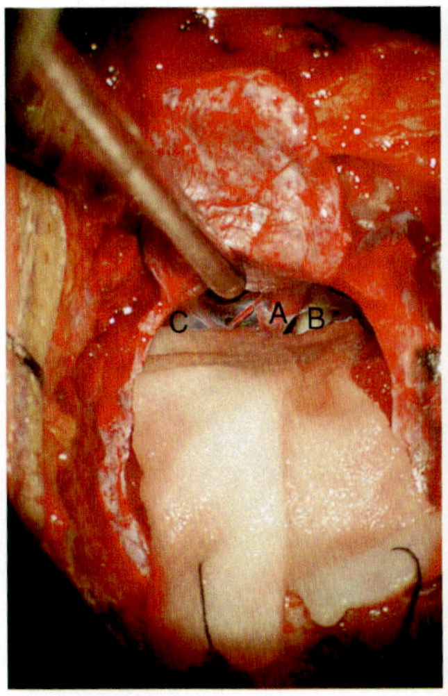

A. Acoustic-facial nerve bundle
B. Trigeminal nerve
C. IX-XI cranial nerves

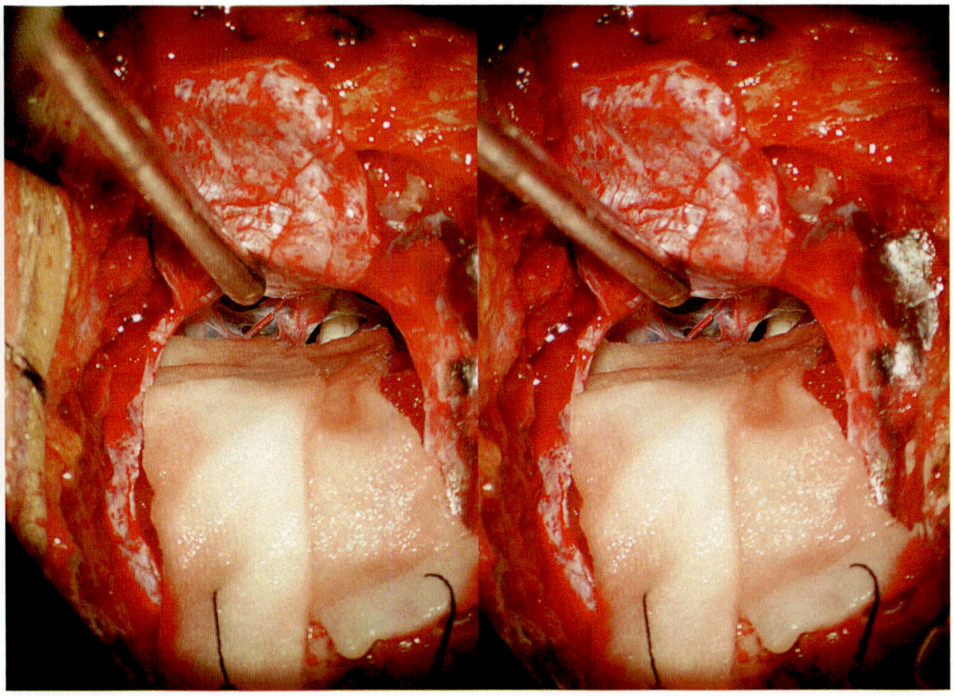

Fig. 5.28 Identify the cranial nerves in the cerebellopontine angle
From superior to inferior, the cranial nerves are trigeminal nerve, acoustic-facial nerve bundle and IX–XI cranial nerves. The tumor can be seen bulging into cerebellopontine angle at the porus of the internal auditory canal

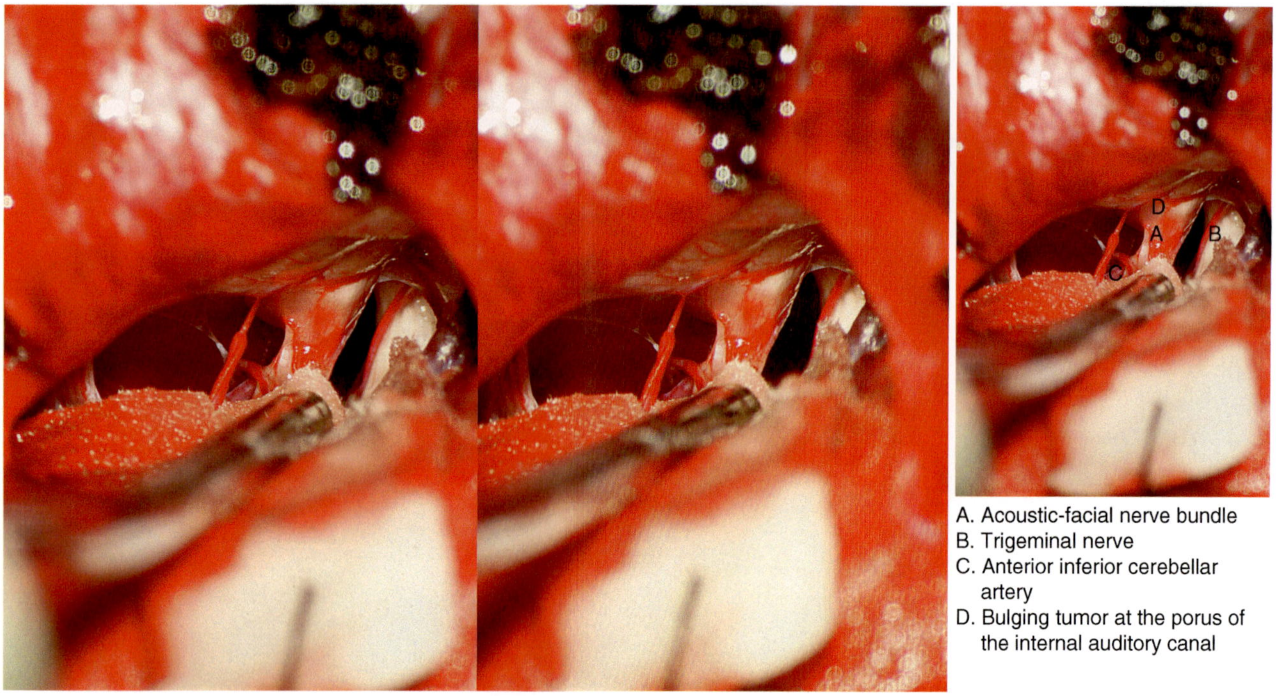

A. Acoustic-facial nerve bundle
B. Trigeminal nerve
C. Anterior inferior cerebellar artery
D. Bulging tumor at the porus of the internal auditory canal

Fig. 5.29 Expose the tumor at the porus of the internal auditory canal
The tumor bulges into the cerebellopontine angle at the entrance of the internal auditory canal seen under high magnification, compressing the acoustic-facial nerve bundle. The anterior inferior cerebellar artery can be seen at the end of the bundle near the brainstem

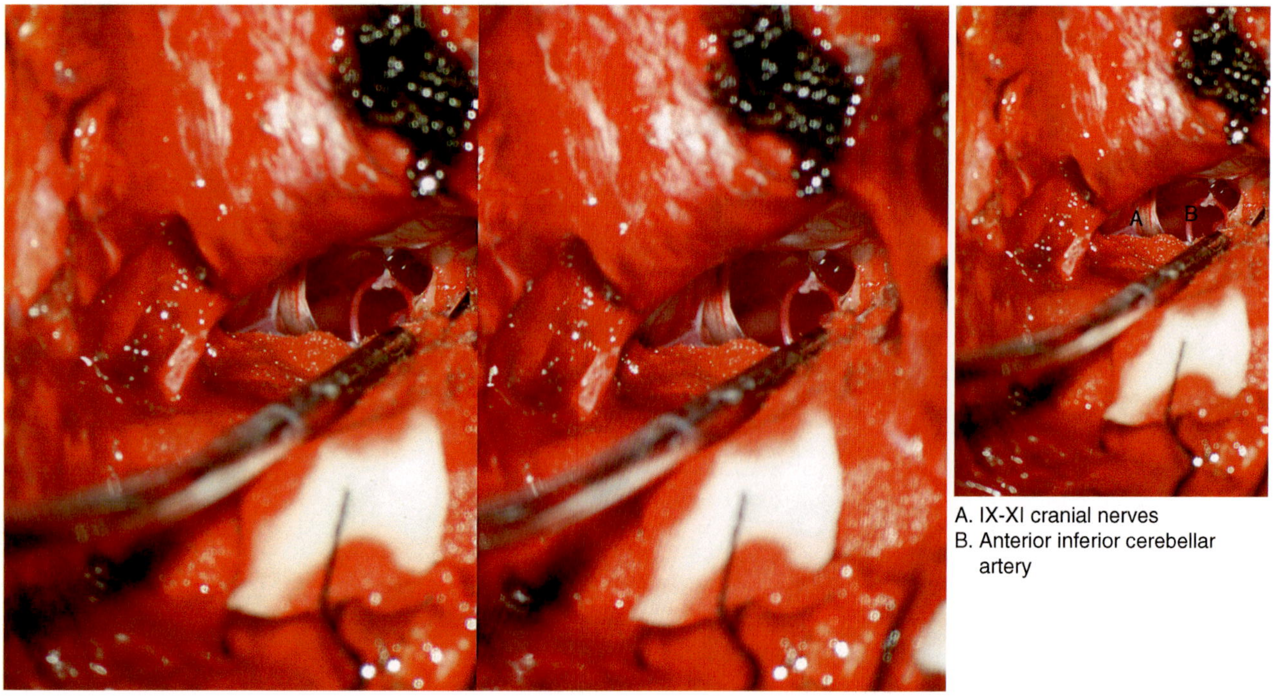

A. IX-XI cranial nerves
B. Anterior inferior cerebellar artery

Fig. 5.30 Expose the anterior inferior cerebellar artery
Angle the microscope inferiorly to observe the anterior inferior cerebellar artery and IX–XI cranial nerve tract under high magnification

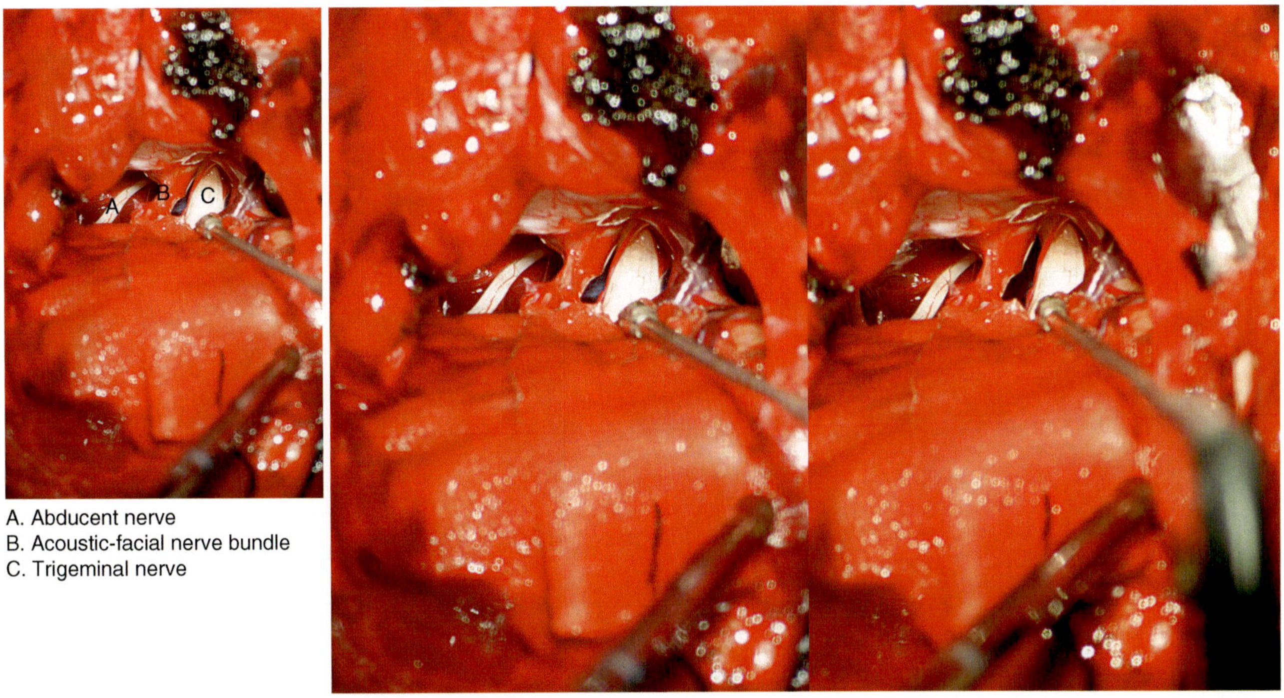

A. Abducent nerve
B. Acoustic-facial nerve bundle
C. Trigeminal nerve

Fig. 5.31 Expose the abducent nerve (VI)
The abducent nerve can be observed by focusing deep to the acoustic-facial nerve bundle. The abducent nerve originates from the brainstem near the midline in the ventral pontobulbar sulcus then passes forwards through petrous apex medial to the trigeminal nerve, traverses the cavernous sinus and passes through the superior orbital fissure into orbital cavity and innervates the lateral rectus muscle

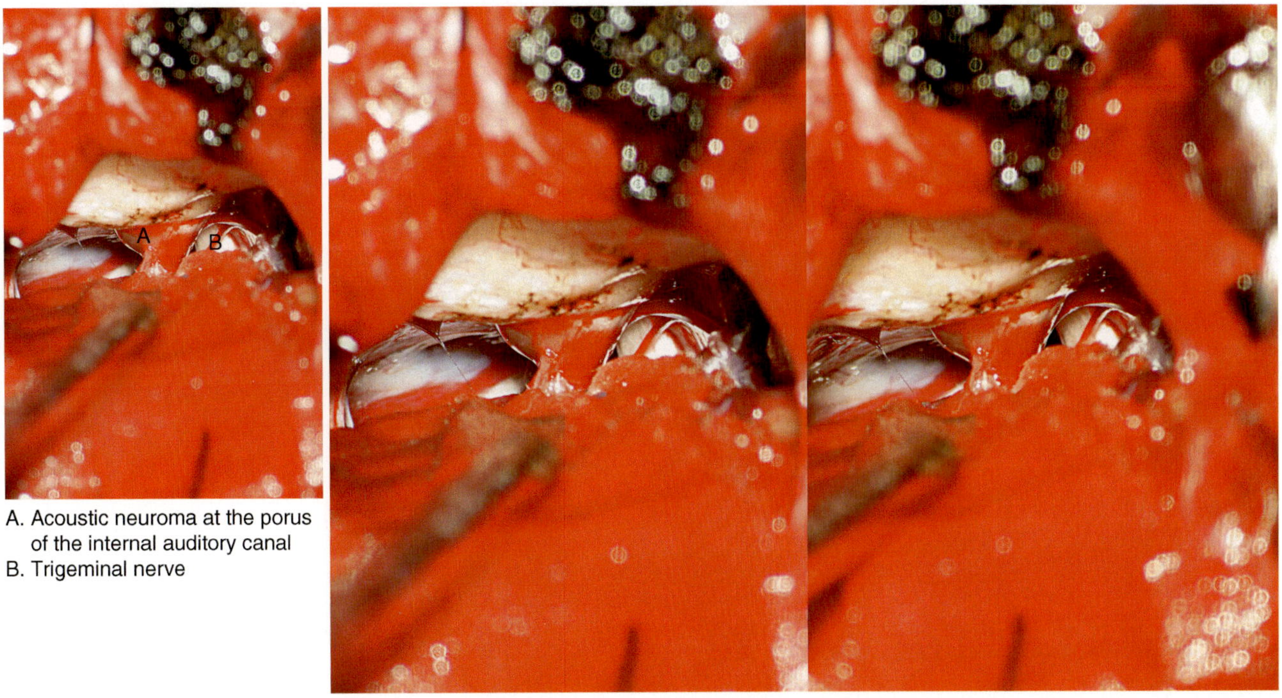

A. Acoustic neuroma at the porus of the internal auditory canal
B. Trigeminal nerve

Fig. 5.32 Expose the tumor at the entrance of the internal auditory canal and prepare to remove it
Increase the magnification to clearly show the tumor bulging into cerebellopontine angle at the porus of the internal auditory canal. The entrance of the canal is expanded and the tumor compresses acoustic-facial nerve bundle. The tumor is ready for removal

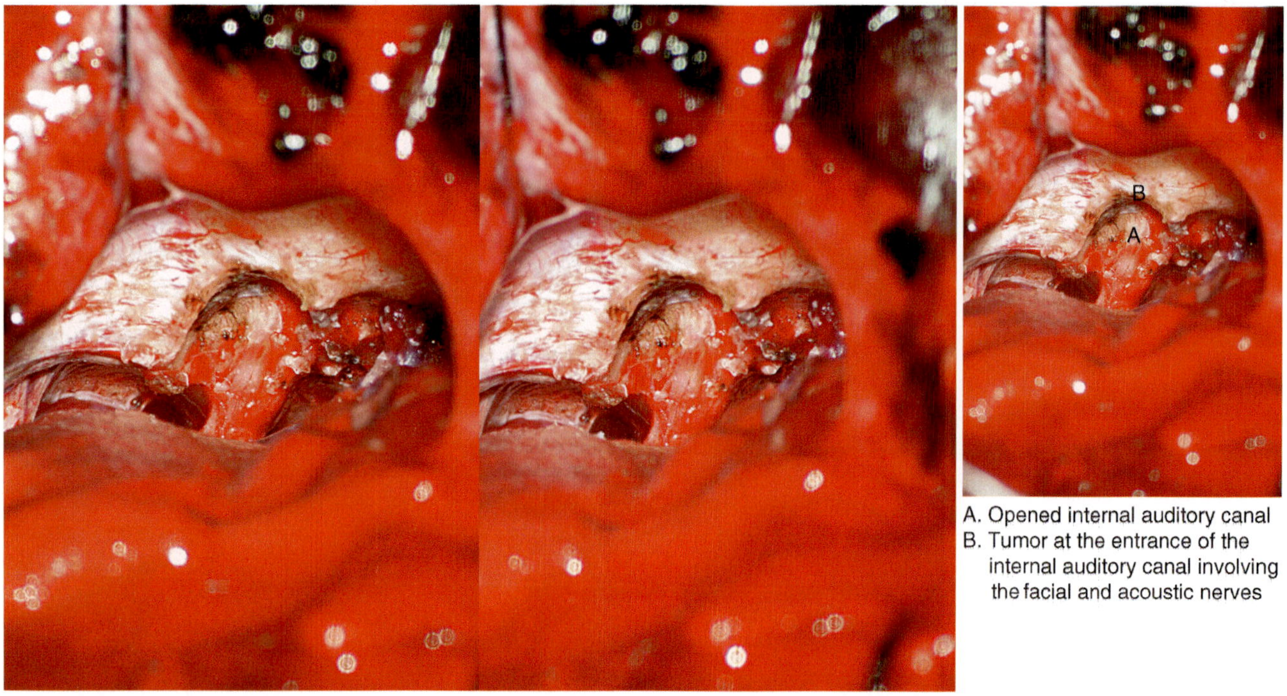

A. Opened internal auditory canal
B. Tumor at the entrance of the internal auditory canal involving the facial and acoustic nerves

Fig. 5.33 Open internal auditory canal
Remove the posterior wall of the internal auditory canal and expose the tumor inside. The tumor involves facial and acoustic nerves

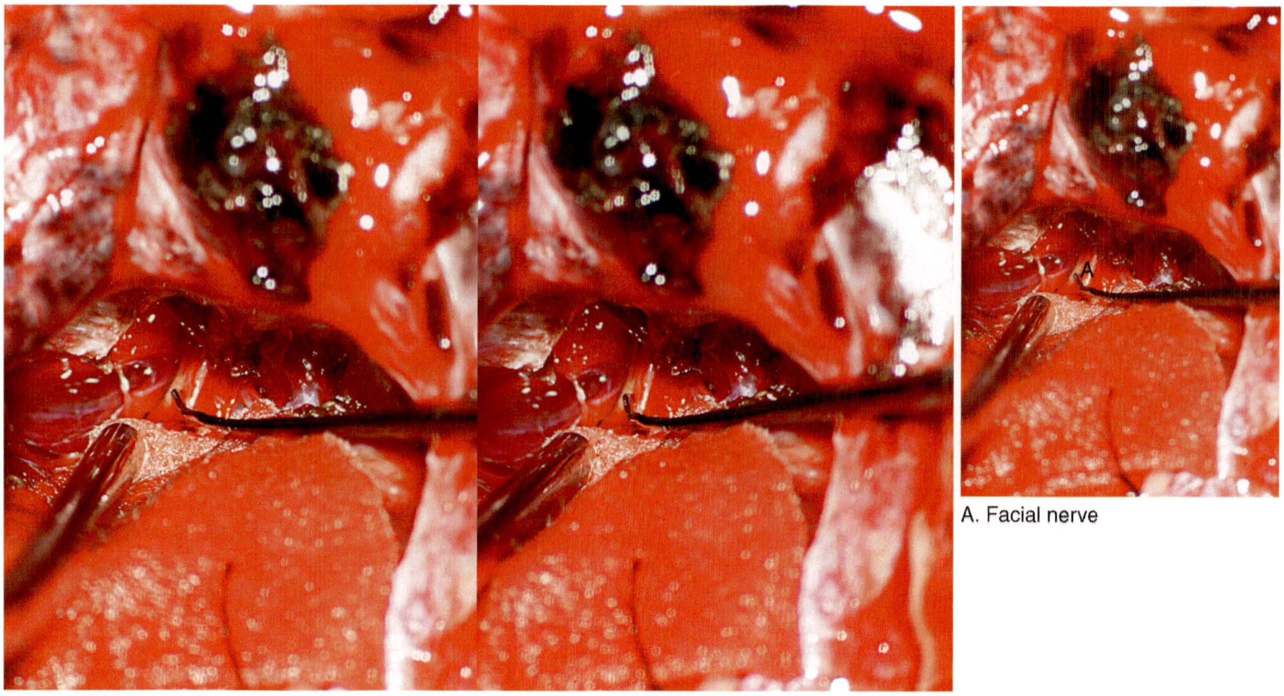

A. Facial nerve

Fig. 5.34 Removal of the tumor in internal auditory canal
Resect the tumor in the internal auditory canal step by step under facial nerve monitoring. In this case, the facial nerve was preserved well while the vestibular nerve was removed with the tumor

Translabyrinthine Approach for Removal of Acoustic Neuroma

Jun Liu and Pu Dai

Indications

The translabyrinthine approach is generally used in patients with poor hearing, normal facial nerve function and small or medium-sized internal auditory canal (IAC) tumors. This approach is used in neuromas that extend into the cerebellopontine angle (CPA) from the IAC. Large tumors may require extension of this approach to the retrolabyrinthine region to allow complete removal from the brainstem and cerebellum.

Contraindications

1. Poor general condition unable to tolerate the surgery.
2. Clotting dysfunction.
3. Normal hearing or serviceable hearing in smaller tumors, where it may be possible to preserve hearing.
4. Surgery may be able to be avoided in the elderly with tumors smaller than 2 cm and no symptoms of brainstem or cerebellar compression.

Operative Procedures

1. Incision: a postauricular incision is made 1–1.5 cm behind the postauricular sulcus, and extended through the subcutaneous tissues. The anterior skin flap and auricle are retracted forward. The deep tissues are incised to the mastoid cortex, exposing the mastoid tip, posterior edge of the external auditory canal, suprameatal spine, cribriform area and temporal line.
2. Mastoidectomy: The suprameatal spine and cribriform area are used to locate the antrum. The short process of the incus, fossa incudis, prominence of the lateral semicircular canal and the digastric crest are used to locate the vertical part of facial nerve. A complete mastoidectomy is performed and its margins are saucerized. The posterior wall of the external auditory canal is thinned but kept intact. The sigmoid sinus and the lateral and posterior semicircular canals are identified.
3. Resection of the semicircular canals and opening the vestibule: the fossa incudis and aditus ad antrum are the initial guides to the lateral semicircular canal. The lateral, posterior and superior semicircular canals are all drilled out to expose the vestibule. The membranous labyrinth structures are exposed. The superior vestibular nerve is located deep to the ampullated end of the superior canal. The labyrinthine segment of the facial nerve is exposed.
4. Opening the internal auditory canal and exposing tumor: the medial vestibular wall gives an indication of the upper and lower limits of the internal auditory canal. The canal is skeletonized with the drill and the dura is exposed. The canal is expanded by the tumor which is seen as a reddish mass through the dura. An incision is made in the dura along the lower edge of the internal auditory canal and extending in an L-shape to the dura in front of the sigmoid sinus. Retraction of the dura exposes the contents of the IAC and the cerebellopontine angle and allows the drainage of cerebrospinal fluid. At the lateral end of the canal, the vertical ridge (Bill's bar) is identified separating the facial and superior vestibular nerves.

   Facial nerve injury is obviated by correctly identifying the nerve's anatomy, careful dissection and electrical monitoring of facial nerve function.
5. The separation and removal of acoustic neuroma: the superior and inferior vestibular nerves are seen after opening the dura of the IAC. The canal is filled with a pink mass and may have a surface membrane. The tumor may be confined to the IAC or extend into the cerebellopontine angle, where it may contact or compress the brainstem. Tumors often originate from the superior vestibular nerve. The superior and inferior vestibular nerves are divided above and below the transverse crest, respectively. The cochlear nerve is also divided medial to the vestibular nerve. The tumor is separated from the brainstem using cottonoids. Intracapsular debulking is performed in larger tumors. The capsule of tumor in the cerebellopontine angle is incised and the majority of the intracapsular tumor is removed to reduce the size of the tumor and allow gradual separation of the medial capsule from the brainstem. The facial nerve is identified medial and lateral to the tumor using the facial nerve monitor. Tumor feeding blood vessels are coagulated with bipolar coagulation. The tumor is separated from surrounding structures. Facial nerve monitoring is used to safely remove all tumor from the facial nerve.
6. Hemostasis: the surgical field is liberally irrigated with sterile saline to remove blood and debris. Bipolar coagulation and absorbable hemostatic gauze can be used to stop bleeding.
7. Cavity closure and isolation of tympanic cavity from surgical field: the aditus ad antrum is bared of its mucosa and packed with a muscle plug to prevent postoperative cerebrospinal oto-rhinorrhea. The front wall of mastoid cavity is covered with fascia placed over the aditus, the posterior wall of external auditory canal and the vertical segment of facial nerve. The posterior fossa dura is apposed with sutures as well as is possible and the mastoid cavity is packed with subcutaneous fat from the abdominal wall.

8. Wound closure and dressing: reposition the auricle, suture the wound in layers and apply a mastoid dressing.

Special Comments

1. A complete mastoidectomy is performed, paying attention to identifying anatomical landmarks and not injuring the sigmoid sinus, facial nerve and middle cranial fossa dura.
2. The labyrinthine segment of the facial nerve should be protected after resection of semicircular canals, by exposing the medial vestibular wall and the inferior wall of the internal auditory canal. The medial wall of bone of the superior semicircular canal is preserved until late in the dissection when the internal auditory canal has been fully opened.
3. Care is taken with the labyrinthine artery which should not be avulsed. It can be bipolar coagulated and divided laterally. The loop of AICA must be preserved, and particular attention is paid when it extends to the IAC.
4. Thorough intraoperative hemostasis must be achieved.
5. The vertical segment of the facial nerve should not be exposed.
6. Avoid thermal damage to the facial nerve when use bipolar coagulation.
7. Remove the mucosa of aditus ad antrum and close the aditus with a muscle plug near the dural incision to prevent postoperative cerebrospinal oto-rhinorrhea. If the incus is removed, avoid fracture or dislocation of the stapes to prevent postoperative cerebrospinal oto-rhinorrhea.
8. The tympanic segment of the facial nerve is located lateral to the outer wall of the vestibule. Care must be taken to avoid damaging it when opening the vestibule.

Complications

1. Postoperative bleeding, epidural or subdural hematoma.
2. Peripheral facial paralysis (temporary or permanent).
3. Cerebrospinal fluid leakage: including cerebrospinal oto-rhinorrhea and incision leak.
4. Wound or intracranial infection.
5. Cranial nerve injury.
6. Brainstem injury.
7. Hemiplegia, ataxia and other neurological deficits.

Surgery 1: Translabyrinthine Approach for Removal of Acoustic Neuroma

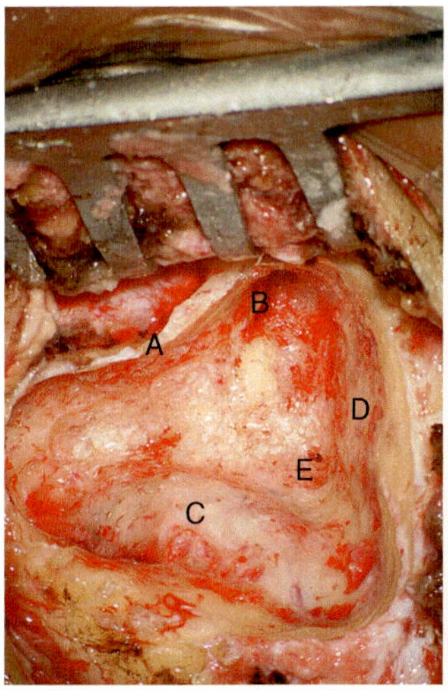

A. Posterior wall of the external auditory canal
B. Incus
C. Sigmoid sinus
D. Mastoid tegmen
E. Sinodural angle

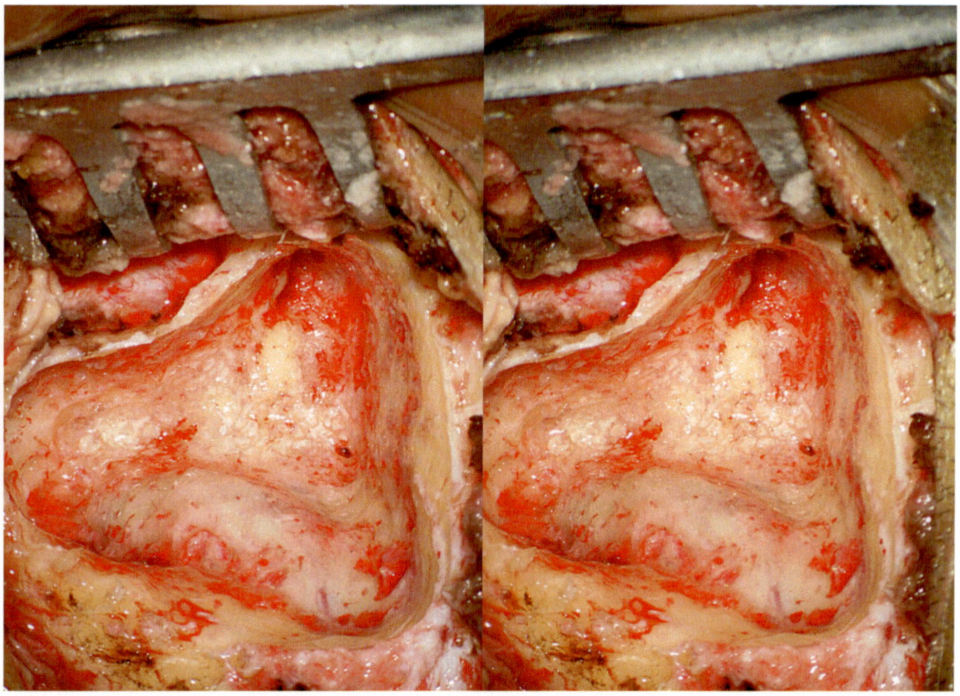

Fig. 5.35 Mastoidectomy
A postauricular incision is made. The suprameatal spine and cribriform area are used to locate the antrum and the mastoidectomy is performed. The fossa incudis, prominence of lateral semicircular canal and digastric crest are used to locate the vertical part of the facial nerve. A complete mastoidectomy is performed and its margins are saucerized. The posterior wall of the external auditory canal is thinned but kept intact. The sigmoid sinus and the lateral and posterior semicircular canals are identified

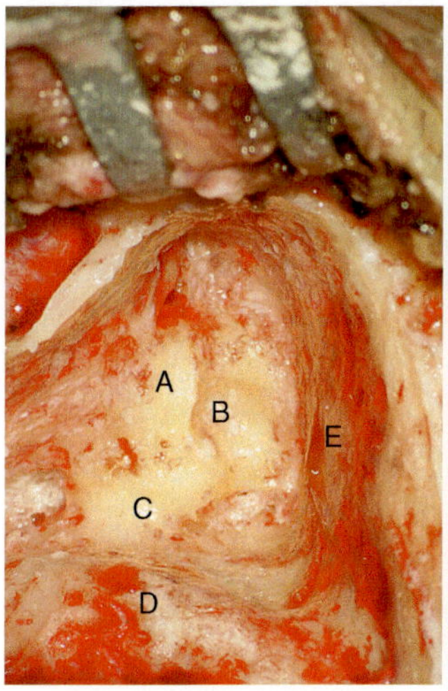

A. Prominence of lateral semicircular canal
B. Superior semicircular canal
C. Posterior semicircular canal
D. Sigmoid sinus
E. Mastoid tegmen

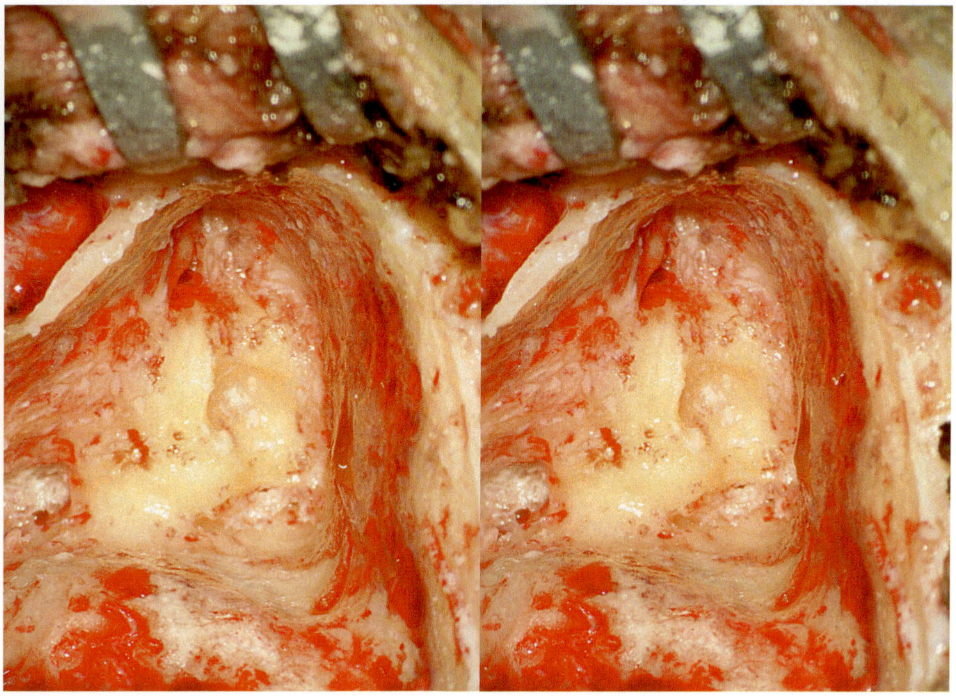

Fig. 5.36 Skeletonizing the semicircular canals
At the depths of the mastoidectomy, the prominences of lateral, posterior and superior semicircular canals are revealed. This picture clearly shows the incus, fossa incudis, the mastoid tegmen, the sigmoid sinus, and the bony contour of three semicircular canals

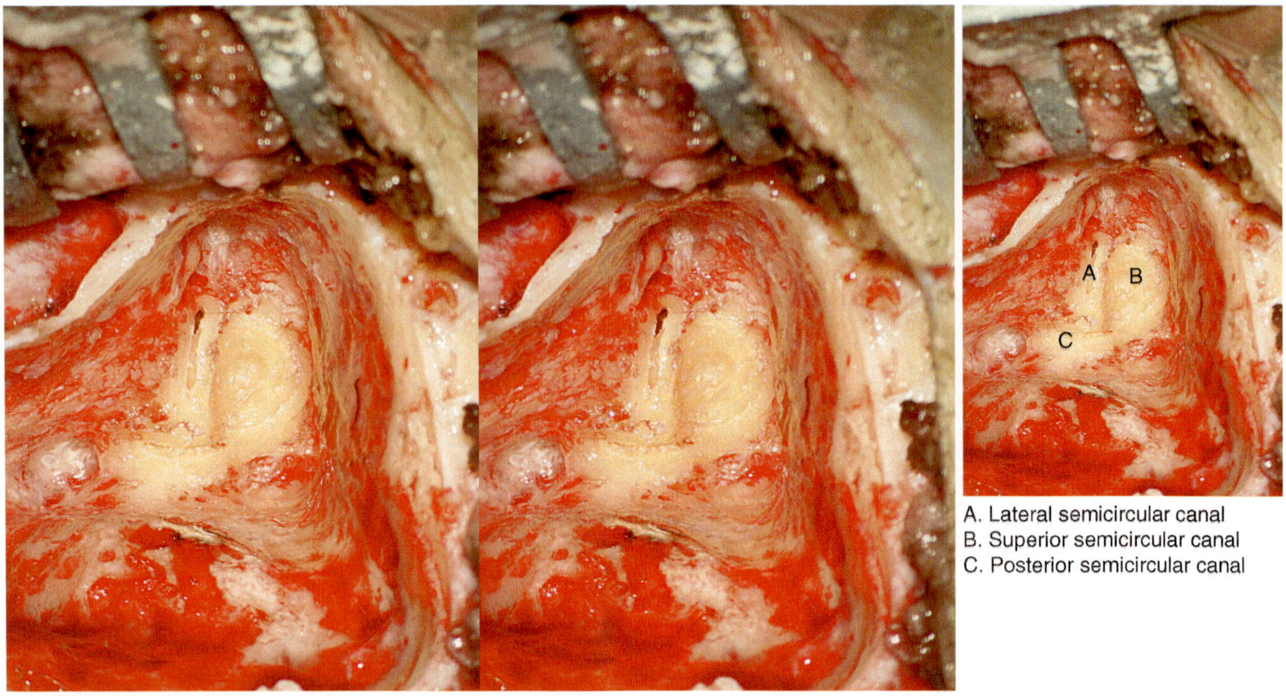

A. Lateral semicircular canal
B. Superior semicircular canal
C. Posterior semicircular canal

Fig. 5.37 Opening the semicircular canals
In the depths of the cavity, the bony contours of the three semicircular canals are seen. The three canals have been opened exposing the membranous labyrinth

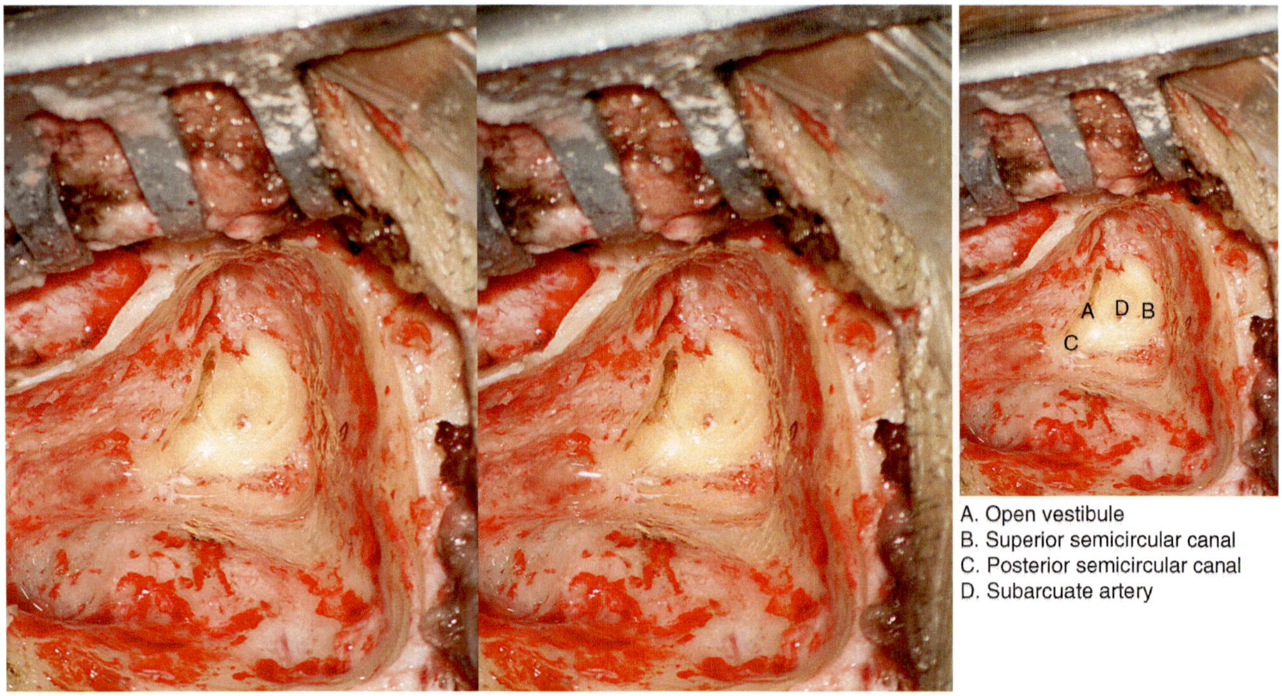

A. Open vestibule
B. Superior semicircular canal
C. Posterior semicircular canal
D. Subarcuate artery

Fig. 5.38 Removal of semicircular canals and opening vestibule
The subarcuate artery is seen in the arch of the superior canal

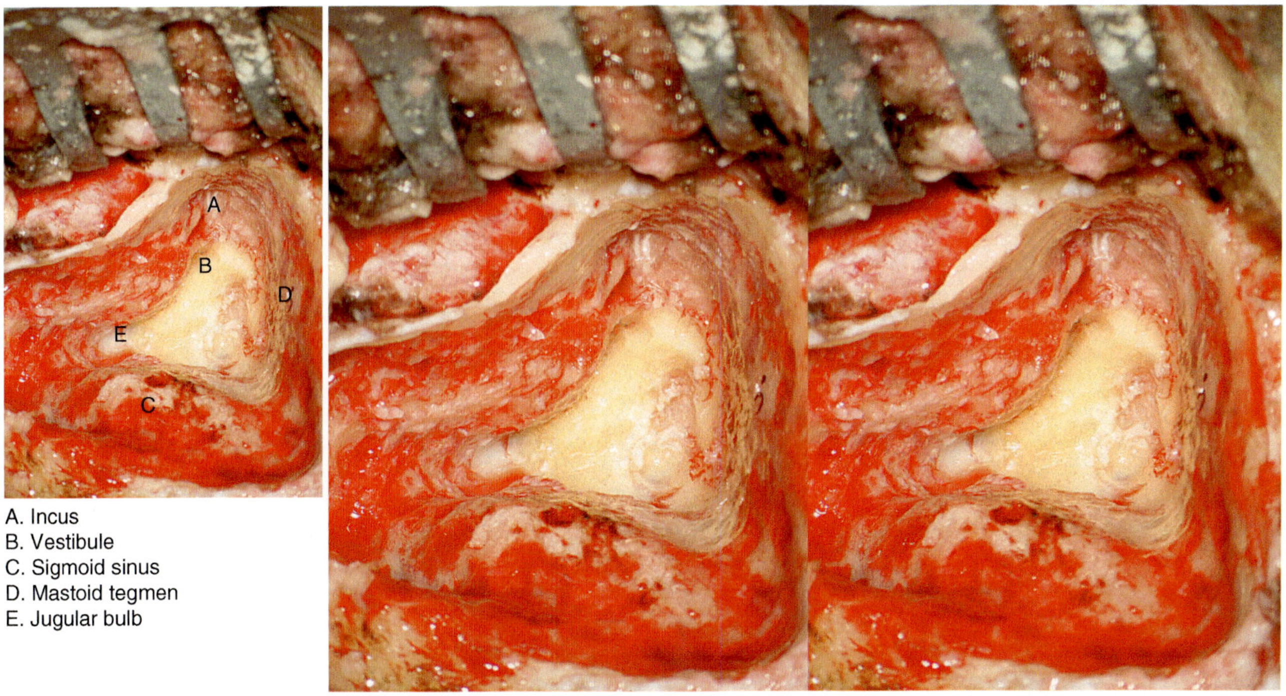

Fig. 5.39 Opening the vestibule
Open the vestibule and expose its medial wall which covers the lateral end of the vestibular nerve. The superior vestibular nerve leads to the labyrinthine segment of the facial nerve leaving the internal auditory canal. Initial preservation of the medial wall of the superior canal ampulla protects the facial nerve. Dissection should stay posterior to the vertical ridge

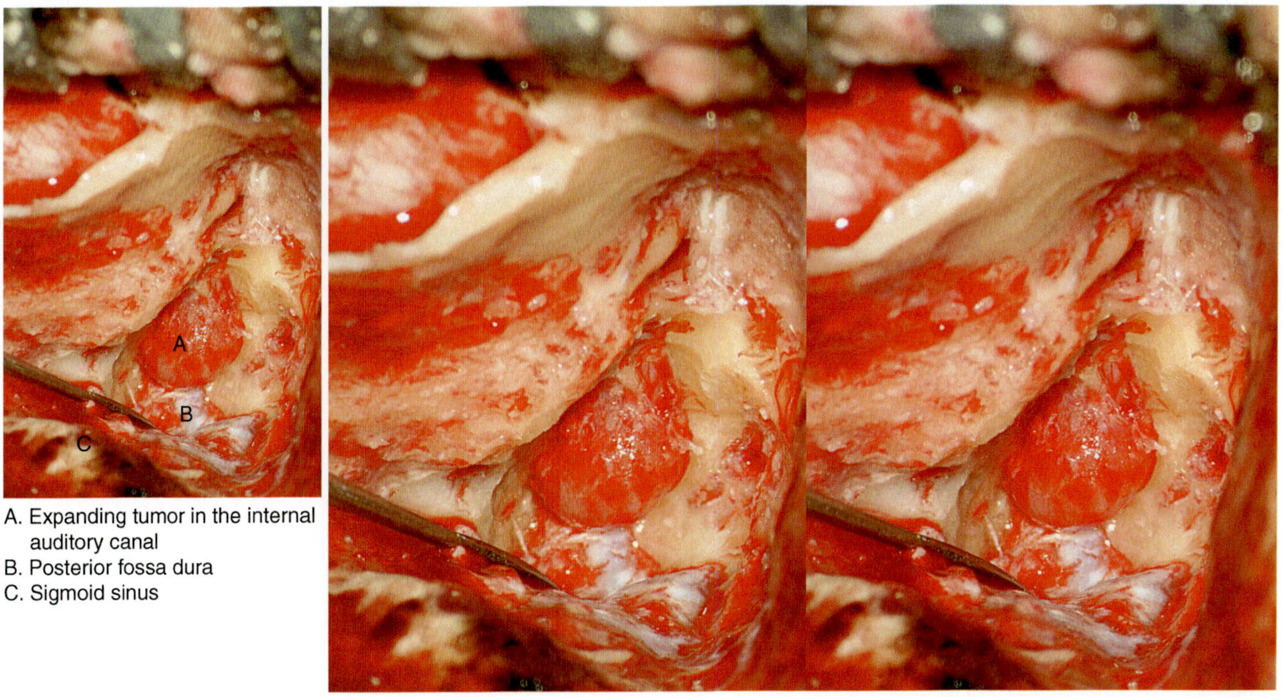

Fig. 5.40 Expose the dura of the internal auditory canal
The cribriform area of medial wall of vestibule is removed with 2–3 mm diamond drill. The bone of the posterior half (180°) of the internal auditory canal is removed. Open the internal auditory canal which is expanded by tumor. Clear cerebrospinal fluid egress is seen as soon as the dura is opened to expose the tumor. Part of the posterior fossa dura is also exposed

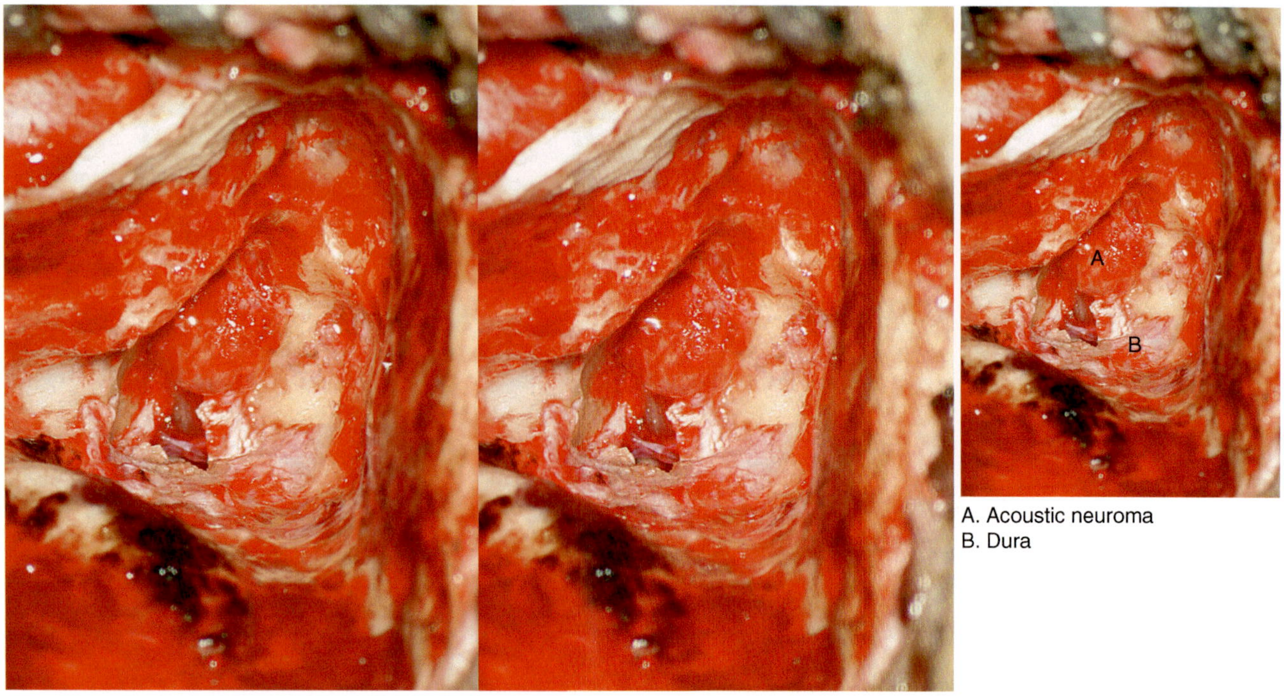

Fig. 5.41 Exposure of tumor in internal auditory canal
The upper, posterior and lower walls of the internal auditory canal are exposed thoroughly. The posterior canal dura is removed to expose the tumor and the posterior fossa dura is opened. The nerves medial to the tumor are just on view. The tumor is mostly confined to the IAC

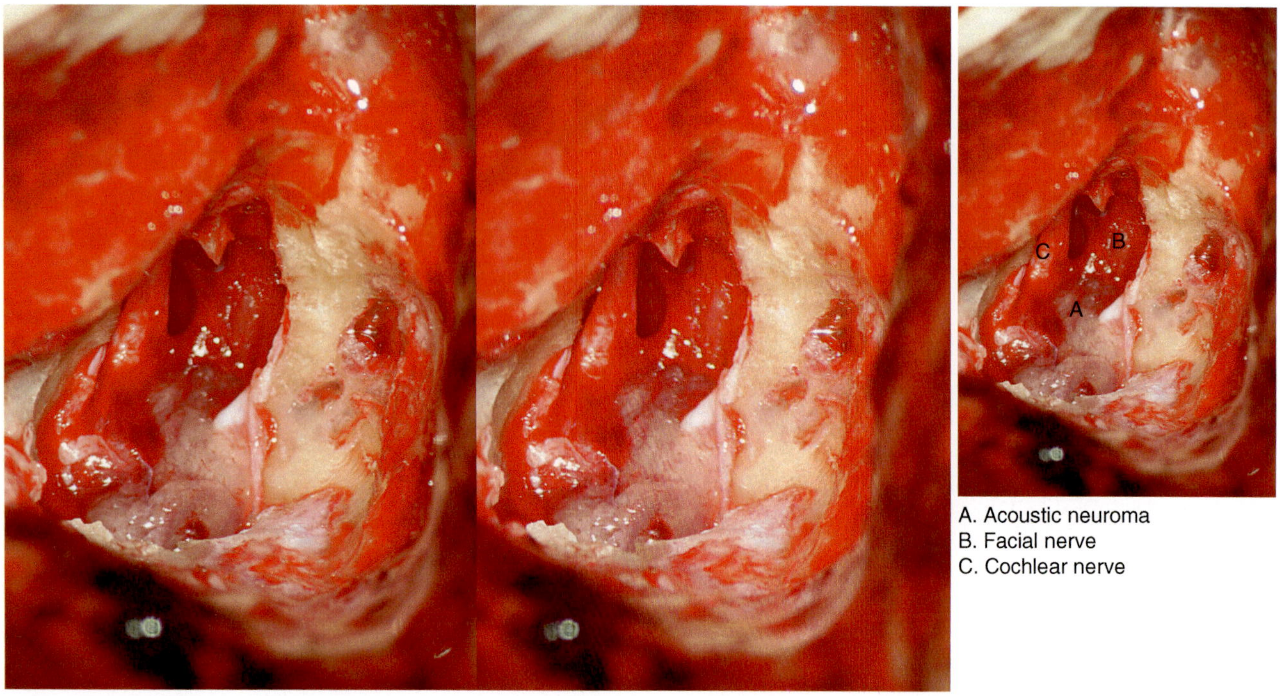

Fig. 5.42 Separation of the facial nerve from the tumor
Separation and removal of the tumor. The facial nerve is adherent to the surface of the tumor and sharp dissection is used to separate them. Attention is paid to achieve good hemostasis. This tumor arose from the common vestibular nerve. Large tumors need intracapsular debulking before complete removal of the capsule. Facial nerve monitoring helps prevent nerve injury. The facial nerve is above and the cochlear nerve below the level of the transverse crest

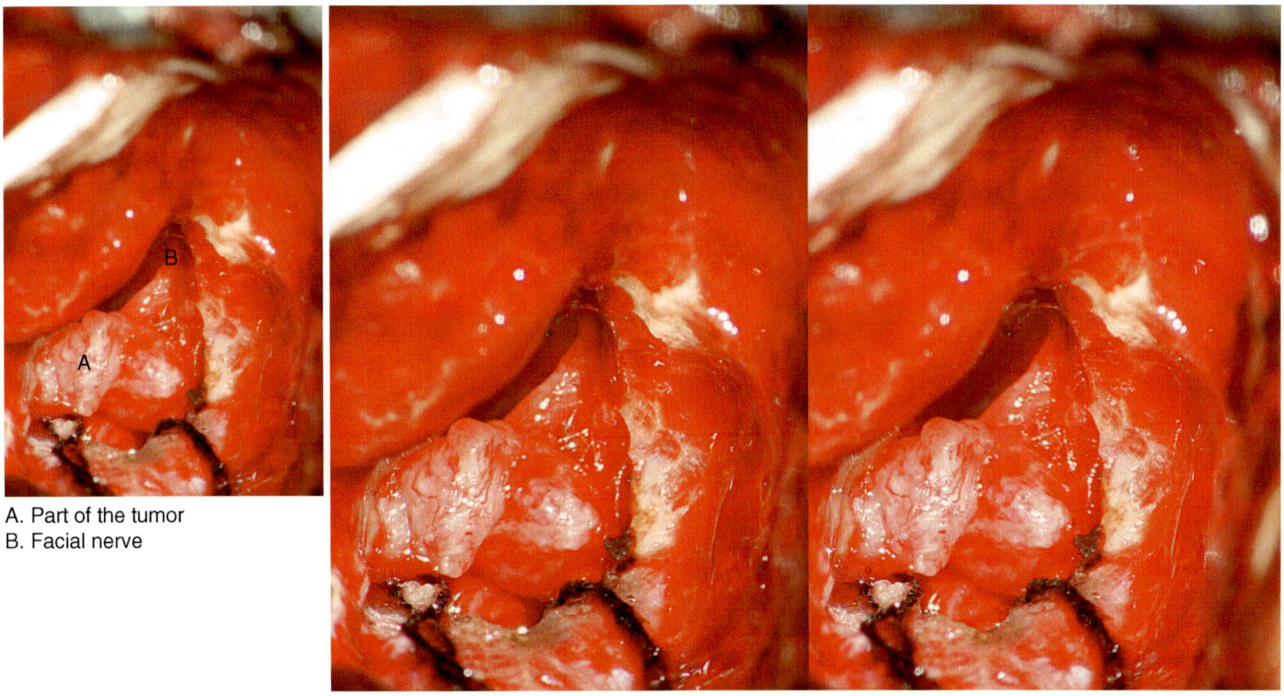

A. Part of the tumor
B. Facial nerve

Fig. 5.43 Resection of the tumor within the internal auditory canal
Remove the cochlear nerve. The tumor is separated and removed in a piecemeal fashion from the facial nerve with the assistance of facial nerve monitoring. This picture shows the tumor being separated from the facial nerve

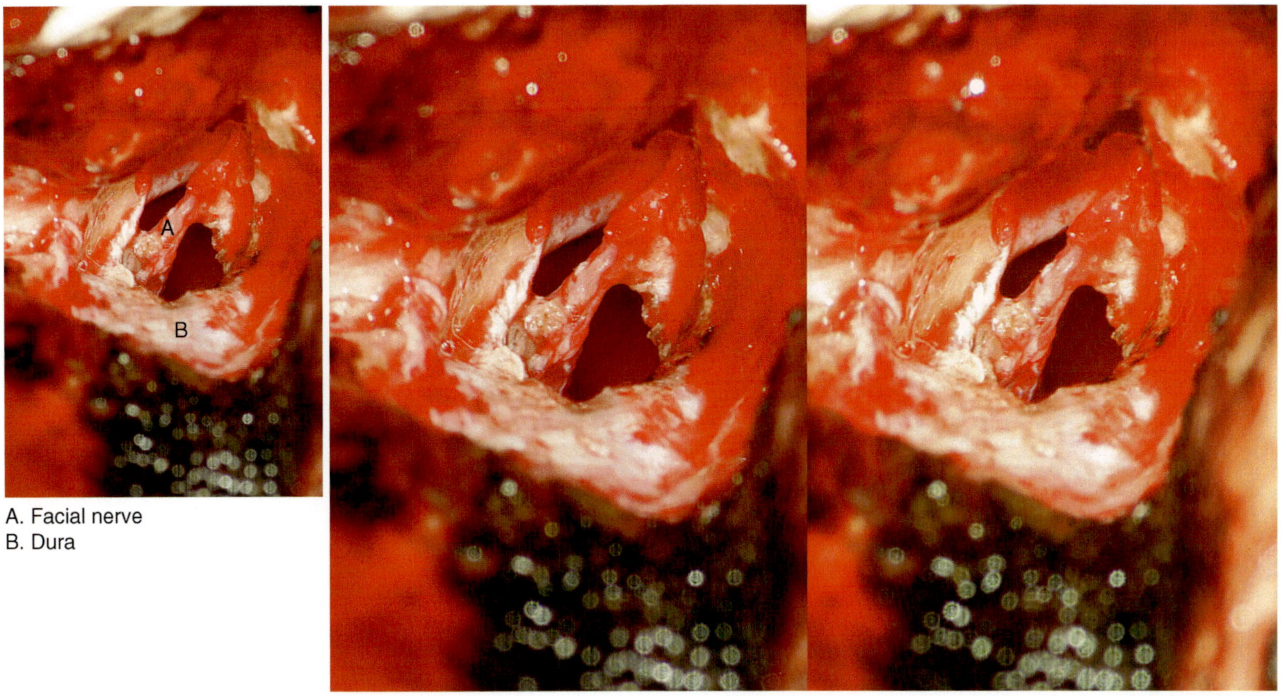

A. Facial nerve
B. Dura

Fig. 5.44 Remove the tumor and preserve the facial nerve
The majority of tumor has been removed successfully. The facial nerve is seen to be in good condition and the monitoring confirmed its good function

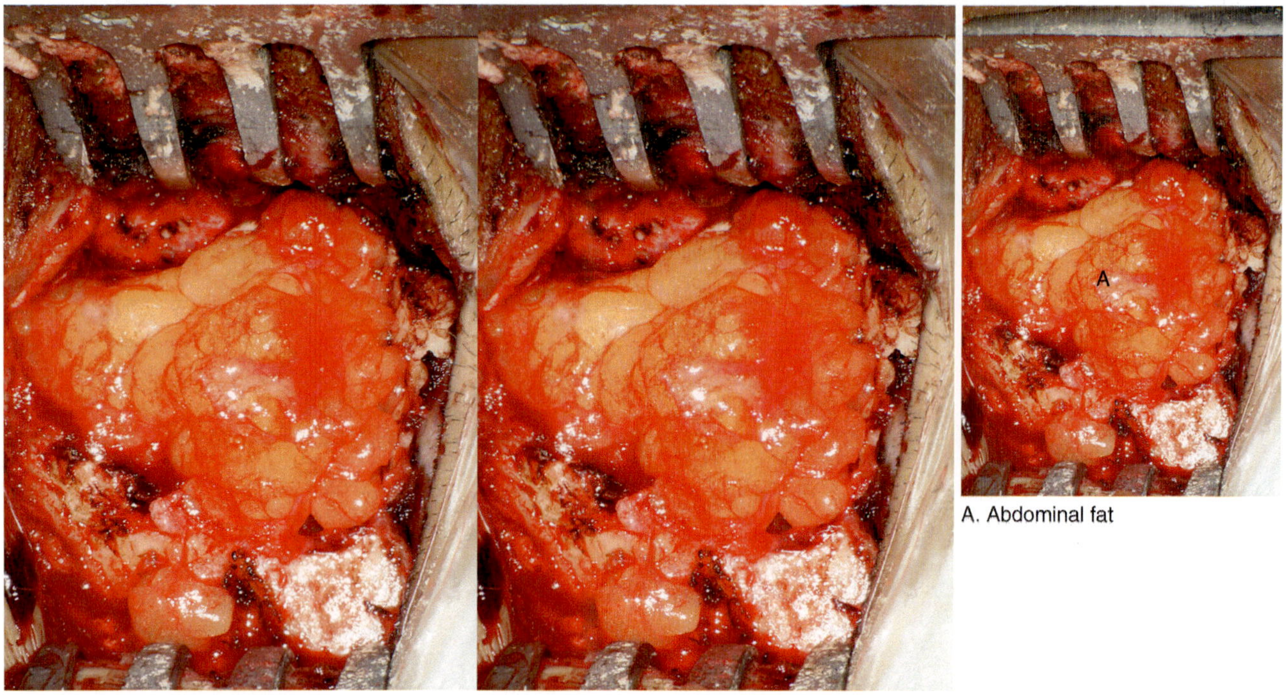

Fig. 5.45 Filling the cavity with fat
The cavity is liberally irrigated after complete tumor resection to clear debris and check for any bleeding which is then controlled. The aditus ad antrum and air space between the mastoid and tympanic cavity will be closed completely with a muscle plug to prevent postoperative cerebrospinal fluid otorrhea. The open mastoid cavity and internal auditory canal are filled with autologous abdominal wall fat. The incision is closed with interrupted sutures and a compression dressing is applied

Surgery 2: Translabyrinthine approach for Removal of Acoustic Neuroma

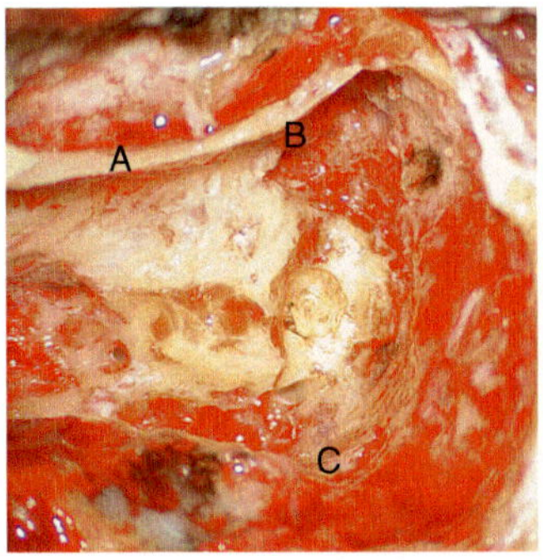

A. Posterior wall of the external auditory canal
B. Incus
C. Sinodural angle

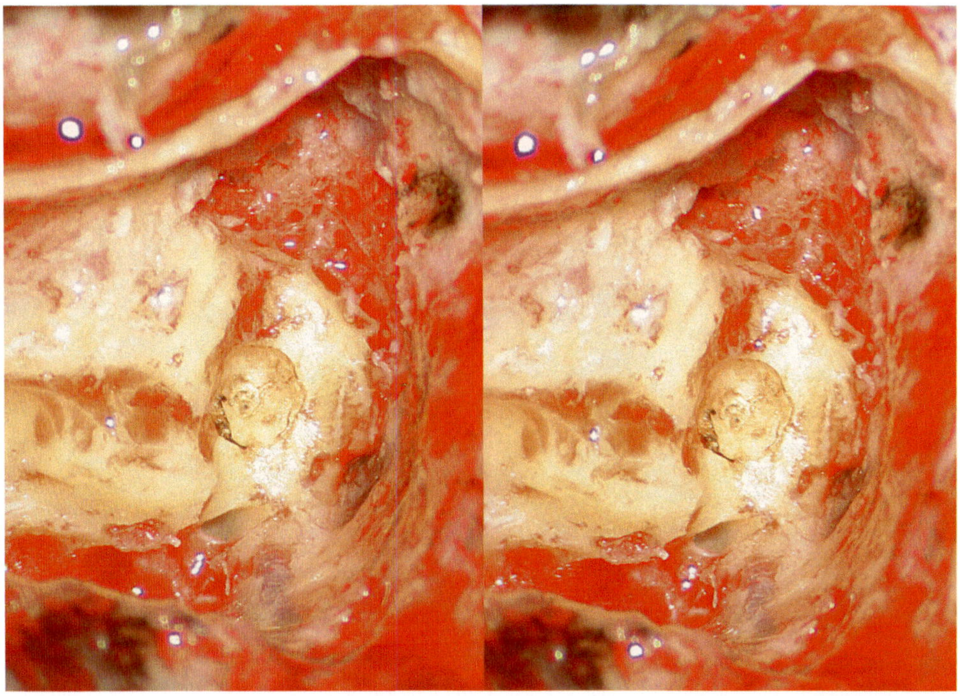

Fig. 5.46 Mastoidectomy and exposed semicircular canals
The mastoidectomy is completed: the posterior bony wall of the external auditory canal is thinned but preserved. The suprameatal spine and cribriform area are used to locate the antrum. The tegmen of the mastoid is skeletonized and the bone over the sigmoid sinus is drilled to a thin shell. Inferiorly the mastoid tip is drilled out and the digastric crest exposed. The bony contours of the three semicircular canals are now apparent

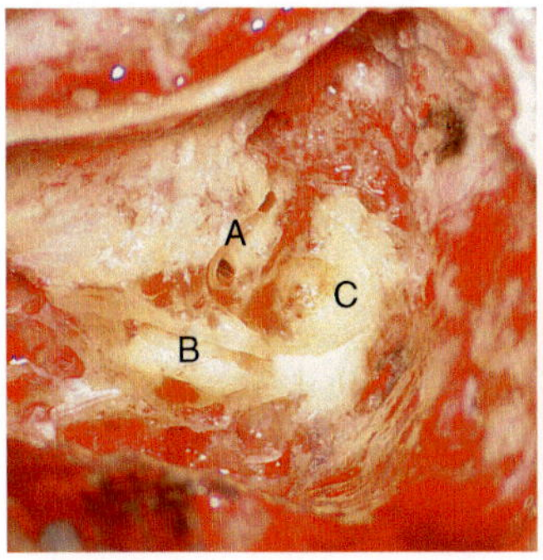

A. Open lateral semicircular canal
B. Open posterior semicircular canal
C. Open superior semicircular canal

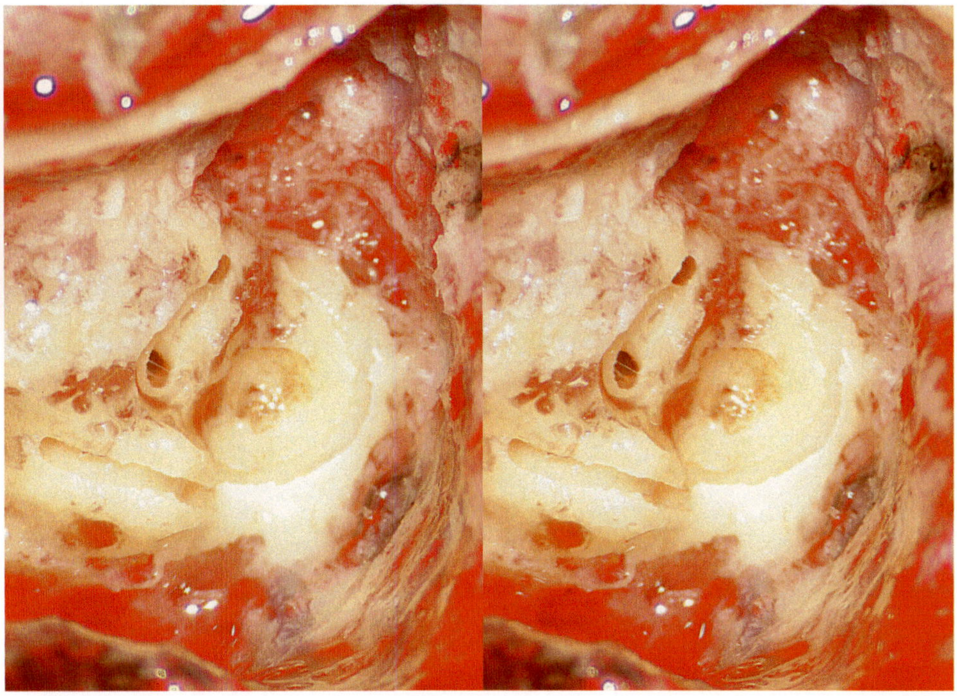

Fig. 5.47 Semicircular canal resection
In the depths of the cavity, the bony contours of the three semicircular canals are seen. The lateral canal is opened first. Initially, a faint blue line can be seen when drilling down the wall before opening into the canal lumen to expose the membranous labyrinth structures. Drilling then continues through the posterior canal, common crus, and the superior canal. The lateral semicircular canal lies immediately above the facial nerve

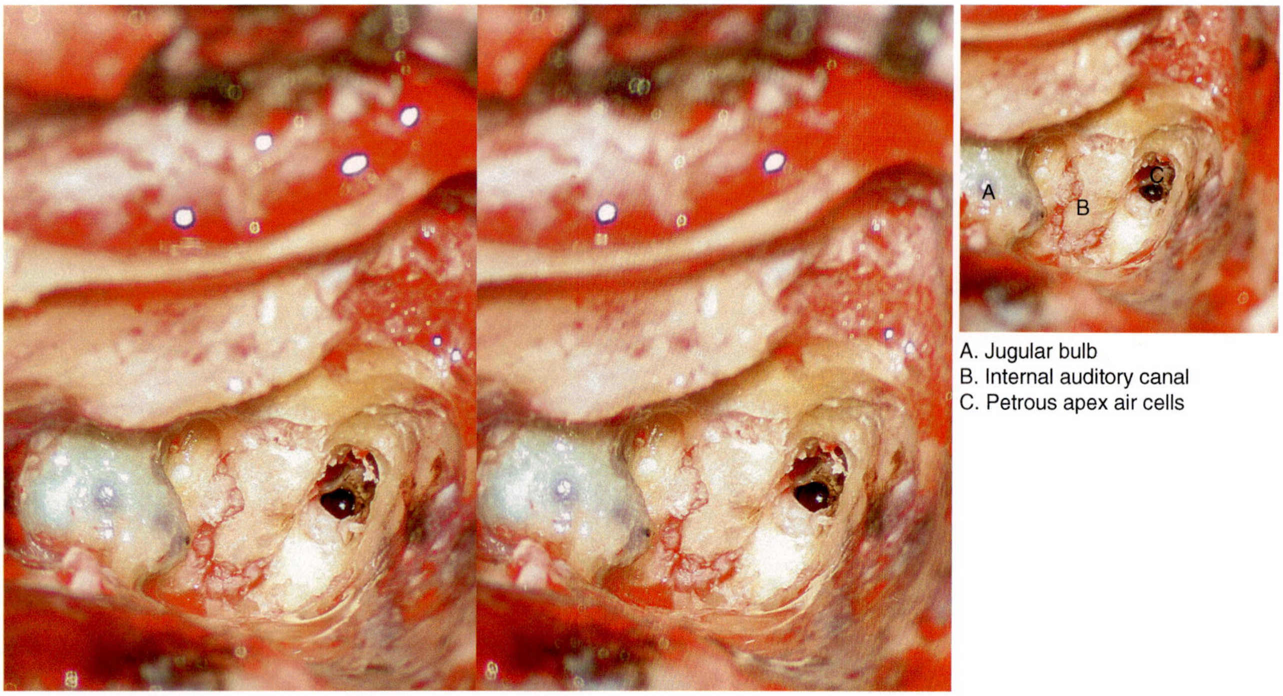

Fig. 5.48 Skeletonizing the internal auditory canal
The position of the internal auditory canal is revealed after removal of the lateral semicircular canal and opening the vestibule. A thin layer of bone is left over the dura of the canal. The air cells of the petrous apex are above the internal auditory canal

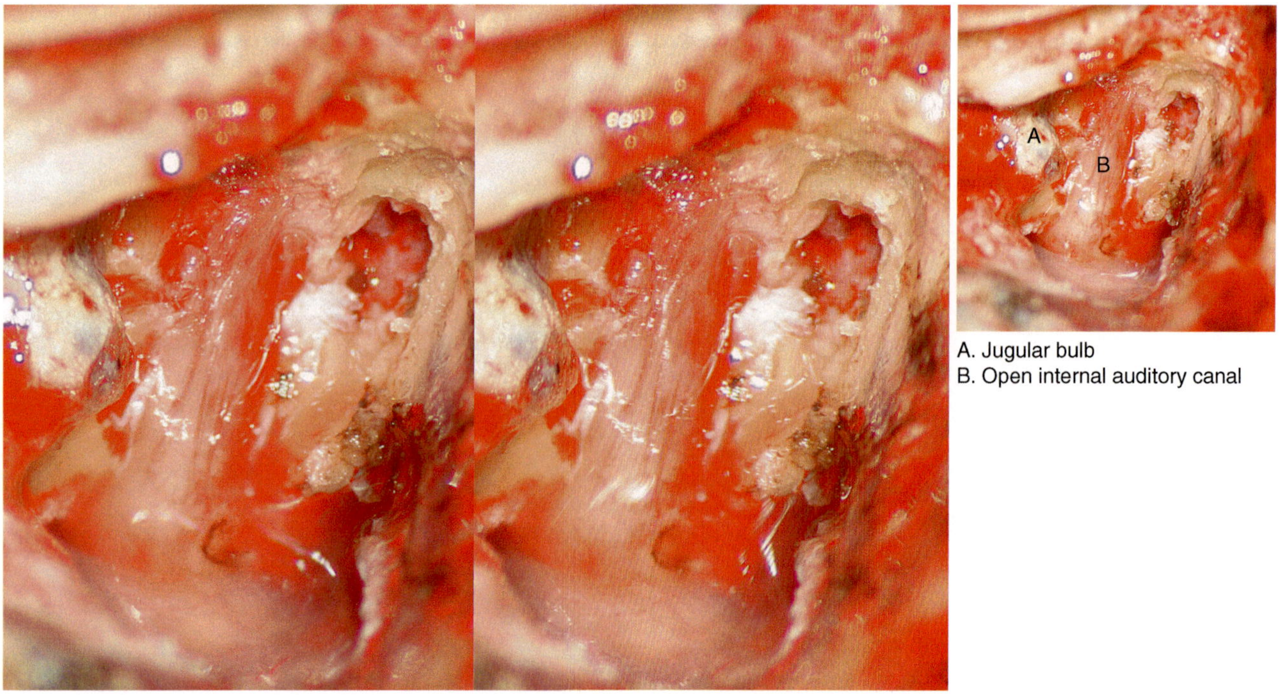

Fig. 5.49 Exposure of nerves and tumor in the internal auditory canal
The shell of bone over the internal auditory canal is removed and the dura is incised at the bottom of internal auditory canal and over the posterior fossa. The dural flaps are retracted to lay open the internal auditory canal and CPA. The nerves and tumor contained in the internal auditory canal can be seen

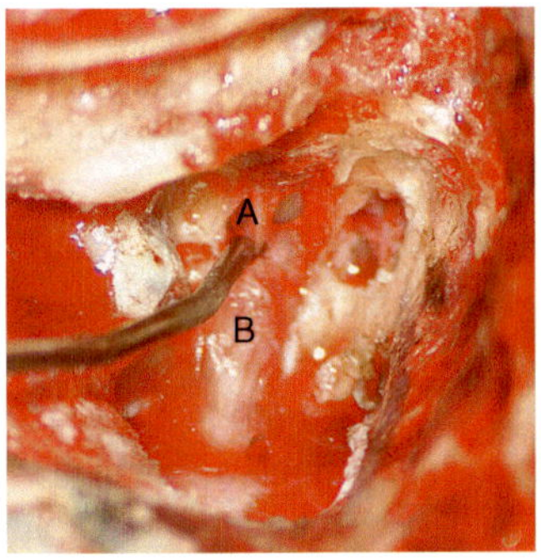

A. Facial nerve
B. Acoustic neuroma

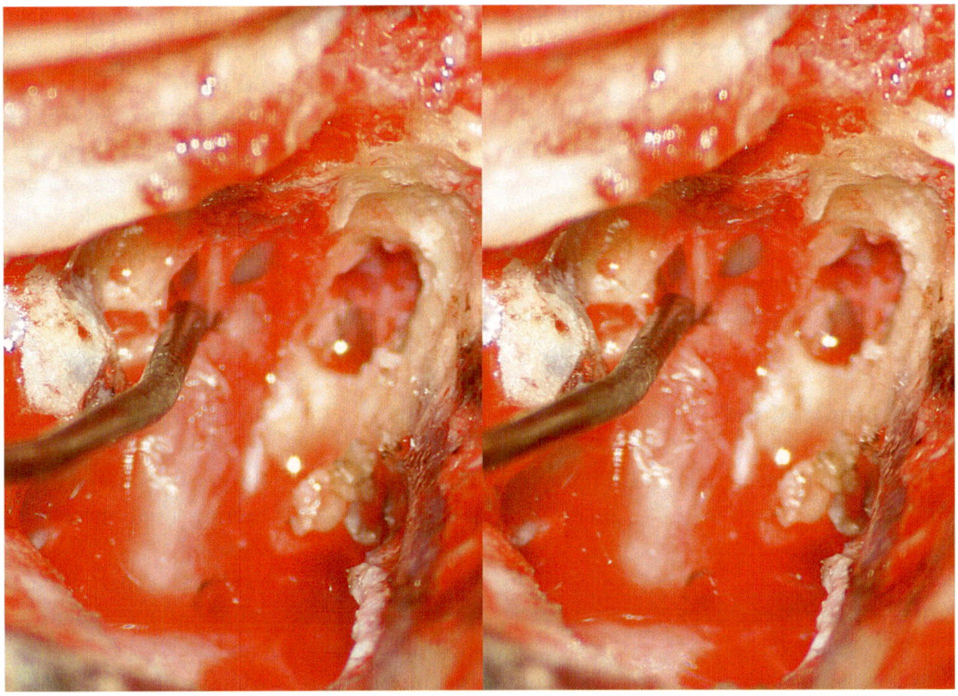

Fig. 5.50 Separation of tumor from the facial nerve
After the tumor of the internal auditory canal is exposed, the facial nerve position is confirmed with the monitor. The facial nerve lies above the transverse crest and the cochlear nerve

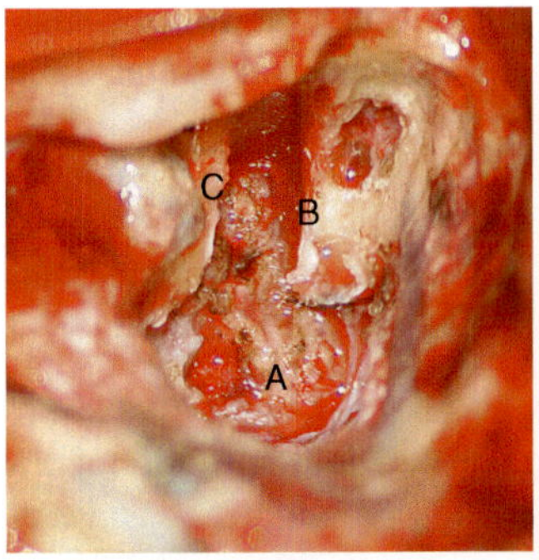

A. Acoustic neuroma in the cerebellopontine angle
B. Upper lip of internal auditory canal
C. Lower lip of internal auditory canal

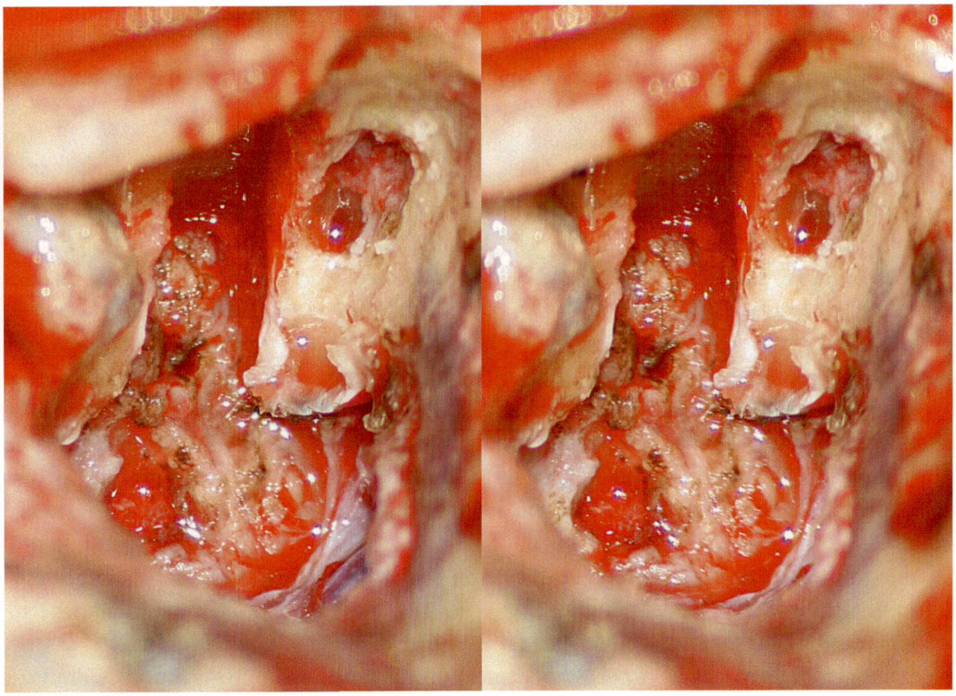

Fig. 5.51 Exposed tumor within the cerebellopontine angle
The tumor in the cerebellopontine angle will be exposed after the nerves of the internal auditory canal are identified. We locate the facial nerve and remove the acoustic neuroma whilst monitoring facial nerve function

Removal of Acoustic Neuroma Middle-Cranial Fossa Approach

Jun Liu and Pu Dai

Indications

Normal facial nerve function, serviceable hearing, less than 1.5 cm tumor of the internal auditory canal.

Contraindications

Larger acoustic neuroma prolapsing into the cerebellopontine angle.

Operative Procedures

1. Incision: an S-shaped incision is begun 1 cm anterior to the upper part of the auricle and extending 8 cm superiorly through skin and subcutaneous tissue to the temporalis fascia. The bottom of the incision is near the temporal line. Blunt dissection is used to elevate the temporalis muscle to expose the squamous temporal bone and held with a self-retaining retractor.
2. A 4×3 cm bone flap is created in the squamous bone and is removed to expose the dura overlying the temporal lobe. The front 2/3 of bone window is located in front of a line through the anterior wall of the external auditory canal bone. Its inferior limit is as close as possible to the temporal line and level with the floor of the middle cranial fossa to minimize temporal lobe retraction during surgery.
3. Elevation of the dura and localization of the internal auditory canal and facial nerve: the dura of the floor of the middle cranial fossa is elevated for the full width of the bone window to expose the facial nerve hiatus, arcuate eminence and great superficial petrosal nerve (GSPN) which will lead to the location of the internal auditory canal. If the geniculate ganglion is not easily identified due to thick bone cover, it may be necessary to drill the bone a little to confirm its position.
4. Exposure of the internal auditory canal: the line of the internal auditory canal bisects the angle between the superior semicircular canal and the GSPN. The roof of the canal is gradually drilled away, starting medially. The anterior and posterior margins of the canal are identified then the dura of the roof is completely uncovered. It usually appears pink and may bulge up a little.
5. Identify and remove the tumor: incise the dura longitudinally along the posterior border of the canal. It is likely to be filled with tumor. The facial nerve runs along the front border of the canal and therefore along the front edge of the tumor. The facial nerve monitoring probe can be used to confirm the position of the nerve. The interface between the tumor and the facial nerve is identified with a hook. The tumor often originates from the superior vestibular nerve. The capsule of the tumor is incised, and the majority of the tumor is removed within it to reduce its size. The tumor is freed up from its connections within the rest of the internal auditory canal. The remaining tumor capsule is completely resected after careful separation from the facial nerve. After tumor resection, the continuity of the facial nerve is confirmed and its function shown to be intact with the nerve monitor. Auditory Brainstem Response (ABR) may be used to confirm preservation of hearing (and therefore the cochlear nerve and blood vessels).
6. Skull base repair. Liberally irrigate the field with normal saline. After complete hemostasis is achieved, the middle cranial fossa defect of the internal auditory canal is closed with fascia, as is any other defect in the floor of the middle cranial fossa to prevent leakage of cerebrospinal fluid (CSF). Any open air cells in the root of the zygoma or mastoid bone posteriorly are sealed with bone wax as well to prevent CSF leak
7. Wound closure: the bone flap is reinserted; a subcutaneous drain tube is inserted; the wound is closed in layers and a compression dressing is applied.

Special Comments

1. The location of bone window must be accurate. The bone window is made in the squamous part of temporal bone with its lower edge at the zygomatic arch and temporal line (the lower limit of the middle cranial fossa). This minimizes the need for temporal lobe retraction. The bone flap is positioned with 2/3 anterior to the front wall of the external canal.
2. When elevating the dura, care is taken to protect the superior petrosal sinus, the middle meningeal artery and geniculate ganglion of the facial nerve.
3. Accurately identify the position of the internal auditory canal; avoid damage to the superior semicircular canal and cochlea.
4. Preservation of the facial and cochlear nerves is greatly assisted with facial nerve and auditory monitoring. The point of opening the IAC dura should be well away from the facial nerve.
5. The vertical ridge and facial nerve are identified correctly when the internal auditory canal is opened.
6. Avoid injury to the facial and cochlear nerves when using thermal coagulation.

7. Take care in preserving the blood vessels supplying the facial and cochlear nerves.
8. The roof of the internal auditory canal must be well sealed at the completion of the procedure to prevent the occurrence of cerebrospinal fluid otorrhea.
9. Open air cells and any other defect in the floor of the middle cranial fossa are also sealed or covered with fascia to prevent the occurrence of cerebrospinal fluid otorrhea.
10. A loop of the anterior inferior cerebellar artery may pass in to the internal auditory canal. Care must be taken to avoid injuring it and prevent bleeding or interruption of blood supply to the facial and cochlear nerves and brainstem.
11. Real-time monitoring of facial and cochlear nerve function is very important in identifying the nerves and separating them and their related blood vessel from the tumor.

Complications

1. Postoperative bleeding, epidural or subdural hematoma.
2. Peripheral facial paralysis (temporary or permanent).
3. Loss of hearing
4. Cerebrospinal oto-rhinorrhea.
5. Wound or intracranial infection.
6. Temporal lobe injury and brain edema

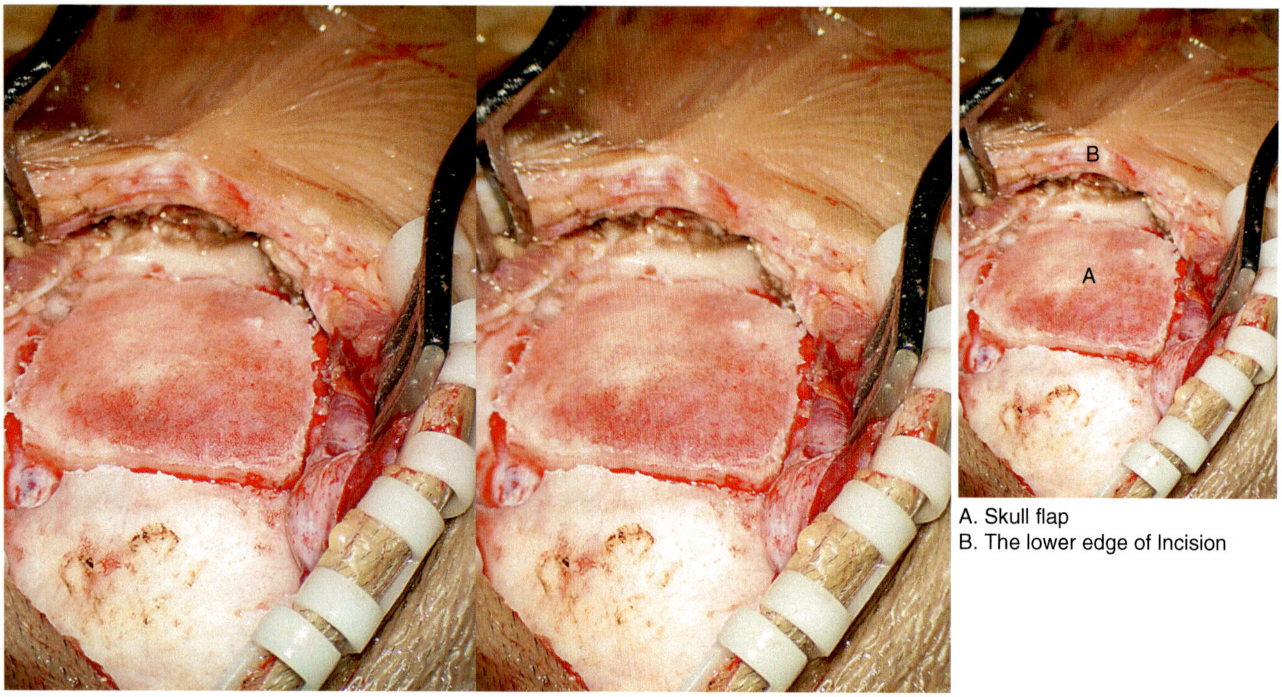

Fig. 5.52 Bone window in squamous part of temporal bone
Open a rectangular bone window in the squamous part of the temporal bone: The front 2/3 of bone window is located at the front of the bony external auditory canal and 1/3 behind. Its lower edge is as close as possible to the temporal line. The flap is 4 cm in width 3 cm in height

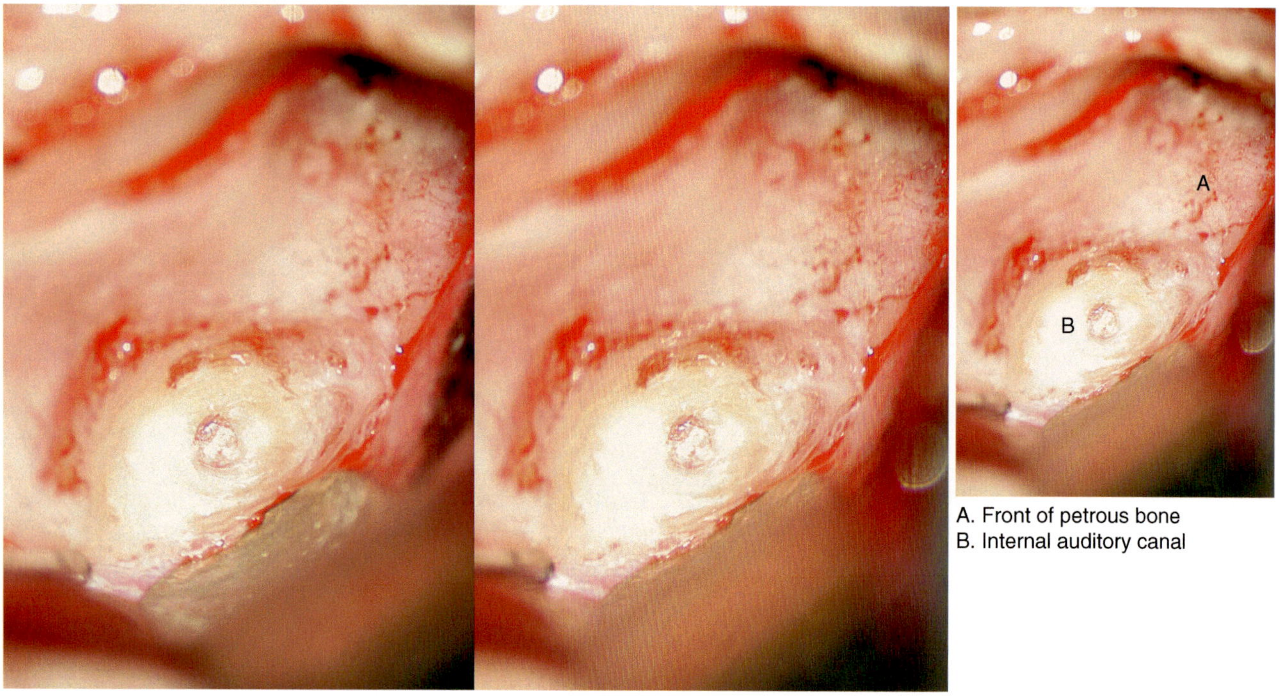

Fig. 5.53 Location of internal auditory canal
Elevate the dura and expose the arcuate eminence, foramen spinosum and greater superficial petrosal (GSPN) nerve to then locate the internal auditory canal and facial nerve. The angle between the GSPN and the arcuate eminence is about 120 °. Drilling to expose the internal auditory canal starts along a line that bisects this angle, and medially near the superior petrosal sinus

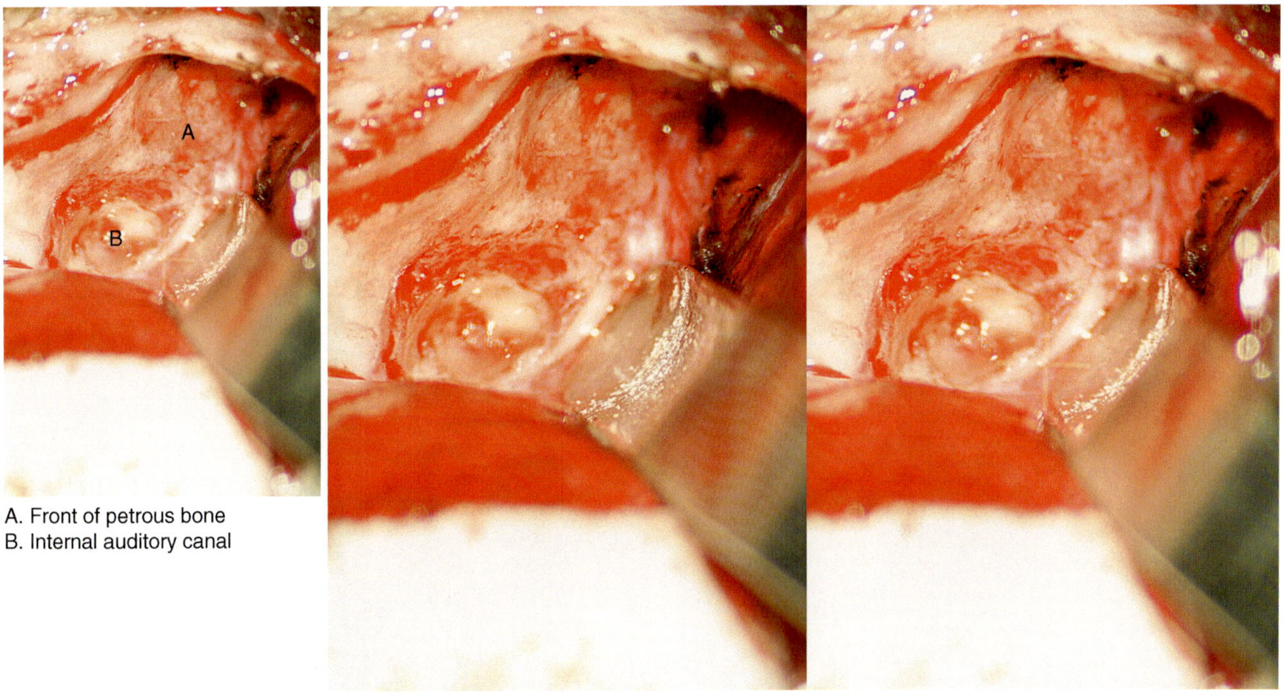

Fig. 5.54 Part exposure of internal auditory canal
Due to abnormal expansion of the internal auditory canal and distortion of the landmarks, it may be necessary to expose the geniculate ganglion and labyrinthine segment of the facial nerve

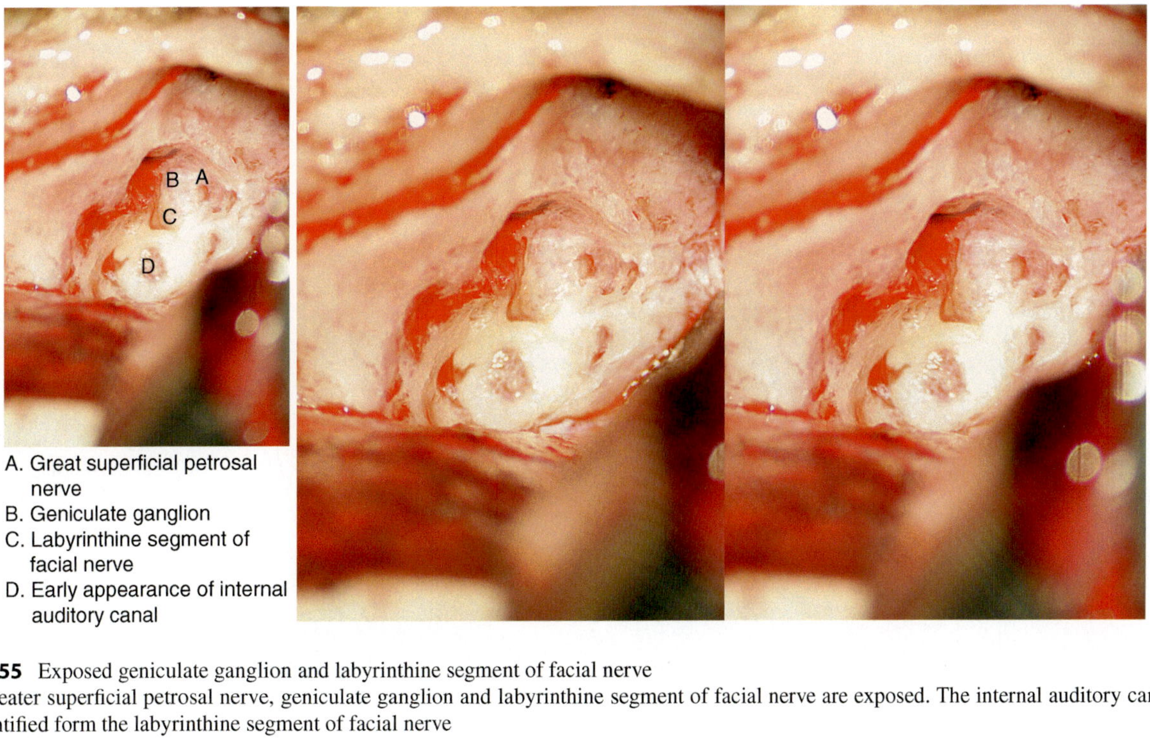

Fig. 5.55 Exposed geniculate ganglion and labyrinthine segment of facial nerve
The greater superficial petrosal nerve, geniculate ganglion and labyrinthine segment of facial nerve are exposed. The internal auditory canal can be identified form the labyrinthine segment of facial nerve

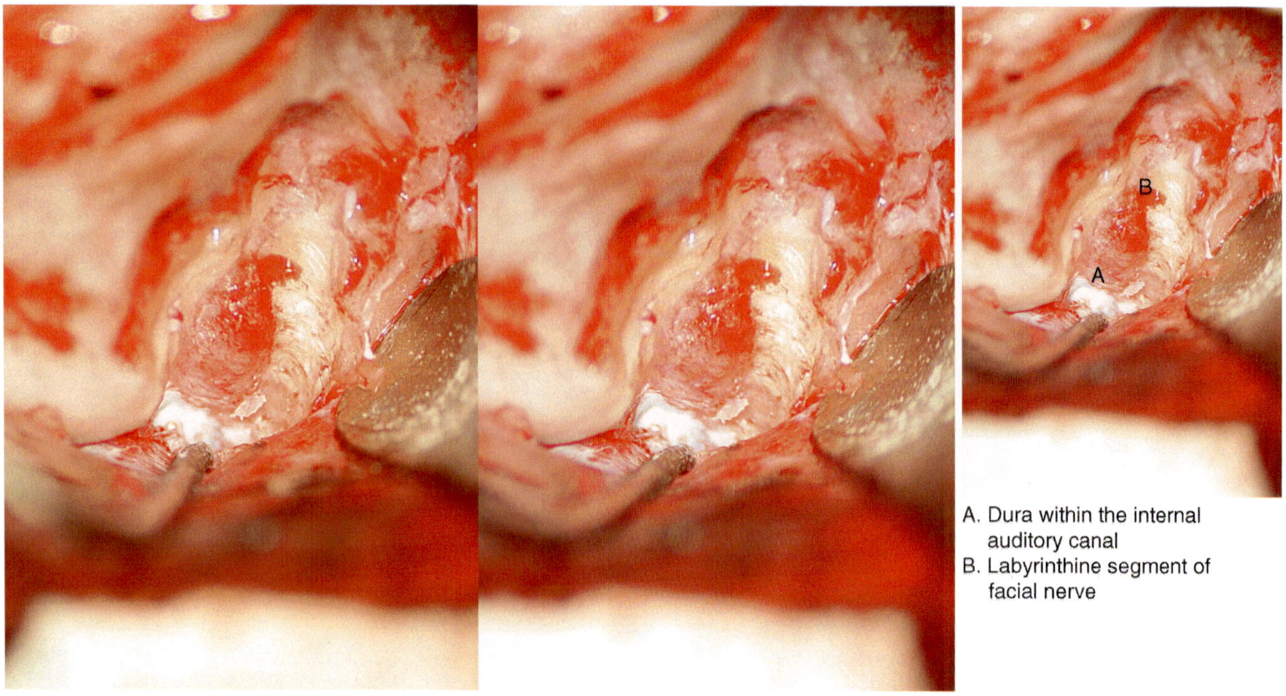

Fig. 5.56 Exposed dura and tumor within the internal auditory canal
Dissect the fundus of the internal auditory canal in relation to the labyrinthine segment of the facial nerve. Then drill medially until the canal is fully opened, exposing dura and tumor within. The internal auditory canal is expanded by tumor

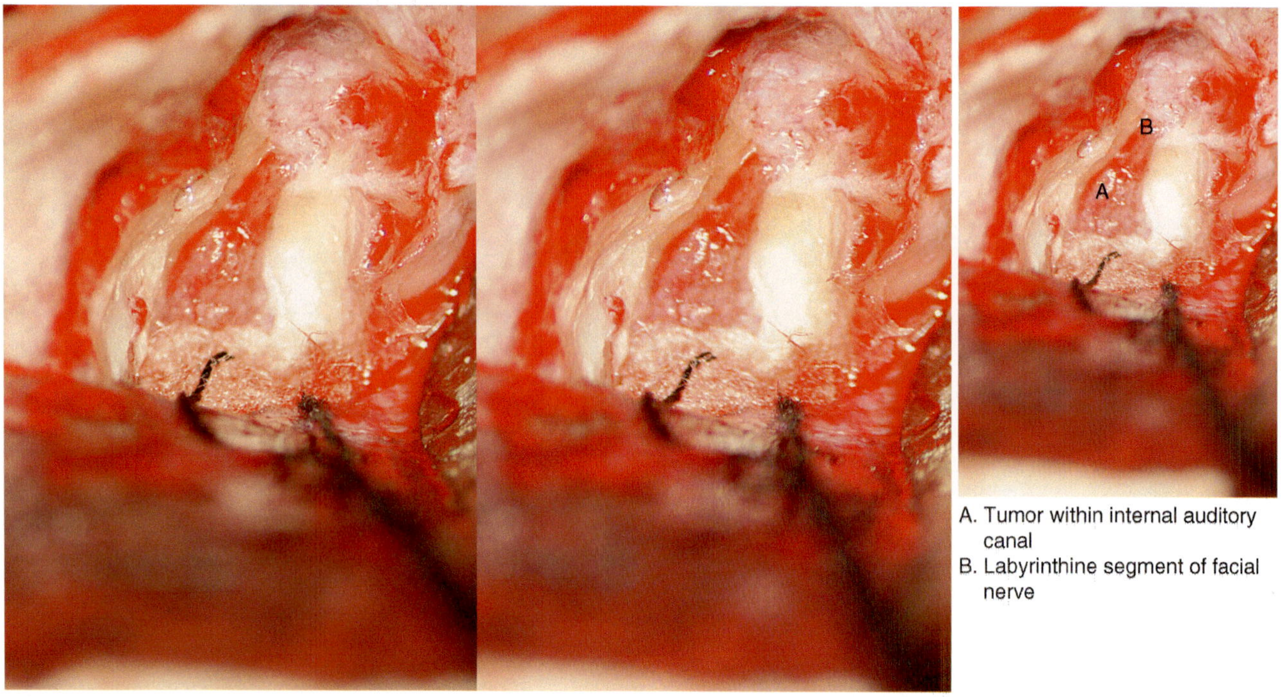

Fig. 5.57 Exposure and resection of tumor
Open the internal auditory canal and incise the dura to expose the tumor within. Total tumor removal is achieved using electrical monitoring to preserve facial and auditory nerve function

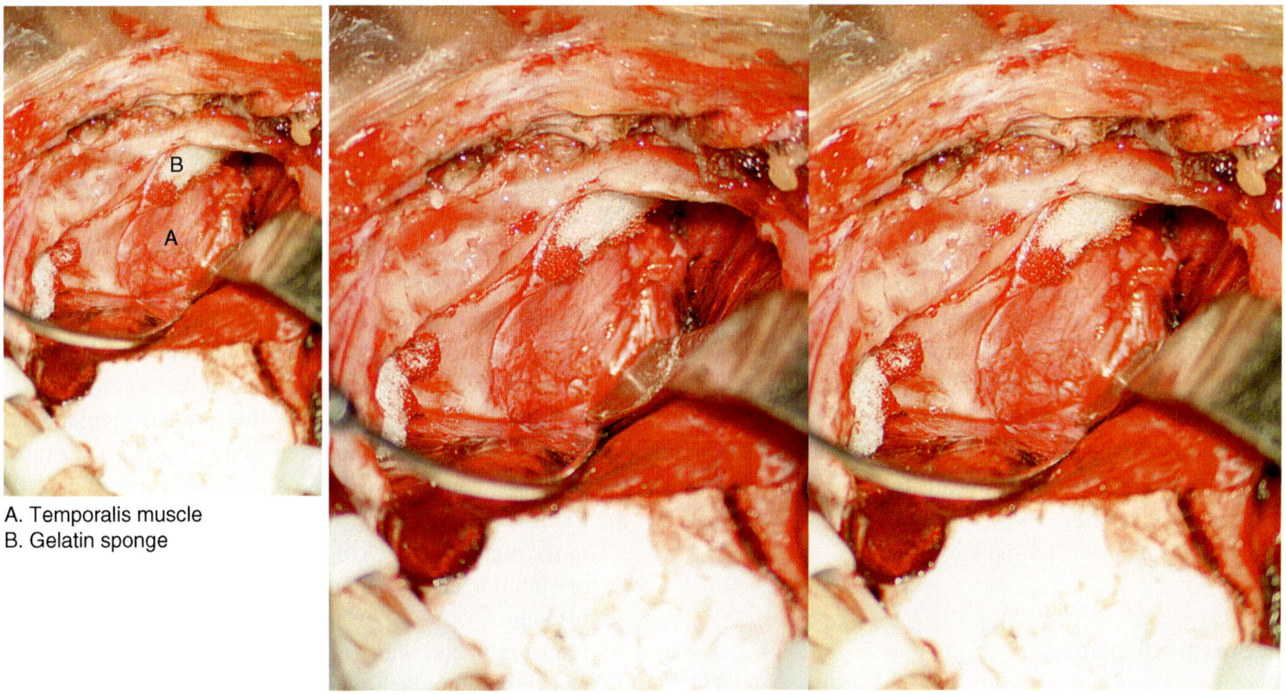

Fig. 5.58 The middle cranial fossa defect of the internal auditory
Once all tumor has been removed, the surgical field is liberally irrigated with normal saline. After complete hemostasis is achieved, the middle cranial fossa defect of internal auditory canal is closed with fascia. Other defects of the base of the middle cranial fossa are also sealed to prevent leakage of cerebrospinal fluid

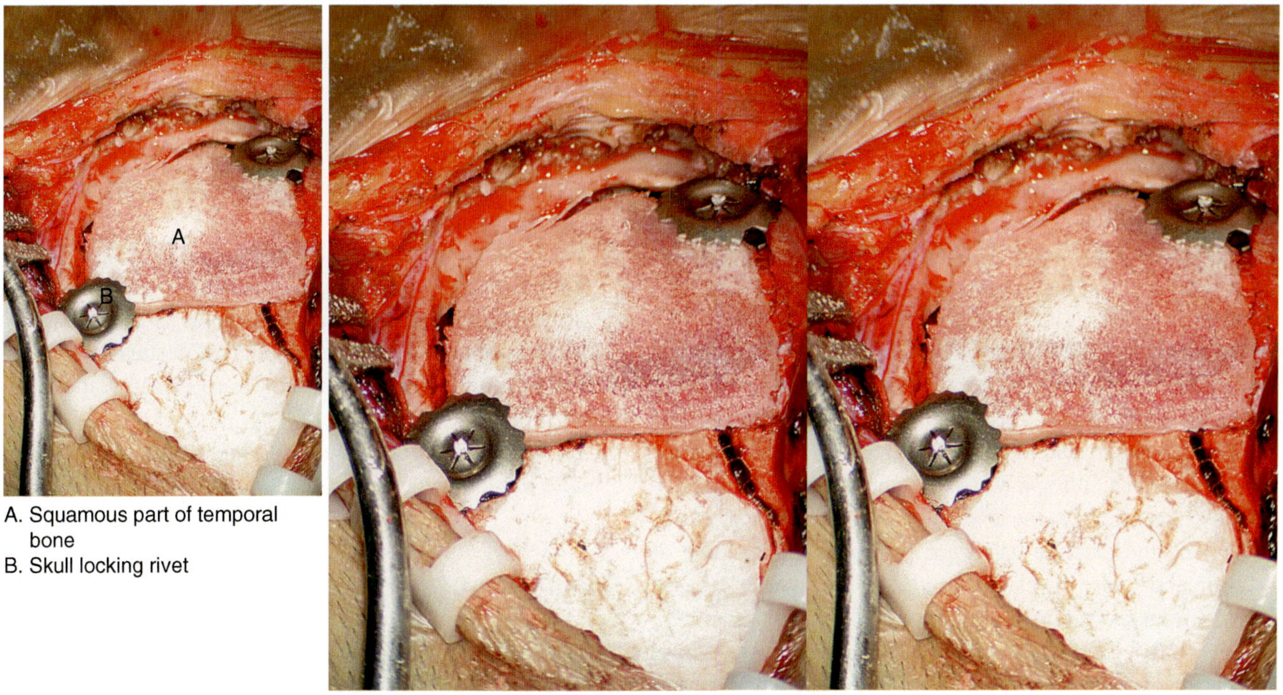

Fig. 5.59 Reposition and fix the bone flap of squamous part of temporal bone
The bone flap of the squamous part of temporal bone is resited and fixed with skull locking rivets; the wound is sutured in layers and a compression dressing is applied

Resection of Glomus Jugulare Tumors Through Postauricular Infratemporal Fossa Approach

Shi-ming Yang, Jia-nan Li, and Vincent C Cousins

Indications

1. Glomus tumor invading the infralabyrinthine and petrous portion of the temporal bone. C1 tumor invades to jugular fossa and the bone around it; C2 the vertical portion of the carotid canal is invaded; C3 petrous portion of the temporal bone and horizontal portion of the carotid canal are invaded.
2. Tumor extending intracranial less than 2 cm.
3. Tumor extending intracranial more than 2 cm some of which can be left for radiation therapy.

Contraindications

1. The intracranial tumor is larger than 2 cm and compressing the brainstem or other important structures.
2. Tumor with rapid intracranial growth despite previous radiation therapy.
3. The patient's general condition is too poor to stand the operation and the tumor is surrounding the internal carotid artery.
4. Possibility of uncontrollable complications.

Operative Procedures

Supine position, General anesthesia with endotracheal intubation.

1. Incision: make a postauricular incision from the temporal region, 5 cm above the apex of the auricle to hyoid bone in the neck.
2. Flap: raise the skin flap superficial to the temporalis muscle and reflect it forward. Create a musculo-periosteal flap based anteriorly at the level of the external auditory canal. Divide the external canal completely, evert the tube of skin and suture the canal closed. Use the anteriorly based flap for a second layer closure of the canal.
3. Exposure of the jugular vein and cranial nerves: expose the external jugular vein at the anterior edge of the sternocleidomastoid muscle and ligate it. Expose the carotid sheath and identify the common, external and internal carotid arteries and the internal jugular vein. Expose the IX, X, XI and XII cranial nerves. Expose the facial nerve and external carotid artery in the parotid.
4. Perform a complete mastoidectomy with an electric drill. Identify the lateral and posterior semicircular canals. Skeletonize the bony covering of the sigmoid sinus. Identify the bony facial canal and expose the nerve completely from the geniculate ganglion to the stylomastoid foramen. Remove the bone over the sigmoid sinus, make small incisions in the posterior fossa dura anterior and posterior to the sinus and ligate it.
5. Elevate the facial nerve from its bony canal and reflect it forward. Drill a groove in the bone of the zygoma and lay the facial nerve in it. Ligate the internal jugular vein. Open the jugular bulb between the two ligations to expose the tumor contained within.
6. Excision of the tumor: Remove the tumor with the wall of the jugular bulb. Drill the bone to clear all tumor. Pack the inferior petrosal sinus with muscle to stop the brisk bleeding.
7. Excision of the intracranial tumor: remove the intracranial tumor completely. Once all tumor is removed from the sinus and the petrous bone, the dura can be closed. Fill the cavity with a sternocleidomastoid muscle flap or abdominal fat.
8. Close the incision: Suture the wound in layers over a drain and apply a compression dressing.

Special Comments

1. The front bony wall of the sigmoid sinus must be completely drilled away. Take care to preserve the facial and vagus nerves.
2. The brisk bleeding from the inferior petrosal sinus is controlled with a muscle plug
3. If the tumor invades the dura or extends significantly in to the cranial cavity it should be excised in stages.
4. If the tumor invades the internal carotid artery, the artery must be preserved.
5. The dura is sutured closely and any defects are repaired with muscle patches.

Complications

1. Trauma to the VII, IX X, XI and XII cranial nerves.
2. Leakage of cerebrospinal fluid and meningitis.
3. Intracranial hemorrhage, hydrocephalus.
4. Incisional hematoma
5. Injury to the internal carotid artery and hemiplegia.

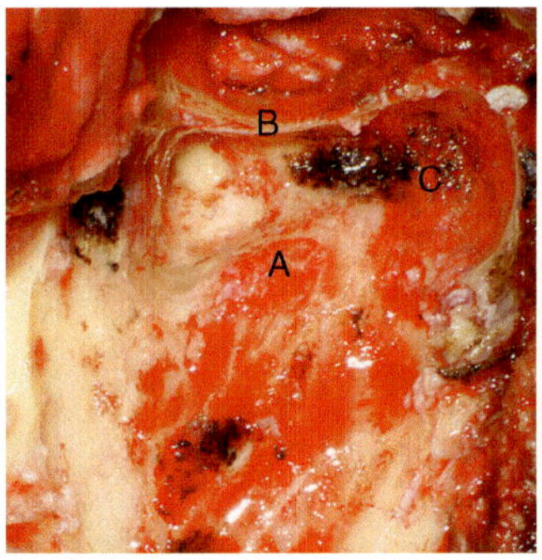

A. Sigmoid sinus
B. Post bony wall of external auditory canal
C. Mastoid tip

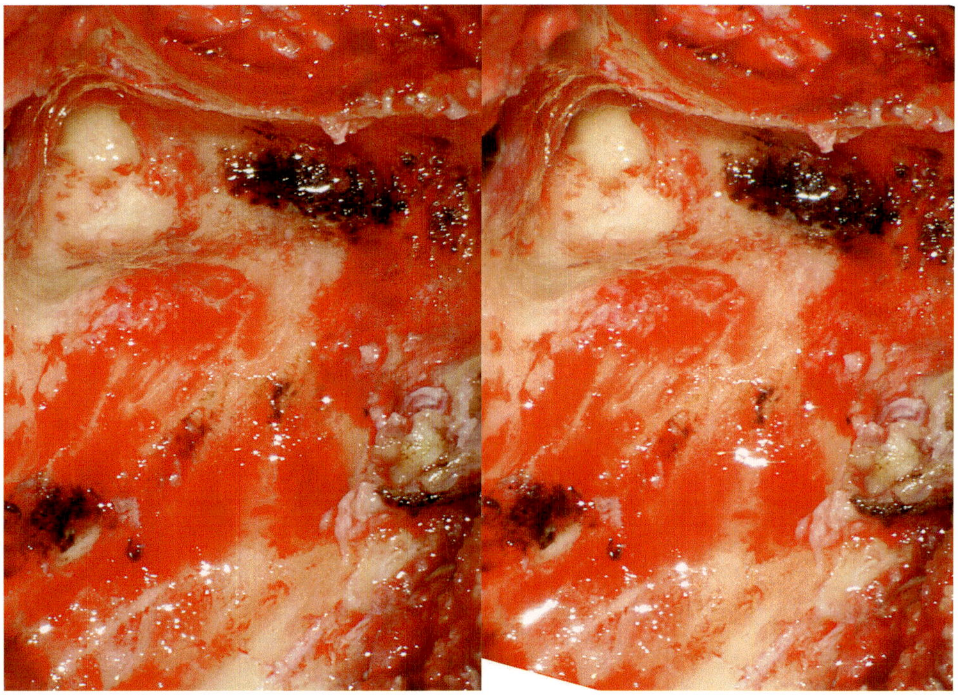

Fig. 5.60 Mastoidectomy
Make a postauricular incision from the temporal region, 5 cm above the apex of the auricle to hyoid bone in the neck. Reflect the flap forwards. Perform a complete mastoidectomy with an electric drill. Skeletonize the sigmoid sinus, sinodural angle, mastoid tegmen, posterior and lateral semicircular canals and the facial nerve canal

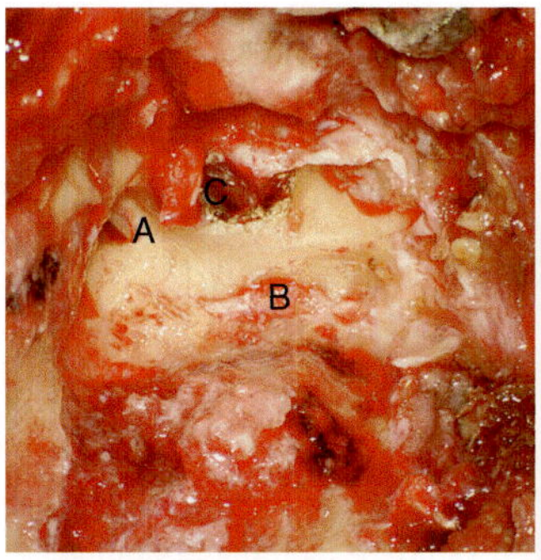

A. Incus buttress
B. The mastoid segment of facial nerve
C. Severed skin of external auditory canal

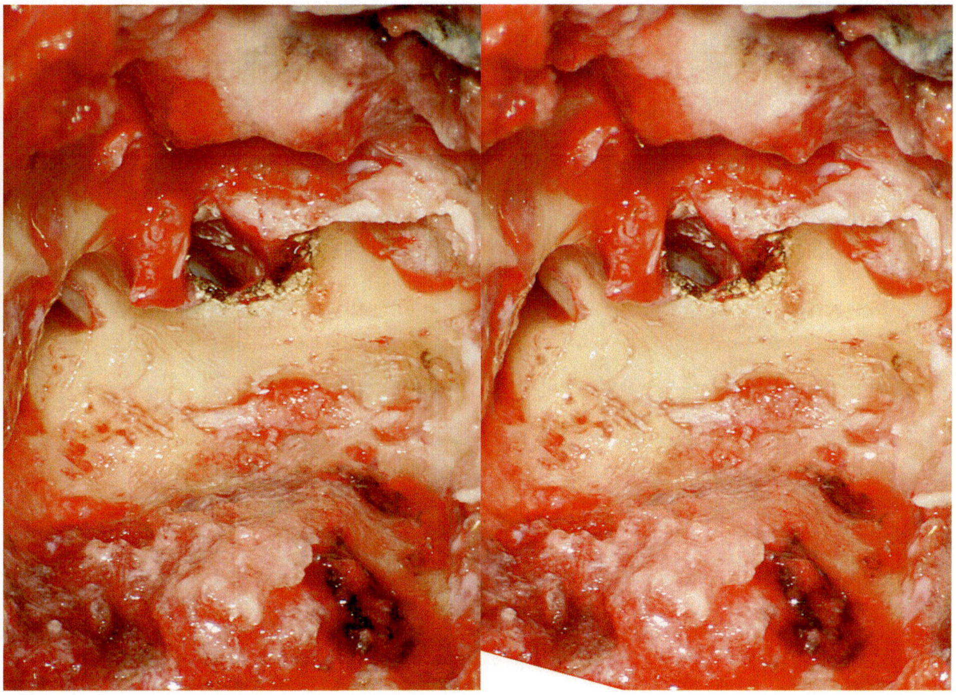

Fig. 5.61 Exposure of the mastoid segment of the facial nerve
The tympanic segment of facial nerve begins at the prominence of the geniculate ganglion. It passes medial to the cochleariform process and inferior to the lateral semicircular canal then turns inferiorly to the pyramidal segment. Open the facial canal from the geniculate ganglion to the stylomastoid foramen. Drill away the posterior bony wall the external auditory canal. Identify the extent of the tumor

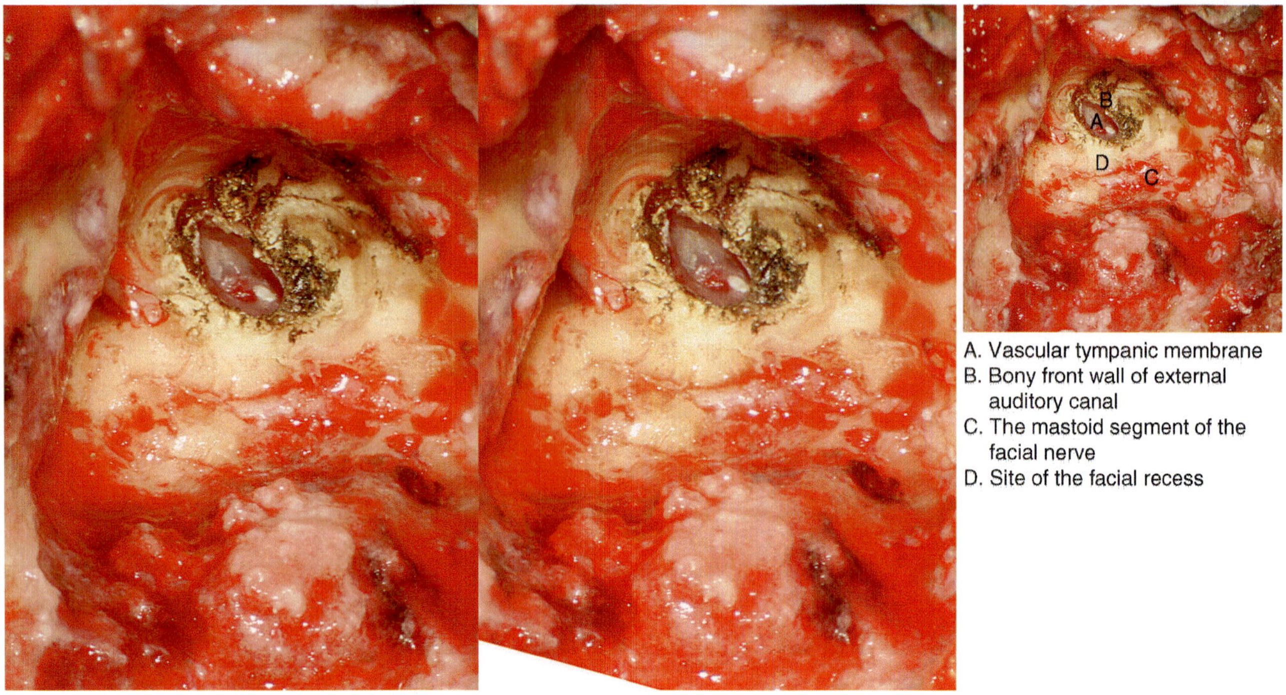

Fig. 5.62 Dissection of the facial recess region
The facial recess is below the fossa incudis, between the facial nerve posteriorly and the chorda tympani nerve anteriorly. Drill out the bone of the facial recess to confirm the extent of tumor in the middle ear

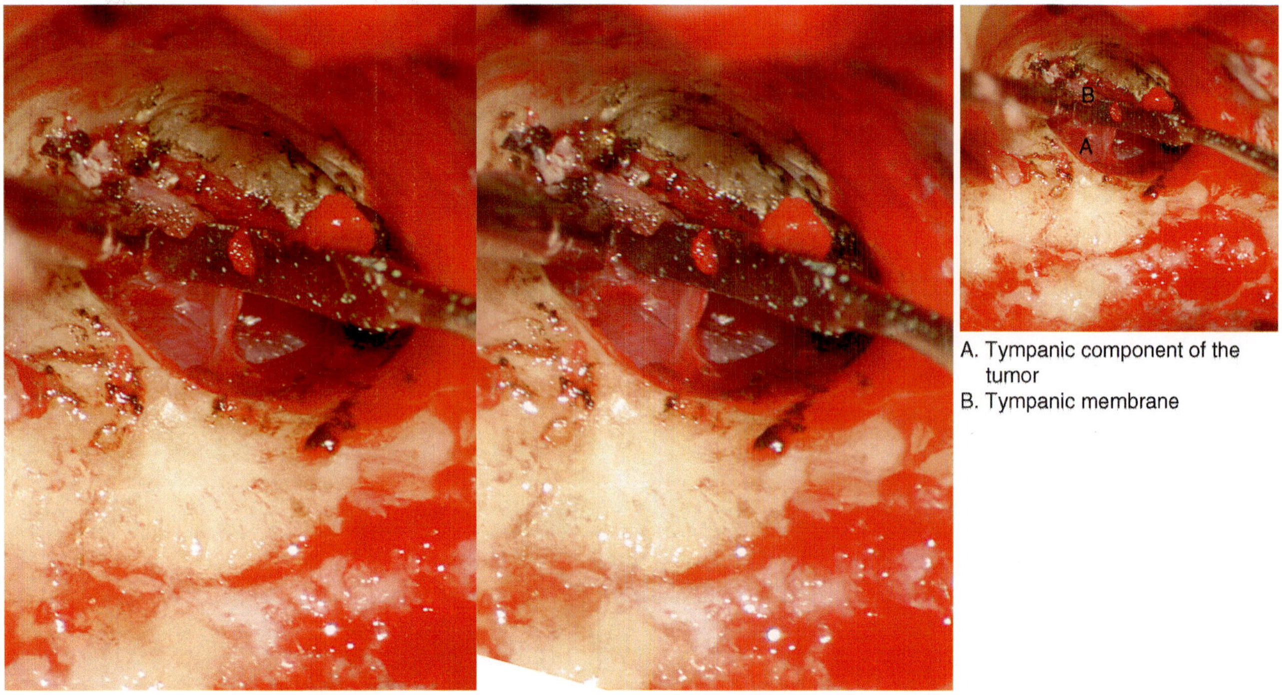

Fig. 5.63 Excision of tumor in the tympanic cavity
Removal of tumor. Take care in dissecting the ossicular chain and facial nerve. Use bipolar coagulation to stop bleeding where required, but avoid the areas of the fallopian canal and round window membrane. If tumor invades bone, it must be burnished with the electric drill

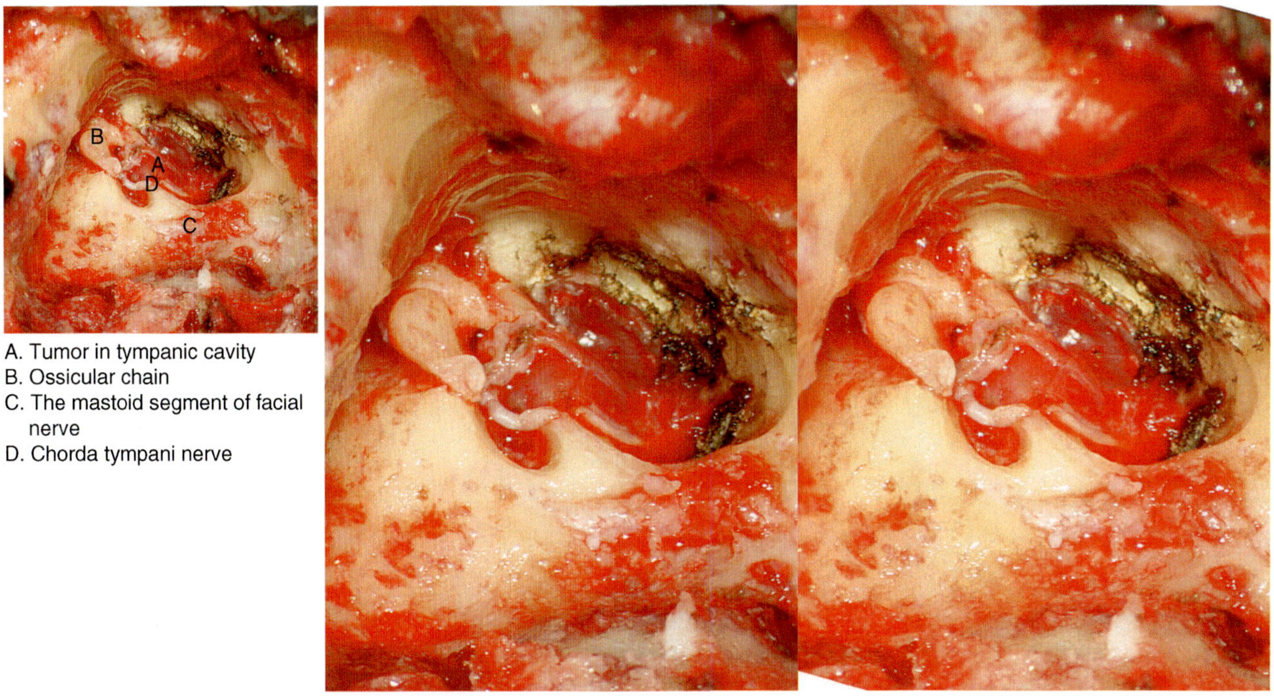

Fig. 5.64 Excision of the tumor in tympanic cavity and ligation of the sigmoid sinus
Carefully drill down the bony canal of the tympanic and pyramid segments of the facial nerve to expose the nerve sheath. Separate the incudostapedial joint. Remove the rest of the posterior bony wall of the external auditory canal, the tympanic membrane, the incus and malleus. Expose the tympanic tumor completely. Open the bone wall of the sigmoid sinus. Make 2 ~ 3 mm incisions in the dura in front of and behind the sinus to allow a suture to be passed around the sinus which is then ligated

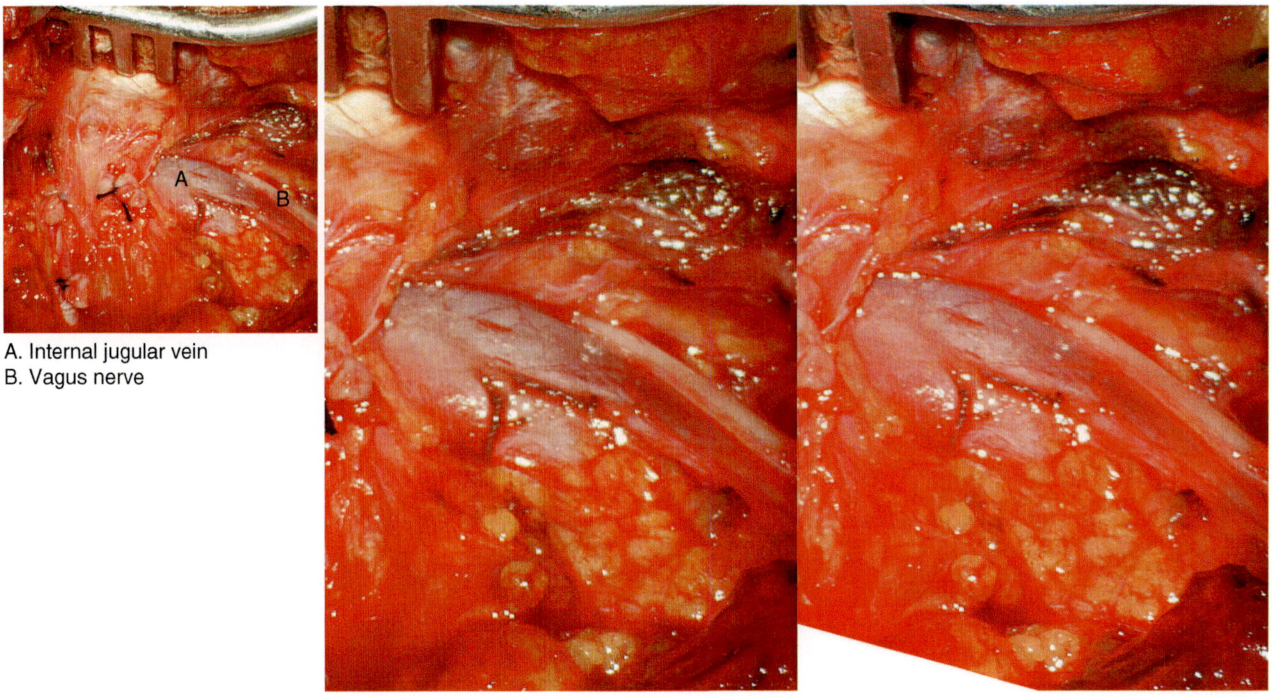

Fig. 5.65 Exposure of the jugular vein and nerves
Separate the external jugular vein in front of the sternocleidomastoid muscle and ligate it. Expose the trunk of the facial nerve after separating the sternocleidomastoid and digastric muscles. Expose the carotid sheath and identify the common, Internal and external carotid arteries and the internal jugular vein. Identify the IX, X, XI and XII cranial nerves

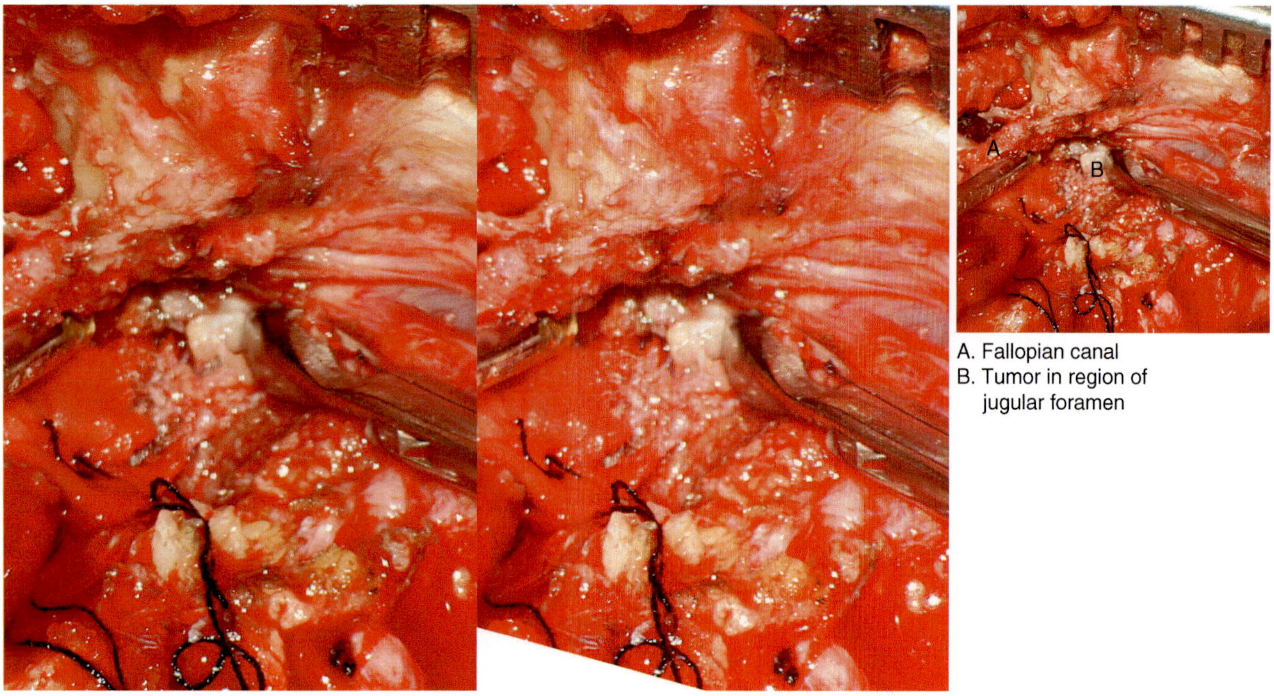

A. Fallopian canal
B. Tumor in region of jugular foramen

Fig. 5.66 Management of the jugular vein and nerves
Ligate the external carotid artery above the superior thyroid artery. Take care to protect the jugular vein and nerves. Drill away the bone of the internal carotid canal whilst protecting the artery. If the tumor is adherent to the internal carotid, it should be gently removed with bipolar diathermy but preserving the integrity of the vessel

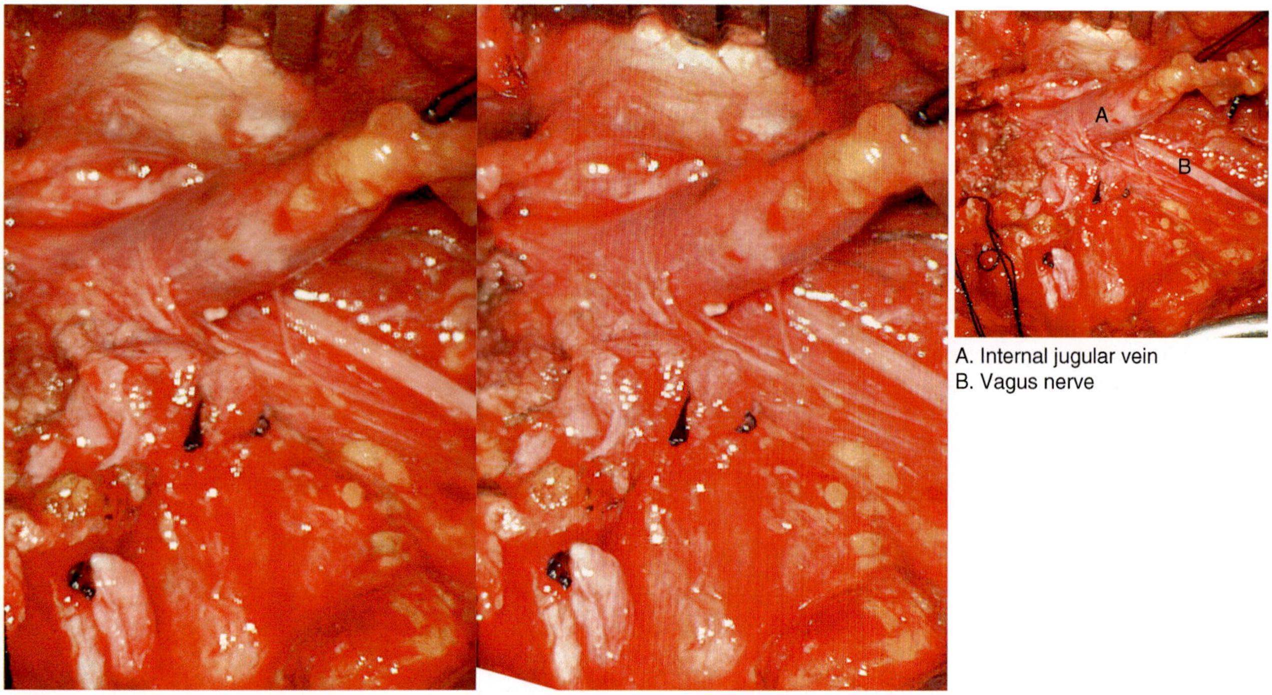

A. Internal jugular vein
B. Vagus nerve

Fig. 5.67 Excision of the tumor in stages
Separate the tumor from the carotid and jugular foramina along the internal carotid artery and internal jugular vein. The sigmoid sinus should be ligated before the internal jugular vein

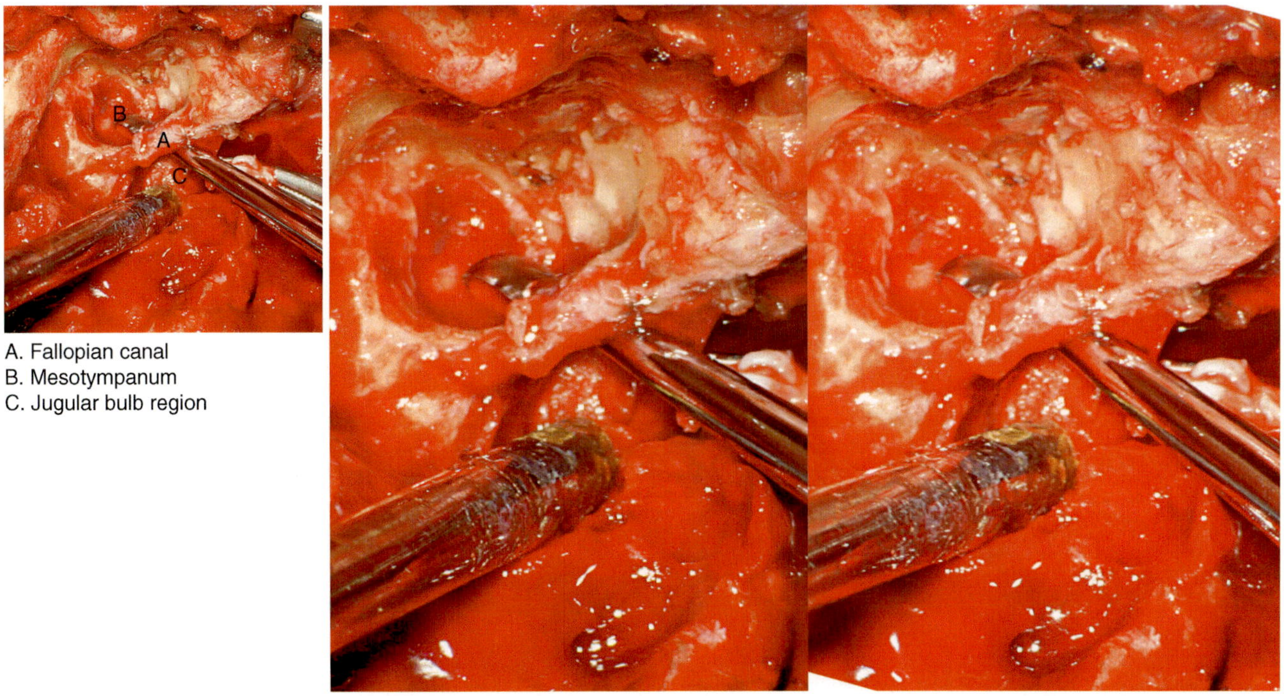

Fig. 5.68 Management of tumor involving the facial nerve
Take care to protect the integrity of the facial nerve and leave it in its position if tumor can be removed completely without re-routing it. Preserve part of bone wall around the facial nerve to reduce ischemia and avoid facial paralysis. The mastoid and tympanic cavities can be connected deep to the facial nerve

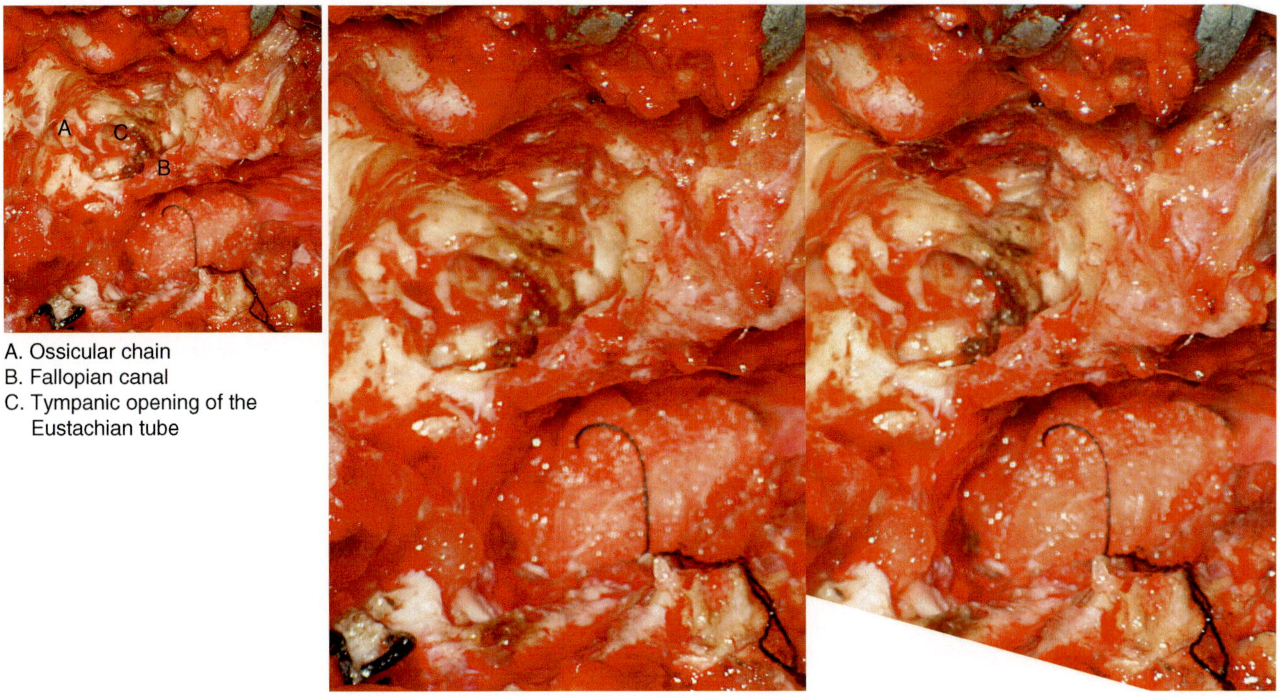

Fig. 5.69 Complete excision of the tumor
The tumor is completely removed including the region of the jugular bulb, and the petrous bone is burnished where necessary. The inferior petrosal sinus is sealed with a muscle plug only after the internal jugular vein has been ligated in order to prevent emboli passing centrally

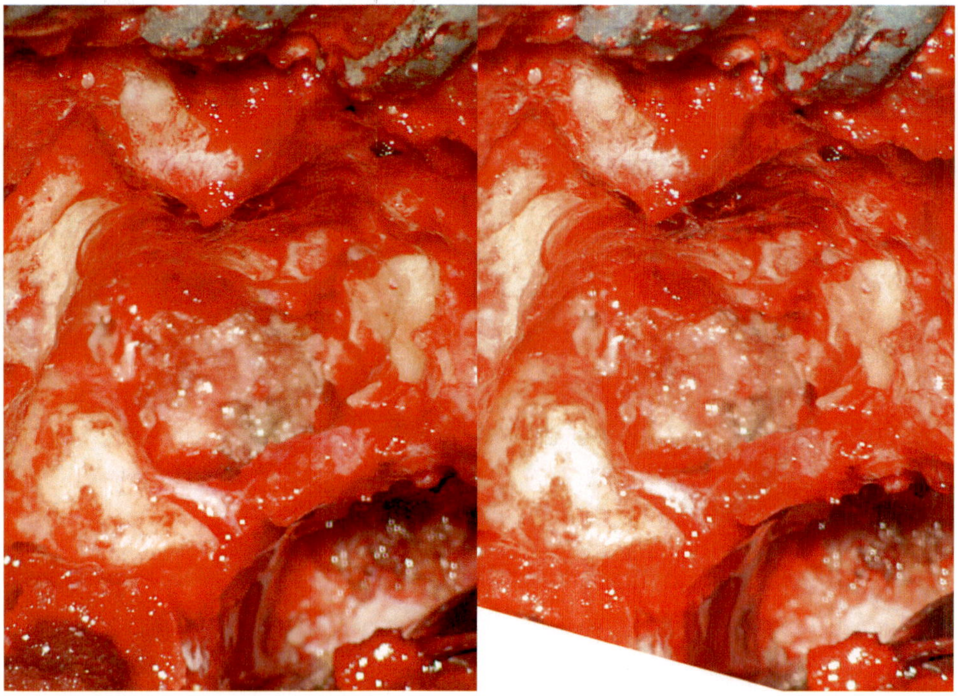

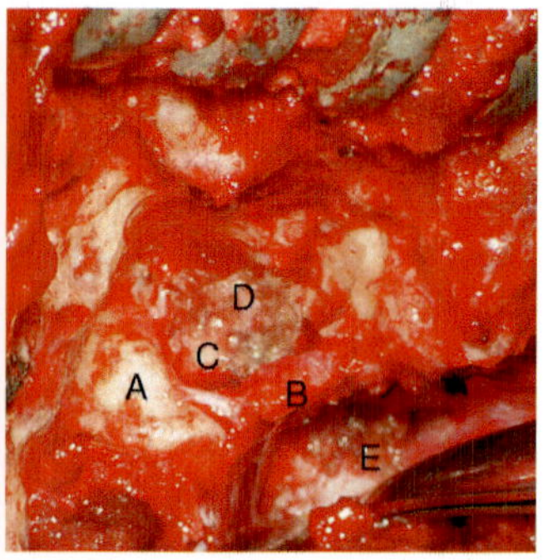

A. Lateral semicircular canal
B. Fallopian canal
C. Head of stapes
D. Muscle Sealing the opening of the Eustachian tube
E. Jugular foramen area (after excision of the tumor)

Fig. 5.70 Closing the cavity
Seal the opening of the Eustachian tube with muscle. Pack the operative cavity with abdominal wall fat or a muscle flap. Biologic albumin gel can be used to assist with sealing the operative cavity

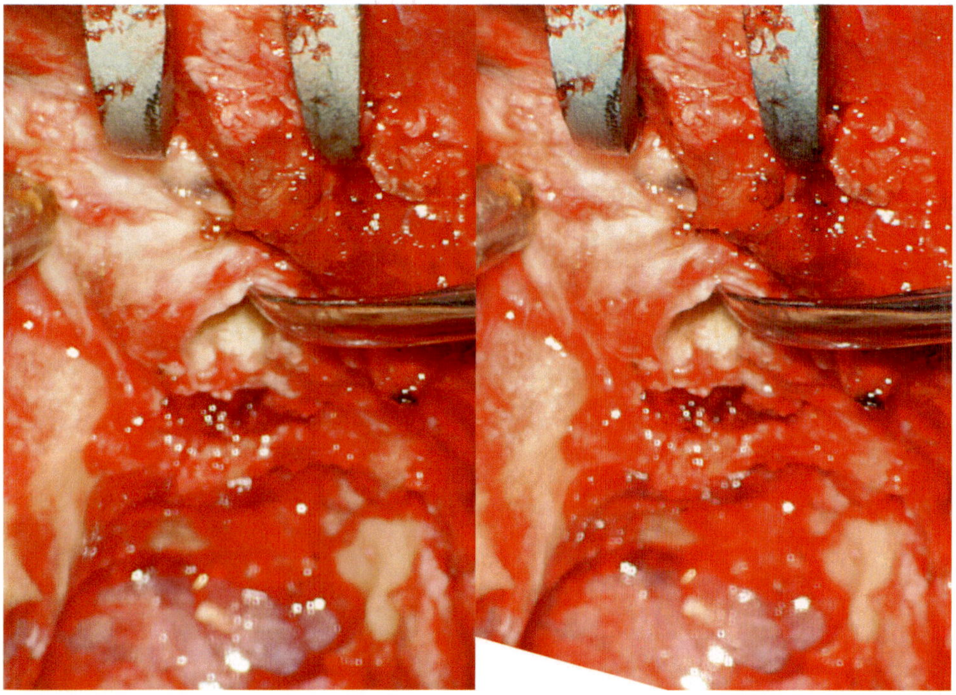

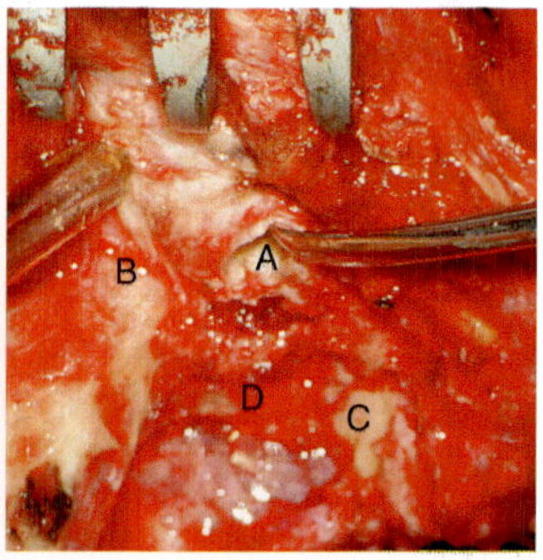

A. Severed medial end of external auditory canal
B. Root of zygoma
C. Inferior wall of external auditory canal
D. Anterior wall of external auditory canal

Fig. 5.71 Management of the external acoustic meatus
Free up the tube of the skin and subcutaneous tissue of the internal opening of the severed external auditory canal. Oversew the tube to seal the canal and reinforce the repair with the anterior based flap created at the start of the procedure

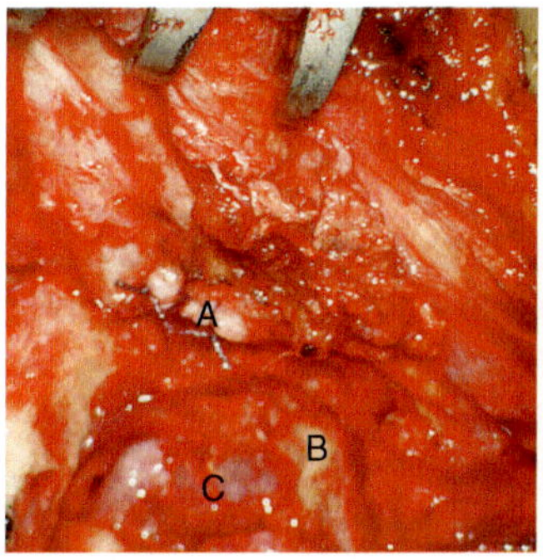

A. Sealed external auditory canal
B. Inferior wall of external auditory canal
C. Muscle Sealing the tympanic opening of the Eustachian tube

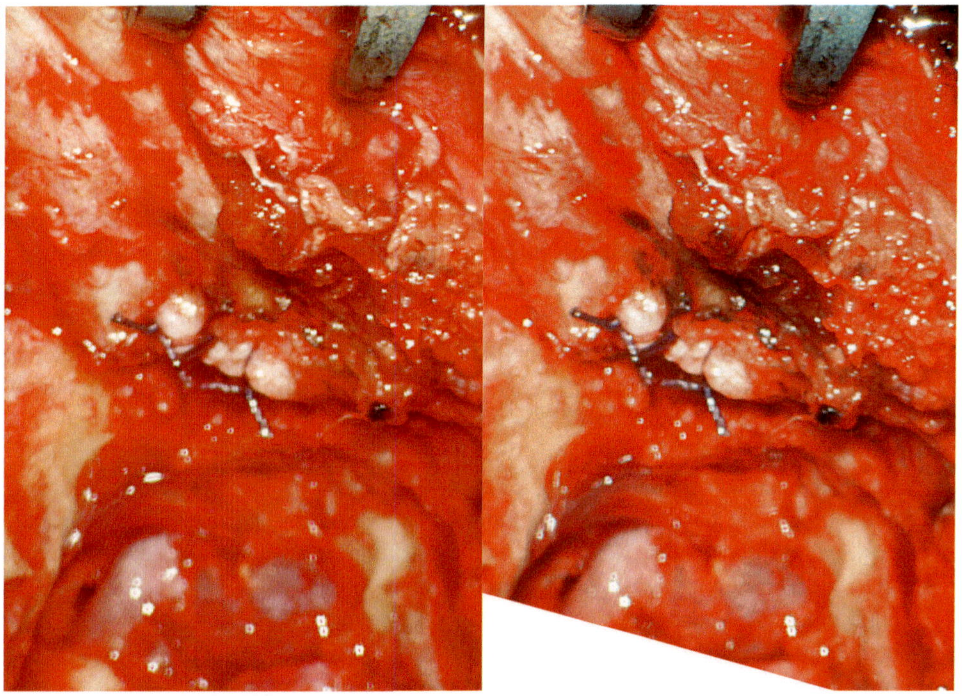

Fig. 5.72 Ligate and seal the external auditory canal
Ligate the internal opening of the external auditory canal. Close the wound in layers over a drain tube and apply a compression dressing

Temporal Bone Resection

Wei-ju Han and Vincent C Cousins

Indications

1. Surgical excision for malignant neoplasms of the temporal bone.
2. Sleeve resection for those tumors truly confined to the skin and soft tissue of the cartilaginous portion of the external auditory canal.
3. Lateral temporal bone resection for tumors that involve the bony and cartilaginous canal but have not violated the annulus or encroached on the tympanic cavity.
4. Subtotal temporal bone resection for tumors that extensively encroach on the tympanic cavity or the mastoid air cells. If necessary, portions of dura, sigmoid sinus, parotid gland, and mandible can be resected with the specimen.
5. Total temporal bone resection for tumors that extensively involve the petrous bone, the cavernous sinus and infratemporal fossa.

Contraindications

1. Patients with malignant invasion of the cavernous sinus, internal carotid artery, infratemporal fossa, and paraspinous musculature are not surgically curable.
2. Although neck dissections can be performed for regional metastases, patients with distant metastases are not surgical candidates.

Operative Procedures

Sleeve Resection

1. An incision is made medially to ensure that the bony cartilaginous junction is not involved.
2. The lateral cut is made so that the resection encompasses the entire lesion.
3. The involved skin and underlying cartilage are removed.
4. The area can be lined with a split-thickness skin graft.

Lateral Temporal Bone Resection

1. The outer canal opening is outlined and an extended postauricular incision is made.
2. The ear is reflected anteriorly and the resulting flap is extended to expose the parotid gland.
3. The facial nerve is dissected from the stylomastoid foramen to the pes anserinus.
4. A cortical mastoidectomy with an extended facial recess approach is performed. The facial nerve should be skeletonized from its second genu to the stylomastoid foramen. The incudostapedial joint is disarticulated and the facial nerve is further exposed anteriorly along its horizontal segment.
5. The superior attachment of the osseous canal must be freed by opening the epitympanum and zygomatic root. The deep plane is created in an anterior, inferior, and medial direction, transecting the tympanic bone medial to the tympanic annulus but lateral to the jugular bulb and facial nerve. This plane is continued anteriorly until the glenoid fossa is skeletonized.
6. The anterior tympanic bone can be fractured free with a medium sized osteotome. The specimen is left attached to the parotid gland and a superficial parotidectomy is performed.
7. The Eustachian tube can be plugged with muscle and the defect closed with split-thickness skin grafts.

Subtotal Temporal Bone Resection

1. The extended postauricular incision is made. The inferior portion of the incision is extended into the neck and connected with a standard S-shaped vertical incision to allow adequate exposure.
2. If a neck exploration is required, the great vessels and nerves of the neck are dissected out.
3. The zygoma is transected. The ramus of the mandible is divided and the head and neck are removed. A subtotal parotidectomy is performed.
4. The facial nerve can be transected, and its distal stump may be tagged for a subsequent hypoglossal-facial anastomosis.
5. The sternocleidomastoid muscle and the posterior belly of the digastric muscle are separated from the mastoid tip. The styloid process is transected.
6. The external carotid artery is identified and divided.
7. A temporal craniotomy is performed to verify that there is no intracranial extension of the tumor. The temporal lobe is retracted medially to expose the petrous bone.
8. A mastoidectomy is performed and the sigmoid sinus is skeletonized to the jugular bulb.
9. The internal carotid artery is exposed anterior to the jugular bulb and separated from the temporal bone.
10. The Eustachian tube is divided anteriorly and the horizontal segment of the internal carotid artery is exposed.
11. The anterior attachment of the temporal bone can be fractured free with gentle rocking and careful use of osteotomes. The entire temporal bone lateral to the petrous segment can be removed in an en bloc fashion.
12. The large defect can be filled either with regional muscle flaps or free vascularized grafts

Total Temporal Bone Resection

1. The auricular and cervical skin flaps are elevated and the great vessels and nerves in the neck are identified.
2. The parotid gland, facial nerve, and ascending ramus of the mandible are resected.
3. The internal and external carotid arteries are divided, as well as cranial nerves IX (glossopharyngeal), X (vagus) and XI (spinal accessory) and the internal jugular vein.
4. The pterygoid muscles are divided. The mandibular division of the trigeminal nerve (V3) is identified and preserved.
5. A craniotomy is performed, and the middle and posterior fossa dura are exposed.
6. The transverse sinus is ligated posterior to its junction with the sigmoid sinus. The superior petrosal sinus is divided anteriorly before it enters the cavernous sinus.
7. The distal portion of the internal carotid artery can be ligated and divided intracranially between the cavernous sinus and the origin of the ophthalmic artery.
8. A chisel is placed just inside the foramen ovale, directed toward the ligated portion of the superior petrosal sinus. It passes lateral to the cavernous sinus through the carotid canal, the skull base, and lateral skull wall, freeing the anterior portion of the middle fossa floor.
9. A posterior cut is made, lateral to medial, directed anteriorly and stopping posteromedial to the mastoid tip and posterior to the jugular foramen.
10. A connection cut is made from the posterior-lateral cut, going medial to the jugular foramen and lateral to the foramen magnum.
11. The inferior petrosal sinus is divided with the final connecting portion of bone and the specimen is removed en bloc.
12. The large defect can be filled either with regional muscle flaps or free vascularized grafts.

Special Comments

1. Although surgical options are available for many temporal bone malignant lesions, the physician and the patient must decide together not what can be done but what should be done.
2. The temporal bone is one of the most complex anatomic areas in the human body. The surgery in this area requires considerable training and experience.
3. These structures are also at risk from the spread of tumors within this area. The concept of en bloc removal of a portion or all of the temporal bone has been established.
4. The appropriate extent of the surgery is still very controversial, with some authors advocating total en bloc removal of the temporal bone surrounding the tumor and others arguing for piecemeal removal of gross tumor with preservation of vital neurovascular structures followed by radiation therapy.
5. For total temporal bone resection, it is important to ascertain that the patient can tolerate the sacrifice of the involved carotid artery. The use of arteriograms with balloon occlusion studies has been advocated for this determination.

Complications

1. Multiple cranial nerves deficits, including VII (facial), VIII (cochleovestibular), IX (glossopharyngeal), X (vagus), and XI (spinal accessory) cranial nerves.
2. For total temporal bone resection with sacrifice of the carotid artery, it is important to ascertain that the patient can tolerate the sacrifice of the involved carotid artery to avoid a stroke.

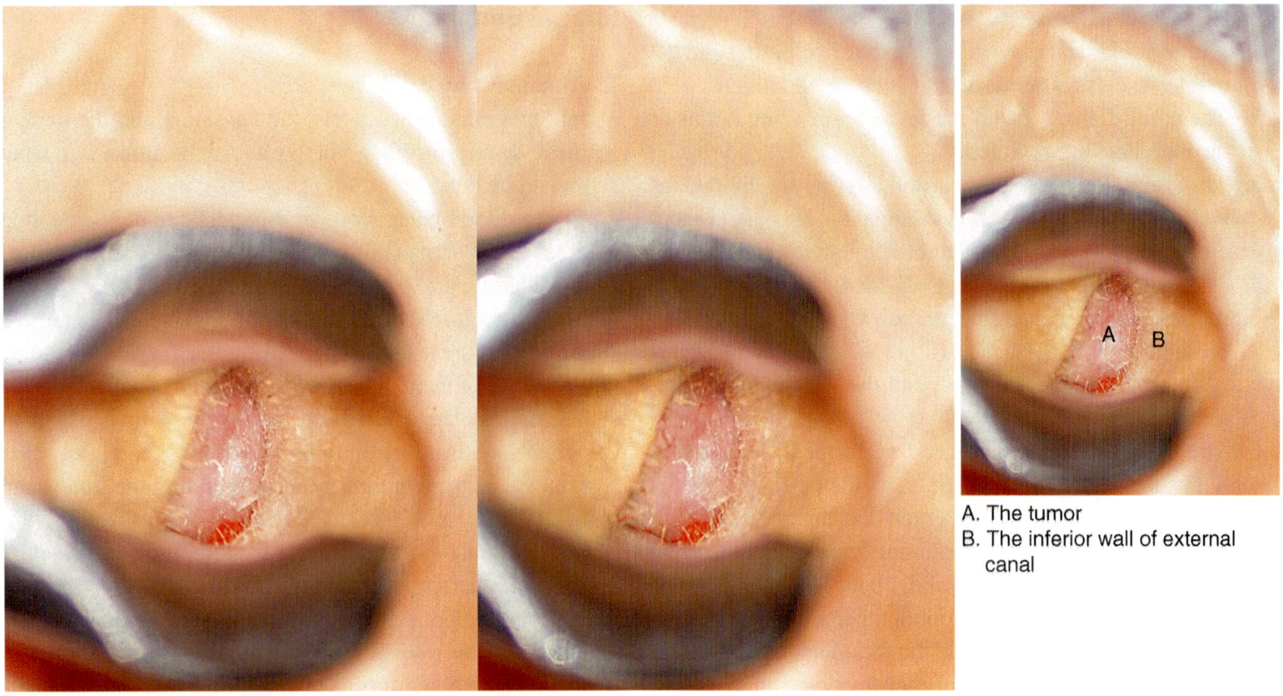

Fig. 5.73 The microscopic examination of the external canal
The external canal dilated with the ear speculum. The tumor is exposed and a piece is taken for pathological examination. The pathological report showed that the tumor is a malignant one

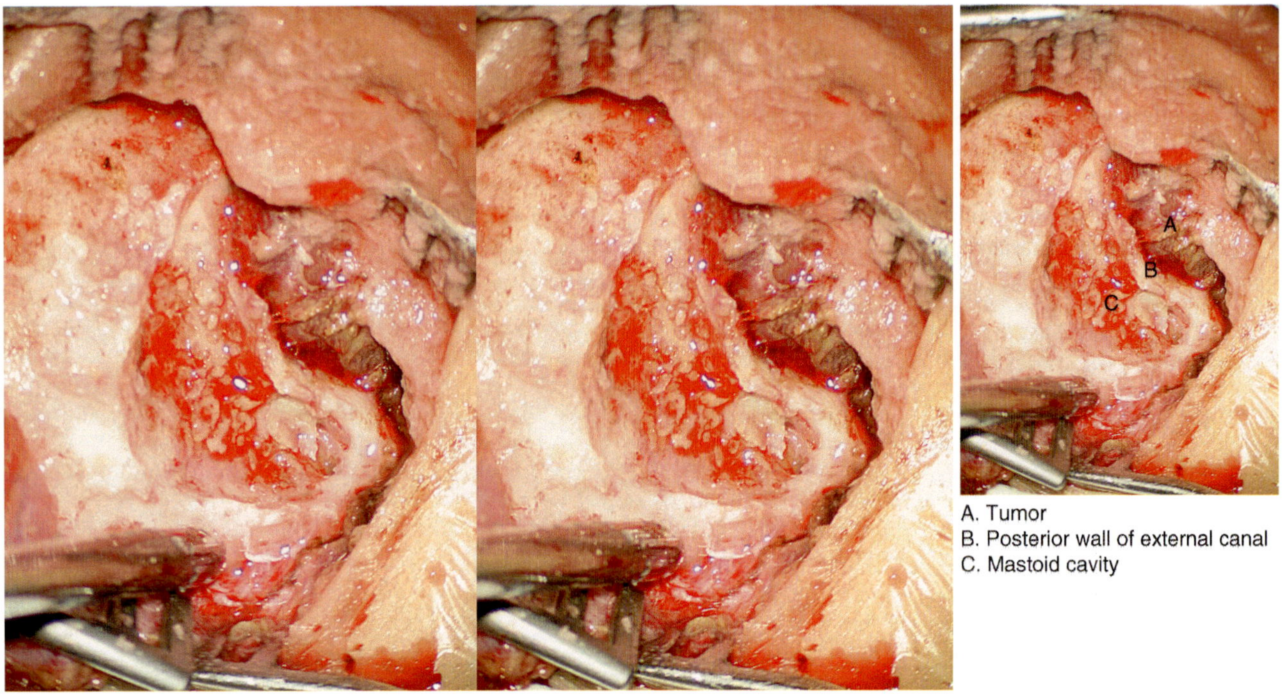

Fig. 5.74 Cortical mastoidectomy
An extended postauricular S-shaped vertical incision is made. The inferior portion of the incision is extended into the neck. A cortical mastoidectomy is performed. The tumor is exposed

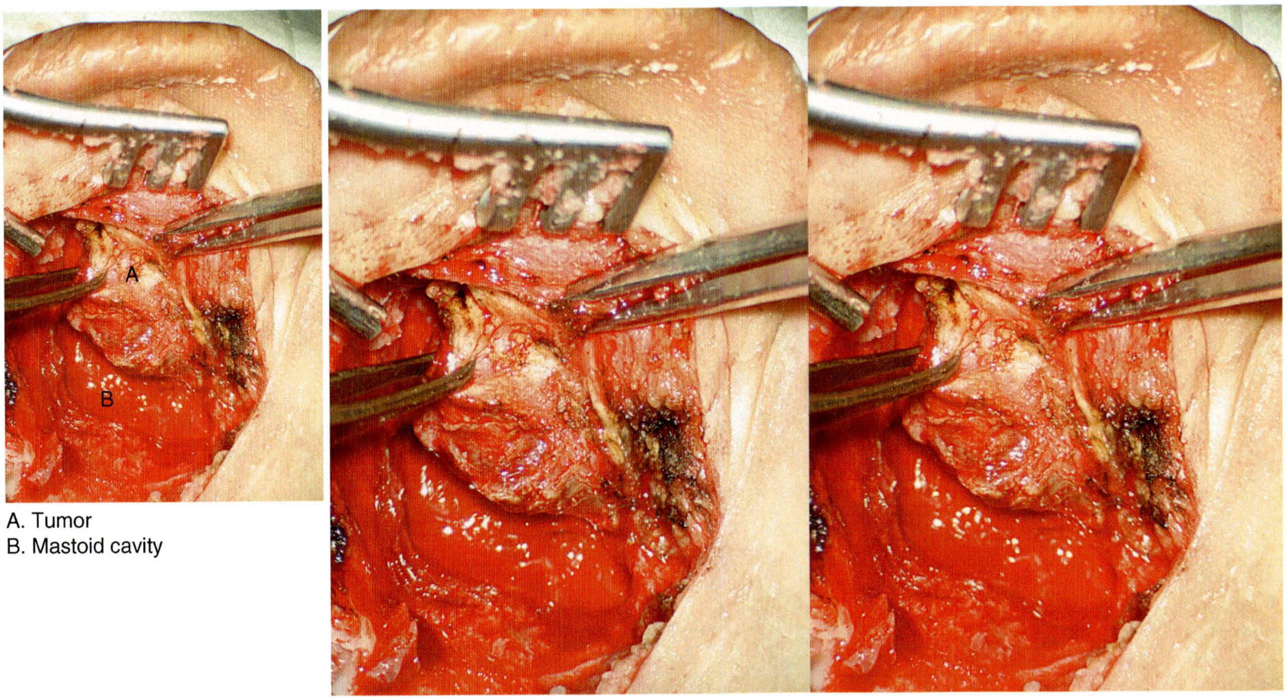

Fig. 5.75 Temporal bone exposure
The ear is reflected anteriorly and the resulting flap is extended to expose the tumor that involves the external canal and encroaches on the tympanic cavity

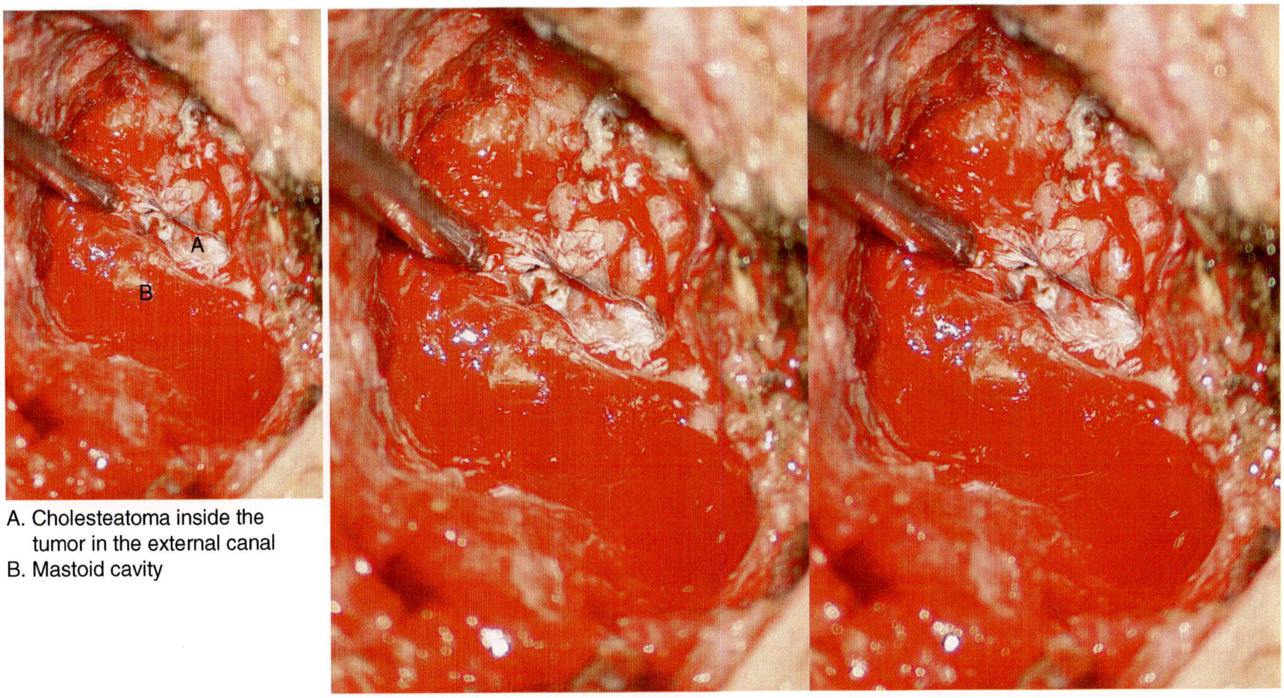

Fig. 5.76 The external ear canal is incised
The external canal is transected lateral to the tumor. The tumor is exposed. The external canal will be closed after the temporal bone resection

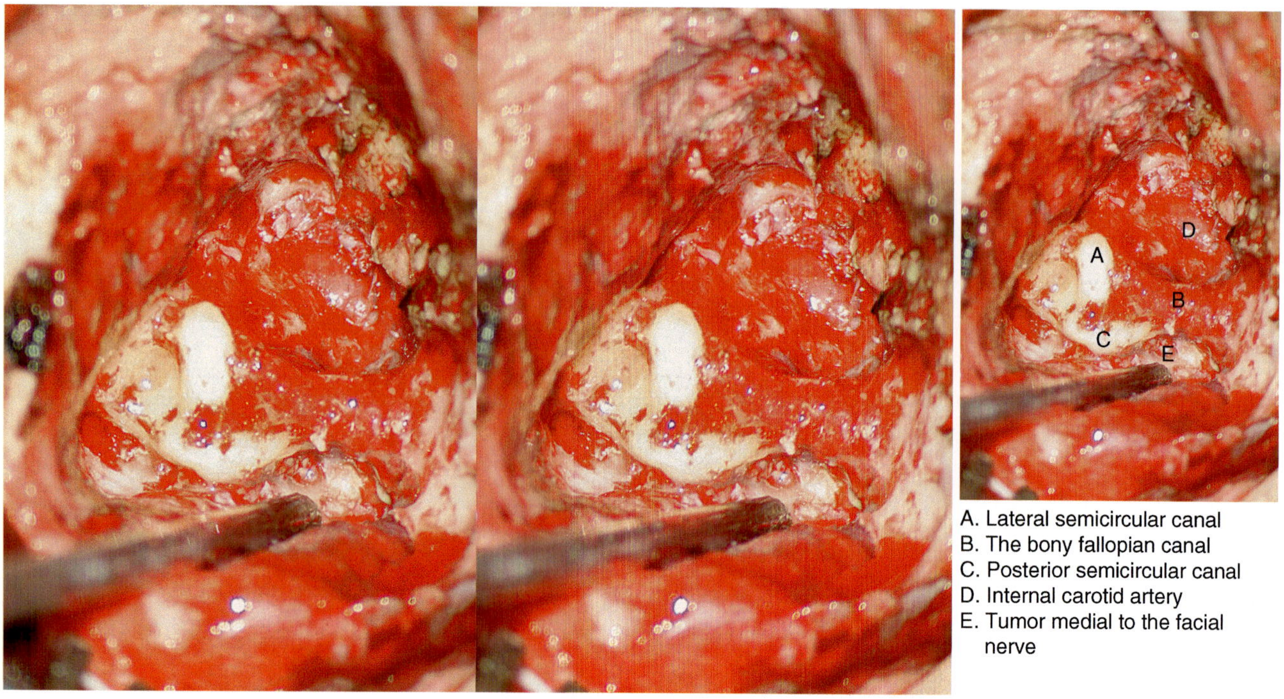

Fig. 5.77 The mastoid cavity and tumor resection
The lateral, superior and posterior semicircular canals are identified and preserved. The facial nerve is skeletonized from its second genu to the stylomastoid foramen. The sigmoid sinus is also skeleteonized

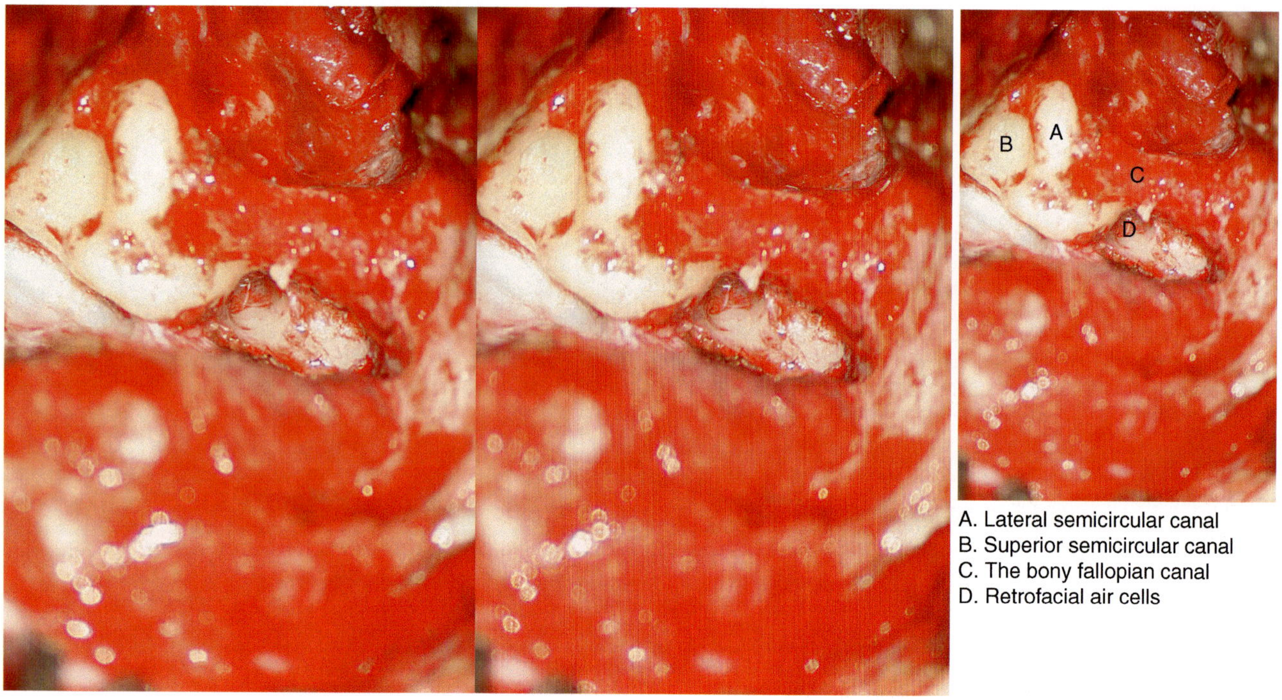

Fig. 5.78 Resection of tumor medial to the facial nerve
The bony fallopian canal is skeletonized. The vertical segment of facial nerve is exposed and preserved. The tumor medial to facial nerve is resected

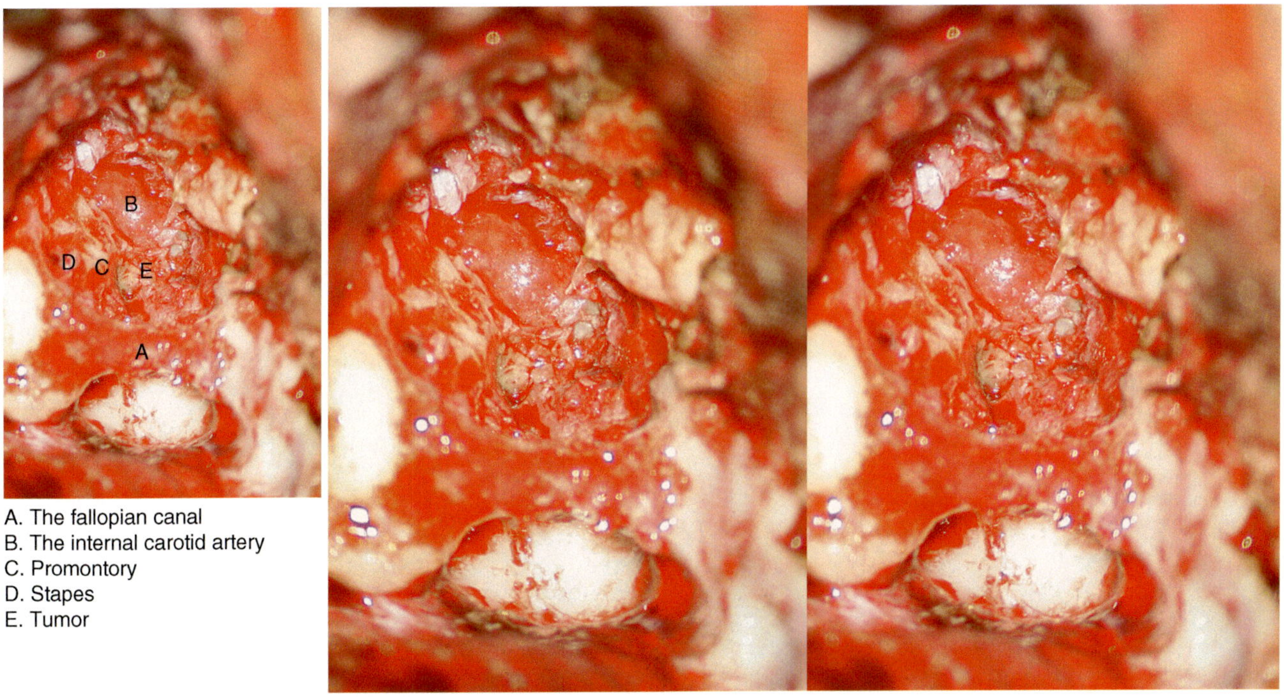

Fig. 5.79 Internal carotid artery exposure
The tympanic cavity is opened. The Eustachian tube is divided anteriorly and the horizontal segment of the internal carotid artery is exposed

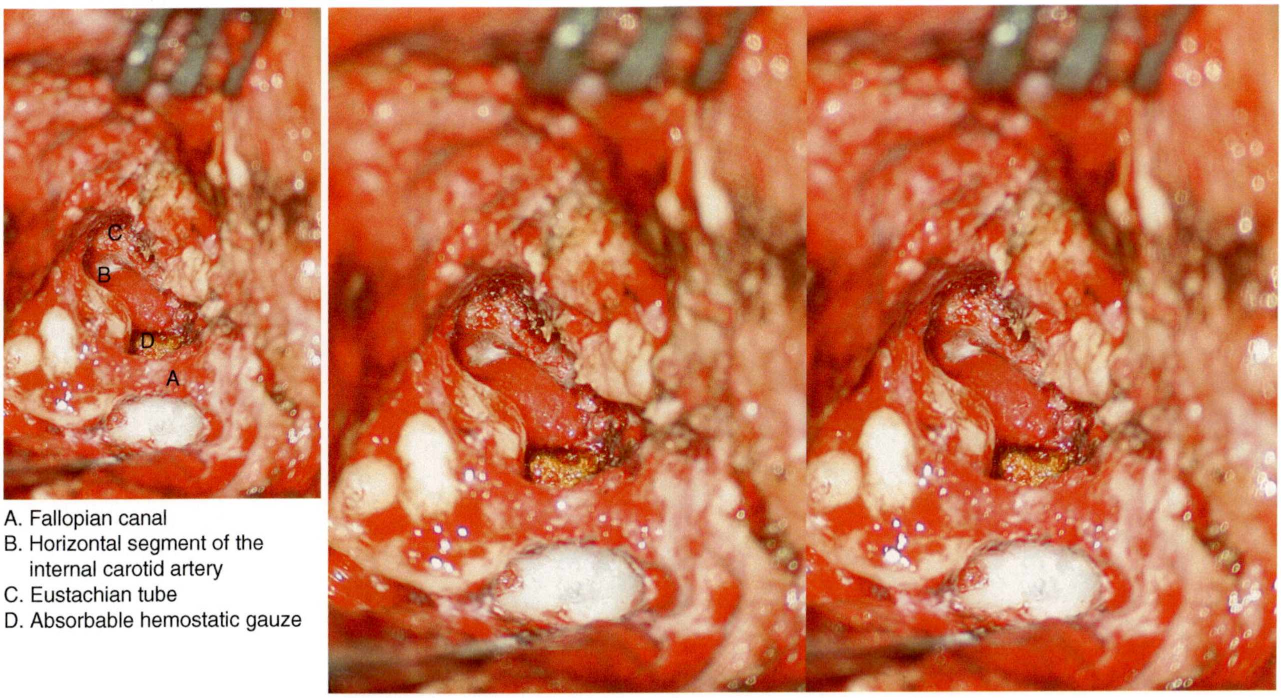

Fig. 5.80 Tumor resection from hypotympanum
The tumor posterior to the internal carotid artery, inferior to the promontory and in the hypotympanum is resected

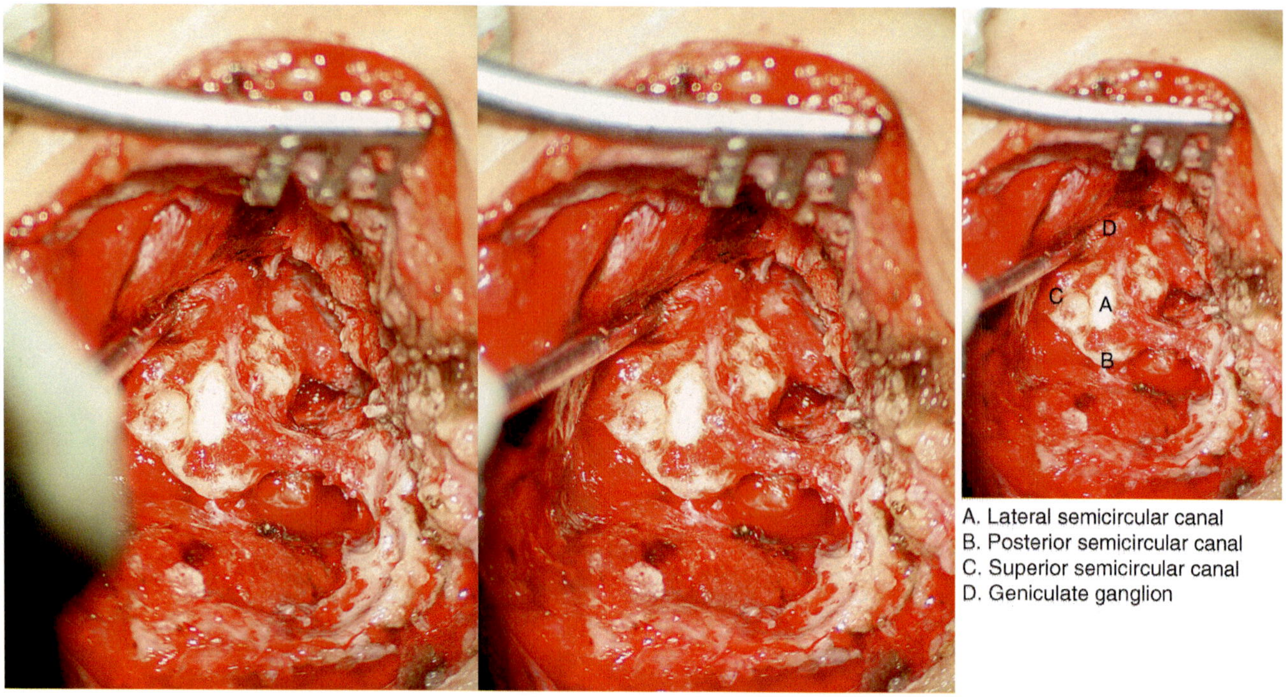

Fig. 5.81 The exposure of the vertical and the labyrinthine segments of the facial nerve
The facial nerve is further exposed anteriorly along its horizontal segment. The geniculate ganglion and labyrinthine segments of the nerve are identified and exposed

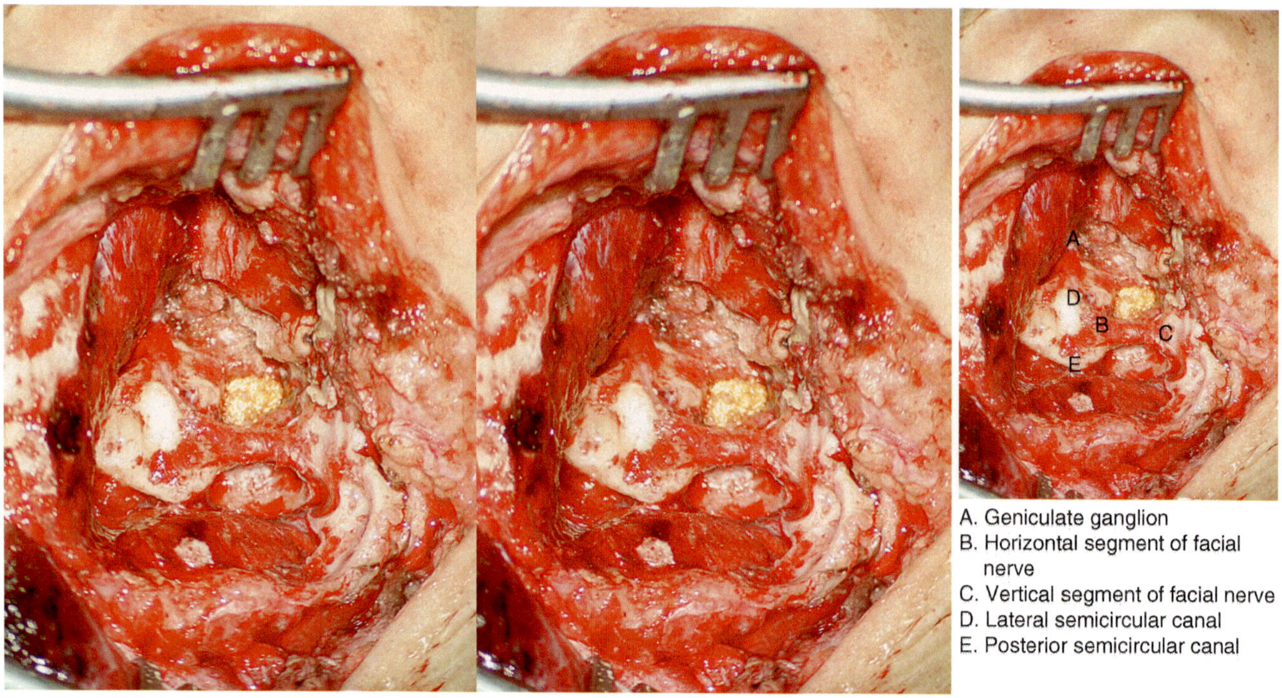

Fig. 5.82 Partial temporal bone resection
The entire temporal bone lateral to the petrous part is removed. The facial nerve is identified and preserved after tumor resection

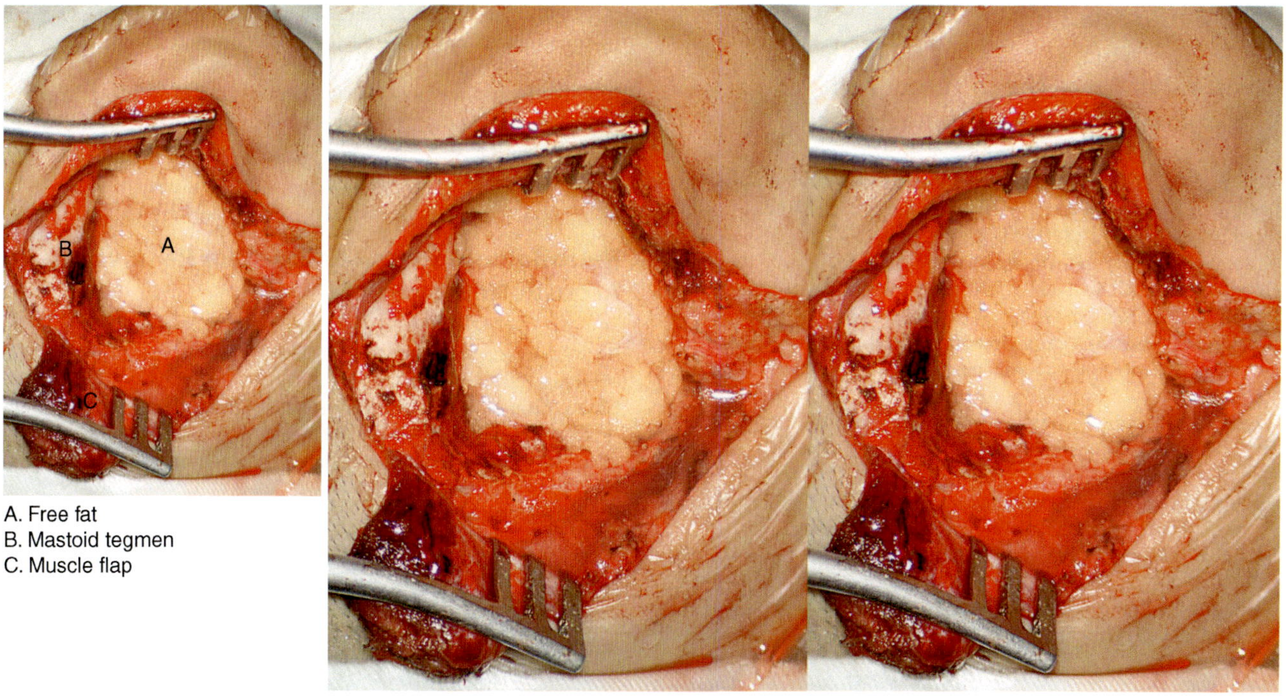

A. Free fat
B. Mastoid tegmen
C. Muscle flap

Fig. 5.83 Obliterating the defect
The large defect can be filled either with regional muscle flaps or free vascularized grafts. We have use free fat from abdominal wall to fill the defect in this patient

Suggested Reading

Removal of Facial Nerve Tumor and Hypoglossal-Facial Anastomosis

Arai H, Sato K, Yanai A. Hemihypoglossal-facial nerve anastomosis in treating unilateral facial palsy after acoustic neurinoma resection. J Neurosurg. 1995;82(1):51–4.

Catalano PJ, Eden AR. An external reference to identify the internal auditory canal in middle fossa surgery. Otolaryngol Head Neck Surg. 1993;108(2):111–6.

Chang CG, Shen AL. Hypoglossofacial anastomosis for facial palsy after resection of acoustic neuroma. Surg Neurol. 1984;21(3): 282–6.

Dongyi H, Shiming Y, Wenming W, et al. Resection of acoustic neurinoma and preservation of function of the facial nerve. Chin J Otol. 2004;2(1):1–3.

Green Jr JD, Shelton C, Brackmann DE. Iatrogenic facial nerve injury during otologic surgery. Laryngoscope. 1994;104:922–6.

Han D-Y. Nerve otology and lateral skull base surgery. Beijing: Science Press; 2008.

Huang X-Z, Wang J-B, Kong W-J. Practice of otorhinolaryngology head and neck surgery. 2nd ed. Beijing: People's Medical Publishing House; 2008.

Jiang S-C. Ear anatomia and temporal bone histopathology. Beijing: People's Military Medical Press; 1999.

Jiang S-C, Gu R, Zheng-Min W. Otorhinolaryngology - otology. 2nd ed. Shanghai: Shanghai Scientific and Technological Education Publishing House; 2002.

Jiang S-C, Yang W-Y, Gu R. The complete works of operative surgery. In: Operative surgery of otorhinolaryngology head and neck department. 2nd ed. Beijing: People's Military Medical Press; 2005.

Kunihiro T, Kanzaki J, O-Uchi T. Hypoglossal-facial nerve anastomosis. Clin Obser Acta Otolaryngol Suppl. 1991;487:80–4.

Pulec JL. Total facial nerve decompression: technique to avoid complications. Ear Nose Throat J. 1996;75(7):410–5.

Rebol J, Milojkovic V, Didanovic V. Side-to-end hypoglossal-facial anastomosis via transposition of the intratemporal facial nerve. Acta Neurochir (Wien). 2006;148(6):653–7.

Tian-hong P, Da-chuan X, Yan-bin L. Anatomic study of the blood vessels and nerves adjacent to tip of the greater horn of hyoid bone. Prog Anat Sci. 2005;23(6):597–9.

Yang W-Y, Zhai S-Q. Head-neck dissection and temporal surgery. Beijing: People's Military Medical Press; 2002.

Yong Z, Xiaofeng M, Hong W, et al. Reasons and prevention of facial paralysis in tympanomastoid surgery. Chin Arch Otolaryngol Head Neck Surg. 2000;7:199–201.

Yu Y-J, Dai P, Liu Z. Stereo anatomical and surgical atlas of temporal bone. Beijing: People's Military Medical Press; 2006.

CPA Microvascular Decompression (MVD) of Facial Nerve by Retrosigmoid Approach

Barker FG, Jannetta PJ, Bissonette DJ, Shields PT, Larkins MV, Jho HD. Microvascular decompression for hemifacialspasm. J Neurosurg. 1995;82(2):201–10.

Lavon H, Cohen-Kerem R, Uri N. Hemifacial spasm associated with otitis media with effusion: a first reported case. Int J Pediatr Otorhinolaryngol. 2006;70(5):947–50.

Moffat DA, Durvasula VS, Stevens King A, De R, Hardy DG. Outcome following retrosigmoid microvasculardecompression of the facial nerve for hemifacial spasm. J Laryngol Otol. 2005;119(10):779–83.

Peitersen E. Bell's palsy: the spontaneous course of 2,500 peripheral facial nerve palsies of different etiologies. Acta Otolaryngol. 2002; 549(Suppl):4–30.

Retrosigmoid Sinus Approach for Removal of Acoustic Neuroma

Bo S-L. Systematic anatomy. 2nd ed. Beijing: People's Medical Publishing House; 2010.

Ciric I, Zhao JC, Rosenblatt S, Wiet R, O'Shaughnessy B. Suboccipital retrosigmoid approach for removal of vestibular schwannomas: facial nerve function and hearing preservation. Neurosurgery. 2005;56(3):560–70.

Gharabaghi A, Samii A, Koerbel A, Rosahl SK, Tatagiba M, Samii M. Preservation of function in vestibular schwannoma surgery. Neurosurgery. 2007;60(2 Suppl 1):ONS124–7.

Han D-Y. Nerve otology and lateral skull base surgery. Beijing: Science Press; 2008.

Huang X-Z, Wang J-B, Kong W-J. Practice of otorhinolaryngology head and neck surgery. 2nd ed. Beijing: People's Medical Publishing House; 2008.

Jacob A, Robinson Jr LL, Bortman JS, Yu L, Dodson EE, Welling DB. Nerve of origin, tumor size, hearing preservation, and facial nerve outcomes in 359 vestibular schwannoma resections at a tertiary care academic center. Laryngoscope. 2007;117(12): 2087–92.

Jiang S-C. Ear anatomia and temporal bone histopathology. Beijing: People's Military Medical Press; 1999. p. 209–12.

Jiang S-C, Yang W-Y, Gu R. The complete works of operative surgery. In: Operative surgery of otorhinolaryngology head and neck department. 2nd ed. Beijing: People's Military Medical Press; 2005. p. 257–60.

Maw AR, Coakham HB, Ayoub O, Butler SR. Hearing preservation and facial nerve function in vestibular schwannoma surgery. Clin Otolaryngol Allied Sci. 2003;28(3):252–6.

Sanna M, et al. The temporal bone a maunal for dissection and surgical apporaches. New York: Thieme; 2005.

Translabyrinthine Approach for Removal of Acoustic Neuroma

Bennett M, Haynes DS. Surgical approaches and complications in the removal of vestibular schwannomas. Neurosurg Clin N Am. 2007;19(2):331–43.

Bo B, Dingbiao Z, Bainan X. Clinical investigations on 110 large acoustic neuromas with multimodality intraoperative monitoring of facial nerves. Chin J Minim Invasive Surg. 2001;1(6):347–8.

Brackmann DE, Cullen RD, Fisher LM. Facial nerve function after translabyrinthine vestibular schwannoma surgery. Otolaryngol Head Neck Surg. 2007;136(5):773–7.

Dongyi H, Shiming Y, Wenming W, et al. Resection of acoustic neurinoma and preservation of function of the facial nerve. Chin J Otol. 2004;2(1):1–3.

Han D-Y, Limei Y. Hearing protection during the operation of acoustic neurinoma. Chin Med Dig Otolaryngol. 2007;22(2):70–2.

Limei Y, Dongyi H. Hearing protection of acoustic neurinoma. J Clin Otorhinolaryngol. 2005;19(10):474–7.

Li-mei Y, Shi-ming Y, Dong-yi H, et al. Preliminary study of intraoperative auditory monitoring techniques in acoustic neuroma surgery. Chin J Otorhinolaryngol Head Neck Surg. 2006;41(5):335–40.

Magliulo G, Stasolla A, Parrotto D, et al. Modified translabyrinthine approach and hearing preservation: imaging evaluation. J Laryngol Otol. 2007;121(8):736–41.

Removal of Acoustic Neuroma Middle-Cranial Fossa Approach

Bento RF, De Brito RV, Sanchez TG, et al. The transmastoid retrolabyrinthine approach in vestibular schwannoma surgery. Otolaryngol Head Neck Surg. 2002;127(5):437–41.

Dongyi H, Weiyan Y, Sichang J. early diagnosis of acoustic neuroma. Chin J Otorhinolaryngol. 1995;30(6):335–7.

Dongyi H, Weiyan Y, Dingbiao Z. Bilateral acoustic neuromas. Chin J Otorhinolaryngol. 1999;34(1):18–20.

Dongyi H, Limei Y, Shiming Y, et al. Hearing protection during the operation of acoustic neurinoma. Chin J Otol. 2004;2(3):174–8.

Han D-Y. Clinical diagnosis and medical treatment of acoustic neurinoma. Chin Sci J Hearing Speech Rehabil. 2007;5:10–3.

Han D-Y. Nerve otology and lateral skull base surgery. Beijing: Science Press; 2008.

Ho SY, Hudgens S, Wiet RJ. Comparison of postoperative facial nerve outcomes between translabyrinthine and retrosigmoid approaches in matched-pair patients. Laryngoscope. 2003;113(11):2014–20.

Huang X-Z, Wang JB, Kong WJ. Practice of otorhinolaryngology head and neck surgery. 2nd ed. Beijing: People's Medical Publishing House; 2008.

Jiang S-C, Gu R, Zheng-Min W. Otorhinolaryngology – otology. 2nd ed. Shanghai: Shanghai Scientific and Technological Education Publishing House; 2002.

Jiang S-C, Yang W-Y, Gu R. The complete works of operative surgery. In: Operative surgery of otorhinolaryngology head and neck department. 2nd ed. Beijing: People's Military Medical Press; 2005.

Kong W-J. Otorhinolaryngology head and neck surgery. Beijing: People's Medical Publishing House; 2005.

Limei Y, Shiming Y, Dongyi H, et al. Recurrence of acoustic neuroma and management after surgery. Chin Arch Otolaryngol Head Neck Surg. 2005;12(11):709–13.

Li-mei Y, Shi-ming Y, Dong-yi H, et al. Management of operative complications in acoustic neuroma surgery. Chin J Otorhinolaryngol. 2006;41(1):26–30.

Mamikoglu B, Wiet RJ, Esquivel CR. Translabyrinthine approach for the management of large and giant vestibular schwannomas. Otol Neurotol. 2002;23(2):224–7.

Yong-qian W, Mei-xiu D. A study on identification of the internal auditory canal in middle fossa surgery. Chin J Clin Anat. 2005;23(1):63–6.

Resection of Glomus Jugulare Tumors Through Postauricular Infratemporal Fossa Approach

Glassock 3rd ME, Jackson CG, Dickins JR, Wiet RJ. Panel discussion: glomus jugulare tumors of the temporal bone. The surgical management of glomus tumors. Laryngoscope. 1979;89:1640–54.

Jiang S-C, Gu R, Zheng-Min W. Otorhinolaryngology – otology. 2nd ed. Shanghai: Shanghai Scientific and Technological Education Publishing House; 2002.

Zheng-Min W. Microsurgery of the ear. Shanghai: Shanghai Scientific and Technological Education Publishing House; 2004.

Temporal Bone Resection

Glasscock III ME, Gulya AJ. Glasscock-Shambaugh surgery of the ear. 5th ed. Hamilton: B C Decker; 2003. p. 743–59.

Jiang S-C, Yang W-Y, Gu R. The complete works of operative surgery. In: Operative surgery of otorhinolaryngology head and neck department. 2nd ed. Beijing: People's Military Medical Press; 2005.

Index

P. Dai et al. (eds.), *Stereo Operative Atlas of Micro Ear Surgery*, DOI 10.1007/978-981-10-2089-6